Optimal Digestive Health

Optimal Digestive Health

A COMPLETE GUIDE

Edited by
TRENT W. NICHOLS, MD,
and NANCY FAASS, MSW, MPH

Healing Arts Press
Rochester, Vermont

Healing Arts Press
One Park Street
Rochester, Vermont 05767
www.InnerTraditions.com

Healing Arts Press is a division of Inner Traditions International

*Note to the reader: This book is intended as an informational guide. The remedies,
approaches, and techniques described herein are meant to supplement, and not to be a
substitute for, professional medical care or treatment. They should not be used to treat
a serious ailment without prior consultation with a qualified health care professional.*

Library of Congress Cataloging-in-Publication Data
Optimal digestive health : a complete guide / edited by Trent W. Nichols and Nancy
Faass.
   p. cm.
  Summary: "A comprehensive and integrative approach to achieving digestive health
using mainstream, complementary, and alternative therapies."—Provided by publisher.
  Includes index.
  ISBN 1-59477-036-0 (pbk.)
  1. Digestive organs—Diseases—Popular works. 2. Digestion—Popular works. 3.
Digestive organs—Diseases—Alternative treatment. I. Nichols, Trent W. II. Faass, Nancy.
  RC801.O687 2005
  616.3'06—dc22

                                               2004022879

Printed and bound in Canada by Transcontinental Printing

10 9 8 7 6 5 4 3 2

Text design and layout by Priscilla Baker
This book was typeset in Sabon with Avenir used as a display typeface

Contents

Preface to the Second Edition   ix

Part I
HOW YOUR BODY WORKS

1   Redefining the Problem • *Jerry Stine*   2

2   How Digestion Works • *Jerry Stine*   13

3   Your Five Protective Barriers • *Scott Anderson, M.D.*   24

4   Immune Defenses • *Michael Rosenbaum, M.D.*   32

5   Friendly Flora • *Nigel Plummer, Ph.D.*   42

6   Harmful Flora • *Len Saputo, M.D.*   49

7   Leaky Gut Syndrome • *Len Saputo, M.D.*   57

8   Effects of Food Allergies • *Michael Rosenbaum, M.D.*   65

9   Harm from Toxins • *Jeffry Anderson, M.D.*   73

10   Stress and Digestion • *Martin Rossman, M.D.*   87

11   Toxic Overload • *Trent W. Nichols, M.D.*   95

12   Damage from Free Radicals • *Jeffrey Bland, Ph.D.*   105

13   How Problems with Digestion Can Cause Illness
Anywhere in the Body • *Jeffry Anderson, M.D.*   112

Part II
TOOLS FOR EVALUATING YOUR HEALTH

14   Testing to Rule Out Disease • *Trent W. Nichols, M.D.*   120

Unraveling the Mystery of Digestive Illness:
Using Antibody Testing • *Aristo Vojdani, Ph.D., M.T.*   126

15   Detecting Microbes • *Omar Amin, Ph.D.*   130

16   Testing in Preventive Medicine • *The Institute for
Functional Medicine*   138

Food Allergy Testing • *Sidney MacDonald Baker, M.D.*   141

17 How to Find Out What's Working and What Isn't •
    John Furlong, N.D., and Great Smokies Diagnostic Laboratory   144

18 Assessing Immunity and Inflammation • *William G. Timmins, N.D.* 153

Part III
NEW STRATEGIES FOR INNER HEALTH

19 Remove, Replace, Restore, and Repair • *Jeffrey Bland, Ph.D.*   162

20 Minimizing Food Allergies • *Michael Rosenbaum, M.D.*   164

21 Clearing Bad Bugs • *The Team*   173

22 The Problem of Viruses • *Richard Kunin, M.D.*   189

23 Minimizing Toxic Exposure • *Jeffry Anderson, M.D.*   193

24 Replacing Digestants and Restoring Flora • *The Team*   209

25 Repairing the GI Tract • *The Team*   218

26 Detox • *Jeffry Anderson, M.D., and Jerry Stine*   229

27 Cleaning Up Bad Habits • *Elson Haas, M.D.*   239

28 Rebalancing Lifestyle • *Elson Haas, M.D.*   248

29 Renewing Immunity—A Checklist • *Michael Rosenbaum, M.D.*   255

30 The Basics of a Healthy Diet • *The Team*   257

31 Managing Blood Sugar and Carbs • *Jerry Stine*   269

32 First Aid for Inflammation • *Paul Lynn, M.D.*   281

33 Nutrients for Repair • *Richard Kunin, M.D.*   288

34 The Role of Hormones in Healing • *Paul Lynn, M.D.*   305

35 Drugs and Nutrition in Combination • *Trent W. Nichols, M.D.* 312

36 Drug Cautions • *Len Saputo, M.D.*   323

37 Benefits of Herbal Therapies • *Timothy Kuss, Ph.D.*   328

38 New Strategies for Digestive Health • *Jerry Stine*   349

39 Medicine for the Future: Bioelectromagnetic Therapy •
    Trent W. Nichols, M.D.   359

40 Improving Digestive Health with Chinese Medicine •
    Efrem Korngold, O.M.D.   366

41 Using Homeopathy • *Nancy Faass, MSW, MPH*   382

42 Ayurveda: A Brief Introduction and Guide •
    Vasant Lad, Ayurvedic Physician   387

43 Gentle Exercise • *Roger Jahnke, O.M.D.*   395

Part IV
THERAPIES FROM MIND-BODY MEDICINE

44 Quality of Life • *Michael Lerner, Ph.D.*   414

45 Meditation in Healing • *Madeline Ko-i Bastis,*
    Jon Kabat-Zinn, Ph.D., Nancy Faass, MSW, MPH, Jim Castelli,
    and H.H. the Dalai Lama   416

46 Guided Imagery • *Martin Rossman, M.D.*   422

47 Self-Care • *Tom Ferguson, M.D.*   432

48 Getting the Support You Need • *Len Saputo, M.D.,*
    and Nancy Faass, MSW, MPH   438

49 Support Groups • *Rebecca McLean*   450

50 Tips for Online Health Searching • *Tom Ferguson, M.D.*   460

51 The Healer Within • *Roger Jahnke, O.M.D.*   462

52 The Proactive Patient • *Nancy Faass, MSW, MPH*   466

Part V
TREATMENT OPTIONS FOR SPECIFIC CONDITIONS
Trent W. Nichols, M.D.

Cancer of the Colon   473

Candida (Yeast Overgrowth)   477

Celiac Disease (Sprue)   481

Cirrhosis   485

Constipation (Chronic)   488

Diarrhea (Chronic)   494

Diverticulosis and Diverticulitis   499

Dyspepsia—Without Ulcers   502

Fibromyalgia   504

Fissures   510

Fistulas   511

Food Allergies   512

Gallstones   512

Gastritis   517

Hemorrhoids   520

Hepatitis (Chronic) 523

Inflammatory Bowel Diseases (IBD): Ulcerative Colitis
    and Crohn's Disease 526

Irritable Bowel Syndrome (IBS) 532

Lactose Intolerance 537

Liver Disease 538

Malabsorption 544

Pancreatic Cancer 546

Pancreatitis 548

Pruritus Ani 551

Reflux and Heartburn—GERD (Gastroesophageal Reflux Disease) 551

Strictures and Structural Conditions 557

Ulcers/Ulcer Disease 560

Resources 564

Index 578

Preface to the Second Edition

◈

More than 90 million Americans suffer from digestive
disorders according to the National Institutes of Health.

To develop a resource for people coping with digestive issues, we invited more than twenty experts to contribute their best treatment strategies. This book reflects the original thinking of these contributors, some of the finest complementary and integrative practitioners in the country.

The importance of digestive health is vastly underappreciated. Without good digestion, one cannot be truly healthy. Impaired digestion can trigger problems ranging from mild stomach upsets to life-threatening cancer. What's more, millions of people struggle with these conditions year in, year out. A number of major problems can result from digestive disorders, including fatigue, weight gain, and food allergies. Poor digestion can also be a factor in attention deficit disorders, arthritis, asthma, chemical sensitivities, eczema, liver problems, and mood disorders.

These conditions can be difficult to overcome, so it is useful to have a range of treatment options available. Our experience suggests that the best strategies for healing include both mainstream and complementary therapies—integrative medicine. Many people with chronic disorders have improved significantly through the use of good nutrition, enzymes, vitamins, herbs, or natural therapies.

It is important to seek the most skilled medical expertise available. This book is not offered as a prescription for self-treatment, because insight alone will not replace good medical care. However, medication alone does not always restore health either. The greatest opportunity for recovery occurs when the patient actively participates in the healing process, supported by the consistent efforts of capable and compassionate healers.

It has been five years since the first edition of *Optimal Digestion* was published. Since that time there have been major advances in both conventional gastroenterology and integrative/complementary medicine.

In testing, capsule endoscopy is now used to provide information on digestive function via video and real-time imaging. New medications are available that are based on functional medicine paradigms, including tumor necrosis factor antibodies and antisense therapy. Courses on complementary medicine are now being taught in more than 50 medical schools, and major urban hospitals have complementary medicine programs for patients and for the training of doctors.

Since the first edition the importance of nutrition has gained broader recognition. New types of treatment, particularly stem cell therapy and bio-electromagnetics, have arrived in the medical arena and we believe will come to be considered the therapy of the twenty-first century—"regenerative medicine." Many alternative therapies are now viewed as complementary and are being incorporated into conventional medical treatment. As the field of integrative medicine emerges, these advances have the potential to further expand the options available to patients.

This book can be used in a number of ways. Part I contains questionnaires that can be used as a tool to evaluate your symptoms and help you gain a better sense of your overall health situation. Part II explains various types of medical and lab testing that your physician may request in order to learn more about your condition. Parts III and IV offer an extensive range of options for self-care. Part V provides information on the causes, symptoms, and mainstream and complementary treatments of more than 25 chronic digestive disorders. The chapters are brief and self-contained so that they do not necessarily need to be read in order.

Whether you are a patient or a physician, there is sure to be information provided here that views health and illness from a different perspective than you may have previously considered. Give these ideas serious consideration. This knowledge is hard won: The driving force for the creation of this book has been the suffering of so many people with digestive illness. The hope is that doctors and patients together, using approaches such as these, can reduce needless suffering.

—Trent W. Nichols, M.D., and Nancy Faass, MSW, MPH

Part I

How Your Body Works

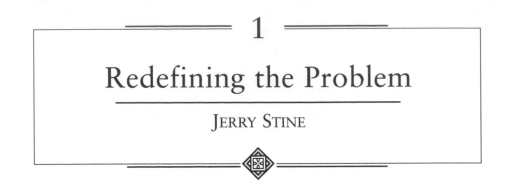

1

Redefining the Problem

JERRY STINE

A NEW PERSPECTIVE

If you have digestive illness, this book was written for you, drawn from the experience of people like you. Your experience holds the clues to solving the mystery of your condition. Ultimately the solution will be based on your health history, symptoms, and responses. The details of your situation are the basis for individualizing treatment to fit your unique circumstances and will enhance your opportunities for healing. The promise of this approach is the freedom to lead a rich life, unencumbered by the pain and distress of illness.

This highly individualized approach is an aspect of integrative medicine, which encompasses both mainstream and complementary therapies. The challenges of chronic illness sometimes require additional options. The benefits of nutrition, acupuncture, functional medicine, and other complementary approaches have been confirmed in research and in treatment. Integrative medicine draws from the best of both worlds.

The information in this book is not just theory—it is the result of years of experience of both doctors and patients. The fruits of this knowledge are presented here as specific techniques and therapies. To those of us suffering from gastrointestinal illness, this information can be precious and critical.

TOOLS FOR HEALING

We want to provide you with key tools and concepts that are the basis of integrative medicine. Let's consider some of the resources that seem to make the greatest difference for patients who are managing chronic health conditions:

1. *An individualized approach.*
2. *Nutritional therapy.* Using nutrition to adjust the body's chemistry and promote healing.
3. *Functional medicine and testing.* New ways of looking at health that focus on how your body works and new lab tests that expand treatment options.

4. *Integrative treatment.* Using different therapies in combination.
5. *Lifestyle.* How lifestyle can become a tool for healing.

These approaches and resources offer hope for many complex conditions, from hidden food allergies to chronic illnesses such as Crohn's disease. This is not to say that all the answers are available yet, but in many cases we can now make real advances toward health by using the latest information and resources.

1. An Individualized Approach

We know intuitively that we're not all the same. You may function quite differently from those around you and experience reactions to foods or medications that others tolerate without any problem. Although your responses may be unusual, that doesn't discount their significance. By fully understanding the very individual nature of your responses, you can come to appreciate their importance.

Your physical and mental reactions reflect the status of your body's chemistry, including your minute-to-minute interaction with the foods you eat and the substances in your environment, such as cigarette smoke. Your biochemistry is essentially the complex interplay that occurs within your body between nutrients, hormones, brain, and immune function, and all the other aspects of your chemistry. Although you have inherited some of these tendencies, other aspects have evolved throughout your life, influenced by your environment and lifestyle.

An important first step in healing involves a deeper understanding of the very individual nature of your physical makeup and your body's chemistry. In clinical nutrition the uniqueness of each individual is described as *biochemical individuality,* a term coined by Nobel Prize–winning researcher Roger Williams. He was one of the first to define the wide range of variations in body chemistry that occurs from one person to the next. Your body and chemistry are as individual as your fingerprints and your DNA.

2. Nutritional Therapy

Deficiencies of vitamins or minerals are as individual as any other aspect of health and can be a major cause of illness. You may know, for example, that vitamin C deficiency can cause scurvy, but did you know that a B_{12} deficiency is an important causal factor in many digestive disorders? These correlations between illness and nutritional deficiencies (and a great many others) have been identified through research. Researchers and physicians have also found that when the missing nutrients are supplied, healing begins to occur.

Nutritional therapy is especially useful in managing chronic illness on a day-to-day basis. Nutrition offers the opportunity to strengthen the body by replenishing depleted resources. In this approach we use the same raw materials that the body uses: foods, vitamins, minerals, amino acids, flora, fiber, and water. New lab tests can guide therapy by identifying deficiencies, and monitor treatment more precisely.

A wide range of nutritional supplements is another of the resources now available to you. These products are skillfully formulated and highly sophisticated, provided through enhanced delivery systems, and better assimilated. As a result an unparalleled level of precision is possible in nutritional prescribing. Using the new lab testing and the incredible range of nutrients currently available, we have additional resources to address the underlying causes of disease.

At this point there is abundant evidence on the effectiveness of nutritional therapy. There are more than 50,000 studies on ascorbic acid (vitamin C) alone. We also have a great deal of research, conducted over long periods of time, on large populations. For example, the Framingham Study has been ongoing for more than 50 years. This research has served to dispel many clinical misconceptions about conditions such as hypertension, glucose intolerance, and diabetes. Our current understanding of cholesterol in all its subtleties also grows out of this work. Recent breakthroughs in research include insight into a number of conditions that can lead to disease:

- Insulin resistance (a prediabetic and diabetic condition)
- Homocysteine (a risk factor for heart disease, stroke, and dementia)
- Microcirculation problems (associated with many chronic conditions)

Although our understanding of these conditions is based on medical research, many of these disorders can be addressed through nutrition (see chapter 38). Since nutrition is one of the cornerstones of an integrative approach, integrative physicians are often among the first to incorporate these clinical strategies.

3. Functional Medicine and Testing

Functional medicine involves another new way of looking at health and illness. This approach applies the concept of biochemical individuality, with a focus on function. This means assessing how well a particular organ or system is functioning—for example, the liver or the adrenal glands. There is an advantage to this approach, because functional testing sometimes identifies problems in organs that might be missed in other types of testing. These tests can also pick up organ malfunction, in some cases before there is manifest disease or a definitive diagnosis. Dysfunction—even subtle dysfunction—can often be detected and defined in detail through functional testing.

By identifying problems in functioning, we can intervene more precisely. When function is restored, healing begins. Balance and healing are promoted by identifying the optimal diet for each individual and by supplementing specific nutrients. Botanicals and/or medications may also be used strategically. Information from testing becomes critically important in developing this individualized nutritional therapy. Functional testing can also guide strategies for prevention, optimal wellness, or antiaging programs.

Functional testing focuses on the kinks, defects, or system failures that underlie any given individual's particular symptoms. For example, the new lab testing makes it possible to evaluate your specific levels of vitamins, minerals, amino acids, and digestive flora. Tests are also available to measure:

- Genetic risk factors for specific diseases
- The vitality of your immune system
- Markers of inflammation
- The levels and interaction of many hormones
- Predictors of illness in the digestive tract and elsewhere in the body
- The overgrowth of yeast or bacteria, or the presence of other harmful microbes
- The success or failure of digestive processes

These new tests can also define and measure how you respond to stress and the impact of environmental toxins. This testing is now available in affordable, easy-to-use at-home kits, which can be requested from doctors who practice functional medicine. The information from these functional tests makes it possible to target treatment to your specific needs.

4. Integrative Treatment

In our experience, an integrative approach can be quite useful in the successful management of chronic illness. We've observed that some of the patients most successful in coping with chronic illness have involved more than one practitioner in their treatment—for example, an integrative physician, an acupuncturist, a nutritionist, and a conventional physician. We have seen patients who used this approach do very well. These patients tended to be proactive in their use of different therapies. Since every major discipline has its own body of knowledge, treatment protocol, and specific techniques, treatment strategies that include more than one modality can amplify healing. We know that no one therapy provides the whole picture, yet the synergy that can result from this type of approach can be exceptional.

5. Lifestyle

It is clear to many of us that lifestyle is also an important factor in our health. Surprisingly, this is a fairly new perspective (actually it's the return to an earlier paradigm). For decades lifestyle was considered a minor aspect in the treatment of any illness. Our current appreciation for lifestyle grows out of the wisdom of traditional therapies. Every major healing tradition throughout history has had lifestyle as its foundation and lifestyle was frequently part of overall treatment.

SELF-EVALUATION

At this moment in time and space, the way you experience your life and your health is the result of thousands of interrelated factors. Different aspects of your life, your physical uniqueness, and your lifestyle are all interacting to produce the health you are experiencing.

If you are currently dealing with chronic illness, this may be the ideal time to reassess your situation. A reevaluation offers an opportunity to start over, to describe where you are right now, and to begin putting together a plan for healing. We have chosen the Health Profile below because it's substantiated by research and provides a reliable basis for self-appraisal. It has been used worldwide in more than one million health assessments.

Approach this self-assessment as if you were evaluating someone else. Note and report everything, no matter how insignificant it seems. Even if a symptom has been with you for a long time, report it. Be honest with yourself and take your time. For the few minutes it takes to do this evaluation, leave behind any preconceptions. A neutral mind-set is also important if you have a genetic predisposition or unresolved illness. You may want to give yourself two scores. To do this, make two columns—one for good days and one for bad days. We encourage you to take yourself seriously—honor your intuitions and observations. You have lived within your body your whole life—no one knows it better than you.

The Health Profile
Immuno Laboratories, Fort Lauderdale, FL

Rate each of the following symptoms based on your typical health profile for:

___ **INITIAL TEST:** *the past 30 days*   ___ **RETEST:** *the past 48 hours*

POINT SCALE: 0 = Never or almost never have the symptom
1 = Occasionally have it, effect is not severe
2 = Occasionally have it, effect is severe
3 = Frequently have it, effect is not severe
4 = Frequently have it, effect is severe

HEAD
___ Headaches
___ Faintness
___ Dizziness
___ Insomnia
___ **TOTAL**

EYES
___ Watery or itchy eyes
___ Swollen, reddened, or sticky
eyelids
___ Bags or dark circles under eyes
___ Blurred or tunnel vision
(does not include near- or
far-sightedness)
___ **TOTAL**

EARS
___ Itchy ears
___ Earaches, ear infections
___ Drainage from ear
___ Ringing in ears, hearing loss
___ **TOTAL**

NOSE
___ Stuffy nose
___ Sinus problems
___ Hay fever
___ Sneezing attacks
___ Excessive mucus
___ **TOTAL**

MOUTH/THROAT
___ Chronic coughing
___ Gagging, frequent need to
clear throat
___ Sore throat, hoarseness, loss of
voice
___ Swollen or discolored tongue,
gums, lips
___ Canker sores
___ **TOTAL**

SKIN
___ Acne
___ Hives, rashes, dry skin
___ Hair-loss
___ Flushing, hot flashes
___ Excessive sweating
___ **TOTAL**

HEART
___ Irregular or skipped heartbeat
___ Rapid or pounding heartbeat
___ Chest pain
___ **TOTAL**

LUNGS
___ Chest congestion
___ Asthma, bronchitis
___ Shortness of breath
___ Difficulty breathing
___ **TOTAL**

DIGESTIVE TRACT
___ Nausea, vomiting
___ Diarrhea
___ Constipation
___ Bloated feeling
___ Heartburn
___ Intestinal/stomach pain
___ **TOTAL**

JOINTS/MUSCLES
___ Pain or aches in joints
___ Arthritis
___ Stiffness or limitation of
movement
___ Pain or aches in muscles
___ Feeling of weakness or
tiredness
___ **TOTAL**

WEIGHT
___ Binge eating/drinking
___ Craving certain foods
___ Excessive weight
___ Compulsive eating
___ Water retention
___ Underweight
___ TOTAL

ENERGY/ACTIVITY
___ Fatigue, sluggishness
___ Apathy, lethargy
___ Hyperactivity
___ Restlessness
___ TOTAL

MIND
___ Poor memory
___ Confusion, poor comprehension
___ Poor concentration
___ Poor physical coordination

___ Difficulty in making decisions
___ Stuttering or stammering
___ Slurred speech
___ Learning disabilities
___ TOTAL

EMOTIONS
___ Mood swings
___ Anxiety, fear, nervousness
___ Anger, irritability, aggressiveness
___ Depression
___ TOTAL

OTHER SYMPTOMS
___ Frequent or urgent urination
___ Genital itch or discharge
___ Frequent illness
___ TOTAL

TOTAL SCORE _____

The Health Profile was modified with permission from the Immuno Symptom Checklist (ISC) copyrighted 1988 by Immuno Laboratories, Inc., Fort Lauderdale, FL (800) 231-9197. Versions of the ISC has been used by more than one million patients and their physicians worldwide to assist in the evaluation of food allergies and IgG-mediated, "delayed" food sensitivities.

Scoring the Health Profile

At this point let's review your scores. The profile can be a useful screening tool and focusing device. The total score can indicate the overall severity of your symptoms, while the individual sections can serve to highlight the problem areas.

A high score of 50 or above may reflect increased intestinal permeability and suggest the need for further testing. There are many causes of hyperpermeability and many associated symptoms throughout the body. Permeability can be checked using a simple at-home test prescribed by your doctor. (See chapters 7 and 17 for further information on this test.)

A high score may also suggest the possibility of food allergies, which can pose a real threat to GI (gastrointestinal) health. Unfortunately food allergies are often difficult to diagnose. Some allergies can cause a direct response in the body, but others cause a delayed reaction and are therefore harder to detect.

For additional information on allergies and allergy testing see chapters 8, 16, and 20. If you got a high score on the profile, you will also want to take a look at the candida questionnaire and the parasite questionnaire, both in chapter 2. Remember that all the symptoms on the test can result from any of a number of causes.

INFLUENCES ON OUR HEALTH

Consider some of the major factors that influence overall health: our genetic heritage, our environment, and our habits.

Genetic Factors

Our genetic heritage is the basis for our uniqueness. We each have our own genetic makeup encoded on the chromosomes of our DNA. However, genetic coding is only one of many influences. The health we each experience is the result of our genetic coding plus thousands of influences from our environment from the moment of our conception.

Recent evidence indicates that we can influence our genetic expression. This refers to the *expression* of our genetic tendencies and whether risk factors actually become expressed as disease. (For infomation on genetic testing see chapter 17.) We now know that the quality of nutrition affects genetic expression. Research has also shown that, for most people, the strongest influences on health are still environmental factors such as toxic exposure and lifestyle. Although we were brought into the world with a certain genetic code, we can significantly influence our health through our nutrition and lifestyle. Genetics are *not* destiny.

Influences from Our Environment

The major environmental factors for most people include the quality of food, water, and air; hygiene; physical and emotional stresses; and exposure to toxic substances and microbes.

As we become more conscious of how environmental factors affect us, we are better able to maintain our health by consciously choosing habits that support us. We can begin by focusing on our own immediate environment, educating ourselves about nutrition and water quality. This knowledge can be translated into action by purchasing organic food whenever possible and drinking the cleanest water available. We can lower our exposures at home, because that is where we have the most control. It's important to make informed choices about cleaning products, pest control, garden and yard spraying, and other details of living that carry subtle risks. (Chapters 9 and

23 on minimizing toxic exposure are particularly important and chapter 26 provides practical information on clearing toxins from the body through detoxification.) Another aspect of coping with our environment involves learning how to minimize the effects of stress in our lives. (See part IV, which offers a variety of resources for stress reduction from mind–body medicine.)

The Importance of Lifestyle and Habits

For anyone with chronic illness, lifestyle is doubly important. The ability to eat and exercise normally is often impaired. Stress is usually higher around all types of issues—work, family, relationships, money. So the challenge is to get good nutrition, exercise, relaxation, and emotional support—at the very time when they are most difficult to obtain. (You'll find useful information on nutrition in chapters 20, 30, and 31; on exercise in chapter 43; on relaxation in chapter 28; and on expanding your support system in 48 and 49.)

Habits are another important aspect of our lifestyle. Much of our lives is composed of the habits that we have absorbed from our families and the social environment. But habits that work for one person may not work for another. Even habits that seem harmless can compromise our health. Good habits strengthen our vitality. (Resources that can strengthen your self discipline to help you create a healthy lifestyle on a day-to-day basis include exercise, which is discussed further in chapter 43 and meditation, discussed in chapter 45.)

COPING WITH CHRONIC ILLNESS

Unresolved illness can be enormously confusing and frustrating. Consider viewing your situation as a complex puzzle. You may have two or more conditions that coexist. There could be a number of symptoms. A domino effect can occur—the original illness may cause other problems. And even your doctor may not be sure of exactly what is wrong.

If your illness is unresolved, you probably already consider it a mystery. View yourself as a detective. The clues are your symptoms, the results of your lab work, and your responses to treatment. Consider all evidence important, including information on what has been successful *and what has not*. Even treatments that don't work provide useful information. Here are some ideas you might find helpful:

Working with Your Practitioner

- Work with the most informed and capable healers available to you.
- Avail yourself of the relevant testing and explore the suspected causes, step by step.
- Become involved in the development of a complete treatment strategy.
- Let your physician(s) know how you are responding to therapy so that adjustments can be made. It is as important for your physicians to know what is not working as it is for them to know what is.
- If you are seeing more than one practitioner, keep them all informed of what you are doing.
- When you see your doctor, ask questions and be sure you understand.
- Remember that the best practitioners want to involve you in the healing process.

Developing a Clear History

- Review your entire history. The assessment questionnaires in this chapter and in chapter 2 can be part of this process.
- Develop and prioritize a list of possible causes.
- Maintain a file of the results from your lab work.
- Integrate the results of the lab work with the clues from your individual history to develop the most complete understanding possible.
- Keep a journal and a record of your progress.
    - Record all the circumstances—when, where, how
    - Create a list of what has helped *and what hasn't*
    - Include everything: diet, supplements, drugs and herbs, exercise, stresses, liquid intake, time of day, and seasonal response
    - Also create summaries so you can stay focused on your primary successes

Expanding Your Resources

- Review the literature at your bookstore, neighborhood library, or medical library.
- Continue to adjust and develop your program in response to your progress.
- Include lifestyle approaches in your therapy.
- Be good to yourself.

Be patient. Not everything you try or every practitioner you see will provide you all the answers, all at once. You may need to explore a number of ideas and see several practitioners before you find all the clues that are required to solve the puzzle of your health situation.

We wish you well.

Jerry Stine is a nutritional consultant and the director of the Lifespan Institute for Antiaging and Functional Nutrition, which he founded in 1987 to develop advanced nutritional programs for life-extension and performance-enhancement. He also founded and directed Health Evaluations, a nonprofit research group with a nutritional consulting clinic and a research lab. For the past 15 years, he has been an independent nutritional counselor with an active private practice and has served as consultant for several respected vitamin manufacturers.

The Lifespan Institute provides nutritional supplements, individual nutritional consultations by phone, and access to a variety of the latest functional testing, including evaluations for allergies, GI health, parasites, adrenal function, oxidative stress, and general screening. For more information, you can reach the institute by phone at (415) 479-3552 or visit its Web site at www.LifespanProducts.com.

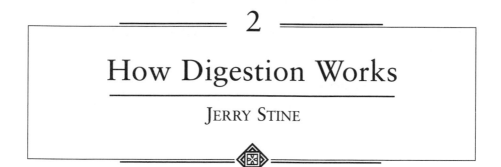

2

How Digestion Works

JERRY STINE

OUR INTERNAL ECOSYSTEM

Our bodies are constructed from the products of our digestion—we literally are what we eat. With that in mind, think of the digestive tract as an entire ecosystem, a self-contained environment supporting a community of hundreds of species of bacteria. This ecology consists primarily of friendly bacteria at work, our digestive flora. Without these beneficial bacteria to ferment and digest our food, we can't have complete digestion or healthy bodies.

Protective Immunity

The immune system in our digestive tract performs the tremendous task of distinguishing friend from foe in this internal world, playing traffic cop to more than 500 species of bacteria. Most of these are friendly, but even in a healthy digestive tract small numbers of destructive microbes are always present. We also consume a wide range of bacteria, yeasts, and molds in our food and water; some of these microbes can be harmful if they survive and flourish.

The protective mechanisms of our GI tract are designed to neutralize these common organisms. A significant portion of our immune function is strategically located in the GI tract to keep a favorable balance between the helpful and destructive organisms. This immune function is so vital that 50 percent of the lymph tissue in the body is located in the intestinal lining and 80 percent of all our protective antibodies are produced there. In short, the body devotes an enormous amount of energy to maintaining the proper balance in the digestive system.

When the Balance Is Lost

A number of influences can upset this elegant balance:

- Overgrowth of yeast, including candida
- Overgrowth of undesirable bacteria
- Microscopic parasites
- Parasites such as worms
- Viral illnesses
- Poor hygiene

- Bad water
- A starchy diet
- Too many sweets
- Excessive alcohol intake
- Food allergies
- Certain medications
- Frequent use of antibiotics

- Radiation
- Surgery
- Physical injury
- Stress
- Genetic tendencies
- Environmental toxins

Friendly Flora

The bacteria in our GI tract number in the trillions. A healthy adult has five to eight pounds of living bacteria in their digestive tract, most of which are beneficial. These bacteria perform an essential part of our digestive function and we are completely reliant on their activities. This huge engine of fermentation produces the nutrients essential to our functioning.

Previously it was thought that the cells lining the GI tract were nourished by our body through the blood supply. However, recent research has shown that it is the beneficial bacteria that nourish the digestive tract (for example, they produce essential short-chain fatty acids). A number of other important nutrients are also available only through the bacterial fermentation of our food. Without the nutrients from these bacteria, there is a loss of function in the lining of the gut. (This can occur whenever we take antibiotics, unless we replenish the bacteria afterward with probiotics.)

Unfriendly Flora

When the flora is compromised or the immune system weakened, destructive bacteria or yeast that happen to be in residence may not be held in check. Then colonies of the harmful organisms (pathogens) can establish themselves in numbers great enough to disturb the intestinal environment and harm the body. This imbalance in the microorganisms of the digestive tract is called *dysbiosis*.

If the friendly flora are compromised, the intestinal lining can become malnourished, because the supply of vital nutrients is diminished. What's worse, the destructive microbes produce toxic chemicals that can cause tissue damage in the GI tract and elsewhere in the body. The immune system may then become further impaired.

Nutrient Absorption

The ultimate priority of the GI tract is to contain (and dispel) the substances that are toxic and to admit the nutrients our bodies require. To accomplish this, the gut membrane acts as a selective barrier. This is the single most important activity of the digestive tract. These functions—containing toxins and

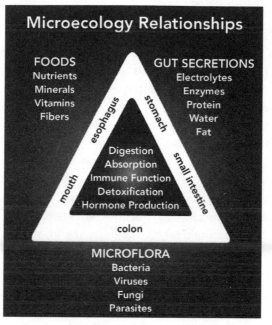

SOURCE: Great Smokies Diagnostic Laboratory, © 1999

absorbing nutrients—use an incredible amount of our energy. Digestive activities include regulating and accepting just the nutrients needed and rejecting everything else. And most of the material in the GI tract is rejected—very little is actually absorbed. You can see why the breakdown of these protective systems can cause a toxic condition in the body, a condition referred to as *leaky gut;* it can also create the potential for illness.

Leaky Gut Syndrome

A form of leakage can occur through the gut lining, compromising the barrier function of the digestive tract. Then some degree of toxins and bacteria can seep into the bloodstream and be passed along to the liver. The leaking of the gut wall—also called leaky gut syndrome or *hyperpermeability*—can be triggered by a number of factors, including food allergies, certain medications, alcoholism, radiation, chemotherapy, infections including HIV, and severe trauma such as burns. Hereditary tendencies can also play a role in leaky gut. As the gut becomes excessively porous or permeable, the bloodstream begins receiving both nutrients and toxins. All this material is picked up by the blood vessels lining the gut wall and is transported to the liver. The increased load must then be detoxified by the liver. Much of this inappropriately absorbed material is a source of metabolic stress and is potentially damaging to the body.

The Work of the Liver: Detoxification

The liver has the job of sorting out and processing all this material. If the substance is a nutrient the liver processes it into an active form the body can use. If the material is toxic the liver's job is to neutralize it (to make it less toxic—to detoxify it). This process is essential because even a perfectly healthy gut will release some toxic matter.

The liver is capable of neutralizing an amazing variety of substances in enormous quantities. However, if it is continually overloaded by toxins, detoxification may be incomplete. These toxins can suppress the immune system and compromise its ability to recognize and defend against infection. This excessive load can also directly damage the immune system and the self-repair mechanisms within each cell. Detoxification stress occurs in a feedback loop: The more toxins that are absorbed, the more the liver's capacity to detoxify can be compromised. At some point, real problems can begin to occur.

CONSEQUENCES OF POOR DIGESTION

The Development of Allergies and Sensitivities

When permeability increases, unprocessed substances can be passed on to the liver, completely undigested. This means that the liver would have to process undigested foods, bacteria, toxic chemicals, or whatever happens to be in the gut. The system could become overwhelmed and release these substances directly into the bloodstream. When this toxic material begins to circulate in the body, the immune system can become triggered, producing allergic responses to foods or other material released from the GI tract. An allergy or a hypersensitivity is typically an overreaction by the immune system, and can cause symptoms anywhere in the body. The food or substance causing the reactions may be relatively innocent—it is actually the overactive response of the immune system that causes the damage.

This dynamic can have a number of causes and result in a wide range of symptoms. For example, eating an allergic food is also a common *cause* of hyperpermeability and can be such a powerful trigger that permeability can increase within a matter of hours. This is a vicious cycle—hyperpermeability increases the absorption of more toxins and food fragments, which stimulates more allergic responses and amplifies the reactions in a snowball effect.

Innocent Foods and Toxic Effects

There are a number of ways in which problems associated with an overloaded liver can cause additional symptoms. One is the hypersensitization of the immune system just described. Another is direct damage to the body's tissues caused by the toxic effects of chemicals in food or digestive debris. For example, certain elements in milk or wheat can have direct toxic effects on the nervous or immune system. Specific sensitivities to proteins in wheat have even been implicated in certain forms of schizophrenia.

Autoimmune Disorders

Constant overstimulation of the immune system can also lead to an autoimmune disorder in which the immune system can mistake the tissues of the body for an invader. The white blood cells and T cells may actually attack the body rather than the invasive bacteria or offending substance. This can be a cause of chronic conditions such as asthma, lupus, multiple sclerosis, and rheumatoid arthritis.

With the development of chronic illness an even greater toxic burden is placed on the liver. Under this increased stress, the liver may no longer be able to perform competently. This sets the stage for a whole new arena of possible problems.

Inflammation

Inflammation is a normal consequence of our immune response. Yet if the immune system is continually on hyperalert, inflammation can become chronic. This is often a feature of digestive disorders, and can be caused by many of the stressors we've mentioned.

If inflammation continues in the long term, changes in the tissue can occur, degrading resilience and function. Over decades more serious tissue damage can occur, manifesting in conditions such as accelerated aging, diabetes, and cancer. For example, research shows that as many as 40 percent of stomach ulcer cases caused by *H. pylori* infection go on to become stomach cancer. The body's attempts to combat infection cause low-level inflammation in the lining of the stomach. If the infection persists, this sets the stage for the development of cancer.

For this reason it is extremely important to resolve inflammation. The best approach is to take it seriously, particularly if it doesn't seem to be improving or if it recurs.

Challenges to the Immune System: Free Radicals

The chronic overwork of the liver's detoxification mechanisms, caused by hyperpermeability, sets in motion a series of stresses. The first of these is the increased production of toxic by-products called free radicals. We hear about free radicals in the media, because they have been identified as a major cause of cancer. The assault of free radicals, also referred to as oxidative stress, further overstimulates the liver, causing it to send out signals that can confuse the immune system. These signals may trigger inappropriate reactions in both the immune and neurological systems and cause inflammation. This can occur even in a liver that is still generally functional.

If the liver's detox mechanisms are held in constant operation, its functions may eventually become compromised. Increased stress on the liver can be caused by even minor but frequent GI complaints, such as chronic constipation or an overgrowth of bacteria or yeast. Continual stress may ultimately compromise the liver's detoxification capacity. At the same time, free radicals (with the potential to cause cellular damage) could be generated in excessive amounts. Their effects are experienced throughout the body in cell membranes, connective tissue, and genetic material. This oxidative stress can lead to serious chronic illnesses such as Alzheimer's disease, diabetes, irritable bowel syndrome (IBS), and Parkinson's disease.

Oxidative stress from free radicals can also cause problems by depleting essential nutrients. This can short-circuit immune function, the activity of the nervous system, and the production of hormones. Over decades these compromises can develop into conditions such as heart disease and cancer. Free radicals have also been identified as a primary cause of aging.

YEAST AND PARASITES

When the delicate balance in the GI tract is lost, an overgrowth of yeast can occur, particularly *Candida albicans*. Candida is an undesirable species of yeast that is normally found in the gut even when we are healthy, but usually in small numbers. However, when candida develops too large a population (an overgrowth), it can overwhelm the beneficial bacteria, like weeds taking over a garden. An overgrowth can also be caused by certain bacteria or microbes in the gut. Imbalance in the flora has the potential to set in motion the entire sequence of harmful effects we have just described. Candida can cause illness and trigger symptoms anywhere in the body.

Parasites are another cause of digestive disorders that are often overlooked. When we think of parasites we tend to think of worms. Here in the United States, most parasites are single-celled protozoa, so small they can only be seen by microscope. Research by the Centers for Disease Control has found that more than 90 percent of all parasites in 80,000 lab tests were microscopic species. These microbes are a growing public health problem. They are now considered one of the important causes (among many) in some cases of chronic fatigue, arthritis, neurological problems, and immune suppression.

The Possibility of a Yeast Overgrowth of Candida

This is a frequently used questionnaire developed by practitioners to assess the likelihood of a *Candida albicans* infection.

SECTION A. MAJOR SYMPTOMS

Choose the score that fits your symptoms:
Mild = 4   Moderate = 8   Severe = 12

Energy/Toxicity

4   8   12   ___ Fatigue or lethargy
4   8   12   ___ Irritability or discomfort when hungry
4   8   12   ___ Headache

Mental/Emotional Functioning

4   8   12   ___ Anxiety, sometimes without apparent cause
4   8   12   ___ Depression
4   8   12   ___ Feeling spacey, lightheaded, or disoriented
4   0   12   ___ Poor memory
4   8   12   ___ Inability to make decisions and to concentrate

Digestive Symptoms

4   8   12   ___ Bloating or gas
4   8   12   ___ Chronic diarrhea
4   8   12   ___ Chronic constipation
4   8   12   ___ Abdominal pain

Reproductive System

4   8   12   ___ Loss of sexual interest or ability
4   8   12   ___ Troublesome vaginal burning, itching, or discharge
4   8   12   ___ Premenstrual tension or cramps

Muscles and Joints

4   8   12   ___ Muscle aches and weakness
4   8   12   ___ Cold hands or feet or physical chilliness
4   8   12   ___ Pain or swelling in joints

___ TOTAL SECTION A

SECTION B. OTHER SYMPTOMS

Scoring: Mild = 3   Moderate = 6   Severe = 9

3	6	9	___ Chronic eczema, rashes, or itching
3	6	9	___ Body odor not relieved by washing or bad breath
3	6	9	___ Chronic sore throat, laryngitis, cough, or tender glands
3	6	9	___ Urinary frequency, burning, or urgency
3	6	9	___ Pain or tightness in the chest, wheezing, or shortness of breath
3	6	9	___ Recurrent ear infections, fluid in the ears, or sinus or nasal congestion
3	6	9	___ Tendency to bruise easily
3	6	9	___ Insomnia
3	6	9	___ Lack of coordination, dizziness, or poor balance
3	6	9	___ Food sensitivity or intolerance

___ TOTAL SECTION B

SECTION C. MAJOR INFLUENCES—PERSONAL HISTORY

Scoring: Yes = number shown   No = zero

Antibiotics and Drugs as Factors

35   ___ Have you taken tetracycline or other antibiotics for one month or longer?

35   ___ Have you taken frequent short courses of other broad-spectrum antibiotics?

15   ___ Have you taken prednisone or other cortisone-type drugs for one month or more?

10   ___ Have you taken birth control pills for more than a year?

Symptoms and Sensitivities

25   ___ Have you had persistent bladder infections or prostatitis, vaginitis, or other reproductive problems?

20   ___ Have you been frequently exposed to high mold environments? Are you sensitive to mold?

20   ___ Do you have severe athlete's foot, nail or skin fungus, ringworm, or other types of chronic fungus?

20   ___ Have you been treated for internal parasites?

10   ___ Do perfumes, insecticides, or chemicals provoke strong symptoms?

10   ___ Does tobacco smoke *really* bother you?

Cravings

10 ___ Do you crave or eat lots of starches, such as pastas or breads?
10 ___ Do you crave or consume lots of sweets?
10 ___ Do you crave or consume alcoholic beverages?

___ TOTAL SECTION C

___ GRAND TOTAL (SECTIONS A, B, & C)

Scores over 100 suggest the possibility of a candida overgrowth. Scores over 175 indicate a high probability of candida and suggest the value of seeing a health care professional.

© 1997, J. Anderson, N. Faass, T. Kuss, J. Ross, and J. Stine.

Scoring the Candida Questionnaire

A high score on the candida questionnaire suggests the possibility of an overgrowth of *Candida albicans* or other microbes. If your score is over 100, you have a number of symptoms often seen in people with a yeast overgrowth. Additional follow-up with your doctor and with relevant lab work could be very worthwhile. A score over 150 reflects the strong possibility of a problem caused by yeast.

If you find that you have candida, it is important not to view that as the primary problem. An overgrowth typically occurs when the digestive tract is no longer able to protect itself. Other stressors may be causing a suppressed immune function, allowing the candida to proliferate. Factors that promote candida overgrowth include the frequent use of antibiotics, a highly sweet or starchy diet, low levels of stomach acid or digestive enzymes, exposure to toxic chemicals, microscopic parasites, or chronic stress.

It is quite possible to score high on more than one of these questionnaires. These problems are by no means separate from one another—frequently they occur as overlapping conditions. If your scores are high on any of the tests, we encourage you to see your health care professional. Information on candida is included in chapters 15 and 17 on testing and in chapter 21.

Symptoms from Microscopic Parasites

The following questionnaire is designed to assess the possibility of intestinal para-sites, particularly the single-celled parasites.

Scoring: 0 = Never   1 = Sometimes   2 = Often   3 = All the time

	0	1	2	3
1. Increased appetite	0	1	2	3
2. Allergies, food sensitivities	0	1	2	3
3. Irritability	0	1	2	3
4. Chronic fatigue	0	1	2	3
5. A tendency toward hyperactivity	0	1	2	3
6. Restless sleep	0	1	2	3
7. Grinding teeth while sleeping	0	1	2	3
8. Night sweats	0	1	2	3
9. Fevers of unknown origin	0	1	2	3
10. Loose stools or bowel urgency	0	1	2	3
11. Constipation	0	1	2	3
12. Diarrhea alternating with constipation	0	1	2	3
13. An itchy bottom	0	1	2	3
14. Bloating or gas	0	1	2	3
15. Abdominal pain	0	1	2	3
16. Stuffy nose	0	1	2	3
17. Wrinkles around the mouth	0	1	2	3
18. Dark circles under the eyes	0	1	2	3
19. Track lines in the soles of the feet	0	1	2	3
20. Swollen or achy joints	0	1	2	3
TOTALS:	___	___	___	___

GRAND TOTAL: _____

Scores over 30 suggest the possible presence of microscopic parasites. The most important next step is testing by a lab with special expertise in this field, and treat-ment by a knowledgeable health care professional.

SOURCE: T. Kuss, Infinity Health Systems, Littleton, Colorado.

Scoring the Questionnaire about Microscopic Parasites

The symptoms described in the questionnaires are associated with any of a number of illnesses. Consequently the scores from the tests point to possibili-ties, but not to a diagnosis.

A test score above thirty on this questionnaire suggests the possibility of infection by microscopic parasites. They can be extremely difficult to detect and can be difficult to treat. Microscopic parasites can actually suppress the immune system and significantly impair digestion—they can also cause other illnesses almost anywhere in the body.

The incidence of microscopic parasites in the United States is increasing rapidly. If you have had long-term, chronic digestive illness and have not been tested for parasites, this may be the next logical step. Even if you were previously tested, retesting is appropriate since new advances in lab detection are improving doctors' ability to diagnose this troublesome problem. Undiagnosed infection can underlie many other illnesses. Note that the symptoms from these chronic parasitic infections may not necessarily occur in the digestive tract.

If you think you have a parasitic infection, it may be tempting to undertake self-treatment. It is vitally important not to self-treat if you do have parasites. Many parasitic infections can only be eradicated by a specific drug or drug combination. Herbs can be very useful in combination with prescription drugs and may enhance the effectiveness of the eradication program. However, we advise against relying on the use of herbs alone. Information on lab work for protozoa and parasites is included in chapters 15 and 17 on testing; treatment information appears in chapter 21 on protozoa.

We also want to emphasize that the questionnaires highlight only a few of the many aspects of digestive illness. The scores may indicate the value of lab testing for food allergies, hyperpermeability, candida, or parasites. These relatively simple conditions can play a role in maintaining the chronic nature of more serious digestive disease. We have included these health issues because they are often overlooked in traditional evaluations and treatments. The tests are also useful because very low scores can help to rule out the presence of these problems. Your responses to the questionnaires will assist you in developing strategies to deal with digestive problems.

Biographical information for **Jerry Stine** appears on page 12.

3

Your Five Protective Barriers

Scott Anderson, M.D.

THE FIRST PROTECTIVE BARRIER: INTELLIGENCE

Intelligence is the first and most important barrier that guards our health. Although we may think of our brains as the source of our intelligence, we can also define intelligence as the way we live, the way we run our entire lives. It is reflected in our capacity to be proactive—to see positive options and to act on them.

We each have a sphere of influence in which we make choices about our lives. We can choose what we bring into our lives—the people we spend time with, the thoughts we think, and the foods we eat. The more intelligent these choices, the better. Although we often take our diet for granted, it's important to be very conscious of what we eat, because if we consume only what tempts us, we may not be very healthy. So we should exercise intelligence on behalf of the entire body.

Eating smart means making wise choices about when, how, and where we eat, and all those other little decisions we make when we buy, prepare, and

---

Anatomy of the Mouth

Why is it so important to chew our food well?

- Chewing well mixes our food with saliva to begin digestion and makes it easier to swallow.
- Chemicals in our saliva (enzymes) start breaking down the food. The better they're mixed into the food, the more thoroughly it will be digested.
- Our food is moved down the esophagus by waves of muscle contractions (peristalsis) that act as a conveyor belt to the stomach.

Doctors have noticed that people who bolt down their food have a greater tendency toward gastrointestinal problems than those who chew thoroughly. Think of chewing as a time to really taste and savor your food.

consume food. This may mean planning ahead to bring a healthy snack to work for an energy boost in the afternoon. It should include eating in a relaxed way, perhaps sitting in the sun or a cozy café. Eating smart means paying attention to details such as chewing our food rather than just bolting it down. And it's wise to know the basics of nutrition.

THE SECOND BARRIER: STOMACH ACID

Believe it or not, our stomach acid (hydrochloric acid, or HCl for short) is one of the most important self-protections the body provides; it destroys the "bad bugs"—microbes that are always trying to invade our systems.

Most of us don't even think about our stomach acid, and when we do, we are more likely to think of it as a problem. But the body invests an enormous amount of energy to produce HCl. If we drew an energy map of the body, the energy used to create this acid would be comparable to the amount of energy it would take to climb Mount Everest. Although we're used to hearing about the dangers of stomach acid on television, these gastric juices are actually an essential and vital protection to our digestion. Here's how they work:

- *Stomach acid basically sterilizes our food.* It destroys microbes such as bacteria or yeast seeking to colonize the warm and nutrient-rich folds of the intestines. As our food is mixed with acid in the stomach, the germs are destroyed on contact by burning them with a solution strong enough to literally burn a hole in this book. Germs such as bacteria, microscopic parasites, viruses, and molds can contaminate anything we eat or drink.
- *Stomach acid begins the process of protein digestion.* Stomach juices contain acid and an enzyme called pepsin. This creates just the right chemical conditions for digesting protein.
- *In the acid mix of the stomach, minerals are processed for absorption.* Without enough stomach acid we'd have poor absorption of minerals. In fact, malabsorption of minerals is one of the tip-offs to doctors that a patient may have chronically low stomach acid. The trace mineral deficiencies that may result can be identified through simple lab tests such as hair analysis.
- *Stomach acid stimulates secretions from the pancreas that are essential to good digestion (enzymes and bicarbonate).* The acidity of the food coming out of the stomach signals the pancreas to pour out its juices. When the acid mix comes in contact with the gut wall, this stimulates the next phase of digestion. If the stomach's output is only mildly acidic, then the pancreas gets a weak signal and the whole digestive process is compromised.

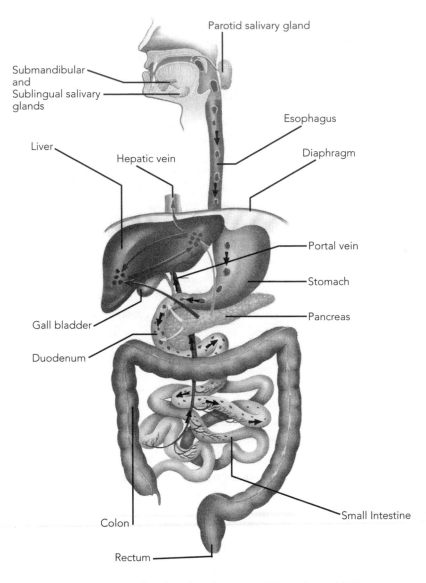

SOURCE: *Know Your Body: The Atlas of Anatomy* (Ulysses Press, 2002), illustration © 2002 Times Media Private Limited.

DIGESTION: THE FOOD PROCESSOR

After we've eaten, food stays in the stomach for a while. How long depends on the size and content of what we've just eaten and how well our digestive equipment is working. During that time (typically at least ninety minutes) food is confined in the stomach under very acidic conditions. Here's what's happening when our food is digesting:

- The food is being churned in the stomach, grinding it to the consistency of cornmeal
- This mixture is "cooking" in the stomach acid
- Germs are being killed
- Protein digestion is beginning
- Minerals are being processed

When this process has been completed, the food is ready for the next phase of digestion, which takes place in the small intestine. There nourishment from our food will be absorbed by the body, to actually become part of our tissues.

As the stomach sends the food into the small intestine, the food-acid mix needs to be neutralized. If this didn't occur, the mix would burn the delicate lining of the small gut. By adding bicarb into the mix, the tender lining of the gut (the epithelium) is protected from the chemical burn of digestive acid. This food mixture (called chyme) is about the consistency of liquid oatmeal and contains saliva, stomach acid, pepsin, bicarb, and enzymes.

A Note from the Doctor

As a doctor, when I identify patients who have frequent indigestion, one of the first things I have them try is an over-the-counter supplement of hydrochloric acid, betaine hydrochloride, which they can get from most any health food store. In some cases, just that addition will resolve their digestive problems. If not the next step is to try adding over-the-counter pancreatic enzymes. So my first strategy is to support natural processes in the body that may be weakened, with supplements such as stomach acid and digestive enzymes.

- If you have any concerns or questions, be sure to talk about them with your doctor.
- When you begin a new supplement, make that the only addition to your diet for at least two weeks so you can more easily identify unwanted effects.
- Start by taking only one capsule a day for about four days—just as you start eating.
- If it agrees with you, then gradually increase the dose every two to four days until you are taking the recommended dose.
- Remember that we're all different—the nutritional requirements of a 100 pound woman are quite different than those of a growing child of 50 pounds or a man who weighs 200.

—Scott Anderson, M.D.

The Pancreas Takes Center Stage

At this point, the pancreas also makes its contribution. This gland is located near the stomach and is a thin organ about 4 to 6 inches long, shaped like a fleshy leaf. It produces a number of important secretions that help us digest. The major ones include:

- Digestive enzymes
- Bicarbonate
- Insulin (which is secreted into the bloodstream rather than the GI tract)

In this next phase of digestion food is moved into the small gut by the action of the pylorus, a thick muscular ring that acts as the gatekeeper, separating the opening leading out of the stomach from the small gut, which is called the duodenum. The pylorus releases the food mix little by little. If it were to open fully and stay open, the entire contents of the stomach would come flooding out all at once. Instead, the contents of the stomach are released in small squirts, every few seconds or every few minutes. At this point the pancreas secretes more enzymes to continue the digestive process, including:

- Lipase to digest fats
- Protease for proteins
- Amylase for starches
- Other enzymes with specialized functions

The Small Intestine: The Source of Our Nourishment

The primary job of the small gut is to absorb nutrients from our food. The breakdown and absorption of proteins and fats and the final digestion and absorption of starches and sugars all occur there.

The small intestine is essentially a tube—25 feet long! Its inner surface is covered with tiny folds that provide the greatest possible surface area for absorption, so we can get the maximum nutrition from our food. If you could unroll and unwrinkle the folds and lay the surface of the tissue out flat, the small gut would be about 60 feet across—at a size of 60 feet wide and 25 feet long, the small intestine has roughly the surface area of a tennis court. The large intestine, in contrast, is only about 5 feet long, with a surface area smaller than the top of a desk.

If you were to view the digestive tract through a videoscope, as gastroenterologists now do, the small intestine has a velvety appearance because its surface is made up of minute folds that are covered with tiny fingerlike structures called villi. The villi themselves are covered with other much smaller hairlike structures (microvilli), which can be seen only through a microscope.

The Incredible Digestive System

- In a cubic millimeter of the mucosal lining (smaller than the size of a grain of rice), there are 6 to 9 feet of nerve cell fibers.
- "Gut reactions" are transmitted by nerve impulses that travel through the gut in a matter of seconds.
- There are ten times more bacterial cells within the gut than there are cells in our entire body.
- Human cells are hundreds of times bigger than bacterial cells.

Although bacteria are microscopic and their DNA is tiny, if we were to take many billions of them and place their DNA end to end, the total length can be huge. For example, there are approximately 75,000 miles of bacterial DNA in a teaspoon of yogurt. And these are the same friendly bacteria that thrive in a healthy digestive tract.

All these structures are exquisitely constructed to absorb nutrients. The villi and microvilli are covered with a layer of protective mucus. The large gut is also lined with mucus, but it has a smooth, glistening surface when seen through the videoscope.

In the small gut the fingerlike villi shrink when chronic irritation is present. As the absorptive area decreases, people usually have problems with malabsorption. In fact, the loss of the villi is one of the findings doctors use to diagnose irritations such as wheat/gluten intolerance (celiac disease, or sprue). If there is infection or irritation, absorption is compromised and the sufferer may lose weight or experience failure to thrive.

After the digested food moves into the colon or large intestine, water is absorbed from the spent food, preparing it to be discarded from the body as stool. Another major function of the colon may be its role as host to a huge population of bacteria, including the friendly flora. Some nutrients are also transferred to the blood here, but the vast majority of absorption has already taken place in the small gut.

THE THIRD BARRIER: THE INNER DEFENSE SYSTEM

We have marvelous safeguards built into our digestive tracts, there to destroy invaders from the outside world, microbes hiding in our food and coming in with our water, waiting to do us harm.

Our protections include microbe fighters (antibodies) concealed in the mucous lining of the gut. Antibodies target antigens, which are anything the body has identified as unknown or potentially harmful. A wide range of substances can be tagged as antigens, from allergenic foods to microbes.

Secretory immunoglobulin A is one of our foremost defenders (sometimes called SIgA). When invading antigens, such as microbes, try to work their way into the folds of the gut, our antibodies attack. Each SIgA molecule resembles a microscopic arrow tipped with a suction cup. Hundreds of these arrows may adhere to the surface of an invader, making it fuzzier and stickier so it will become trapped in the mucous layer.

THE FOURTH BARRIER: THE LIVER

The liver is the Grand Central Station of our metabolism, handling an enormous amount of molecular traffic. The liver is the site of a huge variety of processing, whose vital roles include:

- Breaking down nutrients
- Filtering out toxins that come in from the gut and breaking them down
- Synthesizing important blood components

There are extensive networks of tiny blood vessels around the gut that absorb nutrients from our food. This nutrient-rich blood all flows directly into the larger collecting veins of the portal system and is carried on to the liver. Another network of capillaries comprises the bulk of the liver and surrounds the liver cells. Guarding this system are specialized cells called macrophages, which destroy much of the bacteria that comes in from the GI tract.

All the nutrients and other substances that have been absorbed from our food are processed by the liver and then transported to the rest of the body. Nutrients will be broken down to provide energy and the raw materials from which our body will actually be constructed and maintained. These are the building blocks of muscle, skin, and bone.

The liver also functions somewhat like the oil filter on your car; one of its jobs is to protect the rest of the body from all the debris and gunk that could be harmful. Essentially all the material absorbed from the gut passes through the liver, carried by the bloodstream. The liver cleans the blood before it enters the heart and before it's pumped throughout the body.

So the liver is the center for toxic cleanup in the body. The majority of the toxins are processed and transformed there. Some substances are exiled: If they don't measure up, they may get processed out of the body via the bile, in the urine, or in stool. If the liver is required to process too many toxins, an overload may occur. Then the impaired capacity can limit its ability to monitor incoming traffic and filter out harmful substances, like a police force outnumbered by thugs who then get into general circulation.

THE FIFTH BARRIER: FRIENDLY FLORA

The friendly flora are bacteria that have beneficial effects in the body. They are important because they help keep our immune defenses well tuned and provide valuable nutrients such as vitamin K, folic acid, and the essential fatty acid butyrate. This barrier is so central to our well-being that chapter 5 has been devoted to the subject. Read on to learn more about your inner ecology.

OPTIMIZING YOUR FIVE PROTECTIVE BARRIERS

1. *Intelligence.* Know as much as you can about your food and make healthy choices of what to put in your mouth. There are many foods available that you would be smart not to eat.
2. *Stomach acid.* Know that stomach acid is doing a very important job; avoid antacids and acid-blocking medications. If needed, take supplemental HCl to support this important barrier.
3. *Intestinal lining.* Big as a tennis court, this is the delicate velvet surface across which food molecules enter the inner world of your bodily self. Learn as much as you can about how to keep this healthy. (See, for example, chapter 19 for a brief overview of the options.)
4. *Liver.* Metabolic Grand Central, the liver chemically transforms and detoxifies all the complex chemistry absorbed from the digestive tract through the intestinal lining. Chapters 9, 23, and 26 have useful information on minimizing toxins, detox, and nutritional support.
5. *Friendly flora.* There are ten times as many bacterial cells in your digestive tract as there are in your entire body.

Scott Anderson, M.D., obtained his undergraduate degree in biology from Harvard, a masters degree in genetics (where his thesis focused on human gut microbiology), and his medical degree from the University of Connecticut. During his 20 year career in medicine, he practiced in a variety of clinical settings, including hospitals, outpatient clinics, and medical centers. His areas of focus include preventive, nutritional, and antiaging medicine. Dr. Anderson's current endeavors include research, writing, and consulting; he can be reached at SVAMD@aol.com.

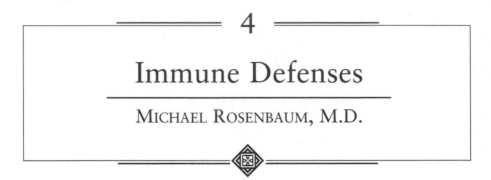

Immune Defenses

Michael Rosenbaum, M.D.

The digestive tract is the most extensive area of immune activity in the body. Although we typically think of the GI tract as the place where food is digested and then discarded, the GI tract is also a very active immune center. For example, it contains more than 80 percent of our antibody-producing cells.

This immunity is different from the immunity elsewhere in the body in general, an entirely separate immune system that was not really appreciated until recently. It's considered the largest of our lymph organs, larger than the thymus and all the other lymph nodes scattered throughout our systems.

A MAJOR SYSTEM OF DEFENSES

- We are constantly under siege. We coexist with a vast population of microscopic armies consisting of viruses, bacteria, yeast, and parasites. The immune system is our major defense against this constant bombardment. To combat a never-ending horde of enemies, our immunity must be dynamic and ever vigilant.

    In the gut, material from the outside environment literally enters the interior of the body as our food and water. They can contain all manner of pathogens. Our trusty immune system is there in the gut to protect us from this outside world inside us.

- Our protective barrier is fairly vulnerable. To penetrate the inner gut lining and get into the blood vessels, invaders need only penetrate the mucous barrier and a layer of cells (the epithelium). This is quite different from the skin, for example, which has several protective layers of cells.

- There is a lot of internal area to be protected. Consider that the small intestine is on average 25 feet long—more than four times most people's height. And the large intestine is typically 5 feet long. So you have about 30 feet of GI tract.

- Resident bacteria have to be kept under control. In that 30 feet of intestine you have an enormous number of resident bacteria. They're supposed to be there—they're normal flora. And it turns out that the normal bacterial population in the human gut is about equal to the number of cells in our entire body.

In the small gut, there are millions of bacteria in each teaspoon of liquid (about a cubic centimeter). In the colon, there are probably at least a trillion. There's just an incredible amount of normal flora. People have no idea that they carry so much bacteria inside them. And if you take an antibiotic, in a sense you're probably wiping out almost half the cells in your body. In fact, some antibiotics literally wipe out all the bacteria, harmful and helpful, all at once.

When things are in balance, we have a symbiotic, harmonious relationship with these bacteria. We need the bacteria for so many reasons. They actually produce vitamins such as vitamin K, which helps our blood clot, and folic acid, which is essential to the female reproductive system. They also preserve and maintain a healthy lining of the gut and they tend to crowd out the bad bugs.

There's rapid turnover. What's even more amazing is that the gut lining is completely replaced about every five to seven days. These cells work very hard and then they die. If our body can't keep up with the effort of destroying and replacing them, we could end up with an impaired gut lining. Then we're subject to intestinal permeability, food allergies, or all kinds of other potential problems.

GUT DEFENSES

Your immune system is a vast military service fighting a never-ending war. The gut marshals several different kinds of defenses to protect us from the outside world that literally comes inside our bodies with food and water. Immune functions can be compared to munitions factories, artillery, hidden attackers, sentries, and even guardsmen that check ID.

- *Chemical warfare*—acid and enzymes. Digestive enzymes in the saliva and throughout the gut help us digest our food and literally dissolve invading "bad bugs." Stomach acid (HCl) also destroys bacteria and other pathogens.
- *The munitions factory*—your lymph tissue. The lymph tissue secretes antibodies, the artillery of our digestive immune system. Oral tolerance performs ID checks on invaders to separate friend from foe, thus protecting our friendly flora and digested food from attack.
- *Immune artillery*—antibodies. Antibodies are the immune artillery that target specific prey. The antibodies can be compared to ballistic missiles with a tracking device that seeks and finds and chases invaders—and never lets go.

IMMUNE DEFENSES

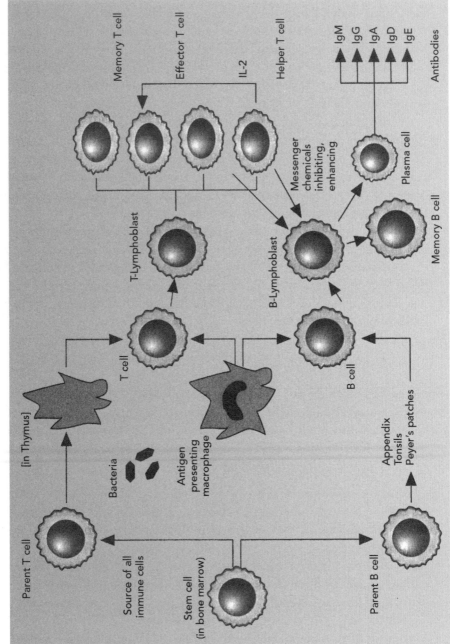

SOURCE: Immunosciences Lab, Inc.

- *The invaders*—antigens. The prey are called antigens; they trigger the antibodies' protective response. Antigens are any kind of invading agent perceived by the body as new, foreign, intrusive, or harmful. Antigens may be bacteria or parasites or even allergenic foods.
- *Killer cells*—cellular immunity. Our immunity also includes components such as T cells, called killer cells and natural killer cells, that police our bodies, targeted to destroy bacteria, viruses, and even tumors by releasing toxic enzymes. Note that there is little cellular immunity in the gut, so the secretory IgA, our immune artillery, are of supreme importance.

THE MUNITIONS FACTORY

The immune response of the gut is generated by a specialized kind of lymph tissue researchers call GALT (gut-associated lymphoid tissue). In general the lymph system is a network within the body that provides certain immune functions. Lymph is a clear liquid that circulates through a series of interconnected spaces and vessels, including the lymph nodes, located between the tissues and organs. The lymph is responsible for removing bacteria and supplying white blood cells (lymphocytes) to the blood, as well as the transport of certain proteins and fats.

The GALT consists of specialized colonies of cells in the gut lining called Peyer's patches and also the lymphatic tissue in the appendix. In the Peyer's patches live the plasma cells that manufacture our antibodies, the immune artillery that protects us from invaders. The antibodies in the gut are primarily the secreted (or secretory) immunoglobulin A (SIgA), our first line of immune defense in the digestive tract.

Most of the gut lymph tissue is located at the juncture of the large and small intestine, near the appendix. This strategic concentration of lymph tissue appears to play an important role in protecting the small intestine against the migration of bacteria or parasites back up into the small intestine from the colon, since there's a much greater concentration of microbes in the colon.

It's probably no coincidence that most inflammation in the gut occurs at this juncture. There is a greater potential for infection here, and that's probably why there is so much lymphatic tissue. This is the area where Crohn's disease, for example, is most likely to occur (in the ileum). Appendix infections are well known. However, removing the appendix or a section of the ileum through surgery can be both a blessing and a curse, because while it can decrease inflammation, a lot of immune tissue is removed in the process. In most cases this seems to decrease immune defenses, and unfortunately, in some conditions such as Crohn's disease, the inflammation may reappear in other parts of the digestive tract. Research has found that people who have the appendix removed more often get Hodgkin's or Crohn's disease.

Your Amazing Immune Defenses

Immunity in the Gut

Type of protector	Where it's made and lives	Its role in our defense
B cells (live for years)	Made in bone marrow and mature in spleen and lymph nodes	Mature into plasma cells
Plasma cells (live about four days)	Reside in Peyer's patches in the lower small intestine	Make all the antibodies: IgA, SIgA, IgE, IgG, IgM
Memory cells (may live as long as twenty years)	Originate in bone marrow, migrate to the thymus where they mature; live hidden away in the spleen and in Peyer's patches	Attack specific microbes encountered in the past

Immunity Throughout the Body

T cells—T helpers, T suppressors, killer and natural killer cells, T cytotoxic cells	Made in bone marrow Mature in the thymus	Roam the body to protect us; some stimulate immunity, and others calm it

DEFENDERS AND PEACEKEEPING

In the barrier lining there are specialized cells, called M cells, that perform a protective function. The M cells can't move, so they can be compared to guardsmen who can't leave their post. They have the ability to bind onto anything considered dangerous—any kind of pathogen or oversized food particle. When an invader approaches them, they latch onto it and pull it underneath the surface to the lymphocytes below in the Peyer's patches. There in the trenches, white blood cells (lymphocytes) screen invaders to determine if they're friend or foe and produce the SIgA antibodies that line the entire tract and act against invasion. Macrophages are there to digest and process the invading microbes and alert T helper cells to the identity of the invader for future reference. Throughout the gut the secretory IgA bombards any and all invaders in a generalized response. When a problem is detected, SIgA secretion tends to increase throughout the gut to bolster our defenses.

The antibodies are tiny little arrow-shaped molecules that are part of our mucous defense barrier. Their role is to attack and detain. If they perceive bacteria, for example, which are typically hundreds of times larger than the antibody, they cover its surface, until it resembles an orange stuck with cloves. Several hundred SIgA molecules may adhere to the surface of a single invading bacteria. The purpose is to create a rough or uneven surface that will catch the microbe in the mucous layer that covers the gut lining. The mucous acts like a slow conveyor belt, gradually sliding the food through the gut and also moving microbes and large food particles out of the gut. The bacteria can then simply be discarded with the spent food in the stool. If you decrease the body's secretions, you decrease immune defenses. Aspirin, for example, decreases the mucous lining, one reason it can cause intestinal bleeding.

Our First Line of Defense: SIgA

In the digestive tract, the secretory IgA is our first line of immune defense. The SIgA antibodies are produced in the lining of the gut in the specialized cells called Peyer's patches. These cells secrete the SIgA into the mucous barrier, so they're called secretory immune globulins (SIgA for short). SIgA is also an important part of the defense system found in the saliva, and lives in the mucous membranes of the nose and the lungs.

Fortunately the entire digestive tract is loaded with SIgA, because there are very few of our protective roving scavenger T cells there. The SIgA is targeted against anything potentially harmful—bacteria, microscopic parasites, even large food particles that might cause inflammation. Note that other kinds of antibodies (IgE, IgG, and IgM) specifically target one subspecies of invader, such as a particular strain of flu or an allergenic food, but they won't attack any others. For example, if I caught the flu this year, I won't catch it again later this year, because I have built up antibodies against it. However, when a new strain of flu comes around next year, I will have no protective immunity against it. My antibodies are so specific, they recognize only illnesses to which I've already been exposed but ignore all others. But our faithful SIgA offers nonspecific immunity—it will attack anything it perceives as potentially harmful.

Peacekeeping Roles: SIgA

SIgA is ingeniously programmed to be tolerant of our friendly flora. Although it will attack anything offensive, it's somehow able to recognize what belongs there and what doesn't—no friendly fire. SIgA targets only microorganisms that don't have the right identifier and binds to them—metaphorically speaking, only those without the right ID or badge. Macrophages in the GALT attach to the invader, consume it, and display its identity. T cells scan the ID to see if the immune system has been in combat with this invader before. The memory cells are checked (they function as a huge database documenting past offenders). If the scan matches the identity of an old enemy, the memory cells begin to rapidly replicate in a cloninglike activity that generates a huge immune response. In addition, SIgA has the ability to bind to particles that aren't fully digested or dissolved, typically large food particles, to minimize the wear and tear on the gut and the potential for problems such as leaky gut syndrome. Basically SIgA targets both pathogens and food.

In the gut secretory IgA acts as a kind of peacemaker through an anti-inflammatory effect. Immunoglobulin A (IgA) in general prevents inflammation. It can reduce the biochemical panic response that can occur when the metabolic alarm system goes off in the body. This warning system includes immune messenger chemicals (the cytokines) that function like sirens sounding the call to respond when a threat is perceived. If the cytokines stimulate too heavy an attack, major inflammation can occur as a protective mechanism. By toning down the metabolic panic and the inflammation that could follow, SIgA maintains the integrity of the lining cells of the gut barrier.

There are some things that promote our body's arsenal of SIgA, and others that deplete it. Some people are just born with less ability to make it. SIgA is reduced in people who have allergies in general, and in children born of parents who are allergic. And as a result, such children may be more prone to food allergy and to gluten/wheat intolerance. This is an important response to monitor, because gluten has the unique ability to inflame the lining of the small intestine, which can cause you to become allergic to everything else.

Vitamin A can significantly increase our ability to produce SIgA. If you are suddenly exposed to bacteria, the secretory IgA production usually goes up, particularly in response to bacteroides and nonpathogenic forms of E. coli. The level of SIgA in our bodies at any given time can now be measured through a simple mail-in lab test. One test is performed on saliva, the other on stool, and there are labs that do both. People with low levels of SIgA in saliva or stool tend to be much more prone to infection and to food allergy.

OTHER IMMUNE DEFENSES

IgM is also found in the gut, although it's not as important as SIgA. It's produced whenever there is a definite infection in the gut. Anything from botulism to salmonella will induce an IgM response.

Lysosomes are another kind of "chemical warfare"—specialized enzymes. They're a very primitive form of immune defense that's present in saliva, tears, and in gut secretions. Lysosomes are also capable of killing pathogens in the gut, essentially by digesting them, just as the enzymes in meat tenderizer break down meat tissue.

Our Immune Artillery—the Antibodies

Type and location	Source	Task	Effect
B cells become plasma cells and memory cells	Develop and mature in bone marrow	Plasma cells produce antibodies; memory cells direct them	Antibodies (immunoglobulins, or Ig) are our immune artillery
SIgA secreted into the mucous lining	Peyer's patches (GALT): lymph tissue in small gut, appendix, elsewhere in the gut	Targets any invader (nonspecific immunity)	First line of defense; tones down inflammation
IgA in saliva and mucus of nose, lungs	From B cells, including lymph tissue in nose and tonsils	Targets any invader	Tones down inflammation
IgE made by plasma cells	Produced by B cells throughout the body	Targets specific invaders	Immediate response
IgG in bloodstream—80% of blood immunity	Like other immuno-globulins, made by plasma cells (mature B cells)	Highly specific (work through a lock-and-key mechanism)	Delayed response that can cause inflammation
IgM—secreted into gut mucous lining	Peyer's patches	Fights specific infection	Immediate response

TELLING FRIEND FROM FOE

The second major immune defense of the GALT is oral tolerance. Oral tolerance is extremely important because it's the mechanism by which your gut immune system tells friend from foe and it deals with both food and microbes.

Our oral-tolerance system has learned to distinguish what we can tolerate and what we can't. As adults we consume about a ton of food a year. If the immune system attacked everything that came into the gut, it would attack all the food we eat, since it's actually all foreign to our body. But fortunately it doesn't. Food that's undigested, in large particles, or allergenic can be attacked by both SIgA and IgM antibodies. Sometimes our oral tolerance doesn't work. When it doesn't we are more prone to food sensitivities.

Oral tolerance has the job of identifying the friendly bacteria again; no small task. There are also ten trillion bacteria in an adult gut. Without oral tolerance, our immune system would attack all of the zillions of bacteria in the gut, even those that belong there. Fortunately this system has learned to distinguish between what should be there and what shouldn't. It identifies normal flora and signals the body not to attack. So the gut immune response attacks only pathogenic organisms.

SUPPORTING YOUR IMMUNE SYSTEM

Any kind of infection, even a flu, can lower our stores of antibodies (our precious SIgA). An infection anywhere in the body, even a tooth abscess, can affect the gut by increasing stress and reducing the secretory IgA.

Stress reduces secretory IgA. Any kind of stress can do this. Two German studies indicate that mental relaxation procedures, such as meditation or biofeedback, can lead to increased secretion of SIgA. To promote this positive effect, stress reduction; moderate exercise such as yoga, tai chi, or Qigong; meditation; or any kind of mental relaxation are very important for a healthy digestive tract.

Poor diet and low nutrient levels generally also lower SIgA. It's been shown that kids in third world countries who have protein calorie malnutrition (PCM) have lower SIgA levels and therefore frequently get diarrhea because they're lacking the SIgA to protect them against it. Once you get diarrhea, you lose even more lining in the gut and it becomes a vicious cycle.

SIgA decreases with age. It seems that there are many more things that reduce secretory IgA than easily increase it, so you really have to be on guard.

The key influences on your immune system are (1) genetics, (2) inherited allergies, (3) nutrition, (4) stress, (5) lack of breast-feeding, (6) age, (7) the integrity of the gut lining, (8) the health of the microflora, and (9) the presence of infection in the gut or anywhere in the body. Research has found that nutrition can actually affect the way your genetic makeup is expressed. Good nutrition can tip the balance toward health.

Vitamin A in particular is critical in replenishing the lining of the gut and maintaining the integrity of the mucosa. Unfortunately the lack of vitamin A happens to be the most common vitamin deficiency in the entire world. Other nutrients that increase SIgA include zinc taken with vitamin A, colostrum (for people who are not dairy intolerant), and probably L-glutamine.

Immune Defenses in the Gut

	Primary Task	Role with microbes	Role with food
Size of the job	Must differentiate friend from foe	Ten trillion microbes in a normal adult GI tract	One ton of food is eaten yearly by a normal adult
Secretory IgA	On the attack— "up-regulates" immunity	Attacks pathogens: yeast, bacteria, parasites	Attaches to larger undigested food particles and allergens
Oral tolerance	Calms the system— "down-regulates" it	Identifies and protects normal flora	Assures the passage of digested, dissolved foods

Michael Rosenbaum, M.D., of Corte Madera, California, has had an active private practice since 1977, focused on immunology, clinical nutrition, and allergy. He is a graduate of the Albert Einstein College of Medicine in New York City and holds an M.S. in clinical biochemistry from the Hebrew University in Jerusalem. He is the author of *Super Supplements* (Viking Penguin and Signet), *Solving the Puzzle of Chronic Fatigue Syndrome* (Life Science Press), and numerous articles on nutrition. A frequent lecturer to professional medical groups, he has participated in numerous television and radio talk shows on the topics of chronic fatigue syndrome, nutrition, and immunity.

Dr. Rosenbaum is available for consultations on nutritional therapy, allergy treatment, and antiaging medicine, which can be arranged by calling his office at (415) 927-9450. For additional information, see his Web site at www.michaelrosenbaummmd.com.

5

Friendly Flora

Nigel Plummer, Ph.D.

You often hear about ecology, the relationship between organisms and their environment. As you read in chapter 2, within your body there is an entire miniature ecosystem, a microecology, that has a major influence on your health. This inner ecology is made up of the microflora, more than 500 species of microscopic living bacteria, creating an internal environment that is diverse, complex, interrelated, and ever changing. This population, although minute, is so enormous that the number of microbial cells in our bodies at any one time is greater than the number of our own cells.

The microflora are essential to our well-being. These bacteria provide very real beneficial effects. They limit the populations of harmful bacteria. They assist in the process of digestion. And they even manufacture some essential nutrients, such as butyrate, an essential fatty acid and a primary fuel for the gut lining. So when our gut ecology is in balance, we thrive.

BENEFICIAL EFFECTS OF FLORA

- *Crowding out the harmful microbes.* It appears that the beneficial flora may actually interfere with the ability of some pathogens to adhere to the gut lining by covering all available surfaces, which is reported to limit the colonization of microbes such as *E. coli,* candida, and giardia.
- *Producing natural antibiotic effects.* Lactobacilli are believed to produce substances that suppress the growth of potentially harmful organisms.
- *Slowing the growth of pathogens.* Many pathogenic microbes require iron in order to be highly active and destructive. Our bodies have a mechanism to minimize microbe growth by ensuring that very little free iron remains in the bloodstream. In the gut bifidobacteria appear to aid in binding iron, making it unavailable to microbes by concentrating it up to a thousand times the normal content.
- *Discouraging destructive organisms.* Most gut pathogens stop growing in highly acid environments, so creating a more acidic environment in the

mucous lining (with a low pH, below 5) potentially stops colonization by pathogenic types.

- *Improving digestion.* Digestive absorption can be enhanced in people who lack the enzyme to digest dairy products (lactose). In some cases, the consumption of fermented milk products or the addition of *L. acidophilus* to dairy products can be quite helpful. The fermenting process reduces the level of lactose and makes it more easily absorbed. Lactose digestion is greatly enhanced by the addition of *L. acidophilus,* whether the milk is fermented or not.

- *Reducing the harmful effects of cholesterol.* Researchers have noticed repeatedly that eating yogurtlike foods is beneficial for health. A study of the Masai peoples of Africa found a very low incidence of heart disease, despite a diet high in animal fat. Diets high in animal fat normally tend to raise cholesterol levels and increase clogging of the heart arteries (atherosclerosis). In another study, a 5 to 10 percent decrease in cholesterol was seen in subjects after they had been eating yogurt for just seven days! This effect was also found to be true in studies of animals and even poultry. So yogurt can be a great addition to your diet if you're not dairy intolerant. When this is the case, use a good acidophilus/bifidus supplement.

- *Increasing the efficiency of the body.* Bile salts can inhibit harmful flora, the bad guys. By recycling bile salts, the helpful flora maximize the levels of bile in the system. This conservation saves the body precious energy, and increases the protection of the gut.

- *Regulating the immune system.* Yogurt has been found to significantly enhance the production of B-interferon in the human immune system. This effect was observed when cultures of *L. bulgaricus* and *Streptococcus thermophilus* were introduced.

- *Protecting against cancer.* Supplementing the diet with *L. acidophilus,* researchers found that levels of potentially harmful enzymes in the gut were reduced. These included the enzymes that convert nitrates into much more harmful nitrosamines, documented to cause cancer in children and adults. They also included enzymes that convert azo-compounds, found in food colors, into potentially toxic products.

- *Suppressing tumors.* Animal studies have found that it took twice as long for cancer to form when fermented milk was part of the diet. *L. bulgaricus* was observed consistently to be more effective than *Streptococcus thermophilus.* A number of studies also found that yogurt had the capacity to suppress tumors or halt tumor growth.

The Benefits of Good Flora

Joel had suffered from inflammatory bowel disease for more than ten years, when he was first diagnosed and treated with standard drug therapy (5-ASA drugs and steroids, the treatment of choice at that time). Following his first episode he had many periods of relapse, most often in the spring and fall. The colonoscopic exam showed nothing unusual, but a comprehensive lab analysis of his stool indicated that he had severe dysbiosis with an overgrowth of *E. coli* bacteria that may have become pathogenic.

Although it was necessary to put him back on steroids, Joel also began a program of nutritional support that included probiotics, a friendly flora product with bifidus and acidophilus. He also began taking vitamins and minerals and replaced one meal a day with liquid nutrition to rest his digestive tract. He was gradually able to taper off the steroids, but continued with the nutritional program. Joel's job took him to another state, but when he returned two years later, he told us that he'd never been in such good health before in his life. He's had no relapses and no longer has to take steroids every spring and fall. He continues to use one medication in low doses, the rice powder supplement, extra glutamine, and the flora products. We are delighted to know he's been "feeling great!"

—Trent W. Nichols, M.D.

FACTS ABOUT FLORA

There are half a dozen types of bacteria present in the gut in large numbers. Of these, *Lactobacillus acidophilus* (in the small gut) and bifidobacteria (in the large gut) are two of the primary strains. Although researchers have identified more than 400 species of microflora that can live in the gut environment, most of them are transient, occur in low numbers, and contribute little to our overall functioning. Friendly flora are:

- Present in children once they begin eating solid food, and in normal healthy adults
- Predictably found in specific areas of the GI tract
- Often associated with the lining of the gut
- Mostly live without air; in ratio, there are 1,000 anaerobes for each of the aerobic bacteria

Types of Flora

Part of the GI Tract	Species	Approx. number in normal adult
Stomach	Lactobacilli	1,000 per gram of contents of the stomach
Duodenum and first part of jejunum (first section of small gut)	Mainly: *Lactobacillus acidophilus Bifidobacterium bifidus Streptococci* Also smaller numbers of *E. coli* yeast, *Proteus spp.*, and Veillonella	10,000 per gram of contents of the duodenum (in the chyme)
End of jejunum Ileum	More complex ecology Coliforms Numerous bifidobacteria	1,000,000 to 100,000,000 per gram of contents of the jejunum (in the chyme)
Large intestine (colon)	Anaerobic bacteria Bacteroides Bifidobacteria	100,000,000,000 to 1,000,000,000,000 per gram of contents of the large intestine (in the stool)

THE ORIGIN OF FLORA

Just before birth, a human infant has a sterile GI tract, with no flora whatsoever. The development of the flora of a newborn depends on whether the child is breast or bottle fed. In breast-fed children the flora of the GI tract quickly becomes dominated by a species of friendly flora called bifidobacteria and a few other types of bacteria. If left undisturbed, this community of flora remains stable until the child is weaned, when the changeover to solid food marks the development of typical adult flora.

In bottle-fed babies a different microflora develops in early infancy. The population is mainly lactobacilli, with a much lower incidence of bifidobacteria. There is a large body of evidence to suggest that this difference in the makeup of the flora is connected with the greater susceptibility of bottle-fed infants to infection by harmful microbes that typically cause mild to severe diarrhea.

Once a child begins solid food, distinct changes occur in the flora of the gut, due to the changes in diet. By midchildhood, the community of microflora that has developed should remain stable throughout most of adult life, under normal conditions. However, this delicate balance can be significantly disrupted by antibiotic treatment, microbial infection (such as traveler's diarrhea), or periods of stress, sometimes leading to overgrowth by other potentially harmful microorganisms.

Since the turn of the century, there have been recurring reports from researchers worldwide that supplementing the diet with viable bacteria, mainly lactobacilli, has beneficial effects on health that range from reestablishing flora to preventing cancer. Elie Metchnikoff is often quoted as the first researcher to identify the benefits of lactic acid bacteria. He suggested that yogurt and fermented milk products in the diet of the Bulgarian people contributed to their longevity. He suggested that the lactobacilli in these foods prevented the overgrowth of harmful bacteria in the gut flora.

THE BALANCE OF FLORA

Our inner ecology can experience distress, just as any other ecosystem can. And like the environment, our internal ecosystem may seem to be intact, but the biodynamics may be stressed and the system out of tune.

What causes imbalances in the microflora? Research has found that stress, a poor diet, or antibiotic therapy can destroy many of the helpful bacteria. The use of certain drugs or the chronic use of processed laxatives can also have a negative effect. When the friendly flora decrease in number, our inner environment is open to invasion and colonization by destructive microbes—harmful bacteria such as *E. coli* and salmonella, parasites including giardia and cryptosporidium, or yeasts such as candida.

- *Stress.* When the mind or body are under stress, the changes in the makeup of the mucous lining can create an environment less favorable to the friendly flora. In addition, motility in the gut (peristalsis) may slow down, and then the food may be colonized by different and possibly harmful microbes, no longer held in check by the lactobacilli and bifidobacteria. *E. coli,* bacteroides, and candida can increase significantly at these times.
- *Your choice of food.* Diet has an extremely important influence on the quality and quantity of the flora. Researchers have found that a diet of wheat meal greatly favored the growth of lactobacilli and decreased the levels of potentially harmful bacteria (such as strep, *E. coli,* and clostridium). In contrast, rats fed a diet of pork developed microflora low in lactobacilli and high in *E. coli.* A diet of easily digested milk protein (casein) produced a decrease in all bacteria types, with the exception of streptococci. This research suggests that a diet high in meat and milk products could depress the levels of favorable flora.

- *Antibiotics.* The widespread use of antibiotics by their very nature induces a dramatic and destructive effect on the microflora in the GI tract. Unfortunately the action of most antibiotics is not specific, so the harmful (pathogenic) organisms and the beneficial ones are often destroyed together. This is especially true of the lactobacilli and bifidobacteria, which are particularly sensitive to a wide variety of antibiotics and whose numbers fall dramatically following therapy.

Stressors That Are Destructive to Flora

Effects	How They Can Be Harmful	Potential Invaders
Stress	Decrease in mucous secretions; causes changes in composition of the gut lining; flora may be unable to cling to the gut lining and can be washed away	*E. coli*, bacteroides, and candida
Diet	Meat-based diet suspended beneficial bacteria Milk-based diet suspended most growth of beneficial bacteria	Meat-based diets can encourage *E. coli* and clostridium overgrowth Milk-based diets can encourage the growth of strep
Antibiotics	Eradicates both helpful and harmful bacteria; leaves the gut open to invasion by harmful microbes	*E. coli*, staph, strep, yeasts, especially candida

This reduction of the beneficial flora leaves the intestine open to invasion by opportunistic pathogens or overgrowth by less desirable components that the normal flora usually keep in check (including *E. coli*, staph such as *S. aureus*, strep, and yeasts, especially candida). It is worth noting that this situation is made worse when the undesirable microbes have developed drug resistance. In that case they survive treatment, but ironically the beneficial flora are killed off—exactly the opposite of what the body requires. Then the "bad bugs" are left to thrive unopposed—like a lawless Western town with no sheriff. In fact, the imbalance that results can allow the overgrowth of normally harmless bacteria such as strep; if their number increase sufficiently, they can become so invasive as to cause severe problems such as inflammation of the heart lining (endocarditis). Yeast are also quite resistant to antibiotics, so an overgrowth of candida in the GI tract following antibiotics is a likely occurrence.

The results of any of these stressors—physical or mental stress, poor diet, or antibiotic therapy—is that the microflora can become unbalanced to such an extent that health is harmed. Symptoms of minor imbalance may include intestinal discomfort, indigestion, gas, and bloating. A major or prolonged imbalance can lead to severe diarrhea or even a bacterial infection in the bloodstream (septicemia).

The most effective way to reestablish the normal microflora is by taking flora supplements of lactobacilli and bifidobacteria, available from many health food stores. (See the Resources for mail-order sources for supplements such as probiotics.)

Nigel Plummer, Ph.D., holds a doctorate in microbiology from the University of Surrey, England. He has worked both in the pharmaceutical and the nutriceutical industries. At Pfizer his research focused on the development of antibiotics. Subsequent research concentrated on the prevention and treatment of genitourinary candidiasis. This work furthered his interest in the beneficial role of normal flora in intestinal health and general well-being. For the past 20 years, he and his research team have been involved in the research and development of probiotic supplements that promote good flora and digestive health. Dr. Plummer is the CEO of the Pharmax Group of Companies.

The Pharmax Group was founded in 1988 and today is the largest branded nutriceutical provider to professional health care providers in the United Kingdom. Pharmax LLC in the United States was formally established in 2000 and sells nutritional supplements exclusively to licensed health care practitioners. The product line of Pharmax LLC encompasses a broad spectrum of nutritional and botanical supplements with an emphasis on products related to intestinal health, in particular probiotics. These products are used by practitioners in evidence-based strategies in nutritional medicine.

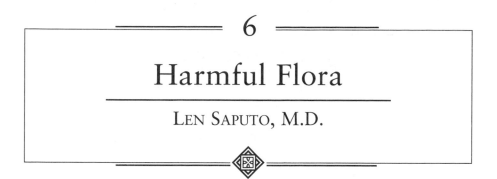

6

Harmful Flora

Len Saputo, M.D.

The balance that exists among our microflora is an example of nature's incredible perfection. When the microflora coexist in harmony, a healthy state of symbiosis results and we thrive. When this ecology is disturbed or dysfunctional, a state of dysbiosis results and a sense of unwellness or even disease can occur.

Our GI flora have been equated to an entire system within itself. There are more than 500 different species of bacteria, which collectively produce more metabolic activity than any other organ system in our bodies. Science also has revealed the many essential functions these flora provide. Although we don't often think about the flora, and their importance, the research shows that even in conditions as serious as AIDS, good flora can enhance health and prolong life.

WHEN INNER BALANCE IS LOST

If the beneficial flora decline, due to heavy antibiotic use or consumption of the wrong foods, the harmful flora can overgrow. These include yeast and numerous kinds of bacteria. Abnormal flora in the GI tract can result in a number of harmful effects. They can:

- Allow infection by microbes
- Deplete vitamin B_{12} and some amino acids
- Short-circuit digestive enzymes
- Transform essential fatty acids into damaging saturated fats
- Encourage conditions such as inflammatory bowel disease
- Interfere with breakdown of bile acids and estrogens, setting up the potential for cancer

The causes of flora imbalance—dysbiosis—occur far more often than we generally appreciate. Many doctors don't really focus on gut ecology. Basically any situation that can alter the physical integrity or the chemical balance of the GI tract can result in changes in the makeup of the microflora by decreasing

How Things Go Wrong

Before Carol entered college, she hardly had a sick day in her life. That first semester at college was really tough. She was up late studying, she gulped down fast foods, and when she partied, she partied! When the cold season hit just before finals, Carol was one of the first to catch a cold, a cold that just wouldn't go away. She saw her doctor, who prescribed several courses of antibiotics because "she just couldn't afford to be sick," and after about three months, the cold went away.

But Carol was never the same again. She began to have recurring vaginal yeast infections, and finally what was called a spastic colon. Her yeast infections were controlled with antiyeast suppositories, but the spastic colon would respond only to muscle relaxants and tranquilizers, and even then she never really felt well. She was finally told to see a psychiatrist, under the assumption that her gastrointestinal problems were probably related to her nerves. I saw Carol a full ten years later, when out of desperation she wanted to try an alternative approach. "There just has to be a better way." By that time, she'd had every test in the book, including X-rays of her GI tract, stool exams for parasites, blood work, and even a colonoscopy, but everything appeared to be "normal."

Carol was beginning to believe that she really was a "head case"! I requested lab tests to analyze her digestive capacity (the CDSA) and found she had a major imbalance of intestinal microflora—a severe overgrowth of yeast and a deficiency of normal beneficial bacteria. We devised a program of nutritional support for the intestinal tract, including mild antiyeast herbs, a very low-sugar diet, antioxidant nutrients, and a rich source of friendly bacteria. Within ten days, Carol's symptoms cleared up, and she has remained free of symptoms ever since. We have been checking her flora levels about every four to six months now for two years, and she's slowly developing a healthy intestinal microflora. Carol has discontinued psychotherapy and is beginning to feel like her old healthy self.

friendly flora and allowing harmful microbes to take over or overgrow. But the harmful microflora alone are rarely the single cause of dysbiosis. The essential questions to ask are: What is happening that enables some of these organisms to overgrow and upset the balanced ecology that previously existed? What makes an organism that is normally not destructive become pathogenic?

Two primary factors determine just how pathogenic an organism can become. First is its ability to overgrow and produce toxins that can injure us. The second factor, our resistance or the strength of our immune defenses, is one that modern medicine acknowledges. But we don't always address it, especially in short-term illness. In fact, it is widely believed that invading organisms are the primary cause of illness and that removing them is the solution. But all the organisms inhabiting the intestinal tract (including friendly bacteria such as acidophilus) can cause serious illness, such as blood poisoning and even death, under certain circumstances.

The treatment goal in combating dysbiosis is often to aggressively kill all the pathogenic microbes in a war between man and germs. We need strategies that also strengthen our own defenses and restore the balance in our inner ecology. In a catastrophic illness such as AIDS, modern medicine honors the fact that host defenses have been weakened. Researchers predict that our increased understanding of immunity will lead to new therapies to strengthen our immunity.

Why Good Flora Go Bad

Overgrowth of flora and dysbiosis are clear signals that something's gone wrong in the GI tract and requires attention. There are at least nine pathways that can lead to dysbiosis. They include:

- Eating too much sweet and starchy food
- Overuse of antibiotics
- Stress
- Poor digestion
- Exposure to toxins
- Inflammation
- Infection
- Lowered immune defenses
- Unknown causes

The Effects of Poor Food and Poor Digestion

What we eat creates the chemical environment in our GI tract. This presents a growth advantage for certain organisms—the microflora have to eat too. Each species of bacteria has specific nutritional needs. If the right food is provided, that species will enjoy accelerated growth. The beneficial bacteria that inhabit the gut survive on high-fiber diets. If we eat adequate amounts of fiber from vegetables and whole grains, these bacteria will have the nutrition they need to flourish.

Meals that are high in fat and meat and low in fiber tend to lead to what's called putrefactive dysbiosis. In this situation, a normal bacteria in the gut called bacteroides overgrows. Its toxic by-products result in the overproduction of ammonia. When this occurs the stool in the large intestine becomes

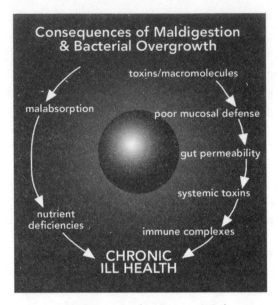

SOURCE © 1999 Great Smokies Diagnostic Laboratory

more alkaline and the production of essential gut fuel (butyrate) falls. As a result nutritional shortages occur throughout the digestive tract. Increased levels of bile acids build, raising the risk of colon cancer; levels of estrogen also go up, which can increase the risk of breast cancer.

Certain illnesses such as Crohn's disease or infections from invading microbes can disrupt the GI lining and cause a loss of normal defenses. Then harmful microorganisms can take advantage of this change in the GI environment and result in a shift in the microflora. When the destructive flora overgrow, their concentration becomes toxic to the gut and can cause other negative conditions, creating a vicious cycle that will be self-perpetuating.

Other factors come into play. Digestion may be poor because there's not enough hydrochloric acid. This can allow more undigested food to reach the lower small intestine and colon, where the microflora typically overgrow. The overgrowth of bacteria can lead to the overproduction of certain enzymes (proteases), resulting in poor digestion. This type of dysbiosis has been called fermentation dysbiosis.

Unintended Side Effects of Antibiotic Therapy

The use and abuse of antibiotic therapy may be the single most frequent cause of dysbiosis today. When antibiotics are taken, profound changes can occur in the microflora of the GI tract and elsewhere in the body where there are flora (such as the mouth, the vagina, the lungs, the skin). If your defenses are adequate and the flora balance is not too deeply disturbed, normal flora are often able to return to their original positive state.

However, repeated or prolonged antibiotic treatment can cause severe and ongoing dysbiosis, especially if our immune defenses are down. This can result in disease. When the beneficial flora have been substantially reduced, the condition is termed deficiency dysbiosis.

How Stress Can Cause Dysbiosis

Stress can have profound effects on our immune defenses. It tends to affect all the systems of our digestive tract—psycho-neuro-endocrine-immune function. This usually has a compromising effect on our immunity.

In addition stress can interfere with our digestion by slowing down the time it takes our food to move through the gut (constipation) or speeding it up (diarrhea). The movement of food through the GI tract (the transit time) affects the completeness of digestion. When these things happen harmful microorganisms shift the ecological balance of the intestinal tract.

Not Enough Fiber

Lack of adequate fiber in our diets can also allow deficiency dysbiosis to develop. Fiber is the major source of nutrition for the normal, health-promoting flora. One of the most dreaded diseases that can develop in this situation is infection due to *Clostridium difficile,* the overgrowth of a gut bacteria that can actually be a life-threatening complication of antibiotic use.

It is ironic that the standard treatment for this condition is to use more antibiotic therapy aimed at stopping the overgrowth of the C. *difficile.* Although this approach is successful at times, we are better assured of healing if we also address the underlying process in the ecology of the microflora and our immune defenses.

I have treated a number of cases of deficiency dysbiosis for patients who've had recurring colitis even though they underwent very aggressive antibiotic treatment for the overgrowth. An alternative approach is to give a short pulse of antibiotic therapy for a few days and then quickly begin replacing the friendly bacteria and the fiber. This can stimulate and stabilize immune function in the intestinal tract. As the flora rebuilds it provides some of the nutritional support so the GI mucosal surface can repair itself. This has worked within a few days in every case I have managed.

Effects of Environmental Toxins

Environmental exposures are increasing at an alarming rate in this era of widespread synthetic-chemical production. Many of these toxins find their way into the intestinal tract through food, water, and products, including toothpastes, mouthwashes, and dental amalgams. These substances can damage the cells of our intestinal tract and lower our resistance. Toxins can also damage the microflora, setting the stage for dysbiosis. A wide variety of drugs are known to have profound effects on the balance of the gut microflora, including steroids, birth control pills, NSAIDs (nonsteroidal anti-inflammatory drugs), antacids, H2 blockers, and some chemotherapy medications.

THE BEST-KEPT SECRET: IMMUNITY

One of the best-kept secrets in health care is that the gastrointestinal tract is the largest immune organ in our body. The intestinal lining has a huge surface area that separates the outer world from the internal milieu of our body. This is a strategic location for our body's defense system. Here is the very site of entry for potentially dangerous organisms or chemicals. It doesn't take a rocket scientist to see that when this large, strategically placed immune system isn't working well, our defenses are lowered. Once our barriers are down, it may not be possible to keep the ecology of the intestinal tract in balance. And it becomes more difficult to defend against invaders.

What If Our Immune Defense Is Down?

The immune system can malfunction in at least three ways. First, it can be weakened so that it can't fight off common illness. This occurs with cancer and AIDS, but can also result from everyday stress. It's called immune suppression. Second, it can overreact and become hyperresponsive to normal stimuli; this occurs in asthma, migraine, and food allergies. These hyperreactions can use up immune reserves of the body, but may also cause defensive immune responses that actually injure the tissue. Third, a malfunctioning immune system can cause autoimmune reactions—antibodies become targeted against our own tissues, as in rheumatoid arthritis or lupus. In any of these mechanisms, the end result is the same: Abnormal body defenses can lead to dysbiosis.

DIAGNOSING THE PROBLEM

Dysbiosis is not a disease per se. As a matter of fact, dysbiosis is frequently found in patients who have no specific symptoms, though they often have a vague sense of not feeling well. The presence of disturbed gut ecology is clearly an abnormal situation. It serves as a warning for the potential of detectable disease.

The diagnosis of dysbiosis centers around three approaches:

- A careful history and physical exam
- A specific test called a comprehensive diagnostic stool analysis (CDSA)
- Testing for yeast, bacteria, and parasites

When dysbiosis is present, other related illnesses often develop as well. Since the primary causes of dysbiosis relate to almost everyone, it is my opinion that a CDSA is a reasonable and cost-effective screening that should be done whenever there is unresolved illness.

RESTORING INNER HEALTH

Treating dysbiosis depends on the strength of one's immunity, the quality of support, and the severity of the infection or overgrowth. In the management of dysbiosis, treat the underlying cause whenever possible. This means carefully evaluating all the possible causes and then finding ways to eliminate them.

The goals in managing dysbiosis are to restore the normal microflora, provide nutrients that will heal the intestinal mucosa, reduce toxic exposures, and increase antibodies in the GI tract (SIgA).

The health of the mucosal lining of the gut is important in maintaining our immune resistance, and this resistance is a powerful determinant that controls which microflora can survive. Nutritional support for the gut mucosal cells is necessary to maintain our most effective defense mechanisms.

The following guidelines can be used to maintain or restore inner health:

- Use a variety of vitamins (A, Bs, C, and E), especially vitamin A
- Use minerals and nutrients (such as L-glutamine and phosphatidyl choline)
- Remember essential fatty acids and bioflavonoids (like quercitin)
- Support with antioxidants (CoQ_{10}, lipoic acid, glutathione, and ginkgo biloba)
- Consume organic food and juice whenever possible
- Minimize toxic exposures

Dysbiosis and leaky gut are often intimately related. They can occur together or exist independently. Or they may be caused by each other, and often coexist. In chapter 7 these interrelationships will be explored more fully.

Len Saputo, M.D., is founder of the Health-Medicine Forum, a nonprofit educational foundation that provides panels and workshops on complementary and alternative medicine for both health care professionals and public audiences. He is also cofounder and medical director of the Health Medicine Institute, an integrative medicine center in Walnut Creek, California, where he has an active private practice.

Dr. Saputo received his medical education at Duke University and his undergraduate degree at the University of California at Berkeley. He has been in private practice in internal medicine since 1971, with a therapeutic focus in the use of nutrition in preventive care and wellness. An avid tennis player, he was a world singles champion in 1995. Dr. Saputo can be reached for phone consultations at the Health Medicine Institute in Lafayette, California, at (925) 962-3799. For more information see their Web site at www.healthmedicineinstitute.com.

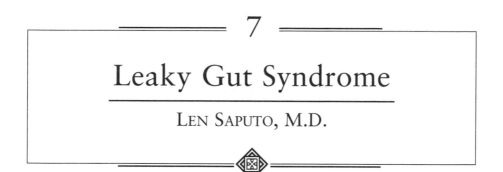

7

Leaky Gut Syndrome

Len Saputo, M.D.

Leaky gut is a surprisingly common problem. Basically it's a condition that occurs whenever there is inflammation and the "pores" lining of the GI tract remain open too long. Then toxic by-products in the digestive tract can be absorbed into the bloodstream and transported on to the liver. The molecules of food and toxins "leaked" through the GI lining may eventually affect systems throughout the body by aggravating inflammation in the joints, expressing toxins in skin disorders, triggering food sensitivities, causing "brain fog" or hyperactivity.

Managing hyperpermeability is definitely preventive medicine. Reducing this toxic load on the liver and the body can prevent illness or improve its outcome. Like dysbiosis, leaky gut is an example of a general process that can lead to disease, rather than being a specific disorder. This condition is far more typical than many practitioners realize and is often overlooked in designing treatment. Resolving hyperpermeability can produce very real benefits.

Leaky gut (or hyperpermeability) is associated with a wide range of general symptoms, such as fatigue, fevers of unknown origin, abdominal pain or bloating, diarrhea, feelings of toxicity, memory problems and difficulty with concentration, and poor tolerance of exercise.

Hyperpermeability can be a causal factor in:

- Attention deficit disorders
- Symptoms resembling autism
- Chronic and rheumatoid arthritis
- Chronic fatigue syndrome
- Eczema
- Food allergies and intolerances
- Inflammatory bowel disease
- Irritable bowel syndrome
- Joint and collagen problems
- Compromised liver function
- Malnutrition
- Multiple chemical sensitivities
- Psoriasis
- Skin disorders ranging from urticaria to acne and dermatitis
- Symptoms like schizophrenia

Hyperpermeability can also be caused by any number of different conditions. Any substance or condition that causes inflammation (such as GI infection), severe trauma (such as burns or surgery), or mechanical overstimulation (such as certain medications or NSAIDs)—anything that overstimulates the pores in the lining and keeps them open too long—is said to cause leaky gut, known as hyperpermeability.

The following conditions sometimes cause hyperpermeability:

- The aging process
- AIDS with diarrhea
- Alcoholism
- Burns
- Cancer
- Celiac disease
- Certain drugs
- Chemotherapy
- Chronic hepatitis
- Crohn's disease
- Cystic fibrosis
- Giardia and other parasites
- HIV
- Intensive illnesses
- Malnutrition
- NSAIDs
- Pancreatitis
- Psoriasis
- Radiation therapy
- Rheumatoid arthritis
- Shock or anaphylaxis
- Toxic shock syndrome
- Trauma
- Ulcerative colitis

DEFINING LEAKY GUT SYNDROME

The intestinal lining has two opposing functions:

- The absorption of nutrients from food in the digestive tract
- A barrier function, to contain microbes or large food particles (potential allergens) so they don't go beyond the gut environment (translocate) and get into our bloodstream

The digestive tract has tiny porous openings between the cells (called tight junctions) so that nutrients can be absorbed from our food. If the porelike structures open too wide, toxins from the gut can flood into the bloodstream, overwhelming the liver and causing allergies or any of dozens of other ailments.

This is known as hyperpermeability because the lining has become too permeable (porous). It's also called leaky gut syndrome because the gut begins leaking larger food particles and toxins from the gut. It's not an illness but rather a natural process gone wrong. Normally all these pores in the gut lining open and close whenever nutrients are absorbed from our food. It's only when the pores open too wide that leaky gut is said to occur.

When the Tests Come out Normal, But . . .

Debbie had complained of stomachaches since she was a child. Sometimes she would double over with cramps and dull, aching abdominal pains so severe she couldn't do anything but lie in bed for hours. Her symptoms seemed to come on a few minutes after eating. She had several thorough medical workups that were all normal. Her doctor prescribed muscle relaxants and tranquilizers, which seemed to help most of the time, and she got along reasonably well until she was in her midforties.

Out of the blue, at a time when Debbie was under enormous stress, she began having repeated attacks so severe they caused intense abdominal pain, explosive diarrhea, vomiting, hives, and a shocklike state in which her blood pressure would drop to almost undetectable levels. She was seen by many doctors and again had extensive testing that all came out normal. This time she was put on steroids, antihistamines, and Tagamet. Since the attacks were potentially life threatening, they had to be stopped.

When Debbie first saw me she was developing additional problems from the steroids. Her physicians tried to taper her off the steroids, but whenever the doses were decreased her attacks recurred. Her symptoms were consistent with a severe form of food allergies. A workup for intestinal permeability provided striking evidence of leaky gut syndrome. In addition she was found to have severe dysbiosis that was associated with both yeast overgrowth and a parasitic infection due to *Blastocystis hominis*.

Debbie was successfully treated with nutrients and diet. She's been off all pharmaceuticals for five years now, and has not had a single attack. Follow-up testing for leaky gut syndrome has been normal, and her dysbiosis is continuing to gradually clear.

HOW LEAKY GUT OCCURS

Here's a blow-by-blow account of how leaky gut occurs. Let's use the example of someone who has an allergy. Suppose Sarah has a dairy allergy and unknowingly eats cheese; this can trigger a reaction in her body. If she has an immediate food allergy, her immune system may begin reacting right away. If she has delayed allergies, the reaction may not occur for as long as three hours, but it could take as long as forty-eight hours to occur.

What is amazing is that no matter when it occurs, Sarah may not even be aware that it's happening. She may have a vague feeling of discomfort that could include a mild stomachache, a headache, even joint or muscle aches. Although she may not notice anything more than vague discomfort at the time, later she may have a flare-up of some chronic problem such as allergies, asthma, or arthritis. And she probably won't link it to this microscopic process going on in her digestive tract as the lining becomes too porous and begins leaking tiny particles.

On the other hand, she may have noticed that if she cheats on her allergy diet and has milk for breakfast, sometime that day or the next her joints may be achy and exercise will become a major effort.

The response of Sarah's body to the offending food also activates her immune system. To alert the system that an invader is present (the dairy food she just ate), her immune system sounds the alarm through chemical messengers, the cytokines. They act like buglers calling out the cavalry, and their job is to bring in the infection fighters (the antibodies). This sets the immune system in motion. While we always have cytokines as an essential part of our system, when there are too many cytokines and other immune chemicals circulating in the bloodstream, the gut will start leaking.

WHEN EVERYTHING IS WORKING RIGHT

When Sarah's system is working properly, absorption is occurring through tiny structures in the lining of the small intestine. All this is happening on a microscopic level. Nutrients are being absorbed through three structures:

- Directly through the cells of the gut lining, called transcellular absorption
- Between the cells, in paracellular absorption
- In the crypts, tiny crevices in the lining of the gut

Each structure is programmed to absorb nutrient molecules of a particular size and electromagnetic charge. Between the fingerlike villi that line the gut are the crypts, crevices at the base of each villi, like the webbing between your fingers. Because of their larger size the crypts absorb bigger molecules, such as the disaccharides, which are complex sugars.

Between every cell in the gut lining is a tiny porelike structure called a tight junction. These tiny pores are also active during digestion. They expand and contract just as other muscles do, opening and closing to release nutrients from the gut into the bloodstream or contain the food mix as it passes through the gut.

WHEN THERE IS INFLAMMATION

Too many immune chemicals can cause the pores to open too wide, causing too much permeability. When there's inflammation or any kind of crisis in the body, if too many of the immune-signaling chemicals are circulating in the bloodstream, they can overstimulate the tight junctions, causing the pores to open too wide. This process can be compared to a house with doors wired to a fire alarm system. If the alarm system malfunctions, it may keep all the doors in the house open and won't let them close. Clearly other problems can result. Intruders could easily enter the house.

Leaky gut can increase the body's vulnerability to intruders, such as bacteria, yeast, or large food particles that would normally remain in the gut. Again, when the pores open too wide, material is inappropriately released into the bloodstream. In Sarah's case, if her immune system detects large food particles in the bloodstream (perhaps other innocent foods, released through the leaky gut), it will assume they're allergens and launch a second attack, flooding her system with more cytokines. Then the whole dynamic just gets worse.

If leaky gut occurs frequently, it can cause chronic conditions. The importance of this increase in the permeability of the small intestine is not to be taken lightly, because two additional serious problems usually develop: liver overload and autoimmune conditions.

- *Stress on the liver.* Leaky gut places an increased toxic load on the liver, producing harmful chemical by-products as the liver attempts to clean up the overload. The free radicals that result form toxic bile, which can directly injure the gut lining. Contamination, caused by bacteria invading the system

LEAKY GUT

SOURCE: Great Smokies Diagnostic Laboratory, © 1999

through dysbiosis, may also be a factor. In the short term this worsens leaky gut, creating a vicious cycle. Over time these toxic by-products can cause gallstones or eventually even cancer. In order to break the cycle, it's important to control the underlying problem that has caused the leaky gut syndrome in the first place.

The liver is the major detoxifying organ of the human body. All products absorbed across the intestinal barrier must pass through the liver before entering the general circulation. There must be a balance between the size of the toxic load presented to the liver and the liver's capacity to metabolize this load. Unless the liver's detoxification system has enough reserve capacity to adjust to an increased toxic load, serious consequences can and often do result.

- *Autoimmune conditions.* Hyperpermeability sets the stage for possible autoimmune complications. When the total load of foreign material (antigens) is increased for a prolonged period, the immune system can become hyperactive, and a hyperimmune state can follow. As the immune system becomes overstimulated, "immune soldiers"—the antibodies—actually begin to attack the cells of the body as if they were the invaders. If one of the invading molecules resembles tissue within the body, the antibody produced to attack the foreign molecule will be unable to distinguish friend from foe, attacking both the original invader and the body's own tissue. This is known as the innocent-bystander phenomenon. In the gut, these conditions include Crohn's disease, food allergies, and celiac disease. Elsewhere in the body conditions such as asthma or rheumatoid arthritis can result.

THE VICIOUS CYCLE

Certain conditions trigger leaky gut and then are made worse as oversized molecules seep into the bloodstream and circulate throughout the body. These include:

- *Allergies.* Food sensitivity can induce leaky gut. The offending food stimulates an allergic reaction in the gut lining that increases permeability. The leaky gut then allows the passage of additional oversized macromolecules that the immune system perceives as invaders (since they are larger than usual) and therefore tagged as "different" or "antigen." This further stimulates the immune system to form antibody complexes that attack the tissue, causing additional aggravation of the leak in the gut lining and further allergic responses. Unless the vicious cycle is interrupted by avoiding the offending food or blocking the allergic reaction, the process will continue to tax the reserves and the functions of the liver, the immune system, and GI tract.

- *Overgrowth (dysbiosis)*. When potentially harmful flora take over leaky gut can occur, allowing bacteria and bacterial fragments across the small intestinal lining (translocation). This can overstimulate the immune system and aggravate intestinal permeability, leading to additional overreaction and further aggravating the leak! Clearing the dysbiosis can break the cycle by removing the bacteria that are translocating across the gut lining. It's also important to increase the beneficial flora, stopping the immune reaction.

- *Malabsorption and malnutrition*. When the gut is starved for nourishment, whatever the cause, within days hyperpermeability can occur. If malabsorption or malnutrition trigger the syndrome, a lack of nutritional supply to the lining of the gut can further limit the vital supply of blood or nutrients. Depriving the lining tissue of nourishment can cause shrinking, deterioration, and increased permeability. This increase in permeability tends to aggravate malabsorption and results in more atrophy and leaky gut syndrome. The cycle can be interrupted by carefully restoring proper nutrition to the cells of the small intestinal lining.

- *Inflammation*. The immune reactions (antibody responses) within the gut wall, although intended to be protective, can create inflammation, further aggravating the leak in the gut, setting the stage for a vicious cycle.

OTHER FACTORS

- *Genetics*. There appear to be genetic patterns of permeability. For example, Crohn's patients frequently have gut permeability; even their relatives with no symptoms also often have increased gut permeability. Although closely related individuals appear to have the same physical structures, some develop the symptoms characteristic of Crohn's disease and others do not. Relatives without symptoms also tend to have small areas of inflammation, not as extensive as fully developed Crohn's disease. These observations imply a genetic predisposition to leaky gut.

- *Mental disorders*. A number of mental conditions have been linked to increased permeability. The elevated toxins that leak into the system from hyperpermeability can produce symptoms that range from spaciness and brain fog to attention deficit disorder. We now know that many children with ADHD have increased gut permeability. In the most extreme form hyperpermeability can cause disorientation resembling autism or schizophrenia. In some cases these disorders are also linked to specific food sensitivities such as gluten intolerance. And a number of stresses can be affecting the body at once: Toxic load on the system appears to affect neurotransmitter production, and specific allergies may directly affect the nervous system as well. Recent research links some allergic responses with brain chemistry and reactions in the receptor sites (see chapter 8).

Clearly the presence of leaky gut syndrome, with its impact on the liver and the immune system, always exacts a metabolic price from the human body. This process is particularly important in patients with existing disease, but even in the absence of specific symptoms, it will tax wellness reserves and can eventually lead to serious consequences.

The widespread frequency and critical importance of leaky gut syndrome has been largely underrated. In one study that tested for leaky gut syndrome in an intensive care unit, all patients studied had leaky gut syndrome, regardless of the condition that originally brought them to intensive care. Because of the incredibly high incidence of chronic diseases today and the high frequency of leaky gut syndrome in patients with chronic diseases, testing for intestinal permeability is worthwhile whenever associated conditions are present. Skillful management of this syndrome will help alleviate the primary illness, regardless of its nature.

Biographical information for **Len Saputo, M.D.,** appears on page 56.

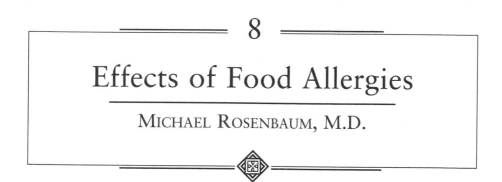

8

Effects of Food Allergies

Michael Rosenbaum, M.D.

Allergies can cause digestive problems. It's that simple. For people who don't have allergies, this is not an issue. For those who do, it's a big deal.

In addition some people have delayed responses that doctors now call food sensitivities. These are even more difficult to detect, because the response could occur even forty-eight hours after the triggering event. Some people go through their entire lives with an allergy, unaware that it's causing them chronic problems.

WHEN TO SUSPECT ALLERGIES

If you have a digestive condition that hasn't gone away, explore the possibility of allergies, food intolerance, and sensitivity. Some aspect of these reactions could be an important component of your illness. Research shows that in some cases allergies are linked to Crohn's disease, colitis, irritable bowel syndrome, chronic constipation, malabsorption, and many other conditions.

It's also important to have a sense of what doctors mean by food allergy and food sensitivity. Although a doctor may find that you don't have an allergy, you may have a food sensitivity, and that can cause problems as well.

What is traditionally thought of as allergy is typically a strong reaction: immediate, obvious, and sometimes life threatening. But this type of allergy accounts for only about 10 percent of allergic events.

In contrast, about 90 percent of the reactions to food seem to be delayed—and these are considered either sensitivities or delayed food allergies. Although the reaction can be observed, the mechanism isn't always known. Delayed reactions may occur from four to forty-eight hours after the offending food is eaten.

Immediate Reactions

Dr. Alan Levin's book *The Type 1 and 2 Allergy Relief Program* (Merla Zellerbach, 1986) was one of the first to describe classic immediate allergies as Type 1 allergies and delayed food allergies as Type 2.

With immediate Type 1 allergies, the same type of antibody that causes hay fever also causes allergies to specific foods. This is a relatively uncommon condition. Type 1 food allergies are *immediate* reactions that can often be life threatening. People who have this condition typically carry adrenaline with them in case of emergency. (So when you think of Type 1 allergies, think of the IgE antibody—E for *emergency*.) The foods that usually cause these reactions are shellfish (such as crab, lobster, or shrimp) or nuts. Cinnamon (used as a spice) and peanuts can also be trigger foods.

People with Type 1 allergies have instant reactions and they know it. Their responses tend to be strong and clear-cut. Type 1 allergies (IgE associated) tend to be hereditary. There is a genetic link, but people don't necessarily inherit an allergy to any specific food. Rather they inherit a general tendency toward strong, specific allergic reactions. When someone tells me he is allergic to shellfish and he has had this problem since childhood, I have a strong suspicion of a Type 1 allergy.

Periodically there are stories in the newspapers about someone suddenly passing out in a restaurant, unable to breathe and having to be taken to a hospital immediately because of something he or she ate. The cause could be as innocent as a trace of peanuts in a sauce! The result can be a sudden, extreme reaction.

Delayed Food Allergies

Type 2 allergies are typically delayed reactions. Alan Levin suggests that Type 2 reactions are associated with the IgG antibody (think of G for *gradual*), but there may also be several other mechanisms involved. There may even be nonantibody mechanisms involved. These responses tend to be much more complicated. The reactions are typically delayed. Foods such as wheat, for example, have been found to cause responses with long delays—as long as two days after the food has been eaten.

In fact, because of the delay it's much more difficult to diagnose delayed reactions to food, which constitute perhaps 90 percent of the responses reported to allergists. These are cases in which there is no obvious immediate cause and effect. There may or may not be a genetic link.

Food Sensitivities

Another category of response is sensitivity to both foods and chemicals, including food additives and coloring, pesticides, and pollutants. With sensitivities you see the response and the symptoms but you don't know the cause. And research indicates that a number of different possible causes and mechanisms are associated with food sensitivities. Some of these processes may not be triggered by antibodies at all. One of the possible causes, for example, is

Food Allergies and Sensitivities

	Type 1 Allergy	Type 2 Allergy	Sensitivity
Response time	Immediate	Delayed	Immediate or delayed
Frequency	10% of allergies	About 90% of allergic responses are delayed	Difficult to identify
Associated antibody	IgE (remember E for *emergency*)	IgG (remember G for *gradual*)	May not trigger immunoglobulins
Severity	May be life threatening	Mild to severe	Mild to severe
Origin	Allergic tendency is inherited	May be inherited or not	Genetic aspect unknown
Cause or trigger	Specific trigger food (antigen)	Food trigger that is difficult to identify because of the delay	A variety of causes, including toxicity to the nervous system

intestinal permeability, leaky gut syndrome (see chapter 7). In these cases, the intensity of the response is influenced by the degree of leaky gut and the levels of protective antibodies (secretory IgA). There's still a lot to be learned about the mechanisms that cause these common sensitivities.

Possible causes of delayed food sensitivities include:

- Stimulation of the nervous system
- Binding to opiate and serotonin receptor sites in the central nervous system
- Direct toxicity to nerve cells
- Foods and substances may have direct hormonelike activity or neurotransmitter-like activity
- Triggered by specific proteins (peptides)

CAUSAL FACTORS

Leaky Gut Syndrome

Food allergies and sensitivities can be made worse by leaky gut syndrome (high intestinal permeability). Many factors can trigger hyperpermeability: GI infection, an overgrowth of yeast or bacteria, viral illness, poor absorption, or genetic factors. In leaky gut syndrome, oversized food particles begin sneaking in between the cells. These particles, which are not fully broken down, enter the bloodstream, and the immune system identifies them as foreign material. At that point, the body mounts an immune response that creates a whole series of symptoms, a symptom complex. This dynamic is believed to be one of the causes of delayed food allergies and sensitivities.

How Allergies Can Affect Digestion

At thirty-seven David had a twenty-year history of abdominal pain, nausea, bloating, and diarrhea. During those years he was seen by many doctors and specialists who diagnosed him as having irritable bowel syndrome. He was treated with a variety of medications, but his symptoms never really improved. David's life also involved a tremendous amount of stress. He was recently divorced and had sole custody of his two children, and he was both breadwinner and a full-time single parent. He often resorted to fast foods as the main staple for the family's diet (which probably didn't help his digestion).

When David's symptoms worsened he consulted a surgeon and his gallbladder was removed. Unfortunately he continued to experience nausea, bloating, and frequent diarrhea. When David was seen for a GI consult in a preventive medicine practice, he appeared to be chronically ill and fatigued. In addition to standard blood tests, stool testing for parasites was ordered and a gastroscopy was performed (scoping the stomach, esophagus, and upper small intestine—the duodenum). The lab studies were normal, but the scope revealed a hiatal hernia and an abnormally smooth texture to the duodenum. Biopsies showed evidence of celiac disease, an allergy to wheat gluten.

Blood tests found antibodies against wheat (antigliadin antibodies), which further confirmed the diagnosis of celiac disease. A low-allergenic and gluten-free diet was prescribed, which David has adhered to faithfully. Within a month his diarrhea and bloating were gone for the first time in more than twenty years! He's being seen monthly for follow-up, and he continues to feel better, look better, and improve.

—Paul Thomas, D.O.

Allergies That Get on Your Nerves

Research suggests that food particles that manage to sneak through the leaky gut into circulation can eventually occupy receptor sites in the brain and possibly in other organs. Fascinating research has shown that particles of foods such as milk and grains such as corn and wheat can occupy morphine or opiate receptor sites in the brain. This may trigger a variety of neurological responses. It can create problems with cognition, mood, or even pain, through responses in the brain described as cerebral reactions.

This receptor mechanism may explain why food allergies tend to obey the laws of addiction. Food particles that occupy morphine and opiate receptors create a craving for the allergenic food. When you don't have the food you go into withdrawal. Then you crave it. And when you eat it you may feel better.

Receptor stimulation does not necessarily depend on having high intestinal permeability. Even with normal permeability research has found that by-products of these foods can still access and occupy receptor sites. But if there is high intestinal permeability, much more rapid absorption can occur. When the "pores" in the gut lining are open too wide, larger undigested particles of foods can be absorbed. Receptors in other organs such as the liver may also trigger responses that lead to other problems.

The processes that have been identified may be just the tip of the iceberg. Researchers have suggested that food particles might occupy not only opiate receptors but also serotonin receptors, affecting mood and sleep. Although there is no definitive evidence at this time, a large body of information links food allergies with mood swings. The specifics of what occurs at the receptor site still need to be detailed, but this mechanism would explain withdrawal, tolerance, and food cravings.

Proteins that Trigger Allergies

Clusters of protein molecules called peptides can stimulate hormone activity. These tiny peptides can be extremely powerful. Some of the hormone activity mediated by peptides occurs in the gut. For example, the intestine releases a powerful peptide called VIP. This potent hormone or transmitter affects gut motility (a vital issue to anyone suffering from chronic constipation or chronic diarrhea). The same peptide is found in certain foods and is now being used in the healing of GI illness. It is included in a product called Seacure, which contains peptides that seem to relax the gut and prevent spasm. Doctors report that such peptides (made from predigested whitefish) can be very useful in treating conditions such as irritable bowel syndrome.

Peptides can also act as neurotransmitters in the brain. Other peptides that control appetite are produced in the intestine and released in the stomach. They appear to control the amount of digestive enzymes that the body makes. They also may control the speed at which food is propelled through the gut. And they may control whether the GI tract is in spasm or not. They are extraordinarily potent in very minute levels.

Researchers have identified CCK (cholecystokinin), a polypeptide hormone that affects the gallbladder by causing the release of bile. As a neurotransmitter in the brain, it appears to shut off appetite. Researchers have been trying to isolate CCK for use in weight-loss programs.

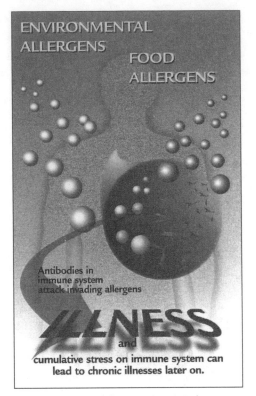

ENVIRONMENTAL
ALLERGENS
                FOOD
              ALLERGENS

Antibodies in
immune system
attack invading allergens

ILLNESS

and

cumulative stress on immune system can
lead to chronic illnesses later on.

© 1999 Great Smokies Diagnostic Laboratory

Some peptides may have adverse effects. Fragments of peptides from undigested food may also have transmitter activity that can cause inflammation or mimic the activity of VIP and cause spasms. These peptides have direct hormonal effects on the gut wall. This is a third mechanism that can cause allergy, but it doesn't appear to be an immune mechanism.

Food Additives and Pesticides

The diet of the average American often contains food colors and food additives that can cause pharmacological actions. Some additives such as MSG have been found in lab experiments to affect the brain, and there are other additives that also act as excito-toxins—brain stimulants. So a lot of food sensitivities may be caused by food additives. Pesticides and heavy metals are also known to have adverse effects on the nervous system and may also stimulate inflammation in the gut. Since the food and water of most industrial nations contain pesticides, industrial chemicals, and heavy metals, these pollutants must also be considered when you're evaluating food sensitivity.

The Connection Between Infection and Allergies

As an allergist I've noticed that there's a connection between having a virus and being more allergic in general. People tell me their food allergies get worse when they have a flu. The interesting connection is that viral infection causes the blood levels of vitamin A to plummet. And when the level of vitamin A drops, the secretory IgA level in the gut goes down as well, so the defenses against allergy are down.

People with low levels of secretory IgA tend to be much more prone to infection and to food allergies. Some people are just born with less ability to make antibodies. SIgA tends to be reduced in people who have allergies and also in children born of parents who are allergic. As a result they're more prone to food allergies and may be more prone to gluten/wheat intolerance, which can cause you to be allergic to everything else.

Lack of vitamin A is the major vitamin deficiency that causes a drop in secretory IgA. Before we had the modern vitamin industry, healthy kids took cod-liver oil. Of course now we can get vitamin A palmitate as a supplement. You have to maintain a balance by keeping up your levels of vitamin A without taking toxic doses. If you have very low nutrient stores in your liver, you can use them up by having a virus, and then it's important to replenish vitamin A.

MINIMIZING FOOD ALLERGIES

Here are some suggestions about how to minimize allergies and sensitivities, digest your food better, and maintain the integrity of your digestive tract.

- *Do everything you can to prevent dysbiosis and high intestinal permeability.* Then you are well on your way to preventing many food sensitivities.
- *Digest your food well.* When food is thoroughly digested, it's less allergenic. It's important that your digestive processes all work smoothly. Is your pancreas functioning properly? Is there enough bicarbonate for the intestine so the pancreatic enzymes can work? Are you eating in a hurry, with no time to really chew your food? Are you eating standing up? Eating under tremendous stress?
- *Do you have enough pancreatic enzymes?* The Chymex Test (from Meridian Laboratories) can actually test pancreatic enzyme levels in the body. This test and other useful lab work can be ordered by your doctor (see Resources for information on Meridian Laboratories).

- *Eat smaller, more frequent meals.* We tend to eat huge meals. Smaller meals usually encourage more thorough digestion.
- *Cook your food if you have a tendency toward sensitivities.* As a general principle, raw food is more allergenic than cooked food. So one way to prevent these allergies is to cook as much of your food as you can, because cooking changes its structure. That explains why applesauce is less allergenic than raw apples. The same is true for tomato sauce as opposed to fresh tomatoes.
- *Use the rotation diet in planning your meals.* Be creative so meals are still interesting and pleasurable.
- *Experiment with food combining.* Food-combining theory is based on not mixing grains and meat at the same meal (or at least not mixing large quantities of both). In this system the main course of grain or protein is combined with vegetables. The idea is to encourage more complete digestion. Minimizing the amount of undigested food moving through the GI tract will decrease the allergic (antigenic) load on the system. Some people report that simpler meals, designed around food combining, are easier to digest.
- *Relax when you eat.* Make mealtime a time of quiet, relaxed pleasure, a refuge from the hectic nature of your day. Do this even if your meal is brief and simple.
- *Keep your immune system strong.* It has been proposed that food allergies are worse in the winter, in cold weather, and better in the summer. Keep your stores of secretory IgA up by taking a moderate amount of vitamin A.
- *Minimize stress.* The concept of stress reduction is important because stress will affect the amount of digestive enzymes you have and the degree of intestinal permeability. Stress is an underappreciated factor in digestion and in allergies and sensitivities. Few of us realize the degree to which stress impairs the lining of the gut.

Biographical information for **Michael Rosenbaum, M.D.**, appears on page 41.

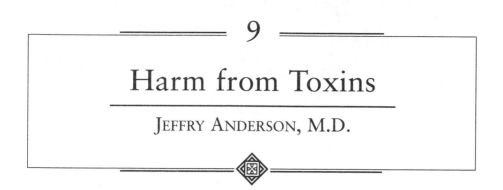

9

Harm from Toxins

Jeffry Anderson, M.D.

TOXINS FROM CHEMICALS AND HEAVY METALS

Most of us don't connect digestive illness and toxic exposure. Yet toxic chemicals can directly injure the lining of the GI tract and interfere with digestion. Symptoms can result from either minimal low-level exposures or intense or long-term exposures. Man-made chemicals, products of our high-tech industrial world, are released into the environment in staggering amounts—thousands of metric tons per year in the United States alone. Toxic spills and new chemical pollutant threats are frequently reported in the media. We may feel a sense of concern when we hear about these pollutants, but few people with digestive illness connect their symptoms with toxic exposure.

Chemicals and heavy metals can trigger inflammation and interfere with the function of the GI tract. These toxins include pesticides, such as everyday household bug sprays; solvents in paint thinner; petroleum products, such as gasoline; industrial chemicals and by-products, including dioxin and PCBs; and heavy metals like mercury and lead.

LOW-LEVEL EXPOSURE

We may be sensitive to chemicals in water, such as fluoride and chlorine. In agricultural areas water often contains pesticides, herbicides, and inorganic fertilizer chemicals. In industrial or military areas water may contain heavy metals, petrochemical derivatives, PCBs, and radioactive compounds, as well as other toxins.

The water supply to many urban/suburban areas contains some of these pollutants from distant runoff contamination, originating in agricultural and industrial areas. This is because water, as well as air, moves over great distances, carrying contaminants with it. In addition chlorine in municipal waters can create new toxins such as THMs by interacting with organic pollutants.

73

THMs have been linked to high rates of miscarriage. Many of these chemicals (particularly pesticides, PCBs, and dioxins) persist for long periods of time in our environment and break down slowly.

- *Pesticides and other chemicals in our food can trigger digestive symptoms.* Fruits, vegetables, and grains may be contaminated by any of the 800 pesticides currently in use. Meat, dairy products, and poultry often contain residues of hormones, antibiotics, tranquilizers, steroids, or other drugs, as well as pesticide residues from feed. Fish and shellfish commonly contain significant levels of heavy metals, particularly mercury, as well as lead, arsenic, cadmium, chromium, and chemicals such as dioxins and PCBs.
- *Low-level chronic exposure to toxins in the home and garden can actually affect our digestion.* Toxic chemicals in everyday home use include solvents such as turpentine, paint and paint thinner, paint and wax strippers, spot removers, degreasers, and gasoline. Pesticides that are found in the home and garden include bug sprays, pet sprays, flea collars, and pest strips.
- *Other unknown low-level chronic exposures include fluoride in toothpaste and chemicals in food and cosmetic products.* Fluoride, for example, is contained in most toothpastes. Researchers have linked conditions such as irritable bowel syndrome (IBS) to toothpaste—fluoride or carrageenan, or both, could be the irritant. Recent studies have found toxic effects from common cosmetic and toothpaste additives such as propylene glycol (a major constituent of antifreeze!), sodium lauryl sulfate, DEA (diethanolamine), and other similar chemicals.
- *The effects of mercury amalgams.* Mercury (along with silver and tin) has been the material of choice for dental fillings (mercury-silver amalgams) in American dentistry and has been used extensively for more than a century. Many scientific studies have documented the toxic effects of mercury on the brain, nervous system, kidney, liver, and GI tract. Tin is also known to cause these effects, especially in the brain, although to a lesser degree.

Toxic processes include the creation of antibiotic-resistant gut bacteria, which contributes to harmful overgrowth (dysbiosis). The antibiotic-resistant bacteria may even become predominant residents in the GI tract. Recent research indicates that some species (*Klebsiella,* citrobacter, and *Proteus*) may play a role in perpetuating ulcerative colitis and Crohn's disease. They can also be communicable to immunocompromised individuals.

Mercury is released from dental fillings continuously in very small amounts, but over a period of fifteen to twenty years can accumulate in the

Digestive Problems Can Be Caused by Toxins in Food

Testing by the Food and Drug Administration (FDA) shows that about half our foods contain some level of pesticides, although legal, while perhaps 5 percent of our foods contain illegal residues (FDA data reported by the Environmental Working Group, 1994). Many toxic chemicals persist in our environment for a long period of time and are said to have a long half-life (period of time before they begin breaking down). They accumulate in our food sources, and because we are higher on the food chain, we get more concentrated amounts of pesticides in our food, particularly from the livestock and poultry we eat and the chemicals they have also been exposed to. The chemicals remain in our tissues and systems, stored in fats and bound to proteins. Researchers suggest that probably every person on earth has some residues of the pesticide DDT in his or her body, despite the fact that it was banned more than thirty years ago.

When one's nutritional status is compromised from poor absorption and poor digestion, combined with the effects of toxins present in the body, then subsequent damage to other tissues is likely, which can result in further illness.

SOURCE: M. Moses. *Designer Poisons*. San Francisco: Pesticide Education Center (1995).

body in dangerous amounts, since most people have multiple fillings by midadolescence. Mercury-silver amalgams have been outlawed in Europe and Scandinavia for several decades, but continue to be widely used by American dentistry. As noted earlier, mercury and heavy metal contamination of foods, particularly fish, can also be a significant contribution to these problems.

LONG-TERM OR HIGH-INTENSITY EXPOSURE

- *Indoor exposure from tight- or sick-building syndrome.* Toxins inhaled or absorbed through the skin can circulate widely in the bloodstream, throughout the body and the GI tract, where they can cause specific damage.

  Sick-building syndrome can occur in commercial or public buildings, including schools and hospitals, as well as in residential buildings characterized by poor ventilation and a high level of synthetic materials. Toxic building materials and commercial chemicals include certain paints, most synthetic carpets and underpadding, adhesives, formaldehyde, sealers, waxes, disinfectants, cleaning agents, photocopier solution and toner, pesticide applications, and PCBs (from older electrical equipment such as fluorescent light transformers). These materials can build up in significantly high concentrations in buildings that lack adequate ventilation and outdoor air exchange.

- *Outdoor and industrial sources.* Occupational exposures have been associated with the use of pesticides (agricultural and pest-control workers and landscapers), solvents (building trades), PCBs, dioxins, and hundreds of thousands of other chemicals (heavy industry, chemical manufacturing), and petroleum and its by-products (the petrochemical industry).
- *Acute, intense exposure from a single incident, an industrial accident, or spill.* This can involve solvents, pesticide spills, agricultural activities such as crop dusting and aerial spraying, petroleum spills, and other sources of exposure.

EFFECTS OF TOXIC EXPOSURE

Any condition that includes inflammation, poor digestion, or poor absorption could be caused partly by environmental toxins or be aggravated by them. Such illnesses include irritable bowel syndrome, peptic ulcer disease, Crohn's disease, ulcerative colitis, celiac disease, and colon cancer.

This can lead to a wide variety of distressing GI symptoms, such as abdominal pain, indigestion, bloating or distention, gas (flatulence), nausea, diarrhea, constipation, and leaky gut syndrome. If the problem in the digestive tract is not cleared up, it can lead to damage and dysfunction elsewhere in the body, which can translate into major illness, chronic illness, or degenerative disease.

This concern can affect anyone to some degree, but people who have greater exposure may also have a more serious problem. On the other hand, people who are highly sensitive, have a genetic tendency toward GI problems, or have an infection may react more strongly to toxins. Any of a number of symptoms can occur. They can occur singly or in combination, and may be constant or intermittent: fatigue, weakness, weight loss, headache, joint and muscle pain/ fibromyalgia, and allergic responses. Repeated infections have been linked to immune system dysfunction, such as frequent colds, coughs, flu, bronchitis, or sinus infections. Other immune system disorders include many types of allergic responses and even autoimmune diseases, such as lupus, Lou Gehrig's disease, or MS (multiple sclerosis). A wide variety of neurological symptoms are frequently seen: migraine; impaired short memory or attention span; difficulty concentrating, brain fog or spaciness; tingling, numbness, and muscle tics; depression, irritability, and panic attacks.

Insight from Environmental Medicine

Susan had a five-year history of chronic illness with what seemed like overwhelming problems—severe fatigue, repeated colds, bladder and GI infections, asthma, chronic constipation with frequent bouts of diarrhea with gas, bloating and cramps, mental fogginess and difficulty with memory, as well as generalized pains in her muscles and joints. Routine medical evaluations had found nothing abnormal, and she was told she was depressed.

An environmental-medicine consultation revealed three significant aspects of her history: a long-standing hobby of silk screen printing that involved the use of numerous solvents, extensive fillings of mercury-silver amalgam present since adolescence, and several episodes of foreign travel prior to her illness. Lab tests revealed a number of significant abnormalities. Stool testing was positive for parasites and yeast overgrowth, as well as high levels of pathogenic bacteria and unusually low levels of normal flora. It also suggested increased hyperpermeability (leaky gut syndrome), abnormally low secretory IgA in saliva, suppression of her immune response (both antibody and white blood count), and major elevations of several toxic solvents in blood specimens (N-hexane, pentane, toluene, and benzene, all used in her silk screening hobby), and abnormally high levels of mercury in the urine analysis. Additional tests also demonstrated an autoimmune condition involving the thyroid gland and many allergic reactions, particularly to a number of foods.

Susan has improved significantly after three years of intensive treatment that involved avoiding the use of solvents; clearing her GI system of microscopic parasites, pathogenic yeast, and bacteria; and restoring normal flora. She has also benefited from the removal of her mercury amalgams (by a dentist with special expertise who performed the work in stages, over a period of months, taking great care not to reintroduce the mercury back into her body). Removal of the amalgams was followed by medically monitored sauna detox therapy and mercury chelation. Susan has experienced a major improvement in most of her symptoms and marked improvement in her daily functioning and general quality of life.

Summary

- Toxins can be the primary cause of illness.
- Most often they coexist with other problems and eventually cause a cascade of chronic illness.

- In some cases, a second condition can develop or be made worse by this exposure. These include GI infections from yeast, bacteria, microscopic parasites, or viruses.
- Other factors can play a significant role in the overall impact of toxins, such as genetic makeup, lifestyle, and nutritional status.

WHEN TO SUSPECT EXPOSURE

In an industrial society almost no one is immune—most everyone has some degree of exposure through the air, water, and food. If you live in the average city or suburb, drink city water, and buy your food at the local supermarket, you are frequently exposed to toxic chemicals. If you live in an area of industry or agriculture, you are probably heavily exposed. Even those of us who live in pristine environments still have some amount of uncontrollable exposure to toxic chemicals. Such chemicals are universally present because they are carried via wind and water, which circulate around the planet.

Although most substances in nature break down and return to the earth, heavy metals and many man-made chemicals do not. Consequently these toxins remain for long periods of time in our environment and in our bodies and break down slowly. Some, such as heavy metals, don't break down at all.

Many of us receive specific exposures at home or at work, in addition to the unavoidable exposure to pollution of the air we breathe, over which we have little control. This may occur frequently, such as the monthly spraying by the exterminator, dusting the garden, using pest strips, starting the barbecue with lighter fluid, or keeping flea collars on our pets. Everyone has some vulnerability.

It's important to know about intentional use, because some exposures can be controlled. We can monitor our health. If we find that we are sensitive to chemicals, we can effectively minimize our exposure by eating organic food, drinking purified water, and using nontoxic pesticides and building materials in our home. (See chapter 23 on cutting toxic exposure for further solutions and strategies.)

When we are exposed to toxins they are absorbed through the skin and mucous membranes of the gut and the lungs and can circulate throughout the body. They can cause damage to almost any cell or organ. Some tissues are more vulnerable than others, due to their unique structure and function:

- Cells that have rapid turnover and repair—gut lining, skin, liver, respiratory tract, and immune system
- Those with exceptionally slow growth, as well as reproductive cells—the brain, eggs, and sperm
- Connective tissues such as muscles, tendons, cartilage, and fat cells are relatively less vulnerable

When digestive problems result from chemical exposure, it can be extremely difficult to discover the actual cause. However, it's important to find the source of the problem in order to eliminate the exposure. Many chronic health problems begin with compromised digestive function.

HOW TOXINS CAN BE HARMFUL

Chemicals and heavy metals can harm the structure and functioning of the GI tract in a number of ways. The gut lining is the focal area where the external environment meets the interior of the body. For this reason the GI tract is one of the most vulnerable organs of the body, where some of the most significant damage can occur. Toxins can directly injure the lining of the digestive tract.

Some of the most important functions of the gastrointestinal tract depend on the integrity of the gut lining and the health of each individual cell. Essential processes include:

- *Communication.* Sending and receiving information occurs through molecules and receptors that coordinate different components and organs in the GI tract to orchestrate digestion.
- *Defense.* Recognizing invading, foreign, or threatening microbes or materials and mounting an immune response.
- *Nutrition.* Identifying and preparing key nutrients for transport and assimilation into the body.

The cells lining the gut have the complex and essential role of defending the GI tract against invading microbes that may enter the body, primarily through ingested materials in food and water. The mucosal cells provide a barrier against microbes by secreting mucus that contains protective secretory IgA antibodies (SIgA). At the same time they provide a barrier against the introduction of large molecules of toxins and allergens from food. The lining cells also have a critical role in the selective transport of essential nutrients into the body.

Damage to the Cells of the GI Lining
Damage to the cells in the delicate lining of the GI tract can be caused by a great many factors, including the following:

- Direct damage by chemicals and heavy metals to the structure of the cell wall, distorting the three-dimensional shape of protein and fatty structures (receptor sites). (This is like distorting a lock so the key no longer fits and the lock no longer works.)
- Free radical or oxidative by-products that cause damage, making essential fatty structures of the cell wall more brittle and rigid. (This is comparable

to the prolonged effects of sunlight and air on rubber or plastic materials—they become oxidized, stiff, and brittle.)

- Direct effects of certain chemicals, particularly solvents and related toxins, on the cell wall, through destruction of the fatty portions of the cell membrane. (This is similar to the action of solvents on grease.)

Interference with the Body's Ability to Absorb Nutrients

One of the ways nutrients are transported into the body is by attaching to receptors in the cell wall. The attachment signals the cell to initiate a complex process in which nutrients are carried into the cell in a series of specific steps. The receptor works through a lock-and-key mechanism, and if the receptor is damaged there's no way for the nutrient to attach to the receptor and initiate the transport process. A second way this process can be interrupted is by damage to specific enzymes essential to the process. In either case essential nutrients are prevented from being absorbed, which can have widespread effects. This is a form of malabsorption and can lead to malnutrition, with symptoms such as weight loss and low energy.

A good example of this is the effect of heavy metals such as mercury (from dental amalgam fillings) or colloidal silver (commonly used as an alternative antibiotic). These metals can bind up a key protein enzyme called glutathione, essential for the transport of trace minerals, so the enzyme no longer works effectively. This disrupts the ability of the body to obtain vital trace minerals. Heavy metals such as cadmium and nickel probably have similar effects.

Damage to Immune Structures and Processes

Some toxins can damage immune structures and processes in the gut lining (the mucosa). Damage to the mucosal layer interferes with the body's ability to produce SIgA and other antibodies such as IgM. Toxins can also damage the white blood cells living within and below the mucosa. These cells come in many forms with multiple roles and include lymphocytes (responsible for sentinel defense and surveillance), macrophages (scavenger cells), and others, which make up our cellular immune defense.

Compromise of immune function can increase our susceptibility to infections—both infections localized in the gut, such as GI viral infections and dysentery, and illness throughout the rest of the body, like colds, flu, bronchitis, and sinus infections. Toxic damage to immune functions can also increase the incidence of allergies, chronic fatigue syndrome, and autoimmune diseases.

Toxins can compromise the gut's barrier and defense functions against microbes—bacteria, parasites, yeast, viruses, and other pathogens. Reductions in SIgA antibodies also diminish protection against the undesirable absorption of oversized macromolecules of toxins and food.

Overstimulation of the Immune Response

Heavy metals such as cadmium and nickel and certain toxic chemical compounds can increase allergic and autoimmune responses. Overstimulation of the immune response can occur in localized areas where tissue is damaged, or generally throughout the GI tract. This can trigger sensitivity to other unrelated substances such as foods, molds, or even bacteria.

This process can also cause autoimmune conditions to develop, for example, ulcerative colitis or Crohn's disease in the GI tract, or general autoimmune disorders such as lupus or rheumatoid arthritis.

Destruction of Beneficial Microflora

Damage can occur to normal beneficial gut flora, leaving the body vulnerable to infection. Unfortunately these flora are often more vulnerable to toxins than the pathogenic bacteria. Beneficial microflora have an essential role in maintaining both normal GI health and general health. For example, maintenance of beneficial bacteria has been found to correlate with keeping the AIDS virus in remission. The flora produce antibiotic-like molecules and enzymes that inhibit the invasion of unfriendly microbes. They also synthesize and process essential nutrients, particularly key vitamins such as B_{12} and essential fatty acids such as butyrate.

In the absence of friendly flora, an overgrowth of harmful microbes can take place, particularly yeast and bacteria. This can result in secondary damage to the integrity of the gut wall, increased fermentation, putrefaction, and toxins.

- *The toxic metabolic by-products of putrefaction* can result in the common symptoms of gas and bloating.
- *Inflammation in the gut can be generated by the toxins.* White blood cells are then mobilized in response to the inflammation, bombarding the tissue with free radicals that produce further inflammation.
- *Carcinogenic by-products can result* from the interaction of free radicals with bacterial toxins and normally nontoxic substances such as nitrates and nitrites, which are transformed into potentially cancer-causing nitrosamines.
- *Chemical toxins and heavy metals bound in the stool for disposal can be released back into the body* when abnormal bacteria flora result in undesirable levels of an enzyme that unbinds toxins (beta-glucaronidase). This allows the toxins to be reabsorbed in a revolving-door process.
- *Certain yeast and pathogenic bacteria produce neurotoxic substances,* which are then absorbed and go to the brain. These toxins are linked to conditions such as attention deficit disorders (ADD/ADHD), autism, panic disorders, chronic depression, and possibly schizophrenia.

Activation of Dormant Viruses

For unknown reasons, chemical damage to the gut lining can result in the activation of viruses such as measles or herpes, which may remain dormant in the cells for years, but which then replicate and spread. The compromise of immune integrity, lowering levels of defending antibodies and white blood cells, can create an opportunity for viruses to more easily flourish. This can lead to either localized inflammation or infection anywhere in the body.

The activation of viruses in the gut may be associated with conditions like chronic fatigue syndrome and irritable bowel syndrome (IBS). Viral activation has also been associated with the mechanism of autoimmunity, both in the gut itself in diseases such as Crohn's and elsewhere in the body.

Induction of Antibiotic-Resistant Bacteria

Recent research has established that mercury, released from amalgam dental fillings, can encourage the development of bacteria that are resistant to antibiotics, particularly varieties of streptococcus. This can occur within two weeks of the amalgam placement. As it turns out, resistance to mercury and antibiotics is encoded on the bacteria's DNA on adjacent sites. Mercury exposure activates the DNA genetic expression for mercury resistance to protect the bacteria from toxic damage, but also induces the expression for antibiotic resistance. This resistance can be passed on to other bacteria of the same or other species. The effect can also be caused by other heavy metals. The implications are profound, considering the major problem that currently exists with antibiotic-resistant pathogens.

THE BREAKDOWN OF COMMUNICATION IN THE DIGESTIVE TRACT

Coordinating Digestion

All the organs of digestion must talk with one another: the stomach, all the parts of the lengthy small intestine—the duodenum, the ileum, the jejunum—as well as the pancreas, gallbladder, and large intestine. They all have to communicate in order for food to make it through the GI tract and get totally processed: all the nutrients extracted, all the toxins eliminated, all the enzymes and digestive juices secreted at the right time and place, and so forth. If that process doesn't occur, food won't be thoroughly digested and toxins won't be thoroughly eliminated. It means there's a much greater likelihood of leaky gut and dysbiosis.

The wrong signals can affect motility, causing diarrhea or constipation. If coordinated communication doesn't take place, it could mean that everything goes through the GI tract so quickly that diarrhea occurs, eventually causing malnutrition. Or it could mean that things move too slowly and there is stasis, excessive fermentation, and putrefaction, encouraging the overgrowth of yeast and bad bacteria. When constipation occurs toxins may actually be reabsorbed back into the body.

Highly Specialized Systems

Messages from the nervous system and endocrine function communicate with cells all over the body, including the gastrointestinal cells that line the mucosa. These mucosal cells carry out all the functions of the GI tract: secretion, nutrient transport, assimilation and absorption, defenses, and motility.

Normally the GI tract is elegantly coordinated by molecules of protein called peptides. They're secreted by specialized cells in the gut lining and released at the cell wall. Signals from the gut and from other distant organs are received by receptors in the cell wall that specialize in identifying these molecules and binding them through a lock-and-key mechanism.

The cell wall has literally thousands of receptors in order to communicate with a wide variety of signaling molecules. Once the molecule binds to the receptor, the cell is instructed to carry out a specific function, such as the production of a particular enzyme. This happens millions of times a day all over our bodies.

Short-Circuited Communication

Toxins can damage the structure of receptors and the ability of cells to produce and release signaling peptides. This damage can block communication to such a degree that the digestive tract becomes nonfunctional. Or it can be overstimulated by too many molecules released too soon, so that they flood the system. Just as when too many people try to dial into the Internet at the same time, the system shuts down because of too much input. In the gut communication can also be misread if the wrong molecule is released at the wrong time or goes to the wrong place. When any of these miscommunications occur the digestive tract no longer functions properly.

Besides communicating within itself, the most critical digestive communication is with the brain. The GI tract is also regulated by peptides secreted by the brain that signal the gut when to move, when to become active. So just as localized miscommunication can cause diarrhea or constipation, so impaired communication with the brain can affect motility. There may be too much communication, like noise. Or there can be too little communication, resulting in lethargy, weakness, and chronic fatigue.

Possible Symptoms and Effects

Many of the peptides secreted in the GI tract have a major influence on brain function. Physical, neurological, and even psychological symptoms can result, including irritability, spaciness, or anxiety. So damage to the gut doesn't affect only the digestive tract because the brain and GI tract have a profound synergistic role in communication and regulation. What happens in the gut doesn't just stay in the gut. When you have stomachache, you may also have a headache. Everything is interconnected.

Some peptides have dual roles. For example, cholecystokinin signals the gallbladder to digest fats and perform other functions. It also controls appetite by notifying the brain that you're no longer hungry, so that you suddenly feel full.

In the GI tract miscommunication can cause numerous symptoms—hypermotility, hyperperistalsis, diarrhea, cramping, spasms, reverse peristalsis, ulcers, pain, nausea, excessive appetite, regurgitation, heartburn, and other derangements. Impaired functioning can result in poor digestion, malabsorption, and poor assimilation, mild or severe.

There is also two-way communication throughout the digestive tract between the gallbladder and the liver, the GI tract and the pancreas, and many other locations. If that communication is interrupted it can lead directly to digestive problems and the malfunction of other organs in the system.

TOXINS AND GI HEALTH

Toxins can damage the regulation of the GI tract by the autonomic nervous system, which runs your body's functions automatically. This can interfere with functions that should happen as a matter of habit, such as motility and the secretion of digestive juices. Since many pollutants are neurotoxic, they can cause these disruptions by damaging junctions between muscles and nerves or damaging the brain centers that control these functions.

Toxins can also inhibit the function of key enzymes within the cell by inhibiting the production of energy in the "engine of the cell," the mitochondria. This can short-circuit the efforts of the cell to defend or repair itself. Certain pesticides that inhibit ATPase can severely inhibit energy-dependent functions. They inhibit mitochondrial ATPase. When these toxins infiltrate the gut lining, they damage the mitochondrial membrane and the cell wall membrane of the lining cells, the epithelium. As a result all the functions of the gut lining that are dependent on energy production through ATP will be impaired.

Toxins and the Liver

Toxins can directly damage the liver in two ways. Toxic buildup can overwhelm the liver's ability to detoxify, leading to a bottleneck and the storage of toxins throughout the body. It can also directly impair the liver's ability to regulate metabolism. This includes the synthesis and breakdown of fats, sugars, and starches and to some degree proteins. Deranged metabolism of carbohydrates can lead to abnormalities in blood sugar levels. This can cause a tendency toward low blood sugar, resulting in fatigue, mood swings, or depression. Impaired fat metabolism can lead to elevated cholesterol and bad cholesterol (LDL), which has been found to increase the risk for heart disease. Damage to protein metabolism can lead to abnormal protein by-products, including the buildup of ammonia in the body that can produce mental impairment.

Toxins and Cancer

Many chemical pollutants have been documented as carcinogens, especially organo-chlorine pesticides, aromatic and chlorinated solvents, and chemicals such as dioxins and PCBs. Some carcinogens are produced by overcooking food, particularly meats done on the barbecue, producing what's called PAHs (polycyclic aromatic hydrocarbons). All these toxins can cause damage to cellular DNA, which can initiate or promote cancerous changes in cells. Cancers of the colon, stomach, esophagus, and pancreas have all been linked with exposure to these chemicals. Of course these toxins can also circulate throughout the body and cause cancers in other organs and tissues.

Leaky Gut Syndrome, Toxins, and Food Allergies

The gut-lining membrane functions as a selective gate or barrier, allowing the passage and transport of small and medium-sized molecules of essential nutrients and communication peptides. At the same time the membrane bars the passage of larger molecules, including many toxins and allergenic substances. The cells of the gut lining play an essential role in this process. Their cell walls are made up of double-layered fatty and protein structures that act as semipermeable membranes, selectively allowing some substances through and barring others.

When nutrients are absorbed, small molecules are actively transported through the cell into the blood vessels beneath (transcellular transport) and other medium-sized molecules are allowed to pass between the cells (paracellular transport). The passage of nutrients between the cells is regulated by specialized structures called tight junctions. Essentially tight junctions are protein structures linking one cell wall to the next in a porelike structure that can open or close selectively to allow nutrients to pass through. The tight junctions are crucial in preventing the passage of large undesirable molecules such as toxins and allergens, as well as whole bacteria.

Toxins can damage or disrupt the tight junctions and their functions. If the tight junctions open too wide, material from the gut can enter the bloodstream directly. This invasive material includes toxins and allergenic molecules, as well as microbes. The malfunction is called leaky gut, and can actually occur within a matter of minutes. Leaky gut can cause infection, allergies, direct toxic damage, or malabsorption and malnutrition. This syndrome can be caused by direct damage from toxins ingested in food and water, but also by toxins produced internally in the gut through fermentation, putrefaction, and inflammation.

This chapter has discussed the various ways in which toxins can damage the gastrointestinal lining and function, leading to a wide variety of diseases. It should be remembered that these mechanisms, although discussed individually, often occur simultaneously or concurrently. Sometimes all of them occur at once to produce a complex chronic condition.

Although our discussion is predominantly about environmental toxins, with dysbiosis a large toxic load is created from within the gut itself by fermentation, putrefaction, and the toxin production of normal flora. These toxins can have an impact that is just as harmful as environmental toxins, if not more damaging. When both conditions coexist the internally generated toxins, in combination with high intake of environmental toxins, can lead to the most serious conditions.

Jeffry Anderson, M.D., is a physician in environmental medicine. His practice has included the treatment of hundreds of patients with environmental exposures, and he has served as consultant on a number of major environmental spills. He received his medical degree from Indiana University, following study at Purdue. Dr. Anderson has provided medical care in a variety of hospital and clinical settings and has been in private practice in Marin County, California, since 1973. He also specializes in allergy-immunology and applied medical nutrition, using an integrated approach to the diagnosis and treatment of chronic disease.

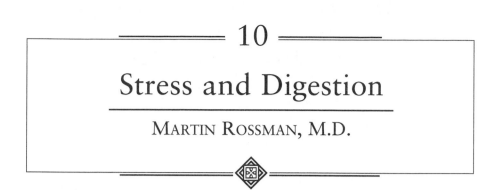

10

Stress and Digestion

Martin Rossman, M.D.

There is probably no system in the body that's more responsive to mind-body influences than the digestive tract. When we get sick, we tend to focus on the physical level, but our emotions and stress can affect digestion fairly profoundly. Problems are often initiated in the mind as well as in the body. Illness typically includes both physical and stress-related aspects.

Health issues can be challenging to sort out. Some conditions (like an overgrowth of yeast or bacteria) have mainly emotional symptoms when they're really a physical problem. On the other hand, research indicates that stress can have a negative effect on our flora and decrease antibody production, both factors in any overgrowth. So stress can directly affect our immune response.

No matter what the diagnosis, stress seems to make everything worse. Stress tends to interfere with digestion, whereas relaxation tends to promote good digestion. In some cases digestive symptoms are simply a response to stress. And doctors report that with conditions such as Crohn's disease, flareups and relapses tend to correlate with stressful life events. This doesn't mean the cause is psychological or emotional, but rather that stress can amplify the level of illness.

We now know that positive emotional factors can promote healing. This has been demonstrated in the work of Dean Ornish on community support and love, Herbert Benson on the relaxation response, Norman Cousins on laughter, and Larry Dossey on prayer.

INSIGHT INTO DIGESTION

Some of the first modern research on the connection between stress and digestion grew out of the work of Dr. William Beaumont, a famous nineteenth-century physician and pioneer in American surgery. One of his patients, Alexis St. Martin, had been shot in the abdomen, resulting in a wound that healed but couldn't be closed. St. Martin's open wound provided a view directly into his stomach through the abdominal wall.

The Powerful Effects of Stress on Digestion

Beverly's situation is an interesting example of the powerful effects of stress on health. Her experience also demonstrates that coping with stress can improve health. I first saw Beverly ten years ago when she was diagnosed with Crohn's disease at the young age of 23. Over the years, whenever she was under extreme stress at home due to a rocky marriage, she would be seen for symptoms of abdominal cramping, diarrhea, rectal bleeding, and weight loss. These relapses would occur about every other year. Otherwise she was generally well and free of symptoms, with the periodic support of medication.

For about five years I saw her very occasionally, primarily to renew prescriptions. Then one day Beverly reappeared, about forty pounds underweight, anemic, and extremely emaciated. She confided that she had recently gotten a divorce and felt her whole life was falling apart. She was overwhelmed by the challenges of dealing with lawyers, an intense child custody battle, unemployment, and a lack of job skills. Her condition was extreme enough to require tube feeding, as well as medication.

Before long we were able to get her back on solid food and supplements, while gradually decreasing the medication. On a program that included vitamin supplements, L-glutamine, and minerals with additional magnesium, she began regaining her weight. Once she developed some work skills and got a job, she was able to piece her life back together. As the stress decreased, she no longer needed most of the medications. At this point her Crohn's disease has been in remission for several years. Although we haven't seen her as a patient, she comes in once a year to let us know how she's doing. She is a perfect example of what stress can do to you—and of the health benefits of coping.

—Trent W. Nichols, M.D.

Alexis St. Martin became a guest in the Beaumont household, where he resided for many years. This provided Beaumont the opportunity to do a lot of observation. In 1833 Beaumont published a monograph, "Experiments and Observations on the Gastric Juices and the Biology of Digestion," in which he detailed 238 experiments that suggested the presence of what we now know to be hydrochloric acids and enzymes such as pepsin. His book marks the beginning of modern study of the digestive system.

Beaumont's experiments included feeding St. Martin foods directly through the opening in his abdomen and then watching the process of digestion and timing how long it took. He noticed that if St. Martin became angry his stomach lining became extremely red; there was a tremendous increase in blood supply and secretions in the stomach that were quite visible. If St. Martin became frightened the stomach wall would blanch, as the blood flow left the stomach lining. So Beaumont was able to see the direct effects of stress and emotions on digestion.

THE STRESS RESPONSE

Research on stress in the 1930s provided additional insight into the interaction between stress and digestion. Studies by Hans Selye, who first named and defined the stress response, found that animals placed under prolonged stress developed physical conditions. Most often, the problems occurred in three primary areas:

- They developed multiple stomach ulcers
- Their adrenal glands became enlarged—four or five times greater than normal—from the effort of producing the tremendous amounts of adrenaline to cope with the stress
- The immune system atrophied; the thymus, lymph nodes, and lymph tissue in the gut became tremendously shrunken

Selye noticed that those same three conditions occurred in both animals and humans whenever continuous stress was present. He decided they were characteristic of a prolonged stress response. Each of these dynamics is relevant to how well the digestive tract is functioning.

"FIGHT OR FLIGHT"

We now know that stress causes other changes in the body as well. During intense stress the blood supply is shunted away from the digestive organs and into the large muscles, so you can fight or run for your life. This is usually termed the fight-or-flight response. Scientists suggest that this protective reaction evolved long ago among prehistoric people in response to the kind of intense life-threatening events hunters must have faced.

Imagine walking out of a cave and running into a saber-toothed tiger! An immediate response is triggered—fight or flight. The senses get very sharp, the heart rate and blood pressure go up, and blood goes into the large muscles so you can either fight for your life or run. This effort is orchestrated by your sympathetic nervous system. As part of this process the blood flow is shunted away from the digestive tract, typically causing digestion and absorption to be less efficient until the stress response is over.

Half an hour later the event is over. After this supercharged period and intense response, you go into a relaxation phase, the opposite kind of response. Your muscles relax, your blood pressure comes down, and your heart rate decreases. All this happens through the action of the parasympathetic nervous system. The focus of the blood flow shifts from the muscles to the internal and digestive organs. This is a time when the body replenishes itself, rebuilds, replaces hormones, and repairs any injuries that may have been incurred. This is basically how researchers now understand the stress response.

MODERN STRESS

Modern people generally experience the stress response much less frequently than our prehistoric ancestors. In contrast, we experience a more subtle form of stress. In fact researchers have identified these different kinds of stress as Type 1 and Type 2. Type 1 stress occurs when there's an easily definable source of stress, there may be a specific action that can be taken, and there's an accompanying physical reaction. Either you run away from the tiger, you kill the tiger, or the tiger eats you for lunch. But one way or another, in half an hour, it's all over, and then the body goes into a relaxation and repair phase. Most modern people don't experience much Type 1 stress, except for people in wartime combat situations.

What we suffer from in modern cultures is a kind of ongoing, multifaceted, vague sense of stress and worry. It's our response to the evening news and "How am I going to pay the bills?" and "Will there be Social Security when I get old?" and "What am I going to do with my aging parents?" and "What am I going to do if my kids get into drugs?" and on and on. You have these worries just as I do—we worry about high school shootings on the news, children dying from hunger overseas, and tragedies in our cities we feel powerless to prevent. There's a constant bombardment of bad news that sets in motion worrying and expectations of the worst. We all worry some, and some of us worry a lot.

The problem is that our bodies tend to respond to this habit of worrying and fearful trains of thought in the same way we would respond to the actual events, but probably at a lower level. Still, when you're worrying about something that is perceived as a potential danger to you, it does tend to stimulate the sympathetic nervous system, the release of adrenaline, and the physical changes that accompany the stress response, such as the redirection of blood away from the stomach. That's why you've probably found that you don't digest so well when you're upset.

STRESS AND DIGESTION

You've probably heard of people having intense, visceral responses in reaction to extreme fear. What that suggests is that responses to fear, anxiety, and stress are directly wired to the gut. People with irritable bowel diseases and syndromes may or may not notice that it's directly related to stress. Some do and some don't. While a significant number of people find that it's not the sole cause of their condition, it's probably one of the common triggers that tends to make most GI conditions worse. Stress seems to sensitize the GI tract to be more twitchy or crampy or to interfere with digestion in one way or another. So there's a real connection wired into our physiology and our nervous systems, linking stress and digestive function. In fact, research has identified nerve fibers in the gut so extensive and complex, they sometimes call it the "gut brain."

This confirms our impression that stress responses and even emotions involve not only mental processes but a series of actual physical changes the body goes through. And many of these changes affect the functioning of the digestive tract, if only temporarily. So it's definitely worthwhile monitoring your own reactions to stress and tracking their effect on your health.

For some people, the digestive tract becomes the sensitized part of the body that functions as a kind of barometer, reflecting stress, worry, or anxiety. Whether we're anxious about a test, a job interview, or a date, we may find ourselves running to the bathroom. Not everybody has that response, but it's pretty common—butterflies in the stomach, nervous diarrhea. For some people the GI tract becomes the target organ; for these people that's the way the body expresses excessive stress.

THE INDIRECT EFFECTS OF STRESS

There's another aspect of the effects of stress on the gut—the indirect effects of stress. When people feel stressed beyond their capacity, they often find coping mechanisms that help to temporarily relieve the stress. Some of these temporary solutions may not be good for their digestion: for example, drinking too much alcohol, drinking too much coffee, overeating, eating junk food, or smoking.

In our attempts to reduce stress and anxiety levels, we often indulge in habits that are more directly damaging to the digestive system. For example, someone who has digestive upsets from a yeast overgrowth will probably find he does better when he eats less sugar. When he's stressed, the cravings for sugar may be intense and the sugar seems to relieve the stress temporarily. In many cases the wave of uncomfortable symptoms that surface within a day make it clear that this is not the best solution.

Learning a more direct way to reduce the stress response can prevent self-damaging or self-sabotaging coping mechanisms that don't really work.

USING STRESS TO YOUR ADVANTAGE

You can learn to use those responses and read them, much as you would notice the oil light coming on in your car and take action to prevent problems. You can use your responses to identify the issues that cause you the most intense anxiety or worry—gut reactions. When emotional reactions affect your digestive system, you can use the same connections with your nervous and immune systems to call up the relaxation response. So if there are nerves that can make your gut feel irritable, crampy, and spastic and upset, you can use these same mind-body connections to send messages to your digestive system that are soothing, relaxing, calming, and stress relieving. And that's something that you can consciously learn to do. Just as we all learn to worry, we can learn to relax.

THE RELAXATION RESPONSE

Learning some form of relaxation technique often has a beneficial effect on chronic digestive symptoms. Although these methods are deceptively simple, they can make a difference. Some people with digestive illness report that these are some of the most important things they do for their health.

- Simple breathing techniques
- Meditation
- The relaxation response (Herbert Benson)
- The body scan, which relaxes different parts of the body (Jon Kabat-Zinn)
- Imagery

Learning how to put your mind and body into a relaxed state allows the body to automatically go into that healing and repair mode. So the regular use of relaxation makes sense. Relaxation is a very direct thing that people can learn to do with a little practice.

When patients come in with conditions that seem to be made worse by stress, I encourage them to learn an effective relaxation technique and practice it diligently for a minimum of three weeks. I give them tapes that can help them learn to relax, and provide information on relaxation classes. If they're having active symptoms and a really difficult problem, I suggest they set aside twenty to thirty minutes twice a day for relaxation, for a three-week trial period. Most of the people I see find that relaxation helps to relieve their symptoms. Some people find it's the most important thing they do. Others notice that it helps them feel better and relieves some of their symptoms, while they and their doctor investigate the other things that affect digestion (like hidden food allergies or undiagnosed infection).

How long does it typically take to integrate these practices? Often people get relief very quickly. But it's something that you learn to do. Accept that it will take a little time, just like anything that's worth doing. I usually ask people to practice a couple of times a day for three weeks. This introductory period provides a very good sense of whether or not this approach is helpful and just how helpful it can be. Knowing that it's a time-limited practice in the beginning gives people a chance to get involved and then decide for themselves, based on their own experience. These techniques are definitely worth exploring and have been used with measurable success in combating conditions as serious as cancer and leukemia.

The Power of Imagery to Promote Healing

Alexandra was 30 years old, active and successful, but worried. She had developed signs of cancer. Several eminent physicians had diagnosed her condition as benign, but she worried that it was precancerous and wanted to know if she could do anything to make it go away.

Alexandra was intensely involved in every aspect of her life. She worked long hours, traveled frequently in her work, and kept a busy social schedule as well. She often felt tense and tired and wanted less stress in her life, though she saw that as a problem separate from her condition.

As part of our consultation, I asked her to relax and let an image of the cancer come to mind. She imagined it as rocks in a stream and was upset to see it was partially obstructing the flow. As she looked more closely, however, her perception of the rocks changed dramatically. She noticed that they were very smooth, shiny, and lustrous, and looked more like pearls than rocks. Alexandra immediately understood that, like pearls in an oyster, these nodules had formed in response to irritation and represented an attempt to protect her from further harm.

When I asked her what would need to happen for the pearls to be able to dissolve, she sensed a need to "remove the source of irritation." She made changes in her scheduling, her traveling, and her diet, and the nodules disappeared within a few months.

By paying attention to her problem in this way, Alexandra not only learned a valuable lesson in stress management but personally experienced the wisdom of her body and mind working together to maintain a healthy equilibrium. Her symptoms got her attention, and her use of imagery allowed her to understand both the meaning of her symptoms and what she needed to do to allow healing to proceed. In her case, the imagery didn't resolve her condition directly, but showed her what she could do to allow that to happen.

Martin Rossman, M.D., is founder and director of the Collaborative Medicine Center, as well as founder and codirector of the Academy for Guided Imagery. With David Bresler, Ph.D., he has defined and developed the therapeutic approach of Interactive Guided Imagery. He received his medical degree from the University of Michigan and is a diplomate of acupuncture. He serves as a faculty associate at the University of California at San Francisco, the California School of Professional Psychology, and John F. Kennedy University. Dr. Rossman is author of *Guided Imagery for Self-Healing* and *Fighting Cancer from Within,* as well as many guided imagery CDs and self-healing programs.

Dr. Rossman can be contacted at P.O. Box 1933, Mill Valley, CA 94942; phone (415) 383-3197; fax (415) 383-0944. For further information, see www.guidedimageryhealing.com.

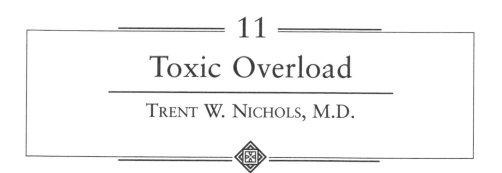

11

Toxic Overload

TRENT W. NICHOLS, M.D.

THE IMPORTANCE OF THE LIVER

As a gastroenterologist, I have noticed that almost half my patients with digestive disorders also turn out to have liver detoxification problems. This is cause for concern, because it is the liver that provides much of our protection against toxins. Everything absorbed from the digestive tract is eventually filtered through the liver—food, alcohol, medication, pesticides, and other toxins. Once the liver becomes overburdened, its detoxification capacity can be compromised.

Many patients with digestive disorders have some degree of liver impairment of which they are unaware. It is difficult to provide effective treatment for patients whose liver function is compromised. They tend to be less able to tolerate medications, many foods, and even nutritional supplements. To begin stabilizing their health, I have found that liver detoxification often needs to be addressed before other forms of treatment are started.

This chapter could be important to you if you have any of the following symptoms or lifestyle issues, which have been linked to compromised liver function:

Symptoms
- Sensitivity or reactions to perfumes, car exhaust, fumes from gasoline or paint, common household chemicals
- Frequent headaches
- Reactions to coffee or MSG (monosodium glutamate)
- Reactions to prescribed or over-the-counter medications

Lifestyle Factors
- Do you take medications on a regular basis for arthritis or chronic pain?
- Do you have a tendency to drink too much, too often?
- Are you exposed to chemicals on the job?
- When you are fasting or have the flu, have you developed jaundice or other more severe symptoms?

• Do you have reactions to detoxification, such as headaches, nausea, diarrhea, aches, or excessive sweating?

Early Detection

The goal is to detect problems early on, while they're still minor. At that point, there are practical steps that can be taken to support the liver and lighten its burden. If the liver continues to be overtaxed, year after year, more serious conditions can develop.

The liver is described as a vital organ because, like the heart, we cannot live without it. It is also one of the secrets to good health. Examples of the liver's essential functions include energy production and the extraction of nutrients from our food. The liver also manufacturers raw materials the body requires to make hormones, immune cells, brain neurotranmitters, and blood clotting factors. It metabolizes proteins, amino acids, and peptides for repair and healing and processes sugars and fats to be stored for future energy.

For information on how you can protect your liver, read on. (Also see chapter 23, on minimizing toxic exposure; chapter 26 on detox; and the sections on liver disease in part V, under treatment options.)

When the Liver Becomes Overwhelmed

Jeff, a drummer in the rock group Toto, died mysteriously one August afternoon in 1992 after using an insecticide spray on the roses in the backyard of his home in Los Angeles. He was believed to have died of a heart attack brought on by an allergic response to the pesticide. The media later reported that this reaction had been aggravated by Jeff's use of drugs and alcohol. This type of response to toxins can occur if liver function is impaired. His death is an example of the unfortunate problems that can result when the liver's ability to detoxify is compromised.

FACTORS IN LIVER HEALTH

Common Causes of Liver Problems

Unfortunately liver disease is on the rise, with a number of major contributing factors:

- Digestive disorders
- Weight gain and obesity
- Genetic predisposition
- Alcohol consumption
- Heavy metals exposure
- Other environmental toxins
- Nutritional deficiencies
- Viral infections
- Stress

Digestive disorders

Many people with digestive disorders tend to have low-grade liver problems that go undetected. These conditions are subtle and may not be diagnosed; currently there is no medical code for detoxification disorders. However, we believe these conditions will become more clearly defined in the future. As a first step, the Human Genome Project has identified genetic information related to the causes of these abnormalities. Genetic testing is also available that can be ordered by physicians, which identifies potential risk for impaired detoxification (see chapter 17).

Leaky gut syndrome (hyperpermeability) is one of the diagnostic disorders sometimes associated with liver disease. Liver impairment can result when toxins are passed on to the liver from the digestive tract. Hyperpermeability is believed to be one of the causes of autoimmune hepatitis. In another example, PSC (primary sclerosing cholangitis) is a liver disorder that often follows Crohn's disease or ulcerative colitis, which both involve hyperpermeability.

Weight gain

Hepatitis or fatty liver can also occur in nondrinkers due to poor metabolism. In those who are prediabetic, this is linked to weight gain—often the result of a high-carbohydrate intake. Eating a diet heavy in starches and sweets triggers the overproduction of insulin. In the short term, this extra insulin serves to maintain blood sugar, but eventually the insulin overproduction can cause a condition known as syndrome X or metabolic syndrome.

Over time these problems can result in obesity and diabetes. A less well-known problem associated with weight gain is the development of a "fatty liver," which slows detoxification. These are risks to be taken seriously—we find that among patients who are overweight, the majority either develop syndrome X or type II diabetes. (See chapter 31 for suggestions on foods that are delicious, healthy, and easier on your body.)

Genetic predisposition

Some patients develop these types of problems because they have genetic disorders. For example, in Gilbert's syndrome the liver is unable to transform toxins into less toxic compounds, because one particular enzyme is missing. In this disorder the liver still functions, but it is not optimal, especially after a prolonged fast or during a viral illness.

Alcohol consumption

Patients who are heavy drinkers can develop hepatitis (liver inflammation) caused by the irritating effects of the alcohol. Others develop fatty liver syndrome. Due to additional fat in the liver cells, energy production is impaired (in the mitochondria, the "engine" of the cell). People with these conditions may experience fatigue resulting from problems with energy production and the burden on the detoxification system.

Heavy metal exposure

We are also seeing a great many patients with heavy metal contamination. Heavy metal toxicity can be closely related to problems with the liver. These disorders can be caused by mercury, iron, copper, thalium, arsenic, antimony, or other heavy metals. Patients often ask me which came first, the heavy metal exposure, the genetic predisposition, or the GI disorders. They are all associated, but differ on a case-by-case basis. Yet we see these three conditions in combination so often that we are beginning to suspect that they are linked.

WHAT YOU CAN DO

As mentioned previously, of the patients we see with digestive disorders, about 50 percent have some degree of compromise in their liver detoxification. Many of my patients have seen other doctors, practitioners, or nutritionists before they come to us. They have already done a great deal, but their health is still not optimal. Although testing is helpful, many of these problems are so subtle they escape detection.

At this point in my practice I assume that patients who've had long-term gastrointestinal problems also have some degree of detox abnormality. So we treat everyone with some form of a nutritional program for clearing the liver. Because we find so many new patients with undiagnosed liver problems, we have come to believe that screening with a liver detoxification profile can be very helpful. The profiles can be used to measure the condition of the liver before and after treatment, to determine progress.

If you suspect that you have a liver problem, there are a number of possible steps you can take:

Consider seeing an integrative physician. See the resources section of this book for the names of national organizations that make referrals to integrative practitioners all over the country. You may want to begin with a consultation with one of the contributors in this book. In any case, look for a physician with good clinical experience in the diagnosis and treatment of liver disorders—one who is knowledgeable about environmental medicine, is familiar with functional tests, and knows how to use them. Referral sources include:

- American Academy of Environmental Medicine
- American College for the Advancement of Medicine (ACAM)
- Bastyr Univesity referral line
- Institute for Functional Medicine, Gig Harbor, Washington

Get your liver tested. (See chapter 17 and the entries in the back of the book under liver disease for more information on testing.) Noninvasive tests that reflect liver health include:

- Liver detoxification test
- Intestinal permeability
- Genetic testing

Minimize exposure to environmental toxins. If you have chronic illness or if you are pregnant, for example, don't pump your own gas or spray your garden. (See chapter 23 for more ideas on how to decrease toxic exposure.)

Eliminate alcohol consumption. If you have moderate or severe liver disease, alcohol should be totally avoided. If you have mild liver problems, it's okay to have an alcoholic beverage occasionally.

Eat clean, organic food whenever possible. Eat whole foods in their natural state to avoid additives and to get the most complete nutrition.

Optimize your digestive health. This is important because one of the major sources of stress to the liver is the digestive tract.

Gradually detoxify your system. If you are quite ill, you should undergo your detoxification in gradual stages. We use a variety of liver-clearing products containing powdered nutrients to support liver function and detoxification. Sensitive patients may begin on half a scoop (rather than the full regimen). These products include UltraClear, UltraClear Sustain, UltraClear Plus, and AdvaClear from Metagenics, and MediClear from Thorne Research.

Patients with severe multiple chemical sensitivities may be so compromised that they are unable to tolerate even nutritional products intended for detoxification. Instead they must begin detoxifying with infrared saunas, to sweat the toxins out of the tissues and the liver.

Enhance the flora in your body. Some people don't do well with certain vegetables, such as broccoli and Brussels sprouts, which are in the cruciferous family. Once you've established good flora using probiotics, and gotten rid of bad bacteria and yeast, you'll probably find that you can eat these vegetables again. Also try taking a digestive enzyme when you eat them.

Begin new supplements gradually. Use a systematic approach to monitor your tolerance. Only start one new thing at a time. Begin with one a day and build up your dosage gradually. For example, silymarin is a gentle herb with an excellent track record in the research literature. Yet even this herb doesn't work for everyone. No matter what you are taking, start small. The more seriously ill you are, the more important it is to proceed one step at a time.

Moderate your fat intake. This is important if you have fatty liver syndrome. You'll also want to monitor your fat-soluble vitamins (A, D, and E). For example, you may not be able to tolerate therapeutic dosages of vitamin A at levels higher than 10,000 I.U. This conservative approach also applies to strategies such as the olive oil flush. Patients (with known or unknown liver disease) can be at risk of a gallstone attack. In addition the increased intake of fat can overwhelm an overburdened liver, creating more toxicity.

Keep your homocysteine levels moderate by taking key supplements. Nutrients that support liver metabolism include the B complex, TMG (tri-methyl-glycine), folic acid, and B_{12}. (One sign of malabsorption is being too thin.)

Get enough nutrients. If you have malabsorption, consider getting your nutrients from different sources.

- At the very least, use capsules rather than tablets. The research shows that frequently only about 30 percent of many tablets are actually absorbed.
- Multiple vitamins are now available in powdered form (such as Total Immune from Allergy Research Group) for better absorption.
- Vitamins are available as sublingual tablets that can be dissolved under the tongue and also come in a spray form or as suppositories.
- Injections can be helpful. If your doctor feels you would benefit from injections such as B_{12} or B complex, you may want to learn to give yourself shots (with instructions from a nurse or practitioner).
- Some patients periodically also receive intravenous vitamins from their doctors, with nutrients such as vitamin C, glutathione, or a multiple-vitamin combination in the form of an IV "Meyers' cocktail."

- The advantage to injected and intravenous nutrients is that they bypass the digestive tract and are absorbed directly into the bloodstream.

Work with your doctor to determine your own individual supplement needs. It will also involve your own careful observation and the use of a diary or a journal. Consider trying no more than one new supplement a week and watching its effects. This will help you determine what is essential to your health and what isn't.

PRACTICAL THOUGHTS ON DETOX

Detoxification is the way our body attempts to cope with toxins—heavy metals, petrochemicals, pesticides, food additives; by-products of infection due to viruses, bacteria, or parasites; allergenic or spoiled foods; by-products of normal food metabolism; alcohol, drugs, and even medication.

What is detoxification? The term *detoxification* literally means "to make less toxic." The liver detoxifies both internal and external toxins in a two-stage process. In Phase 1, liver enzymes disarm toxic substances, making them less harmful. In Phase 2, the liver combines antioxidant nutrients—vitamins or amino acids—with the toxins to form new compounds that can be excreted without damaging the body.

How your nutrition supports detoxification. The nutrients you obtain from your food provide the raw materials your body uses to eliminate toxins. Without the necessary materials—vitamins, minerals, amino acids, and other nutrients—detoxification capacity is limited. When we have sufficient antioxidants (from fresh fruits and vegetables) and amino acids (from protein), we can resist the effects of toxins. (This is why your mother told you to eat your vegetables.) For some people it's important to take vitamin supplements to be sure they get enough nutrients.

What happens when nutrient levels are low. Without the necessary antioxidants to do the job, the liver can become overwhelmed by toxins. The result is usually the production of free radicals—unstable molecules that can damage cells, tissue, and even genetic material. The free radicals that result from poor detoxification are a contributing factor in many forms of chronic illness. Free radical or oxidative damage also plays a major role in cancer, heart disease, and the aging process.

THE PROCESS OF DETOXIFICATION

Phase 1

The primary role of the liver in Phase 1 is to neutralize toxins. Through the action of specific enzymes, toxins are modified and made less harmful. The enzymes take part in an electrochemical process that neutralizes the toxins by electron transfer (via oxidation/reduction). This neutralizing process transforms the toxins so they no longer have a free radical charge, and are no longer a source of oxidative stress. If this phase of detoxification is impaired, our tolerance to medications or toxic exposure is reduced. The Phase 1 enzymes that perform this task are extensive; to date more than sixty variations of cytochrome P450 have been identified.

Phase 2

In this stage, a series of processes prepare the toxins for elimination. At least eight types of detoxification occur in Phase 2. Each of these different processes focuses on clearing specific types of toxins. Consider the importance of a few of these processes and the essential nutrients that serve as the raw materials.

Phase 3

Researchers have recently identified a third phase of detoxification, described as the ABC Transporter system, because it involves transporting toxins out of the cells. Rather than occurring in the liver, phase 3 takes place in the small intestine. This localized detoxification is necessary because cells in the intestinal lining are constantly exposed to toxins in the gut. To minimize this toxicity, the cells contain microscopic pumps (called export pumps) that clear the cell of toxins.

This process is extremely important. When it's working properly, it clears toxins from the gut lining so they won't be absorbed into the bloodstream. This localized detox system is vital because the potential for toxicity is so much higher in the gut. It's necessary to clear the gut before the toxins are absorbed by the extensive network of capillaries and blood vessels that carry nutrients and other material from the digestive tract to the liver.

To gauge the health of the gut lining, the test for intestinal permeability can reflect whether this barrier function is intact. If this barrier is damaged, some of the protective effect of the transporter system can be lost. The test is not a direct evaluation of the transporter system. However, if problems with permeability are detected, this suggests that the function of the transporter system may be compromised to some extent as well.

Protective Efforts of Phase 2

Substances Detoxified	Pathway	Supportive Nutrients
Water-soluble toxins	Glutathione couples toxins with biochemicals to produce water-soluble compounds that can then be excreted via the kidneys. Cases of chronic fatigue have been linked to problems in this pathway, particularly when a great deal of energy is being diverted for detox.	Vitamin C, N-acetylcysteine, glycine, and methionine
Fat-soluble toxins	Glutathione also eliminates toxins stored in body fat, such as mercury and lead. Glutathione has such a vital role in this process that it is now used in IV form to treat patients with heavy metal exposure in environmental-medicine clinics.	An herb that can be used therapeutically to support this pathway is silymarin (milk thistle)
Drug metabolism	Amino acid coupling is another process in which nutrients combine with toxins and neutralize them, particularly important in drug metabolism	Glycine, taurine, glutamine, arginine, and ornithine; vitamin B_6 and magnesium
Estrogen detoxification	Methylation involves coupling methyl-group biochemicals with toxins such as estrogen. When methylation is poor, homocysteine builds up in the blood. This amino acid, in excess, is now recognized as a major factor in strokes, heart attacks, Alzheimer's disease, Parkinson's disease, and osteoporosis.	SAMe
Toxins from food, bacteria, and the environment	Sulfation couples toxins with sulfur-containing compounds, important in detoxifying drugs, food additives, environmental toxins, and toxins from gut bacteria. This is also the main pathway for detoxifying steroid and thyroid hormones.	Cruciferous sulfur-containing vegetables: broccoli and Brussels sprouts
Sulfa drugs and related medications	Acetylation couples or conjugates medications such as sulfa drugs and their derivatives.	Vitamin C, thiamine (B1), and pathothenic acid (B5)
Medications and food additives	Glucuronidation combines glucuronic acid with toxins. This process is important because many commonly prescribed medications are detoxified through this pathway, including aspirin. Food additives such as benzoates and menthol are also detoxified.	Citrus fruits

Your liver is the one of the keys to your energy and stamina. Consider using the suggestions in this chapter to enhance your diet and supplements with the support of your liver in mind. If you suspect that you have any type of liver problem, we encourage you to be seen by an integrative physician and seek functional-medicine liver testing. We consider this one of the most frequently overlooked and underappreciated aspects of good health.

===

Trent W. Nichols, M.D., is a board certified internist, nutritionist and gastroenterologist who is a fellow of the American College of Physicians and American College of Nutrition. He additionally is an active physician/scientist involved in pharmaceutical, nutritional, and bioelectromagnetic research. He is a graduate of the University of Denver with a BS in Chemistry and of the Northwestern University Medical School. His residency in internal medicine and gastroenterology fellowship were also at Northwestern University. He is a member of the Institute of Functional Medicine, the Bioelectromagnetic Society, Tissue Engineering Society International, the Society for Neuroscience, and is vice president of the North American Academy of Magnetic Therapy. Dr. Nichols has been in private practice in Hanover for over 26 years. He was recently selected as one of America's Top Physicians by Consumers' Research Council of America, 2004-5.

The Center for Nutritional and Digestive Disorders is a functional-medicine practice dedicated to helping patients with chronic disorders. The center sees patients with gastrointestinal disorders and those with other types of chronic conditions. Among the digestive disorders treated are celiac sprue, Crohn's disease, food allergies and sensitivities, irritable bowel syndrome, and ulcerative colitis. Treatment is also provided for a range of metabolic and toxic syndromes, including autism, heavy metal exposure, diabetes, obesity, and polycystic ovary syndrome. CNDD is located in Hanover, Pennsylvania, and can be reached by phone at (717) 632-0300 or on the Web at www.gutdoc.org.

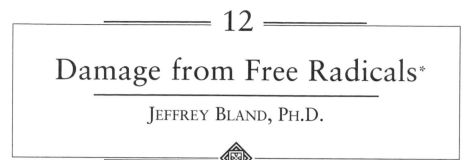

12

Damage from Free Radicals*

JEFFREY BLAND, PH.D.

The cascade of events that begins in the digestive tract and culminates in the liver can generate a particular kind of risk due to reactive and destructive molecules called free radicals. If these dangerous reactions are not detoxified, they can ricochet through the cellular materials of the body. Oxygen-free radicals have the potential to affect the immune system and initiate heart disease, cancer, or genetic damage.

By identifying the presence of free radicals, we can work to prevent the diseases they might initiate. Preventive measures against free radical damage involve a commonsense lifestyle, with good nutrition as part of the bargain. These protections include eating a diet rich in fresh fruits and vegetables and good-quality protein (vegetable or animal), then supplementing it with antioxidant nutrients and sufficient sleep.

WHY FREE RADICALS MATTER

Free radicals are by-products of oxygen metabolism. We know that oxygen is essential to life. Yet it can also be a reactive chemical substance, and in certain forms can cause harm to the body. We know that combining oxygen with iron produces rust and eventually causes the breakdown of objects made of iron. In much the same way certain forms of oxygen can combine with the biological materials of the body, causing them to deteriorate.

Although our bodies don't rust, they are subject to damage from a subtle form of stress due to the effects of oxygen, called oxidative stress. Oxygen can cause harm by breaking down cells and tissues, including fats, structural proteins, enzymes, and genetic material (DNA). Fats can become rancid, cell walls become brittle, and enzymes no longer work. Genetic blueprints are damaged or lost. Since the DNA is the master plan for repairing and rebuilding the body, this is like losing part of the instruction manual for the system. The breaking down of all these processes accelerates any potential for heart disease, cancer, hardening of the arteries, or Alzheimer's disease.

---

*This chapter is adapted from *The 20-Day Rejuvenation Diet Program* (1999) by Jeffrey Bland, Ph.D., and is reprinted by permission of the McGraw Hill Companies.

MINIMIZING FREE RADICALS

By understanding the sources of free radicals generated within the body, we can make efforts to minimize them. We can also buffer our bodies against the effects of oxidative stress through good nutrition and lifestyle. Important sources of free radicals that are initiated *within* the body include:

- The by-products of fighting infection
- The domino effect of free radicals, which amplifies their impact
- Biochemicals produced in the liver
- Effects of the aging process
- Stress due to extreme exercise or physical trauma
- Reactions to oxidative stress from the environment

By-Products of Fighting Infection

Activated forms of oxygen are released by white blood cells as one of our immune defenses against microbes, to poison microbes with bleach or peroxide. The bleach secreted by white blood cells is just like the bleach you use to brighten your clothes. Called hypochlorite, it is chemically converted in our bodies into potentially harmful forms of oxygen, including hydrogen peroxide. The forms of oxygen most likely to damage tissues and cells are called oxygen radicals or free radicals. Within the body, processes that stimulate free radical production include infection by viruses, bacteria, and other harmful microbes, or overstimulation of the immune response. This is a case in which the solution to one problem leads to another, the creation of oxidants. There are numerous other stressors that generate free radical production as well.

A Story with a Happy Ending

At 36 Michael was successful and prosperous, a self-made entrepreneur. What wasn't apparent was his constant struggle with low-grade pain since adolescence, due to fibromyalgia. He also suffered from chronic fatigue so serious it left him little energy for much of a personal life. Each day he had just enough energy to manage the thriving business he had developed, but nothing more. Michael's life was limited by his ever-present health problems. Unfortunately his condition gradually continued to worsen.

Michael's case was so complex that we scheduled a series of functional tests to evaluate the issues. His pancreatic enzymes were low, which meant that he wasn't fully digesting his food. His pH reading indicated that his body was too acidic. A test indicator of inflammation in the colon was high (elevated alpha-antichymotrypsin), suggesting a possible irritation or infection.

Initial stool testing indicated the presence of the yeast *Candida albicans*, which raised our suspicion of other pathogens in the digestive tract. We scheduled another test that evaluates chemical markers to identify a variety of pathogenic microbes. This test, which measures organic acids, found signs of the bacteria *Clostridium difficile* and the parasite *Giardia lamblia*, and confirmed the candida. The first part of the treatment protocol we designed for Michael was aimed at settling down his GI tract, and within ten days, he showed the first significant improvement he had experienced in more than fifteen years.

Given the presence of so much possible inflammation, we also scheduled tests for oxidative stress, as well as testing for LDL, probably one of the best indicators of cardiovascular risk. This test reflects levels of oxidative stress, and his levels were very high. We knew that large amounts of antioxidants, especially vitamin E, would be required to bring these levels down to a safe range. Consider that this is a very active person in his midthirties, with an extremely good diet, yet he is still showing a significantly high marker for oxidative stress. A logical question to ask would be, What is occurring to cause oxidative stress in someone this young, particularly since he has a good diet?

We believe the answer may relate to his intestinal infections, leaky gut syndrome, and liver stress. In response to the toxic overload, his liver apparently was producing high levels of free radicals. We also found cellular DNA adducts, which measure the amount of potential DNA damage that might be resulting— this is an issue related to oxidative stress. However, when we measured his T cell activity, we found the levels to be low.

The immune suppression (low T cell count) in combination with high levels of oxidative stress placed him at risk for more serious illness. Fortunately he may be able to prevent potential problems before there are signs of any form of degenerative disease. The goals are to continue to lower his oxidative stress by clearing problems in the GI tract, to increase protective factors by ensuring antioxidant intake, and to lower his stress.

—Jerry Stine

The Domino Effect of Free Radicals

To understand the intense and random action of free radicals in the tissue, imagine a Ping-Pong table covered with mousetraps. All the traps are set, baited with carefully placed Ping-Pong balls. Then imagine tossing another ball onto the table. As that ball springs a trap it bounces and begins a reaction that triggers a nearby trap, and then the next and the next. Eventually all the mousetraps on the table have been impacted with balls bouncing in all directions. This is similar to the chemical reactions initiated by free radicals.

Biochemicals Produced in the Liver

There is a tremendous potential for free radical damage in the liver. In the first phase of detoxification, some of the toxic load is converted into substances that have free radical activity and are potentially cancer promoting as well. As long as the second phase of detoxification can quickly metabolize these free radicals and carcinogens, there is no problem. Then the transformed, inert by-products are simply secreted into the bile, pass into the stool, and are excreted from the body.

However, when the reserve capacity of this second phase is exhausted, the liver can no longer buffer the body against free radicals and carcinogens. Then they may overflow and cause damage locally or leak into general circulation, where they can create profound biochemical damage in distant parts of the body.

Oxidative stress can occur anywhere in the body. Wherever and whenever oxygen is being used by the tissues in metabolism, there is the potential for oxidative stress. (For example, in bone this effect can take place as part of the process of osteoporosis.) This means that without adequate antioxidant protection, damage can occur to muscles, blood vessels, lungs, kidneys, the brain, joints, or any other tissue.

Minimizing the Effects of Aging

Free radicals are also generated at increased levels as we age. Although this process is beyond the scope of our discussion here, it's encouraging to report that good nutrition can counter these effects. In a study of exercise performance and age, vitamin E was shown to minimize age differences. Male volunteers ranging from 22 to 74 years old were tested for muscle trauma by running downhill on an inclined treadmill. The performance of volunteers who received daily supplements of vitamin E (two 400 IU capsules) was compared with those who received a placebo (containing no vitamin E). Researchers found that supplementing with vitamin E tended to eliminate age differences in performance.

Countering the Effects of Exercise

The protective effect of antioxidants has also been demonstrated in a remarkable study of elite mountain climbers in the Himalayas. During a climb of Annapurna, one of the highest mountains in the world, professional climbers were evaluated for levels of vitamins C and E and the effects on their performance.

The athletes were climbing at altitudes above 20,000 feet without oxygen, under extreme conditions. Some climbers received vitamin E supplements of 200 milligrams twice a day for four weeks, while others received a placebo of no nutritive value. The study confirmed that antioxidants have an important protective effect. Climbers who received supplemental vitamin E were able to engage in strenuous physical activity for longer periods of time without damage, apparently because they had much better resistance to oxidative stress during the climb.

Minimizing Oxidative Stress from the Environment

Major environmental stressors can also stimulate the development of free radicals in the body. They may involve unintentional exposures such as climate or intentional exposures such as those that occur when doing heavy cleaning or painting the house. Common sources of oxidative stress include:

- Air pollution
- Extreme cold
- Radiation
- Heavy metals and other toxins
- Pesticides and various chemicals
- Alcohol consumption
- Smoking
- Medications
- Poor diet

The increased oxidative stress that can result from these types of exposures can cause chronic health problems. When the body is producing excessively high levels of oxygen-free radicals, it is essentially in the process of breaking itself down. The more toxic the burden or the greater the psychological or physical stress, the more potential there is for damage from free radicals—unless there are high enough levels of antioxidants available.

At times of high oxidative stress, pay particular attention to your nutrition. Make sure you don't skip meals, fast, or diet. Don't eat junk food. Take extra care of yourself when you're exposed to any of the stressors that can trigger free radicals in your body.

Reducing Free Radical Stress—A Summary

Health and Lifestyle

- Seek treatment for digestive disorders, since they can generate free radicals.
- Get enough rest and sleep.
- Don't smoke. Consider trying the patch or acupuncture. The benefits of quitting are clear from the research. Those who quit for several years have risks as low as those who have never smoked.
- Minimize toxic exposure and indoor air pollution, including secondhand smoke. There are one hundred trillion free radicals in each puff of cigarette smoke.
- Avoid eating refined and processed foods.
- Use only fresh, quality vegetable oil.
- Minimize alcohol consumption. If drinking is an issue, consider trying acupuncture detox and/or a nutritionally oriented program.

Increasing Antioxidants

- Eat fresh fruits and vegetables because they're good natural sources of antioxidants. Use organic produce whenever possible.
- Supplements can provide basic antioxidant protection, particularly vitamins A, C, and E, coenzyme Q_{10}, and bioflavinoids such as quercetin.
- Include B complex vitamins in your diet, especially B_2.
- Supplements also ensure the benefits of trace minerals such as manganese, copper, zinc, and selenium, and the sulphur-based MSM (methylsulfonyl-methane).
- Beneficial herbs include ginkgo and the pycnogenols such as grape seed extract, silymarin, green tea, and lipoic acid.
- Consider working with a nutritionally oriented physician who can test your levels of these vital nutrients. Your doctor can also have you retested periodically to make sure you are maintaining your protective levels of antioxidants.

Jeffrey Bland, Ph.D., has been actively involved in nutrition-related research for more than twenty years and has served as director of the Bellevue-Redmond Medical Laboratory, as a professor of chemistry at the University of Puget Sound, and as a senior research scientist at the Linus Pauling Institute of Science and Medicine. In 1992 Dr. Bland cofounded the Institute for Functional Medicine, which provides CME-approved continuing medical education courses for physicians (see www.functionalmedicine.org). In 2000 Dr. Bland became the president and chief science officer of Metagenics. Under his guidance Metagenics has become a leader in nutrigenomics research and product development. He is the author of many widely read works on nutrition, including *The 20-Day Rejuvenation Diet Program* (Keats/McGraw-Hill, 1997), *Genetic Nutritioneering* (NTC/McGraw-Hill, 1999), and *Clinical Nutrition* (Institute for Functional Medicine, 2004). Dr. Bland can be reached at Metagenics in Gig Harbor, Washington; phone (800) 843-9960; Web site www.metagenics.com.

The Institute for Functional Medicine provides continuing medical education for physicians and other health care professionals through seminars and an annual symposium. They also publish books; a monthly audio subscription series, *Functional Medicine Updates;* and other educational materials on emerging research and clinical applications. The mission of the Institute for Functional Medicine is to improve patient outcomes through the prevention, early assessment, and comprehensive management of complex chronic diseases. The institute can be reached at (800) 843-9660 or on the Web at www.ifm.org.

13

How Problems with Digestion Can Cause Illness Anywhere in the Body

JEFFRY ANDERSON, M.D.

If you have digestive illness, whether it's severe or mild it's important to know that there are new treatments available. Decades of research have resulted in new understandings of how the body works. In complementary medicine, this expanded understanding is applied to treatment through the strategic use of nutrition, nutrients, and herbal medicine, often in combination with drug therapy.

New information on the dynamics of the body make it clear that conditions in the digestive tract affect the entire system. Folk wisdom reflects this interconnectedness: The saying in India is "Constipation is the mother of all ills."

Recent research suggests that degradation of the gastrointestinal environment is one of the primary points at which health is lost. What we now know is that the same toxins associated with GI dysfunction are frequently absorbed and distributed to other parts of the body. First they place a burden on the liver and the immune system. If liver overload occurs there will be spillover, and some of the toxins will be passed on to other organs or tissues.

Often it's the weak link in the system that will be hit by the damage—affecting the organ or tissue anywhere in the body that is the most vulnerable. The vulnerability may be inherited or caused by physical injury, toxic exposure, or poor diet. If the sensitive system is the lungs, toxins that originate in the gut and circulate in the bloodstream may manifest as asthma or allergies. Sooner or later this toxic overload comes to the attention of the immune system.

- Circulating toxins can trigger a hyperactive immune response, leading to allergies or inflammation with their associated pain and swelling.
- Toxins can short-circuit the immune response, resulting in infection.

At this point, corrosive toxic free radicals are released. Hopefully there are enough antioxidant nutrients to protect the cells and key cellular structures, such as the cell wall and the energy-producing "battery" of the cell, the mitochondria.

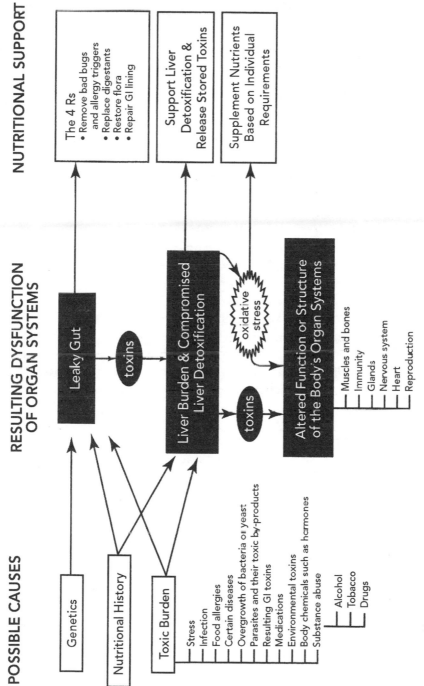

POSSIBLE CAUSES

RESULTING DYSFUNCTION
OF ORGAN SYSTEMS

NUTRITIONAL SUPPORT

Genetics

Nutritional History

Toxic Burden

Stress
Infection
Food allergies
Certain diseases
Overgrowth of bacteria or yeast
Parasites and their toxic by-products
Resulting GI toxins
Medications
Environmental toxins
Body chemicals such as hormones
Substance abuse

Alcohol
Tobacco
Drugs

Leaky Gut

toxins

Liver Burden & Compromised
Liver Detoxification

oxidative
stress

toxins

Altered Function or Structure
of the Body's Organ Systems

Muscles and bones
Immunity
Glands
Nervous system
Heart
Reproduction

The 4 Rs
• Remove bad bugs
  and allergy triggers
• Replace digestants
• Restore flora
• Repair GI lining

Support Liver
Detoxification &
Release Stored Toxins

Supplement Nutrients
Based on Individual
Requirements

SOURCE: HealthComm International, 1999.

THE DOMINO EFFECT

Upstream Activities in the GI Tract and Liver

Envision your body as a complete ecosystem with toxic wastes that must be processed to restore its pristine state. Imagine the liver as a toxic waste–disposal plant. It clears toxins by breaking them down, decreasing their toxicity, linking them to transport molecules, and dispatching them out in urine and stool. If we begin having problems with toxic overload in the liver, it's essential to look at what is going on upstream—at the factors creating problems for the liver.

Are excessive amounts of toxins being created in the gut? The gut is the starting place for major toxicity in the body because much of what goes through the gut is absorbed, whether by design, accident, or pathology. These include:

- By-products of poorly digested food or chronic constipation (such as ammonia)
- Toxins produced by overgrowth of yeast, bacteria, or invasive parasites (endotoxins such as alcohols and aldehydes)
- Chemical pollutants, pesticides, and heavy metals in our food and water

Leaky gut syndrome can cause the absorption of any of this material, all of it potentially harmful and intended for disposal by the body. The by-products of these malfunctions in the gut are all passed on directly through the major blood vessels into the liver portal system. There can be health consequences from the overload on the detox mechanisms of the liver. Toxic spillover can occur throughout the body and the system.

Downstream Effects of Toxic Overload

A bottleneck effect can occur if the liver is overburdened because of chronic or persistent toxicity beyond the capacity of the detoxification pathways to handle. The liver detox machinery may become stressed and compromised. It's trying to do its job, but the process may be creating even more free radicals and even more toxic intermediate chemicals. Here are the events in the liver that can result from overload:

- Increased oxidative stress from the liver's detoxification process
- Impaired carbohydrate metabolism
- Increased immune activity and the production of biochemicals that promote inflammation
- Failure of Phase 1 detoxification or accelerated Phase 1, which can cause increased production of free radicals
- The bottleneck effect if Phase 2 detoxification is slow

Effects on the cells and tissues:

- The body needs to remove these toxins from circulation.
- If the system can't excrete them, it will store them.
- Chemicals and pesticides will typically be stored in fat.
- Heavy metals will be stored in protein tissue—in muscles, bones, cartilage and organ tissue such as the brain and the liver. Nerve cells and enzymes can also be damaged.

Eventually some of these toxins are rereleased and then stored again. When they are released, they eventually go to the liver, and the liver has to cope with them again. The liver either detoxifies them or recirculates them. If this occurs it may cause more damage as they move through the system and then get redeposited. The increasing accumulation of toxins can cause cellular damage. It is critical that you begin detoxifying by starting with first things first, which is the gut.

DIGESTIVE SYSTEM OVERLOAD

Possible Causes

- Genetics
- Stress
- Lifestyle factors
- Environmental toxins
- Medications
- Contaminants in food and water
- Poor absorption
- Food allergies
- Impaired nutritional status
- By-products of poor digestion
- Overgrowth of yeast or bacteria
- Parasitic infection
- General infections
- Inflammatory conditions
- Degenerative diseases

Potential Symptoms

- Widespread chronic fatigue or weakness from compromised energy production, even in the energy-producing unit of the cells (the mitochondria).
- Compromise of the immune system, less resistance to infection, autoimmune disorders, allergies, sensitivities, colds and flu, bronchitis, sinus infections, chemical sensitivity.
- Problems in the muscles and joints, from aches and swelling to pain or arthritis.
- Skin disorders, including acne, dermatitis, eczema, psoriasis, and urticaria.
- Consequences to the central nervous system and brain function: mild problems including difficulty with concentration and memory, coordination, headaches or migraines, attention deficit disorder, and in severe cases, symptoms that resemble autism.

- Circulation of chemical toxins, causing more serious neurological symptoms ranging from seizure disorders to damage of the nervous system.
- Decrease in hormone production caused by toxins in the body.
- Liver damage, with compromised detox functions, possible hypoglycemia, and mood swings.
- Specific conditions such as arthritis, asthma, or allergies that can result from the constant circulation of toxins. This can be due to toxins that compromise the immune system, causing inflammation or aggravating existing conditions. The toxins stimulate the release of an immune response with biochemicals that can set in motion a full-blown reaction.

The presence of conditions caused by leaky gut syndrome indicate that toxins have been released from the GI tract and are out in general circulation. Then degenerative diseases such as cancer or autoimmune conditions can eventually develop.

STRATEGIES TO RESTORE HEALTH

When we talk about strategies to restore health, we mean cleansing and supporting the GI tract, the liver, and the entire system.

- First detox the GI tract.
- Then improve the function of the liver detox systems.
- Finally, the downstream consequences must be addressed. This means detoxifying the body to remove accumulated toxins from the cells and tissues.

So cleaning up the gut is the starting point.

- Make sure that you are not constipated.
- Make sure that you're digesting everything thoroughly. Determine if there's a need to supplement digestive enzymes, hydrochloric acid, or botanicals.
- Clean house. Get rid of bad bugs. Be sure you don't have toxins from an overgrowth of yeast or bacteria or some invasive parasite.
- Restore the good flora by taking probiotics.

Then you can start addressing the liver detox issues.

- The point is that you can't deal with the downstream conditions until you've treated the upstream problem in the gut and liver. For people with a highly toxic system, it is necessary to address the liver as well as the gut simultaneously. If you start mobilizing heavy metals and chemicals out of the tissue, unless you have dealt with the liver first, then you're just putting more demand on it.

- In order for you to be more fully healthy, these concerns need to be addressed in the digestive tract, throughout your entire system, and as symptoms elsewhere in the body.

Doctors observe that some of these conditions resolve naturally as a result of clearing the GI tract and liver. When you clean up the upstream issues and the liver, then the downstream consequences tend to just go away. At that point, stored toxins can also be detoxed from the tissues and cells. If you have any of these concerns, we recommend that you seek a qualified, compassionate health care professional who is familiar with detoxification concepts, and work with your practitioner on resolving your digestive issues.

Biographical information for **Jeffry Anderson, M.D.**, appears on page 86.

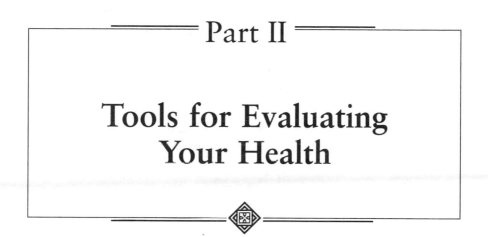

Part II

Tools for Evaluating
Your Health

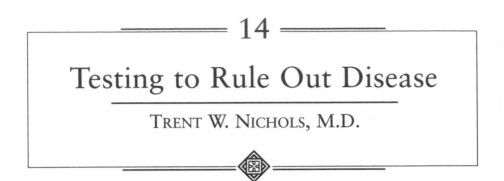

14

Testing to Rule Out Disease

TRENT W. NICHOLS, M.D.

Testing to rule out disease is a sensible way to approach a health problem. If a condition is chronic or long-standing, even if the symptoms are mild, it's important to be sure there is no major underlying condition or pathology. This means ruling out a tumor or a structural problem that could be causing illness.

Diagnosis is essential. When a major condition exists, treatment can't really proceed without a diagnosis. Of course the more exact the diagnosis, the more focused the treatment. Developing an accurate diagnosis involves a kind of systematic "detective work" on the part of the doctor and the patient. In many cases more than one test is necessary to define the problem as exactly as possible. Once the problem is located and defined, treatment can be selected and begun.

BARIUM SWALLOW

The barium swallow is a technique that provides a means of X-raying the upper GI tract. While this is not the most comfortable test in the world, it is a relatively low-cost basic test that can be used to check for any type of gross abnormality in the digestive tract, including disorders of the esophagus, hiatal hernias, and tumors.

In this test the patient drinks a solution that produces an image when X-rayed. A series of X-rays are taken that allow a view of the digestive tract from the mouth to the small intestine. The X-ray is read during the test by a technician and reviewed later by a radiologist and the physician. This test is useful for identifying anatomical and motility problems. It can also detect gastric or peptic ulcers. In some versions of this test, a fizzy tablet is also taken, which helps produce a clearer X-ray by providing air contrast in the image. Glucagon, an antimotility hormone, may also be taken in conjunction with the test. Although this test can be quite uncomfortable, it typically lasts less than half an hour.

BARIUM ENEMA

The barium enema is a procedure used to image the lower GI tract. This is also a rather uncomfortable test, one which involves the slow injection of a highly pressurized enema into a cleaned-out colon to examine the area from the rectum to the beginning of the small intestine. These X-ray images can be used to rule out or evaluate ulcerative colitis, tumors (both benign and cancerous), diverticulosis, strictures, and misshapen, prolapsed colons (often the result of many years of poor diet and constipation). Before and after these tests, cleansing the digestive tract is important. Initially a purge solution is taken (GoLytely or CoLytely); following the test, patients are encouraged to drink a lot of water and take an antioxidant supplement to counter some of the effects of the radiation exposure.

ENDOSCOPY

Endoscopy is the gold standard of GI testing because it allows a direct look at the digestive tract, providing a view of the condition of tissues and structures. Upper endoscopes, colonoscopes, and sigmoidoscopes are performed to view various areas of the gastrointestinal system.

Upper endoscopy is performed using a flexible fiber-optic tube, which may include a videoscope (with a video chip on the tip). The tube is inserted through the mouth to view the esophagus, stomach, and pyloric area, as well as the first portion of the small intestine (the duodenum). The colonoscope is inserted through the anus and travels around the colon into the small intestine. The sigmoidoscope is a flexible instrument used to assess the rectum, the sigmoid (segment of the colon), and the descending colon.

All the major GI conditions discussed in this book can be evaluated to some degree through the use of endoscopy or barium swallows. The scopes are used to search out inflammation, polyps, tumors, diverticulitis or diverticulosis, strictures, a dilated colon, or ulcers. One obvious advantage of the scopes for testing is the total avoidance of any exposure to X-ray radiation. Biopsies or even complete polyp removal can be performed using these instruments, often avoiding more invasive surgery. The procedures are typically performed under conscious sedation from which patients generally recover within about an hour.

VIRTUAL COLONOSCOPY

Virtual Colonoscopy uses a spiral CT scanner to visualize the colon, but is more painful than colonoscopy because there is no sedation and air insufflation is needed to distend the colon. If abnormalities are found colonoscopy for biopsies or surgery will be necessary.

M2A CAPSULE

The M2A (mouth-to-anus) capsule is a new imaging technique available to view primarily the small intestine. This device uses a video chip at the end of a capsule complete with transmitter that sends the data seen back to a computer, which stores the images. After transversing the GI tract, the data is played back for viewing.

ENDOSCOPIC ULTRASOUND

This instrument is an endoscope with an ultrasound transmitter on the tip that provides information through the use of sound waves, producing data that is read by specialized technicians. This type of endoscope can be used on the esophagus, stomach, colon, or rectum. The information gained from this test gives us an idea of the thickness of the muscle in the wall of an organ and whether there are any defects present. The ultrasound device can define the extent of a polyp invasion or show tumors in the muscle wall and indicate their size. If treatment is necessary this information can help the physician plan a surgical resection or radiation therapy. The rectal ultrasound can be used to define problems in the pelvic floor for conditions such as fecal incontinence, constipation, and pelvic pain. This is particularly important in patients who have had unsuccessful surgery for urinary or fecal incontinence or multiple obstetric or gynecological surgeries.

CT SCANNING AND MRIs

These sophisticated imaging techniques, frequently used by doctors today, have now become highly perfected and refined. The MRI is based on a signal from a large magnet that interprets the density of tissue to create X-ray-like images. The CT scan utilizes multiple X-ray beams at different levels, interpreted by a computer to give cross-sectional images. The information gained from these procedures now often replaces exploratory surgery.

Both techniques rely on obtaining cross-sectional images of the anatomy that create a series of sequential images of the patient being X-rayed. The image produced provides detailed information that enables physicians to find problems that could not be detected by normal two-dimensional X-rays such as barium enemas or barium swallows.

To be evaluated, the patient lies in a tunnel-like chamber while the test is being performed. The open MRI, a newer design, doesn't require lying in a closed chamber. Basically the MRI measures the spin of your atoms in a very sophisticated procedure that requires no radiation. The information is generated through a signal from a large magnet that changes proton spin.

In an evaluation of the digestive tract, the MRI is sometimes limited because it's much more sensitive to movement. For images of the abdomen, CT scanning is often still better because the peristalsis of the bowel creates constant motion that can blur the image. While it takes longer to do an MRI than a CT scan, the MRI is useful in areas of the body where there is little movement, such as the liver. Consequently the MRI is probably the test of choice for the liver because it's able to give a little more definition. One of the problems with the CT scan is that metallic objects can distort the image. For instance, surgical staples give off artifacts, an image caused by reflection on the metal, that can blur a portion of the X-ray.

LAPAROSCOPY

This procedure uses a surgical instrument that functions like a telescope, about the thickness of a Magic Marker, inserted in a small port incision in the abdomen. When diagnostic laparoscopy is performed the abdominal cavity is first filled with air or carbon dioxide to create a space in which the organs can be visualized. Surgery can be performed using this same method, through the use of more than one port. With this technique surgeons are able to perform fairly sophisticated surgeries without an incision, such as the removal of a portion of the colon (resection). Laparoscopy can also be used surgically in the treatment of ulcerative colitis and in the removal of colon tumors. The use of this instrument eliminates the necessity of large incisions in the abdominal wall, promoting more rapid healing.

Laparoscopy can allow the surgeon to gently shift organs within the abdominal cavity through the use of probes. This technique can be used to move, manipulate, or remove tissue. In abdominal surgery, binding scar tissue (adhesions) that may be causing pain and interfering with intestinal motility can be freed using this technique. In gallbladder surgery, an instrument can be inserted to move the liver and remove the gallbladder.

In fact, laparoscopy is now widely used by general surgeons for gallbladder removal. The apparent ease with which this procedure can be performed and the promise of quick recovery may be contributing to its overuse. If you are advised to have your gallbladder removed, seek a second opinion from a gastroenterologist. In some cases what has been diagnosed as delayed gallbladder emptying turns out to be irritable bowel syndrome (IBS). In these situations removal of the gallbladder will not fundamentally correct the condition.

TESTING FOR MOTILITY

The esophageal motility test is used for patients who have trouble swallowing (dysphasia) or frequent heartburn. Patients swallow a small nasogastric tube that measures the pressure at various points in the length of the esophagus.

Another test for motility is called colonic transit time. We use this test most often for patients who are troubled by constipation. The test can be performed by having the patient swallow a number of radiopaque rings in a gelatin capsule. The markers contain a material comparable to barium that creates an image visible on X-rays. The patient is then X-rayed for several consecutive days, depending on the protocol being used. The test is usually performed until all the markers are passed. The pellets go right through the digestive tract; they're not absorbed. The length of time it takes for them to move through the gut can reflect problems with colonic inertia, in which the colon has difficulty moving the stool along. If the test shows that the rings remain in the system for five or seven days, this will indicate a slowing of motility, an outlet disorder, or a generalized condition, depending on where the markers are seen. This test can also be used to measure transit time.

MEASURING HYDROCHLORIC ACID AND BICARBONATE

Doctors now measure hydrochloric acid using an endoscope to draw a sample of gastric juices from the stomach and measure the degree of alkalinity or acidity. Another way to perform this test is to use gastrin to stimulate acid secretions and then measure the response.

The test for gastric acid stimulation is most frequently used to detect hyperacidity, which is problematic in cases of *H. pylori* infections. Hyperacidity can cause ulcers or suggest the presence of gastronoma, a pancreatic tumor that causes the secretion of too much gastrin (a neurohormone secreted by the stomach) as a result of hyperacidity. In this test Pentagastrin (a synthetic gastrin) is given by injection and the acid is measured through a nasogastric tube.

In the use of the Heidelberg capsule, the patient swallows a capsule that sends back data via radiotelemetry, reflecting the relative acidity or alkalinity of different areas in the lumen. The information on acidity is used to detect or diagnose low output of hydrochloric acid (called hypochlorhydria) or a total lack of HCl production (called achlorhydria).

The pancreatic secretion of bicarbonate is measured by testing secretin stimulation. Secretin, a synthetic hormone, is given intravenously, and the physician measures the bicarbonate produced in a duodenum over a sixty-minute period. This tells how well the pancreas is performing. The procedure is also being used therapeutically in cases of autism, to improve pancreatic production of this enzyme and stimulate brain function by balancing secretin output and neurotransmitters.

The Comprehensive Digestive Stool Analysis is another practical test for measuring acidity and other aspects of digestive function. (See chapter 16 for a more thorough description of this test.)

FUNCTIONAL TESTING

There is enormous value in the new functional testing. Functional assessment makes it possible to evaluate how various organs are actually performing. With this information treatment can be designed, even if no definitive diagnosis can be made. This is particularly important in minimizing conditions at an early stage or preventing mild illness from becoming more serious. The testing typically involves small, inexpensive, noninvasive samples that can be taken at home and mailed to the lab, once they're ordered by a health practitioner. This testing can provide useful information on disorders for which conventional therapy has no readily available answers.

Biographical information for **Trent W. Nichols, M.D.,** appears on page 104.

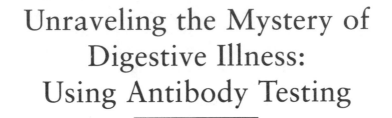

Unraveling the Mystery of Digestive Illness: Using Antibody Testing

Aristo Vojdani, Ph.D., M.T.

Antibody testing is an important recent development in lab technology, a resource that is proving helpful to many people struggling with the riddle of digestive illness.

Antibody tests are performed through samples of saliva or blood. The results reflect the state of immunity within the body. Testing measures the levels of antibodies, which are proteins produced to defend against microbes, allergenic foods, and other foreign substances. Antibodies provide a record of immune activity against specific organisms and an accurate reflection of exactly which microbe is triggering an immune response and causing illness. With this information therapy can be targeted much more specifically than in the past, increasing the possibility of successful treatment.

Laura's Story

Laura had been sick since childhood with low-grade GI complaints. It seemed to begin soon after she got the measles when she was four. As an adult she contracted giardia on a trip to the mountains and suffered severe digestive distress for several years. Repeated lab tests provided no clues to her situation. When antibody testing was performed, both the giardia and a viral infection were identified. Armed with a specific diagnosis, her doctor prescribed the drugs, nutrients, and herbs that helped her clear these microbes almost completely within six months.

SPECIFICS OF ANTIBODY TESTING

Detecting Hidden Microbes

In evaluations for digestive disease, labs have traditionally found it difficult to detect pathogens. Inflammation or infection can be caused by numerous species of bacteria, yeast, parasites, or viruses.

Microbes can be harbored anywhere in the GI tract. The area of the tissue surface within the digestive tract is immense. If all the layers of the tiny ridge-like villi were unfolded and spread flat, it would cover an area the size of a tennis court. Imagine the number of potential hiding places for microbes. Some opportunistic organisms take full advantage of this terrain. For example, cryptosporidium can lodge and remain in the crypts (the deepest crevices between the villi). Due to this type of problem, many pathogens are not detected in lab tests. Yet the need for reliable testing is very real, as anyone with digestive illness can confirm.

Testing the Strength of Immunity

Our understanding of the immune system holds the key that will unlock the mysteries of many diseases and disorders. Although there is tremendous variation in the causes of disease, illness usually develops only when the immune system malfunctions. One of the greatest challenges facing medicine today involves unraveling the complexities of the immune system and finding better methods to diagnose and treat its disorders.

In the last decade the science of immunology has greatly expanded the scope of lab diagnosis. Advances in protein chemistry, the study of bacteria, and cell biology have increased our understanding of the body's natural defenses. Much more accurate testing of immune function is now possible as new biological materials and methods are developed.

An example of these innovations are the tests now available that specifically identify IgM antibodies. IgM are the first antibodies produced in our initial encounter with an invader (an antigen). Elevated levels of IgM are strong evidence of immediate acute exposure. Testing for IgM has gained recognition as an important diagnostic approach.

New technological advances have also enabled the development of a wide range of antibody tests. A variety of sensitive and specific assays have been designed that offer great accuracy and precision. These evaluations reflect reactivity to drugs, proteins, polypeptides, and large molecules. Researchers can link antibodies to radioactive tracers, enzymes, or fluorescent tags. This makes it possible to find evidence of infectious agents, even at very low concentrations in different clinical specimens.

The Role of Antibodies

The foreign molecules from bacteria or other invaders (antigens) are the ultimate target of all immune responses. Immune function is provided by a complex network of specialized organs, cells, and cell products that protect the body from microbes and other infectious agents. When a threat is detected, the body marshals a diverse army of cells and molecules that work in concert. Antibodies are generated in reaction to the antigens, to neutralize them—producing our immunity against microbes or their toxins.

Specialized protective cells roam the body, consuming the antigens they find. This process also involves chemical messengers that activate T cells. The stimulation of T cells results in the production and cloning of an entire army of various T cells and additional messenger chemicals. This in turn can escalate the mounting immune defense to a higher level of intensity.

Many antibodies are "programmed" to react to one specific invader (a particular bacteria or virus). The body has a vast database in memory of earlier invaders and can produce antibodies to match a great number of antigens. When antibodies attack an antigen, great numbers of these microscopic proteins bind to the invader to form a clustered mass called an immune complex. This serves to neutralize the action of the bacterial or viral condition and clear it from the body.

Testing for Antibody Levels

Tests are now available to document antibody levels that reflect the presence of invasive microbes or allergenic foods.

Antibody testing is highly relevant in the diagnosis and resolution of many disgestive disorders. It is also a useful tool in treating autoimmune diseases. While bacteria and food antigens can directly induce disease processes, they can also cause indirect effects as autoimmune disorders. About one in four Americans suffers from some form of autoimmune condition such as ileitis, colitis, asthma, chronic respiratory problems, arthritis, lupus, diabetes, multiple sclerosis, AIDS, or immune deficiency. Physicians who use antibody testing have found that it provides profoundly useful information. It has been suggested that this approach has the capacity to change the way medicine will be practiced in the future. Antibody testing makes it possible to intervene earlier in the disease process. Armed with this type of results, doctors can target treatment very specifically, using natural compounds and powerful medications. Early treatment can reverse problems before more serious invasive conditions develop.

Antibody Tests

Bacteria Panel

- Aerobic bacteria: *E. coli, Lactobacillus, Enterococcus, H. pylori*
- Anaerobic bacteria: *Clostridium perfiringens* and *difficile, Bacteroides fragilis, Klebsiella*

Parasite Antibody Panel

- Antibodies for protozoa: *Blastocystis hominis, Cryptosporidium parvum, Dientamoeba fragilis, Entamoeba histolytica, Giardia lamblia, Toxoplasma gondii,* and others
- For helminths: Ancylostoma, Ascaris, Taenia, Toxocara, Trichuris, and others

Viral Screens

- Epstein-Barr virus, cytomegalo virus (CMV), herpes 1 and 2, HHV-6, human papilloma virus, Lyme disease, *Mycoplasma* species, chlamydia

Additional Evaluations—Intestinal Diseases and Immune Function

- Differentiation between celiac disease, Crohn's disease, and ulcerative colitis
- Gastrointestinal evaluation panel
- Infection and neuroimmunity panel
- Infection: cardiovascular and autoimmune panel
- Intestinal barrier function test
- Saliva secretory IgA

Aristo Vojdani, Ph.D., M.T., can be contacted at Immunosciences Lab, Inc., 8693 Wilshire Boulevard, Suite 2000, Beverly Hills, CA 90211; phone (800) 950 4686 or (310) 657-1077; fax (310) 657-1053. Web site www.immuno-sci-lab.com

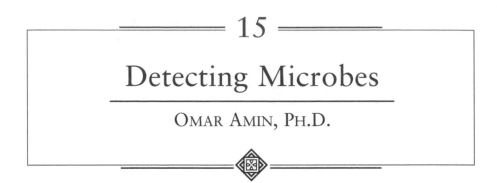

15

Detecting Microbes

OMAR AMIN, PH.D.

Many of us have heard about illnesses caused by giardia and other parasites, but we tend to overlook connections between these microbes and digestive disease. According to the Centers for Disease Control, microscopic parasites probably cause more than 90 percent of all parasitic infections in the United States. Many doctors believe we may be seriously underestimating parasites as contributors to disease. Worldwide, infectious diarrhea due to cholera, amoebas, giardia, and blastocystis, among others, is the second leading cause of death, fatal to 3 million people a year.

JUST A TROPICAL DISEASE?

We consider this type of problem an exception in America, a rarity. Most doctors and patients don't usually think of parasites as a common cause of illness. We assume we've eradicated these problems with modern sanitation and water treatment. But research shows that parasitic infection is common, and the incidence is increasing. In many cases these infections underlie familiar digestive illness and other conditions as well.

Symptoms of intestinal infection are not isolated or unusual. Opportunities for exposure to and transmission of parasitic infection increase as overseas travel and immigration expand. Parasites are also transmitted in food processed through mass methods of farming, food manufacturing, and shipping from sources all over the world. Water treatment in huge urban systems is unable to totally eliminate contamination and periodically makes it worse.

Giardia, for instance, is often waterborne, and these infections are on the rise. In 1997, *The Wall Street Journal* reported an average of 2 million cases annually in the United States. Giardia is also a problem worldwide, even in some modern cities (via the public water systems).

Cyclospora, a parasite in the news, is tracked as a new or emerging pathogen; sometimes it is transmitted on imported fruit. In 1996 it was found on Guatemalan strawberries and raspberries. However, it is also domestic and

A Case of Undetected Infection

When he was about 6 Tony started having problems connected with his digestion. Tests for parasites came out negative. The doctor said it was ulcerative colitis and put Tony on a variety of medications, including steroids. However, his condition did not improve; in fact, it actually worsened. More tests were performed and a stool sample was sent to a lab specializing in the detection of parasites. A infection with *Entamoeba histolytica,* a common but virulent amoeba, was detected. Based on the information from the test results, another of Tony's doctors prescribe medication targeted at clearing the parasite, and his symptoms resolved.

It is impossible to determine if the *E. histolytica* infection caused the ulcerative symptoms (which it often does) or if an earlier intestinal condition compromised the integrity of the GI lining, paving the way for the *E. histolytica* to become established. It is clear that the host-parasite relationship was a causal influence, since the elimination of the parasite was instrumental in resolving the ulcerative condition. The key component here is the proper identification of the specific parasite in the test sample.

common in the United States; like all infectious agents, it can be transferred in stool, on human hands, and as contaminants in food, especially fresh vegetables and fruit, and water.

Cryptosporidium, another waterborne parasite, caused illness in more than 400,000 people in Milwaukee in 1993. More than 4,000 were hospitalized, and more than 100 died. Cryptosporidium is found in the public water systems and reservoirs of many American cities. In some places, such as the San Francisco Bay Area, it is known to be transmitted by the runoff from hillsides where cattle graze, upstream from unprotected reservoirs.

What happened in Milwaukee drew the attention of the media and the public because so many people were affected. But doctors are coming to believe that all over the country this kind of infection happens every day. Most of us live crowded together in big cities, many of us travel overseas, we frequently have contact with people from all over the world, and we have many opportunities for exposure.

In a survey of 5,792 samples received at the Parasitology Center, Inc., in 2000, of 2,896 patients, 916 (32 percent of) patients were infected with parasites; higher than the previously reported national average of about 20 percent.

A Sample of Intestinal Infections, in the U.S. (2000)

A survey of 5,792 samples from 2,896 patients,
received at the Parasitology Center, Inc., Tempe, Arizona

Pathogen—Percentage of Samples Infected	Digestive Symptoms	General Symptoms
Blastocystis hominis—72%	Flatulence, bloating, diarrhea, cramps, constipation, poor digestion/poor absorption	Fatigue, nervous and skin disorders, pain, skin conditions, nausea, allergies, muscle problems
Entamoeba histolytica—7%	Diarrhea, constipation, cramps, bloating, flatulence	Fatigue, nausea, allergies, pain, weight loss, insomnia
Entamoeba coli (E. coli)—5%	Diarrhea, cramps, flatulence, bloating, constipation, irritable bowel	Fatigue, allergies, headache, nausea, depression/irritability, joint/back pain, skin problems
Cyclospora—2%	Symptoms that come and go, bloating, flatulence, diarrhea, cramps	Fatigue, itching, nausea, anemia, headache, muscle aches, depression
Entamoeba hartmanni—1%	Diarrhea, bloating, cramps, flatulence, irritable bowel	Nervous system, respiratory, and skin disorders, allergies, pain, nausea

SOURCE: O. M. Amin. "Seasonal prevalence of intestinal parasites in the United States during 2000." *American Journal of Tropical Medicine and Hygiene*, vol. 66, no. 6 (2002): pp. 799–803.

Among this sampled population, we noticed a number of typical characteristics.

- More than half the people with infections had traveled overseas in the past five years.
- People traveling to Mexico and Europe had the highest risk of infection.
- People living in households where someone was infected had twice the risk of infection.
- Of people who were infected, some had no symptoms.
- This implies that some people unknowingly act as carriers. Since they

have no symptoms, they might be unaware of the problem, go untreated, and unknowingly pass it on to others.

- People infected by more than one parasite had symptoms similar to those with single infections.
- Women were twice as likely to be infected as men and to be more heavily infected.
- The most prevalent pathogen was *Blastocystis hominis* (72 percent), with cryptosporidium (13 percent) and *Entamoeba* species (8 percent) ranking second and third, respectively.

Greatest Risk Factors

Primary Factors

- Foreign travel
- Having a partner or someone in the household with a parasite problem
- Previous parasitic infection (implying relapse or reinfection)
- Not washing fresh vegetables adequately

Other risks

- Drinking tap water
- Poor hygiene
- Dining out often
- Frequenting salad bars
- Having pets
- Going camping (or drinking the water from streams or even fountains)
- Working at an infant-care center
- Living in an institutional setting or group home

PARASITES AND DAMAGE TO THE BODY

Parasitic infection can be damaging to humans by direct injury to the tissue of the digestive tract or the liver, among other organ systems. In addition the most destructive effects may not be caused by the parasite itself, but by its toxic by-products, which are produced unintentionally as a part of its living process. Parasites can disrupt digestive activity, can cause malabsorption, and can interfere with the action of digestive enzymes and nutrients. In addition parasites can compromise the human immune system in order to promote and ensure their own survival.

DIFFICULTIES IN DIAGNOSIS

Parasitic infections have long been considered diseases of the tropics, so physicians often don't consider them when diagnosing common illnesses. Parasitology is seldom discussed in the mainstream medical journals, and traditionally there has been little reporting of parasite incidence. For example, giardia has been widely tracked by the Centers for Disease Control (CDC) only since 1987. When physicians receive their training, very little information is provided on parasitology in medical school and in professional journals. Given the lack of information and minimal clinical exposure, doctors don't usually consider parasites as a possible cause of illness, especially when the symptoms aren't confined to the digestive tract.

Difficulties in Detection

Parasites have complex life cycles and are often not shed at regular intervals. In fact, three of the major parasites in the United States and worldwide (amoebas, giardia, and cyclospora) tend to be shed at irregular intervals. This means that the parasite may be present in the stool for two, three, or four days a week, but not the rest of the week. *Entamoeba histolytica* is active for one or two days, and then is not typically active or detectable the next day or two. When *E. histolytica* migrates to the liver it disappears from the gut and becomes undetectable in fecal specimens. If the stool sample is collected from a patient with one of these cyclical parasites on a day when the pathogen is not active, it won't be in the stool and obviously won't be detected by testing. However, this doesn't mean that there's no infection present. At the current time this is a limitation for which no modem technology can compensate. Consequently repeated samples are very important. Generally, to make testing practicable, we recommend at least two or three samples be taken on different days.

Emerging Pathogens

Another problem we encounter in detection is the fact that there are so many emerging pathogens. These are new parasites, which remain insufficiently studied. For example, cyclospora was formally classified as a human parasite for the first time just a few years ago. Before that the labs were probably seeing it, but didn't know what it was because it hadn't been described as such. Other pathogens are reclassified as they become better understood or as their virulence is observed to change. Only in the 1990s has *Dientamoeba fragilis* come to be considered capable of causing disease (pathogenic). In addition there are some life forms in nature that make detection extremely difficult. Bacteria have been identified that can exist without a cell wall and therefore can take on many shapes. These elusive pathogens make diagnosis extremely difficult.

OPTIMAL DETECTION

The most effective method of detecting parasites continues to be stool sampling. The optimal approach involves taking samples every other day, a minimum of 48 hours apart, collecting at least two or three samples.

Although some microbes such as *E. histolytica* reside in the large intestine, many are harbored in the small intestine. Pathogens such as giardia reside primarily in the small intestine, where they strongly adhere to the intestinal lining and therefore cannot usually be detected in samples from stool further down the digestive tract. For this reason the test must include matter from the small intestine in order to test as accurately as possible. The best specimen is a sample of soft stool taken during the occurrence of a diarrheal episode, because it usually contains material from the small intestine. In the patient who has constipation, the purge test is most optimal.

Other Methods of Testing

- Elevated white blood count (eosinophil level) may be used as a screening tool to indicate the need for further testing.
- Antibody testing is also available. Antibody levels for immunoglobulin G (IgG) can indicate infection, but not whether the infection is current or previous. Repeated testing for IgM levels will show if the infection is currently active.
- Samples of blood serum can be evaluated to detect parasites found in the blood. However, this method is useful only for parasites of the circulatory system, not those most typically found in the GI tract.
- Tissue samples from biopsies of the colon or duodenum can be tested for parasitic infection, as well as tumors or pathology.

Testing For Yeast

A correlation exists between the presence of parasites and the presence of candida (and other forms of fungus as well). In addition when there is excessive candida present, the levels of beneficial bacteria tend to be lower. If there are factors present such as parasites that promote the growth of candida, it consumes the resources and the space that would have originally been allotted to the beneficial microflora (the lactobacillus and bifidus). Yeast overgrowth is also documented as a significant factor in some cases of attention deficit disorder and autism (based on the work of Dr. William Shaw and others).

Dental Toxicities

Digestive health starts in the mouth: For many patients, dental and digestive health seem to go hand in hand. Currently there are a multitude of procedures and materials that have been developed by the dental industry to promote dental health, not to mention to ward off infections and improve oral hygiene. Manufacturers of dental materials spare no effort to provide dentists with the widest array of amalgams, composites, sealants, varnishes, cements, adhesives, pastes, etc. We all know about mercury and heavy metal toxicity; see, for example, Ziff (2002). What we did not know about is the involvement of dental sealants (liners) in the causation of a newly discovered disorder called neurocutaneous syndrome (NCS) (Amin, 2003, 2004).

NCS is a disorder that degrades the skin (cutaneous tissue) and neurological system of patients who have been treated with sealants during filling or root canal procedures. Patients sensitive to sulfa are especially susceptible to experiencing the neurological and dermatological toxicity symptoms of NCS. Neurological symptoms include but are not limited to pinprick and/or creeping, painful, and irritating movement sensations, often interpreted as parasite movement in body tissues or cavities, including the head. Brain fog, loss of memory, and light sensitivity may also be experienced. The cutaneous aspects include the development of small itchy sores or inflamed, elevated, pimples that may eventually evolve into painful, open lesions with a tendency to spread. General symptoms include compromised immune system, fatigue, and psychological trauma.

A complete description of NCS symptoms, the syndrome, compounding factors, and the toxic sealants, with case histories and treatment protocols, is given by Amin (2003, 2004). Dental practitioners should be aware of the adverse effects of using sealants, and employ this knowledge to safeguard the well being of their patients.

SOURCES:

Amin, O. M. "On the diagnosis and management of Neurocutaneous Syndrome (NCS), a toxicity disorder from dental sealants." *Explore*, vol. 13, no. 1 (2003): pp. 21–25.

Amin, O. M. "Dental sealant toxicity: Neurocutaneous Syndrome (NCS), a dermatological and neurological disorder." *Holistic Dental Association Journal*, no. 1 (2004): pp. 1–15.

Ziff, S. *Silver Dental Fillings: The Toxic Time Bomb*. Santa Fe, Aurora Press, 2002.

A NOTE FROM THE LAB

It has been our experience that some people with symptoms of digestive disease may also have an underlying parasitic infection.

Detecting and treating parasitic infections can be a complex process. For example, some organisms are classified as commensals, microorganisms that are present but don't actually cause disease (nonpathogenic). In the past, parasites thought to be harmless have included *H. pylori, Blastocystis hominis, Dientamoeba fragilis,* and even *Giardia lamblia.* In the past ten years they have been reclassified, because we now recognize that these organisms and numerous others can cause serious infections. In fact, some can contribute to illness that can linger for years if untreated. Once the infection is found and treated, patients often improve quite rapidly.

We've also noticed that parasitic GI infections don't cause symptoms in the digestive tract alone. The effects of many pathogens are experienced throughout the body, in any of the major organ systems. Associated illnesses can include fatigue, difficulty with mental concentration, depression, and neurological symptoms, as well as allergies, asthma, arthritis, skin disorders, and other chronic health problems.

Omar Amin, Ph.D., is founder of the Parasitology Center, Inc., in Tempe, Arizona. He is a professor of parasitology and a Ph.D. graduate of Arizona State University, where he relocated after teaching at the University of Wisconsin for twenty years. He is an internationally recognized authority, with more than 145 major publications, extensive worldwide field research, and international teaching experience. He has been a Fulbright scholar and has received numerous research grants for his work. Dr. Amin is available for professional consultations with health care practitioners and will also answer patients' questions directly.

The Parasitology Center, Inc., offers laboratory testing for the detection of human parasitic infections and toxicities from neurocutaneous syndrome; practitioners and patients can contact the lab at 903 South Rural Road., No. 101-318, Tempe, Arizona, 85281; phone (480) 767-2522; fax (480) 767-5855; e-mail OmarAmin@aol.com; Web address www.parasitetesting.com.

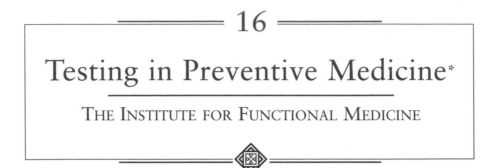

16

Testing in Preventive Medicine*

THE INSTITUTE FOR FUNCTIONAL MEDICINE

Functional medicine focuses on evaluating and treating the dynamic processes of the body. How are each of these systems functioning? How can we assess them? How do we intervene to correct them when they are out of balance? This approach provides a rational, thoughtful way of practicing medicine.

The goal is not just to heal symptoms, but to normalize function—to restore the capacity of organs, tissues, and cells. In this context health is seen as more than the absence of disease. It's the state of positive vitality unique to each person; health on every level from the cell to the whole person.

Functional testing evaluates and measures this physical and biochemical functionality. Those problems that can be detected earlier, when they're less serious, can be addressed through less invasive means. Treatment often involves changes in nutrition and lifestyle to restore health.

BIOCHEMICAL INDIVIDUALITY

We are each unique. It's obvious that we have unique personalities, fingerprints, and genetics. And while it's apparent that your shape, size, and capabilities are your own, so the functioning of your chemistry and organ systems have characteristic patterns individual to you. For example, your liver may be large or small, with an extensive or a more limited functional capacity. It may be highly active or sluggish, healthy or struggling. A familiar example is the highly individual capacity to handle alcohol.

In addition these patterns of functioning aren't static and don't always remain the same. Shifts in function often occur long before disease is apparent. Functional laboratory testing looks at your unique patterns and provides a snapshot of how you're functioning at any given time. For example, a person who is never troubled by liver problems might find himself or herself challenged after heavy exposure to chemicals.

---

*Adapted from *The Fundamentals of Functional Medicine* (1997). Written and published by the Institute for Functional Medicine, Gig Harbor, WA. Used by permission.

The liver is frequently called on to detoxify a wide range of substances, including digestive by-products, toxins from bacteria, alcohol, hormones, medications, caustic chemicals, and heavy metals. Functional liver testing can show how well the detoxification process is working. When problems are detected before major damage has occurred, specific nutrients and herbs can be recommended to heal tissue and restore function.

EARLY DETECTION

Functional testing can provide doctors with the information they need to intervene before disease develops. Traditionally diagnosis has been defined as "the art of distinguishing one disease from another." Clinical diagnosis has been described as "diagnosis based on the symptoms . . . irrespective of the changes producing them." In contrast, many functional tests explore the changes that precede illness, and thus enable clinicians to intervene earlier.

For example, a test to assess the barrier function of the intestinal lining can diagnose the leaky gut syndrome that occurs when the gut becomes too permeable. This particular test answers the question, Is the GI barrier intact and able to keep out harmful microbes and allergens? The goal is to reduce hyperpermeability and slow the leakage of bacteria or oversized food molecules that could trigger allergies or intolerances. Minimizing such reactions and calming inflammation can also help to prevent many symptoms and conditions that can result from leaky gut, such as allergies, arthritis, or asthma.

You can see from this example that a functional approach focuses not only on the end result but also on the dynamic processes that precede and underlie illness. Functional testing provides diagnostic tools that can locate many subtle problems in functioning. Like a good mechanic running a diagnostic on your car, once the practitioner understands what's malfunctioning and why, repair can begin.

FUNCTIONAL TESTING AND TREATMENT

Tests have also been developed to assess digestion, find signs of serious allergies or inflammation, and measure levels of free radicals and the status of metabolism. In addition functional testing can track many aspects of your body chemistry: actual levels of hormones and nutrients or body chemicals that serve as signals of malfunction or disease (biochemical markers). You can imagine how useful it is to have this kind of specific information available through simple testing.

The emphasis here is not only on treating disease but also on raising the capacity of the organ systems, with special emphasis on the systems where illness is first initiated—the GI tract, the liver, and the endocrine glands. Strategies often include rebuilding GI flora and barrier function, reducing the toxic burden on the liver, and restoring the rhythm of the glands that produce essential hormones.

This testing empowers your clinician to address small imbalances before they cause major problems. Getting this information early makes it possible to intervene earlier in the disease process. Harmful dynamics in metabolism and organ function can be shifted using food and nutrients, lifestyle, environmental factors, and mind-body medicine prescribed to fit your unique needs. Restoring function can rebuild inner health.

The Institute for Functional Medicine provides continuing medical education on nutrition and functional medicine for health care professionals through seminars and an annual symposium. They also publish books; a monthly audio subscription series, *Functional Medicine Updates;* and other educational materials on emerging research and clinical applications. The mission of the institute is to improve patient outcomes through new strategies to the prevention, early assessment, and comprehensive management of complex chronic diseases.

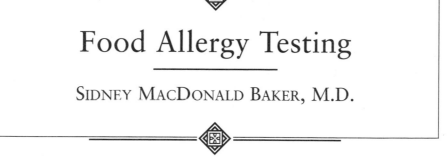

Food Allergy Testing

SIDNEY MACDONALD BAKER, M.D.

When using nutritional medicine to treat digestive illness, two simple questions are key in understanding health problems: Could there be a deficiency or an unmet need for an essential nutrient? Could there be a toxin or allergen that should be avoided or eliminated?

Avoid is the key word in the second question. If our bodies are burdened by the metabolic costs of detoxification, it makes sense to lighten the burden on the system. Wash your hands before dinner. Minimize your exposure to toxins. Eliminate allergens from your diet.

ELIMINATION DIETS

Using an elimination diet means avoiding the offending substance (or substances) before it has a chance to become a burden to your body. Not only may we be challenged by food intolerance, but most of us also suffer some consequence from eating apparently healthy foods against which our immune system has taken a "negative attitude."

One way to discover whether or not the elimination of certain foods may be the key to feeling better is to just avoid them for at least seven days. Foods we eat frequently that can be allergens include cereal grains and milk products, breads and fermented foods, oranges and other citrus fruits, spices, eggs, coconut, fish and shellfish, tea, coffee, and so on.

But what if you go to all that trouble to eliminate foods and miss something that just happens to be your problem, such as potato or tomato or peppers? Sometimes a test can be quite useful in sorting out the problem and giving you a short list of likely possibilities. It's also important to know that there is no perfect test. None will identify foods that could trigger your symptoms throughout your lifespan. That said, there is testing available that can take away some of the guesswork.

The test I find the most useful measures IgG antibodies to foods. Antibodies are proteins produced by the body to combat bacteria or harmful microbes, offending foods, or other threatening substances. IgG antibodies are associated with responses to foods that we sometimes call food sensitivities or delayed food allergies. The reason for testing for IgG is that abnormally high levels of the antibody are an indication that the immune system is responding abnormally and too aggressively to a particular food. This type of evaluation is known as an IgG ELISA test.

We have found that this test is quite valid when done at a laboratory with reliable methods. In certain medical situations, it is an essential tool in the treatment of patients with complex chronic illness. However, this test is technically tricky and lab directors have told me that they have tried to set it up and could not get consistent results. John Rebello of Immuno Laboratories in Fort Lauderdale, Florida, has perfected a technique that produces results that are reliable by the strictest definition of laboratory dependability. Moreover, his tests are the only ones subjected to scientific clinical studies in which patient success is based on the lab results (*Townsend Newsletter*, January 1998).

RESEARCH ON ALLERGY TESTING

Proper scientific studies are based on the assumption that all participants are the same. From this standpoint, it can be difficult to design research that looks at the very different reactions of individuals in response to allergens such as food, pollens, or molds.

To study food intolerances, we posed the question, Do tests for IgG antibodies accurately reflect the reactions caused by particular foods? In order to answer the question, we conducted a series of double-blind, placebo-controlled studies. Reactivity was evaluated for each individual through blood tests that measured their particular levels of IgG antibodies. Then we divided patients into two groups and randomly assigned avoidance diets based on real scores, or diets in which participants avoided nonproblematic foods. In summary:

- Group A avoided foods to be *reactive* through allergy testing
- Group B avoided foods found to be *nonreactive* through the testing

The study was arranged so that neither the patients nor the doctors knew which participants were really on a real allergy avoidance diet. To learn which group did better, we asked the study participants to report their symptoms. The symptoms included problems typically associated with food sensitivity, as well as any and all general health concerns, such as:

- Digestive concerns
- Headaches
- Skin disorders, including eczema or inflammation

- Respiratory problems like wheezing or congestion
- General symptoms—anything from fatigue or sleep problems to hyperactivity or other issues

As patients began feeling better, the scores that reflected their symptoms began to drop. The group who avoided the foods identified as reactive by testing improved by one-third. For those who avoided nonreactive foods, symptoms dropped by only one-fifth. Here's how the symptom scores looked after the first four weeks of the study.

	Initial average symptom scores	Scores after 4 weeks on the diet
Avoided reactive foods	5	3
Avoided nonreactive foods	5	4

All the participants in the study did a little better! The intention to heal is powerful and accompanies any change we make. Since diet is one of the biggest lifestyle changes most people ever commit to, big results can occur. However, the patients who did better were those who were avoiding actual food intolerances that had been confirmed by the antibody testing. They fared far better than those who were avoiding nonreactive foods. The experiments were an elaborate way of showing that allergy testing really works.

It is understandable that an elimination diet has some powerful nonspecific effects in relieving symptoms. If you want to feel better, go on a diet—any diet! If you want to approach the problem of food sensitivities seriously, testing to see which are your reactive foods and which are your safe foods before changing your diet can save you some confusion.

The test also identifies foods that are nonreactive, which may be especially important in chronic illness with excessive and inappropriate immune activation. This type of condition has been associated with conditions such as autoimmune disease, chronic fatigue syndrome, and hyperactivity. In these cases it seems important to know which foods tend to trigger the least immune reactivity. For some health conditions IgG testing can provide so much information on the origin of the problem that it is definitely worth considering this diagnostic option.

Sidney MacDonald Baker, M.D. has worked as a family practitioner, served as director of the Gesell Institute of Human Development, and taught at Yale Medical School and Southern Connecticut State University. He is the author of a number of books, including *Detoxification and Healing, The Circadian Prescription,* and *Folic Acid.*

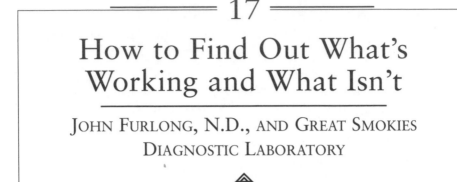

17

How to Find Out What's Working and What Isn't

JOHN FURLONG, N.D., AND GREAT SMOKIES DIAGNOSTIC LABORATORY

In a truly preventive approach to health, timely intervention is the key. We need to know when to intervene. We need to be able to determine that crucial period when health is beginning to slip away, before the damage has been done.

We have identified many pieces of the puzzle—factors leading to health and those leading to a greater likelihood of illness. A range of new laboratory tests are now available that clarify the meaning of various symptoms. These lab tests are based on the biochemical functions of the body:

- Interactions between the body and inputs from the environment, including diet
- Markers that show how the immune system, the digestive tract, or the liver is responding at any given point in time
- Specific information on individual genetic makeup

For example, through genetic evaluation, test profiles can even predict the potential for problems before symptoms develop. The safety and effectiveness of these approaches are clear to both patients and doctors.

THE GENOMIC PROFILE

The recent completion of the Human Genome Project has made possible simple genomic tests that can reveal individual susceptibility to specific diseases. This highly accurate testing can clearly pinpoint health risks that would previously have gone unnoticed until disease developed. With this new information, physicians and patients can make more informed health care decisions, lowering the risk for certain diseases.

Genetic Testing

Alex sought a new type of genetic testing to help explain his sensitivity to chemicals and medications. He seemed to have little tolerance for chemical exposures at work, and he also reacted to certain medications. His doctor explained that the test would provide information on his liver's ability to detoxify substances in food or medication. Since the liver's job is to clear toxic compounds from the body, this is usually the key factor whenever there is chemical sensitivity.

In Alex's case a pattern of testing showed that he is deficient in one of the enzyme systems of the liver that is vital to detoxification. The test also indicated variations in two other related genes, suggesting further impairment. His particular genetic pattern implies that his liver is less effective in clearing toxins. This explains a great deal about Alex's chemical sensitivity. It may be why he feels so uncomfortable when he's spray painting his antique car in the garage or why his newly refinished hardwood floors give him nausea and a headache.

Alex's doctor has advised him to make a careful assessment of his lifestyle and minimize his exposure to chemicals and other types of toxins. He has also recommended a program of antioxidants to support his liver function—particularly vitamins C and E, lipoic acid, glutathione, milk thistle, and selenium.

For Alex the results of the test continue to have practical applications. Knowing that his liver is not particularly efficient, he has changed his habits to minimize toxic exposure. He buys more organic foods and nontoxic household products. He's thinking about changing jobs and considering a move—but in both cases he'll be factoring in the effect of his environment on his health, based on what he has learned from his genomic profile.

The work of the Genome Project has identified millions of variations in human DNA, the differences that determine our biochemical individuality. These variants or polymorphisms have come to be known as "snips" (SNPs, short for *single nucleotide polymorphisms*). SNPs are essentially typographical errors in the DNA code. Although they don't directly cause illness, SNPs appear to play a role in almost every type of human disease.

Common conditions that can be caused by such genetic errors include cancer and heart disease, as well as arthritis, asthma, hypertension, hormone problems, and osteoporosis. Genetics can also be a factor in digestive disorders such as food allergies, various cancers, chemical sensitivities, and liver disease.

Preventive Strategies

Many of us have come to believe that genetically based diseases are inescapable. Yet recent studies suggest that the "expression" of genes in disease is not inevitable. Genetically caused diseases may or may not occur—depending on your lifestyle. We also know that environmental influences need to be factored in. These influences include everything from food, air, and water to lifestyle and smoking. If you live a healthy lifestyle, exercise, eat right, and keep your stress down, your genetic errors may never be "expressed."

The genomic tests provide information a doctor can use to counsel patients on how to minimize their health risks. The testing provides a personalized profile of risk factors—read directly from the DNA. With this information in hand the practitioner can make specific individualized recommendations on diet, supplements, and lifestyle. This can support more informed choices. For example, people who eat more fruits and vegetables have about one-half the cancer risk of the general population.

Disease that occurs frequently in a particular family often turns out to have a genetic component. Genomic testing can identify the specific factors that pose a risk. If one family member finds that they have a modifiable genetic variation, others can be tested to learn whether they also have that error. Since it takes both genes and lifestyle factors to trigger most diseases, these are practical steps that anyone can take to minimize their risk of disease.

Treating Chronic Illness

In some cases the SNPs can be a major factor in a long-standing illness. When a chronic condition hasn't responded to treatment, this type of information can be vital. Sometimes the patient is doing all the right things, but there seems to be no progress. In these cases genomic testing can help identify some of the contributing factors, and this information can be used to focus nutritional interventions or targeted drug therapies.

COMPREHENSIVE DIGESTIVE ANALYSIS

Information on digestive function can be obtained through a basic test known as the Comprehensive Digestive Stool Analysis (CDSA), which provides some twenty different evaluations. It assesses how well food is utilized, the absorption of fats, and the level of digestive enzymes. It includes markers of inflammation and allergic activity in the digestive tract. The test also checks for the presence (or absence) of parasites, levels of bacteria and yeast, and measures important by-products (both good and bad) in the colon.

The CDSA indicates if symptoms are likely to be due to inflammation, caused by conditions such as Crohn's disease, colitis, infections, or food allergies. The current expanded version of the test also assesses pancreatic function and markers for potential colon cancer. The test results can be used to develop a personalized diet and supplement plan to enhance digestion, avoiding unnecessary and ineffective guesswork.

Markers of Infection or Inflammation

Calprotectin and Eosinophil Protein X (EPX) are two enzymes evaluated in the CDSA. These are products released by certain types of protective white blood cells—their level in the stool reflects the degree of immune activity or inflammation. For example, the EPX level will typically be elevated if there is a parasitic infection. Calprotectin levels are elevated in cases of Crohn's disease, colitis, colon cancer, colon polyps, infections, and food allergies. In general, the higher the level of these markers, the more severe the condition. Clearly these markers provide extremely valuable information via a noninvasive test.

The measurement of calprotectin can be used as a first line of investigation for people who have symptoms of a digestive disorder. The test can determine if symptoms reflect a disease process such as Crohn's or another inflammatory process, such as postinfectious irritable bowel syndrome. Extremely high levels of calprotectin indicate that a more serious process is occurring and warrants further investigation. In addition to its use as a form of screening, periodic testing can be used to monitor response to treatment. When levels drop on future tests, this is an indication that there is less inflammatory activity and/or less infection.

Pancreatic Enzymes

This test measures levels of elastase, a particular enzyme from the pancreas. If this enzyme is low it indicates a general deficiency of pancreatic enzyme production, affecting the digestion of protein, fats, sugars, and starches. This results in incomplete digestion, which can cause bloating and gas or the inability to sustain normal weight. Incomplete digestion can also be a factor in conditions such as arthritis (see chapters 7 and 13). This test can also be important to older people whose digestion is impaired, since most people experience a decrease in pancreatic enzyme production as they age. Fortunately these disorders can be corrected by providing the right diet and supplementing with a combination of enzymes and flora.

A Marker of Harmful Bacteria

Another of the markers assessed in the CDSA is beta-glucuronidase, an enzyme produced by certain harmful bacteria. When this enzyme is present in the GI tract in excessive amounts it can accelerate the release of internal toxins. High levels of the enzyme have been found in some cases of colon cancer. Although the test is not telling us that cancer is present, it does indicate an environment in the digestive tract where cancer may be more likely to develop.

Capacity for Repair and Regeneration

The body regenerates the lining of the gastrointestinal tract about every five to seven days. This process is supported by n-butyrate, a short-chain fatty acid that provides energy to the lining cells of the gut. A low level of n-butyrate indicates that these cells are in a state of semistarvation, which makes it difficult for the body to repair the colonic lining. In some cases low levels of n-butyrate also serve as a warning sign of increased risk for colon cancer.

A Clean Bill of Health

When Jim's father died of colon cancer and one of his uncles also developed the disease, he contacted my office. He was concerned that a genetic risk for cancer might run in the family. He had recently found blood in his stool and this was taking a toll on his peace of mind.

We spoke at some length about his symptoms and concerns. After his physical exam, we decided to order a complete digestive analysis, including the calprotectin markers. In Jim's case we found that these markers provided critical information: The calprotectin level was in the low-to-normal range—a very good sign. This indicated that most of his symptoms were "functional" in nature and unlikely to be a sign of colon cancer. While no test can provide 100 percent insurance (not even a colonoscopy), studies suggest that measuring calprotectin levels may be a reasonable first step in deciding if a colonoscopy is required.

The test also showed that Jim's digestive enzymes were low, indicating a moderate deficiency in pancreatic enzyme production. In response we began supplementing his diet with a digestive enzyme preparation. We added a strong probiotic (friendly flora) and adjusted the type and amount of fiber he was getting in his diet (adding in three tablespoons of oat bran a day).

After three weeks Jim returned in a much happier state. His cramping and diarrhea were 90 percent resolved and his peace of mind was greatly improved. Given the high incidence of cancer in his family, he had decided to have a colonoscopy, just to be sure, and had gotten a clean bill of health, confirming the results on the CDSA.

INTESTINAL PERMEABILITY

Many factors can affect the integrity of the lining in the small intestine. We know that the lining of the small intestine is normally porous, selectively allowing nutrients to be absorbed into the bloodstream while keeping out toxins and bacteria. In someone who is sensitive, simply eating certain foods can trigger an allergy and affect the lining's barrier function, causing increased permeability. This can also occur when we're under stress. Stress can cause the minute pores in the intestinal lining to open too wide, allowing toxins, food particles, or even bacteria to enter the bloodstream. This is known as leaky gut syndrome (see chapter 7).

The test of the integrity of the barrier function evaluates the degree of leaky gut—intestinal permeability—in the small intestine. Stress of any kind can cause leaky gut syndrome—physical trauma, shock, burns, or surgery, as well as a number of medications, including commonly used pain relievers. Increased permeability also occurs when the intestinal wall is compromised or damaged in inflammatory disorders such as colitis, Crohn's disease, infections, cancer, and other conditions. The permeability test assesses the integrity of the small intestine to determine if it is still acting as an effective barrier.

Testing

This procedure involves drinking a solution containing two nondigestable sugars, lactulose and mannitol. One compound consists of small molecules, and the other is made up of larger ones. Since these molecules pass through our system undigested, a urine collection tells us whether an increased number of large molecules are passing through the intestinal wall, into the bloodstream, and then through the kidneys. This shows the degree of permeability in the intestinal barrier.

Treatment Strategies

The information gained from this test can help a physician determine if the small intestine has been damaged and if this is a factor in overall poor health. Periodically during treatment, the test can be retaken to gauge how well a person is responding to the treatment. If the test results show improvement, the physician is on the right track.

CANDIDA CULTURES

Yeast overgrowth in the GI tract is important to identify because it can be a factor in a wide variety of illnesses—fatigue, allergies, changes in menstrual cycle, difficulty with concentration or learning, and irritation in the GI tract.

It is important to differentiate an intestinal overgrowth of candida from a systemic infection of yeast or fungi. Systemic infections are usually found only in people whose immune systems are impaired due to conditions such as AIDS, cancer, or the use of certain immunosuppressive medications. A low level of yeast is normal and for most people presents no great problem.

It is also possible to develop an overgrowth of candida in the gut or the mouth. Many women tend to have yeast infections in the vaginal area. Often this is the result of antibiotic treatment and a diet high in sugars and low in fiber. Since yeast is already normally present in the digestive tract, yeast infections do not typically invade the body as a bacterial infection would. However, an overgrowth can occur, overtaxing the immune system in its efforts to keep the yeast in balance. Testing can be performed by culturing the yeast from stool, through yeast by-products in the urine, or by sampling the blood to look for antibodies that combat the yeast.

Stool Testing for Candida

Since yeasts tend to grow easily in the digestive tract under certain conditions, sampling the stool is a practical means of determining the level of yeast present. The stool culture measures the relative abundance of yeast in the lower gut.

The efficacy of antifungal medications and herbs can also be tested in the yeast culture. This "sensitivity testing" enables us to determine the medication or herbal product most likely to eradicate the yeast. This type of testing avoids a trial-and-error approach. It's also important because some yeast, like bacteria, are resistant to drugs that were once effective. In short, culturing tells us which organisms are present, at what levels, and which drugs and herbs are most likely to eradicate them.

Blood Tests for Candida

We know that in some cases an overgrowth of yeast can be problematic. In other situations the immune system has overreacted to the yeast, causing a second issue. We can determine these problems by examining the blood for antibodies—proteins that the immune system sends out as a form of "artillery" against the yeast. (The antibodies are like thousands of Velcro balls that coat the yeast cell to immobilize it.) Blood tests are available to measure levels of several different antibodies. Each type of antibody has a specific role in our defenses.

- IgA antibodies are our first line of defense. These antibodies serve as a marker for yeast infections on the mucous membranes such as the gut, mouth, vaginal, or urinary tract.

- IgM antibodies reflect a more immediate response to yeast. Typically this is the body's early response when candida enters the liver and bloodstream from the gut. Generally speaking, this is the body's initial response to new infection. If the infection persists IgM levels drop and IgG becomes more prevalent, indicating a chronic infection.

- IgG levels, elevated in the blood, reflect an ongoing *exposure* to yeast that has activated the immune system. Higher levels of IgG might also indicate a smoldering or chronic yeast infection.

- Antigen-antibody complexes (immune complexes) can reflect a situation in which the liver is overburdened or the immune system is suppressed. Normally these clusters are consumed by the immune cells of the liver. When a blood test shows a high level of immune complexes, we know that the liver or immune system is overtaxed and unable to perform its job adequately. When the complexes are allowed to circulate in the blood, immune cells throughout the body are engaged to clear them. This can cause inflammatory problems, such as arthritis and other autoimmune diseases.

These tests indicate how much immune activity is necessary to control this normally harmless microbe. It also suggests the degree to which the liver is stressed in the process—and whether the candida overgrowth is a recent or long-term problem. This information helps the practitioner shape the most effective approach, using the least possible amount of medication or botanicals.

TESTING FOR OXIDATIVE STRESS

Free radicals are potentially harmful chemicals that are generated from day-to-day activities such as heavy exercise or food metabolism. They are also created in greater numbers whenever there is infection, inflammation, exposure to toxins, or impaired liver function.

Free radicals do not generally create a problem as long as there are adequate levels of antioxidants, consumed in the diet or from supplements. If you are obtaining your antioxidants from a supplement, it's important to remember that they're best taken in a balanced combination formula, which should include vitamins A, C, and E and the mineral selenium.

Measuring Free Radicals

Free radicals and oxidative stress occur as a result of activated toxins, immune stimulation, and liver detoxification. Lab testing can measure the amount of free radical production, as well as the actual levels of key antioxidant enzymes such as glutathione peroxidase and superoxide dismutase.

Treatment Strategies

If the markers for oxidative stress are abnormal we know that the patient is susceptible to free radical damage. When these levels are normal we know that the patient has adequate stores of antioxidants and that the liver is coping effectively with free radicals in the body. This provides a well-rounded picture of the level of protection available against oxidative stress. It also indicates if the patient needs to increase the intake of specific antioxidant nutrients.

In conclusion, there are a variety of tools now available to help us assess important information about the ecology of the GI tract, the effects of diet and the environment in determining health, the vital status of detoxification, and each individual's genetic predisposition to disease. These factors, when considered together, help us to understand when and how to redirect the body toward health and well-being.

John Furlong, N.D., is a naturopathic physician, trained at Bastyr University in Seattle. His experience in medicine ranges from hospital care to holistic health care. He was a founding member of a collaborative health center in Connecticut, where he provided services in nutritional, homeopathic, and botanical medicine, and detoxification. He also founded the People's Health Alliance, a nonprofit organization promoting public education in natural approaches to healing. After more than six years in education and research at Great Smokies Diagnostic Laboratories, Dr. Furlong has returned to full-time clinical practice.

Great Smokies Diagnostic Laboratory offers a variety of diagnostic testing, including tests described above. Educational materials are available to both patients and practitioners on health, preventive medicine, and functional testing through their Client Services Department, 63 Zillicoa Street, Asheville, NC 28801-1074, by calling (800) 522-4762 or visiting their Web site at www.gsdl.com.

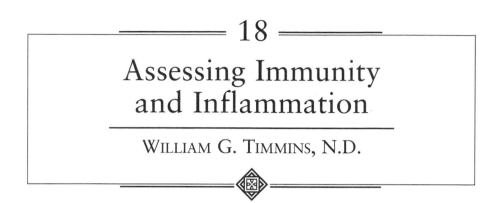

18

Assessing Immunity and Inflammation

WILLIAM G. TIMMINS, N.D.

Functional medicine and testing are based on the view that the body's chemistry can reflect important information on how our systems are functioning. The concept of biochemical individuality suggests that each person has somewhat unique metabolic patterns that can be interpreted to determine his or her nutrition and health needs. Functional treatment involves carefully evaluating personal history, testing to assess the body's capacity to function, supporting the body with optimal nutrition, minimizing harmful environmental factors, and restoring metabolic balance.

TRADITIONAL DIAGNOSIS AND TREATMENT

Traditionally physicians have used lab tests to confirm the source and degree of illness. However, many symptoms can't be associated with a specific disease, particularly in the early stages of an illness. So there are situations in which disease can't be diagnosed using the traditional model of evaluation.

The word *disease* means "without ease." People with undiagnosed and untreated conditions are truly without ease. A patient's chief complaint may be only that he or she has no energy and is unable to carry out day-to-day activities. Until recently doctors have lacked the tools to identify the underlying causes of these types of health problems. As a result it's been difficult to develop treatment for conditions that weren't linked to specific diseases, but were associated with processes in the body that were malfunctioning. Even patients whose illnesses have been accurately diagnosed may not fully heal if only the symptoms of their illnesses are being treated. The ultimate underlying cause may remain unidentified.

FUNCTIONAL DIAGNOSIS AND TREATMENT

The goal of the functional medicine practitioner is to measure the body's processes and treat the dysfunctions that are causing the disorder. If normal functioning is restored throughout the system, symptoms can resolve as the body naturally heals and returns to a state of wellness. The degree of healing may also depend on whether functional diagnosis and treatment are provided before serious damage has occurred.

Only a few years ago the scientific tools needed to accurately assess various aspects of body function did not exist. Functional medicine was correct in theory, but lacking in diagnostic science. Today we have the practical ability to measure a wide range of processes vital to every system in the body.

After taking a careful health history and reviewing symptoms, testing is done to determine whether a particular process is within normal physiological range. If this function is not within normal range, it's viewed as the cause or a contributing factor of illness. When indicated, additional testing can be done to measure other related factors.

MONITORING THERAPY

Functional diagnostic testing strongly influences the way treatment is carried out. This approach provides the information needed by the practitioner to develop a viable course of treatment. Further testing helps the practitioner monitor the progress of the patient's response and guides the adjustment of treatment.

MEASURING IMMUNE DEFENSES

Have you ever wondered why food contaminated with bacteria such as toxic *E. coli* can cause severe illness in some people and not others? In part the answer is found in the ability of our digestive systems to defend against infection.

Many people are amazed to learn that the digestive tract, throat, and mouth hold our defense against potential pathogens, including bacteria, viruses, parasites, fungi, and invasive forms of yeast. The saliva in the mouth and the mucus throughout the entire digestive system contain protective antibodies—secretory IgA (SIgA). These antibodies play a key role in blocking the invasion of unhealthy organisms; they function as our first line of immune defense.

Testing for Secretory IgA

In recent years functional tests have been developed to assess the strength of our secretory IgA. A simple saliva test can be used to measure SIgA levels in the mouth/throat, and a stool test can be used to measure them in the gut. Although SIgA in each area can be evaluated independently, lab testing has shown that there's a strong correlation between antibody levels registered from the mouth/throat area and from the intestinal tract. Since saliva testing can be performed with relative ease, this is a good first step in assessment.

Using Functional Testing and Treatment

Jeanette came to us soon after cancer surgery, seeking help to rebuild her immunity. Functional testing showed poor absorption and also inflammation in reaction to gluten (a component of wheat). In addition her adrenal glands were struggling and her vital hormones were clearly out of balance, due to stress, blood sugar imbalance, and the GI condition. When we tested her adrenal function, the results indicated that her cortisol was far too high and her DHEA was depleted. This type of pattern is known to compromise antibody production, as well as cellular immunity (typically NK killer cells), and this was confirmed in Jeanette's test results. Her hormone levels reflected an elevated cortisol at night, which indicated that her body wasn't shutting down, unable to shift fully into a rest-and-repair cycle. Her melatonin production was also out of cycle, further disturbing her sleep patterns, which wasn't helping her immunity either.

Based on this information we first elected treatment to heal the inflammation in the GI tract from the gluten intolerance. Our other initial goal was to restore normal adrenal function. Jeanette showed marked improvement in the following months. Because of the seriousness of her history we have continued to monitor her progress for the past two years. A summary of the changes in her cortisol levels and DHEA during this time are summarized below. You'll notice the skewed hormone levels when we first saw Jeanette. We've been especially encouraged by the improvement in her DHEA function.

Test	Normal Range	1996	1997	1998
Total Cortisol	23 to 42	44	28	30
DHEA	2 to 10	2	7	8

In Jeanette's case normalizing adrenal function has allowed the return of normal immune response. Supplements and changes in diet and lifestyle have recovered the healthy function of her GI tract. Normal adrenal/melatonin function has restored her to a positive sleep cycle.

Treatment Strategies

If the SIgA level measured in oral saliva is depressed, there is a high probability that it will also be low in other mucus-producing areas of the body. Low levels of SIgA suggest the value of additional testing to rule out infection or inflammation, which can cause nutritional deficiencies and toxicity.

TESTING FOR INFLAMMATION

Inflammation in the Small Intestine

Why this test is important: Testing for alpha-antichymotrypsin reports a marker that indicates if inflammation is present, primarily in the small intestine. High levels of this marker reflect the need for further testing to determine the cause of the inflammation.

Measuring this metabolic marker: A stool sample is used to detect and measure this metabolic marker.

How the results can be applied: Whenever inflammation is present, it is important to find the cause and prevent further problems. Inflammation in the small intestine can be triggered by reactions to gluten, lactose, or sucrose; delayed food allergies; or upper GI parasites such as giardia, cryptosporidium, or amoebas (for example *Dientamoeba fragilis*).

Inflammation in the Large Intestine

Why this test is important: This marker (lysozyme A) typically indicates whether inflammation is present in the large intestine. It can reflect a number of conditions, including irritable bowel syndrome (IBS), inflammatory bowel disease (IBD), and colon cancer.

Evaluation: Lysozyme can be measured through a stool test.

How the results can be applied: The information from this test can be used to direct follow-up testing or treatment. The test can be repeated to monitor progress and evaluate the success of treatment.

Testing for Infection (Nitric Oxide)

Why this test is important: High levels of nitrate (nitric oxide) reflect the presence of infection in the body. Nitric oxide is released to enable our white blood cells to attack invading organisms. Although this biochemical has a beneficial function, excessive nitric oxide can promote generalized inflammation and can cause damage to muscles and joints.

What it measures: The test measures levels of nitric oxide as a metabolic marker in urine.

How the results can be applied: Elevated levels of nitric oxide indicate the need for further testing to determine the source of the infection or inflammation. They also suggest the importance of supplementing with antioxidants to reduce inflammation. Decreasing nitric oxide levels will reduce the potential for damage to muscle tissue and joints.

It is very important to point out that the number one cause of inflammation in the body is infection. A comprehensive diagnostic workup utilizing blood, stool, saliva, and urine samples is necessary to accomplish this. With advanced immunology, in regard to both humoral and mucosal antibodies, Polymerase Chain Reaction (PCR) DNA testing, and next-generation microbiology techniques, we can detect not only acute but chronic, long-term infections. This is essential to identifying the cause of inflammation and directing the appropriate treatment.

EVALUATING THE STRESS RESPONSE

Testing for DHEA

Why DHEA is important: DHEA is often referred to as the mother hormone of the body, and we produce more of this essential hormone than any other. In combination with cortisol, it's involved in the regulation of virtually all aspects of body function. Both are secreted by the adrenal glands, the source of our defense response to the stressors of life (both external and internal). In order for us to cope with digestive illness and support immune defenses, DHEA levels must be maintained so healing can proceed.

How DHEA can be measured: This test is performed through simple saliva specimens.

How the results can be applied: Abnormal DHEA levels can interfere with immunity, energy production, skin regeneration, bone health, sleep quality, and thyroid function. If we have evidence of adrenal hormone levels, that can provide the basis for developing a therapeutic program. The levels can easily be rechecked through future saliva tests, guiding strategies to promote or supplement DHEA gradually until it returns to the normal range.

Measuring Cortisol Levels

Why cortisol is important: Cortisol is the primary hormone that directs immune function, and it works in harmony with DHEA. These hormones also regulate the production of the cells that secrete SIgA (the immunocytes). If cortisol and DHEA values are out of balance, a depression of SIgA can ultimately occur. Therefore when SIgA levels are low, it's important to look at adrenal function. This can reflect excessive physical, mental, or emotional stress.

Stress is handled by the sympathetic system, in response to both intense events (the fight-or-flight mechanism) and low-grade ongoing stress. The parasympathetic system does the repairing, restoring, and rebuilding. A critical balance exists between the two systems. When we are responding to stress too much of the time, it can overload the sympathetic system and lead to adrenal exhaustion. If illness is present it's essential to identify and correct any depression of our adrenal hormones, to maintain our body's ability to heal.

How cortisol is measured: One way to measure cortisol levels is through a simple home test that samples saliva. This provides us with a real-life assessment of the effects of stress on the adrenals.

How the results can be applied: Restoring the normal balance of cortisol and DHEA will help the body produce more immunocytes and therefore improve secretory IgA levels. Measuring cortisol and DHEA can also identify adrenal dysfunction, and treatment strategies can be developed to restore normal function, optimizing health and immunity.

DETERMINING DIGESTIVE STATUS

Measuring Reactions to Gluten

Why this test is important: Reactions to gluten can be devastating for anyone who has inherited gluten intolerance. This condition is especially common in people with northern European and Scandinavian heritage. The body's response can cause severe inflammation in the small intestine, a breakdown in the mucosal lining. The damage from gluten may be so extreme that it can create allergies to numerous other foods, and secondary illnesses may develop. The number one problem that results from gluten intolerance is malabsorption, which can lead to severe nutritional deficiencies and resulting illness.

Measuring gluten intolerance through gliadin antibodies: This test, using a saliva sample, measures the immune response to gliadin (gluten protein). Positive test results indicate gluten intolerance.

How the results can be applied: Gluten intolerance is known to be associated with inflammation of the small intestine and with malabsorption. People with a gluten intolerance often find that once they're on a 100 percent gluten-free diet, within as little as two months there can be a normalization of the SIgA defenses and a major reduction in inflammation. As inflammation decreases, the ability to absorb nutrients will increase, improving nutritional status.

Measuring Milk/Dairy Intolerance

Why this test is important: This test provides essential feedback regarding a person's ability to handle dairy products in general. Allergic reactions to milk and other dairy-based foods have been associated with symptoms such as diarrhea, constipation, chronic fatigue, and arthritis, and can lead to leaky gut syndrome. It can also cause irritation and inflammation of the GI tract, damage to the villi in the gut lining, and the reduction of the immunocytes that produce SIgA. People who are sensitive to milk proteins (casein and lactalbumin) are usually also lactose intolerant. Dairy allergy that's not addressed can lead to illness elsewhere in the body, including respiratory problems and sinus infections.

How dairy proteins are measured: This is a saliva test that measures the response to mixed milk proteins. If an immune reaction is detected (the presence of antibodies), this means the body is mounting an attack against milk protein in an allergic response.

How the results can be applied: A positive result on this test means there is an allergy or a sensitivity to dairy products. In that case it's important to avoid all milk and dairy products. With the complete avoidance of dairy the symptoms subside quite quickly.

The Metabolic Profile

Why this test is important: This diagnostic test assesses the status of our own unique body chemistry. At any given time our chemistry reflects the stability or compromise of our health. If our biochemistry is brought back into balance through the use of nutrients, the foods we eat, and our lifestyle, healing can occur naturally.

What the test evaluates: This test measures body chemicals that reflect:

- Energy production and oxygen metabolism
- Deficiencies in B-complex vitamins, amino acids, and minerals
- Brain function reflected in neurotransmitter metabolism
- Liver function, particularly how well a person is able to neutralize and expel toxins
- Specific needs for antioxidants and other nutrients
- Digestion and absorption problems
- How efficiently the body is metabolizing and using the nutrients from food
- How effectively the body is metabolizing carbohydrates

- Markers for dysbiosis where there is an overgrowth of yeast, microscopic parasites, or bacteria
- Signs of damage to cells

How the results can be applied: This test can be used as a key diagnostic tool for chronic health problems. It is helpful in customizing individual treatment programs. This view of the body's processes at the level of the cell allows us to look at problems that might interfere with our ability to take the fuel from the food we eat and convert it into energy.

The test's chemical markers may reflect nutritional deficiencies. This information can be used to address specific needs for vitamins, minerals, antioxidants, amino acids, and dietary changes. Diet therapy and supplements can play a vital role in restarting or rebalancing the metabolism.

The metabolic profile provides clues about where to intervene in complex problems, by giving an overview of how the metabolism is functioning. It can show whether cells are being destroyed, are malfunctioning, or are functioning normally. With this information more serious health problems can often be prevented or reversed.

William G. Timmins, N.D., is founder and director of San Diego's BioHealth Diagnostics. He received his degree in naturopathy from the International University of Naturopathic Sciences and cofounded two of the nation's first integrative health care centers. A lecturer, author, and former host of two weekly radio programs, he has also appeared on TV shows such as *The Wellness Hour, Serving San Diego,* and *Healthy Living.* A national physicians' consultant for clinical and research laboratories, Dr. Timmins maintains a busy patient practice in nutritional consulting while conducting independent research and providing professional training on functional diagnostic testing. More than a decade of helping his patients has enriched and confirmed his theories in the real-life measurement of his work's success.

Dr. Timmins and BioHealth Diagnostics provide nutritional consulting and individualized wellness and longevity programs for professionals. A wide array of audio- and videotapes are available, as well as seminars and patient and doctor educational programs in the clinical applications of functional diagnostic testing. BioHealth Diagnostics in San Diego can be reached at (800) 570-2000. For more information, see their Web sites at www.biohealthinfo.com and www.biohealthcenters.com.

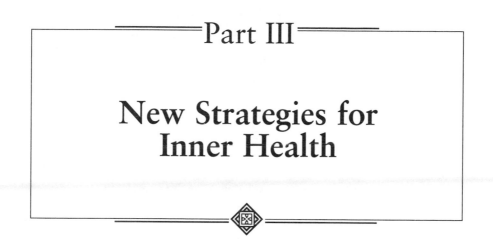

Part III

New Strategies for
Inner Health

19

Remove, Replace, Restore, and Repair*

JEFFREY BLAND, PH.D.

THE 4R SUPPORT PROGRAM

A comprehensive approach to normalizing gastrointestinal function, referred to as the "4Rs," involves four basic steps: Remove, Replace, Restore, and Repair. "Remove" focuses on eliminating pathogenic bacteria, viruses, fungi, parasites, allergens, and toxins from the gastrointestinal tract. The second step in the 4R program, "Replace," replenishes enzymes and other digestive factors that may be lacking, such as pancreatic enzymes, hydrochloric acid (HCl), or intrinsic factor. The third step, "Restore," refers to restoring the beneficial bacteria that are commonly found in a normal digestive system but may be missing from a dysfunctional one. It is an important step in restoring healthy function to the gut. A variety of supplemental resources may be considered helpful in this phase, including cultured and fermented foods and supplements containing live beneficial bacteria. The fourth and final step in a 4R approach, "Repair," addresses intestinal permeability through the use of nutritional supplements known to be critical in intestinal function.

Each of these steps, listed below, includes references to chapters of the book that provide additional information on this approach to good digestive health.

Step 1. Remove
- Common food allergies or sensitivities (see chapter 20).
- Bad bugs—candida or bacterial overgrowth or parasites (see chapter 21).
- Problems from viruses (see chapter 22).
- Minimize environmental toxins and also digestive toxins (see chapters 23, 26, and 27).

---

*Adapted from *Clinical Nutrition: A Functional Approach* (2004). Written and published by the Institute for Functional Medicine, Gig Harbor, WA. Used by permission.

Step 2. Replace
- Betaine hydrochloride (hydrochloric acid)(see chapter 24).
- Enzymes (animal-based or plant-based)(see chapter 24).
- Bicarbonate (which enables the enzymes to work)(see chapter 24).
- Intrinsic factor (see chapter 33, vitamin B_{12}).

Step 3. Restore
See chapter 24.

- Probiotics—*L. acidolphilus* and other probiotics.
- Provide prebiotics if starches and sugars are tolerated. Nourishment for the beneficial microflora such as FOS (fructo-aligo-saccharides) and inulin (in Jerusalem artichokes, dandelion greens).
- Increase fiber and monitor the response. Soluble fiber such as oat bran increases butyrate and other essential fatty acids. Nonsoluble fiber such as cellulose is best tolerated by some.
- Increase resistant starch in the diet to reduce acidity, and raise fatty acids. See *Breaking the Vicious Cycle* by Elaine Gottschall.
- Monitor level of starches and sugars (see chapter 31).

Step 4. Repair
- Provide nutrients to heal the GI mucosa: vitamins A and C, B_5 (pantothenic acid), B_6 (pyrodixine), the amino acid L-glutamine, and the mineral zinc (see chapters 24, 32, and 33).
- Support the immune functions of the GI tract: vitamin A to nourish antibody production (see chapter 25).
- Continue to avoid allergens and irritants: certain drugs (such as NSAIDs), alcohol, and foods that trigger allergies (see chapter 25).

Biographical information for **Jeffrey Bland, Ph.D.**, appears on page 110.

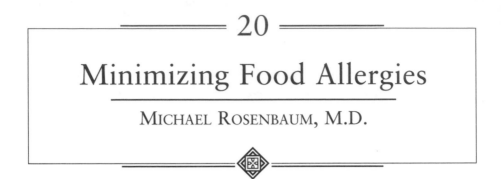

20

Minimizing Food Allergies

Michael Rosenbaum, M.D.

Why are we concerned about allergies? Allergies and sensitivities are often linked to digestive problems. When the offending food is discovered and removed, people improve. So a small investment of time and effort can produce big results.

This process basically involves discovering and then eliminating the food that triggers allergies. The primary self-care strategies include:

- Identifying Allergies: The Food Challenge and The Pulse Test
- Managing Allergies: The Elimination Diet, The Rotation Diet, and Using Digestive Enzymes

Once people see how great they feel without the symptoms, it becomes almost effortless to give up the foods that cause symptoms, because they know how they'll feel if they go back to eating them.

IDENTIFYING AND MANAGING FOOD ALLERGIES

Identifying Allergies: The Food Challenge

The home food challenge test is often considered the gold standard for food allergy testing and it's something you can do on your own that is free. It's best done when you have enough time and attention. This process involves avoiding suspected foods for a week and then reintroducing them one per day. Although this will not always identify delayed food allergies (see chapters 8 and 16) it can alert you to many of the major allergenic foods.

In this test people often go through a brief period of withdrawal from any allergenic foods they have eliminated. We usually wait until the seventh day before introducing suspected foods so that they have had four days of withdrawal and then perhaps three positive days after that. From the seventh day on people can test one food at a time by reintroducing it into their diet.

Typically this test is done at lunchtime, when a large amount of a particular food is consumed as the only food in a "mono-meal." Or, if it is your day off, you can eat the food first thing in the morning on an empty stomach so no other foods are suspected. If there are no obvious symptoms within thirty minutes to an hour, you can repeat half of the amount of the meal again and then wait three to six hours. The food should be tested at a time when you are not at work and your attention is not being diverted, when you can focus on yourself.

A markedly exaggerated reaction can occur, which could include almost any kind of response, but usually is unmistakable.

- It could be a skin rash or even hives
- It could be a rapid pulse
- Extreme fatigue may come on abruptly
- Intense muscle aches and pains or headache could occur suddenly
- Mental symptoms may occur—your mind may suddenly go totally blank
- The symptoms could be anything abdominal, from nausea and vomiting to diarrhea or extreme gas

If there's no clear reaction after three to six hours, often the reaction will manifest on awakening the next morning. People may feel even worse upon awakening and feel very much hungover. If the response does not occur until the next day, yet is very powerful and uncharacteristic, that could also be a sign of delayed food response.

Dealing with Reactions

In these situations wait until the reaction has completely subsided before testing another food. If you want to expedite your recovery, then you can take something like milk of magnesia to force the food out of your system completely. Otherwise you may have to wait two or three days until you are totally over the first reaction and ready to test something else. Allow your system to clear thoroughly.

Bicarbonate (baking soda) can also be used to treat an accidental food allergy reaction. When feeling unwell after food allergy testing or a restaurant meal, you may find it helpful to take Alka-Seltzer Gold, buffered vitamin C, or take 1 tablespoon of baking soda in a cup of water with 500 or 1000 mg of vitamin C. This can be repeated in half an hour if necessary.

Identifying Allergies: The Pulse Test

The pulse test (or Coca Test) can be a practical method for self-testing. The test is named after Dr. Coca, a famous allergist at Columbia University in the 1920s. He found that when people with food allergies ate an allergenic food they could experience an increase in their pulse rate of at least 12 beats a minute.

The first step is to determine your baseline pulse over a period of a week. Then consume a suspected food and check your pulse 30 minutes later. If you find that your pulse has gone up to least 12 to 16 beats per minute, that serves as a positive test. You can become more certain about your response by avoiding the food for a week and then performing the test again, first thing in the morning on an empty stomach. Most people will not get all the symptoms of allergies at once, but often they will get some of them within an hour of ingesting an allergenic food and usually within three hours.

Managing Allergies: The Elimination Diet
Unmasking the Allergy

When an allergenic food is eliminated, a process of unmasking occurs in which people sometimes feel worse rather than better. They may actually go through a period of withdrawal very similar to the withdrawal experienced by people with alcohol or drug addiction. This period of time usually lasts about four days. Often on one or two of those days, patients will crave the very foods that have been removed from their diets and may have uncomfortable symptoms such as diarrhea, aches, pains, a runny nose, or fatigue. That is the unmasking or the withdrawal effect.

Often I can predict the foods someone will be allergic to if he or she says something like, "You can take anything out of my diet, Doctor, but please don't ask me to give up chocolate." It is possible to crave bread or corn or peanuts—any food. When I take a medical history for food allergies I usually ask people about the foods they love and crave the most and what they would miss the most if they had to give it up. Foods that are craved the most are often the offending foods.

Overcoming the Allergy—What to Do and What Not to Do

When we eat an allergenic food every day, the body masks our reaction. In a sense we become numb to it, so we may be unaware of any reactivity. This is described as "tolerance." If the allergy is unmasked and we become sensitive once again, then a strong response can be elicited. We may become as sensitive as we would have been as a baby.

After the four days of the withdrawal period one enters a supersensitive state. For the next three weeks or so—usually until the end of the month—there are another twenty-six days of hyper-sensitivity. During that period, if a person eats the food he or she is sensitive to, there will be an exaggerated reaction to the allergenic food that is much greater than when the person was eating the food on a regular basis.

It's important to be very strict in eliminating an allergenic food for the first four weeks. I have had people who were very careful for two weeks, then said, "Well, I've been invited out to a dinner party and I've been so good for two weeks. I'll treat myself—after all, it's only one meal." At that stage of the elimination diet they could become extremely ill. This period of heightened sensitivity typically lasts at least four weeks. Once it is over it is usually possible to rotate these foods back into the diet without creating a reaction.

Managing Allergies: The Rotation Diet

One practical solution to managing food allergies is the rotation diet. This means eating the offending food(s) on a limited basis. Some foods may be tolerated if they are only eaten periodically—every fourth or seventh day. However, this may not always be possible. For example in cases of celiac sprue (a sensitivity to gluten) the offending wheat or grain must be avoided on a long-term basis.

The rotation diet offers major benefits: it allows you to minimize your exposure to any one food and it makes it just a little easier to identify foods you may be reacting to.

Four-Day Rotation

When people are reactive to a wide range of foods it's not enough to simply eliminate one or two foods. The best solution is to rotate many different foods to make sure that no one food is repeated too often and to ensure a variety of foods in the diet. In a rotation diet any food that is eaten one day is usually not repeated for another four days. One devises a diet with foods that are eaten together for day 1, day 2, day 3, and day 4. Then day 1 is repeated on the fifth day and day 2 is repeated on the sixth day, and so forth. In that sort of diet you'll want to put foods together that you like to eat together. So you have a list of compatible starches and protein foods and vegetables and beans and fruits. And you make sure that whatever is consumed together stays together on that day.

Another important aspect of these diets is the rotation of food families. The principle here is that foods fall into biological families. For instance, lemons, grapefruits, oranges, and limes are all in the citrus family. There is a percentage of the population whose allergies are more severe and who must do a more careful food rotation. In these cases foods can be grouped by food family. Lemons and oranges might be eaten on Monday and Friday, but limes and grapefruits would be taken on Wednesday and Sunday. In that way you can actually eat food in the same family four times in one week.

People with a great many allergies or very severe allergies may find that some of their allergies are permanent. In this case they need to completely eliminate these foods from their diet so that they are not even in the rotation. Then they can eat everything else on a rotation basis. Again, most foods would be taken every four days. However, a few foods might be eaten on an every-seven-day basis, depending on the level of sensitivity.

Seven-Day Rotation

People with severe food allergies may find that they can tolerate many more foods if they use a seven-day rotation. These are people who are still reactive to food on a four-day rotation diet. In one sense the seven-day rotation is much easier because the days of the week never change. What you eat on Monday is always what you eat on Monday. If you require this diet, it can be used to your advantage. For example, you can devise a menu so that the foods you eat on Saturday and Sunday are always the same, and that way you can design very nice meals for the weekend. Within this framework you can be creative. For example, if you always eat chicken on Saturday it could be grilled, roasted, prepared Chinese-style in a stir-fried dish, Italian-style in sauce, or East Indian-style in a curry.

It's helpful to remember that cooked food is less allergenic than raw food. For example cooked tomato sauce tends to be less allergenic than a raw tomato. The same is true for applesauce in comparison with an apple. That may explain why some people are allergic to apples but can eat applesauce. And another basic principle is that people tend to be more allergic to foods in cold weather than in warm weather. So there may be more reactivity in the winter than in the summer months.

Managing Allergies: Using Digestive Aids

Some food allergies may result from incomplete digestion. When large molecules of protein that are not totally digested are absorbed into the bloodstream they can potentially trigger an allergic response.

Apparently some people with food allergies do not produce enough hydrochloric acid, pancreatic digestive enzymes, or perhaps not enough bicarbonate. If you replenish vital digestants and nutrients, digestion can improve, the food particles are broken down more finely, and fewer reactions result (for more information about digestants see chapter 24).

- *Hydrochloric acid.* For some people the tendency to low stomach acid production may be genetic. Others find that digestion is impaired following an illness. Hydrochloric acid (and vitamin B_{12}, which indirectly supports its production) can be supplemented using capsules, labeled "betaine hydrochloride," available at any health food store. (For more information see page 27 and chapter 24.)

- *Pancreatic digestive enzymes or pancreatin.* Depending on the strength of the product, from one to three digestive enzymes can be taken either toward the end of the meal or even fifteen or twenty minutes after the meal. The goal here is to supplement pancreatic enzymes if their production is low. (Note that the most effective pancreatic enzymes come in an enteric-coated tablet so they survive the stomach acid and dissolve further down the digestive tract.)
- *Bicarbonate.* Taking bicarbonate after enzymes helps the pancreatic enzymes work by creating the necessary alkaline environment. Bicarbonate is simply baking soda, which can be taken 1 teaspoonful in a glass of water. As mentioned bicarbonate can often be used to treat an accidental food-allergy reaction. When feeling unwell after a restaurant meal, consider taking Alka-Seltzer Gold or bicarbonate and vitamin C, which can sometimes dispel the symptoms completely within five minutes.

LEAKY GUT SYNDROME AND ALLERGIES

It is likely that some people have food allergies that are *caused* by leaky gut syndrome. (For more information on leaky gut, see chapter 7.) Food allergies can also *trigger* leaky gut syndrome. This is a condition usually diagnosed and managed by an integrative physician using a simple test obtained through the doctor (see chapter 17 for information on testing).

In some cases of leaky gut oversized food molecules are absorbed directly into the lining cells of the GI tract. In other instances the food molecules penetrate between the cells. If the lining is damaged, these molecules can enter the bloodstream. Either of these malfunctions could contribute to food allergies

Healing Leaky Gut Syndrome

There are various ways to correct leaky gut syndrome. In some cases it is believed to be caused by dysbiosis: by parasites, by yeast, or even by a major overgrowth of normal bowel bacteria. There are a number of nutrients you can take for leaky gut syndrome that might result from food allergies.

Zinc is one of the primary nutrients I use because it's critically important for growth and wound healing. Zinc is essential to the cells that have rapid turnover, particularly the lining cells of the GI tract. These cells are replaced about every five to seven days, so zinc can be rapidly depleted in the body. In addition zinc levels tend to be decreasing in the American diet. In older people especially it is not unusual to find evidence of zinc deficiency. Among its many functions zinc also increases the release of vitamin A from the liver. If you are zinc deficient, you may actually have a nice storehouse of vitamin A in the liver and be unable to utilize it.

Vitamin A is the other vitamin essential to digestive health. It is responsible for the integrity of lining cells of all the mucosal surfaces of the body, including the entire digestive system. It is also necessary for the production of the secretory IgA, the antibodies that protect the GI tract.

Glutamine is one of the hallmark nutrients now used to treat leaky gut. It raises the levels of growth hormone vital for wound healing and new protein synthesis and may play an essential role in restoring the lining of the gut. Glutamine is also used as a fuel by many of the cells in the body in place of glucose.

MSM, a form of the mineral sulfur, is another useful nutrient that produces encouraging results. It tends to be very soothing and healing to the entire digestive tract. MSM helps to prevent oxidative stress throughout the GI tract and it's also supposed to prevent pathogens (potentially harmful bacteria, yeast, and parasites) from adhering to the gut wall.

DGL (deglycyrrhizinated licorice) is a type of licorice that has been processed to remove glycyrrhizinate, the fraction that can be upsetting to the stomach. DGL is very soothing to the upper GI tract and in some cases helps to promote healing and overcome leaky gut.

Growth factors are another type of substance that is gaining wider recognition. They have been used to treat all kinds of GI disorders, including colitis, Crohn's disease, and irritable bowel syndrome. Growth factors are found in DGL, glandular products, and peptides (the building blocks of protein). Seacure is a peptide product extracted from predigested white fish. The effect on conditions such as irritable bowel syndrome can sometimes be very profound.

The other important aspect of any leaky gut program is stress reduction. Stress raises cortisol output, and excess cortisol can cause ulcers and impair the lining of the gut. So stress can be a factor in leaky gut and in some allergies as well.

MEDICAL TESTING AND TREATMENT OF ALLERGIES

There are a number of ways to medically test for food allergies, which is especially helpful for those who lack the time or inclination to do home testing.

Antibody Testing for Allergies

Food allergies can be evaluated using a lab test that measures the immune system's antibody reactions to different foods. The vast majority of food reactions are thought to be caused by IgG antibodies. (It is believed that only 10% of food reactions are "classic allergies" caused by the IgE antibody, which can result in acute and even life-threatening reactions.) IgG reactions are often delayed and therefore difficult to diagnose with an elimination diet, but can easily be measured in a blood test. Tests are available to evaluate both IgG and IgE antibodies. The response is usually graded, using a rating scale from 0 to +4, to indicate the intensity of the response (the evaluation scale used depends upon the lab).

When preparing for antibody testing it is important to know that if a food has been out of the diet for a month or more, the blood test result may be low and will not provide a true measure of your reactivity. If you know that you are allergic to a particular food and have totally eliminated it from your diet, when you take the test this can skew the results. My own suggestion to patients who are preparing for these tests is to eat allergenic foods for two or three weeks, three times a week, preceding the lab test (as long as those foods will not harm them).

Intradermal Testing

This type of evaluation involves injecting a very small amount of a suspected allergen underneath the skin (rather than just scratching the surface of the skin as in a scratch test) and observing the skin surface for signs of reactivity. (This method tends to be more accurate than the scratch test, which often does not correlate very well with what we see clinically in the food challenge tests.)

One form of intradermal testing can be used to determine the degree of individual sensitivity. This type of test was devised by the famous allergist Dr. Rinkel during the 1940s and further developed by Dr. Joseph Miller of Alabama. The idea here is to determine not just whether a person reacts to a particular food or not, but also to identify the exact level of sensitivity that an individual has to that food, so a specific treatment dose or antidote can be created for that person. In this type of evaluation intradermal skin tests are performed, but varying dilutions are used for each allergenic food. As part of the test two or three or more injections of each specific food are given—each injection in a different concentration using dilutions of one to five. This particular technique of testing is used more by ear, nose, and throat physicians than traditional allergists.

Treatment for Food Allergies Based on Intradermal Testing

Once intradermal testing for allergens has been completed, an antidote for all foods causing allergies can be put together in one formula.

- *Taking antidotes by injection.* Injections of the antidote can be given on an individual schedule, depending on the severity of the allergy. Some people take them every day or even several times a day. Others get injections twice a week.

- *Taking antidotes by mouth.* Another technique is to give these doses under the tongue (sublingually). In that case the doses are usually taken two to three times a day. The length of treatment depends on the individual. The therapy may be given for one or two years, or it may be required indefinitely.

People are usually retested about once a year to see if their dosage has changed. This type of treatment is used by many integrative physicians today. Doctors and patients report that this approach can be quite effective in addressing food allergies.

Biographical information for **Michael Rosenbaum, M.D.,** appears on page 41.

21

Clearing Bad Bugs

THE TEAM

If you've been sick for a while and don't have a diagnosis, review this chapter carefully to see if any of the symptoms or patterns here match your experience.

Doctors of nutritional medicine are now finding that microbes are often the underlying and undiagnosed cause of many health problems. The microbes may be an overgrowth of yeast or bacteria, or could be parasites or viruses. They can cause illnesses that don't seem to relate to the digestive tract, including allergies, asthma, arthritis, or even neurological problems. These problems are difficult to detect and diagnose. An integrative approach involves:

- Lab testing to identify any existing problem
- Treatment with medication to clear infection, possibly followed by herbs
- Strengthening immunity to guard against future infections

COMMON MICROBES

- *Parasites* in food or water (such as giardia) can invade the body and take up residence.
- *Yeast, such as candida, normally found in the GI tract,* can overgrow and consume too many of our resources. (Also see the information on candida testing in chapter 17 and treatment in part V.)
- *Bacteria that normally reside in the body (aerobic, oxygen-loving types)* may overgrow due to imbalances caused by antibiotic overuse or misuse, or acute viral or bacterial infections that kill off some of the more vulnerable beneficial species, leaving others that are more hardy.
- *Other internal bacteria (anaerobes, the kind that thrive without oxygen)* may overgrow; these are less well known and more difficult to diagnose because they don't survive in the presence of oxygen.
- *Bacteria in food or water that cause food poisoning and dysentery,* such as salmonella, shigella, or *E. coli.*
- *Viruses* can also invade the body, including the GI tract, and survive in the cells for years (see chapter 22).

All They Did Was Drink the Water

Helen and Dave went camping for a long weekend and brought the children. They noticed the warnings in the park not to drink the water in the fountains (giardia, it said). But they never dreamed the water served in the roadside diner would cause problems. After all, they were in America, not the tropics. When they got home everybody got sick. A flu, some kind of bug. After a few days they all got better. Except Helen.

Helen had Montezuma's revenge—diarrhea that just wouldn't stop. She counted the days. Surely it would stop in a few days. She went to the doctor. No apparent cause.

Days stretched into weeks, and weeks into months. She went to another doctor and another. Then she went to a psychiatrist who had a lot to say about her childhood. But none of that had any effect on the diarrhea.

She couldn't digest anything but oatmeal, so her weight dropped pretty low. She could no longer work; in fact, she couldn't really leave the house for very long. Her energy was gone. She still cooked for the family—as it turns out, a major mistake. Her world had telescoped down into a narrow little life—no job, no travel, no dinner parties. No food, no alcohol, no sex.

The months turned into years. Surely she'd get better! But the diarrhea continued. She looked like a death-camp victim—skin and bone, 82 pounds. The doctor had run a stool sample. Dave asked him to do another, just in case. It had been more than two years. The report came back with "Giardia. Known to cause persistent diarrhea."

Helen took the prescribed drug and within ten days things started to turn around. The diarrhea slowed, then stopped altogether. And she could eat again. She didn't have those constant stomachaches and that awful feeling of being toxic that she couldn't really explain to anybody. Dave did some research at the medical library and found that there was another drug that was useful as well. Three months after the first medication, Helen took the second. Within another three months she was almost well! She could eat anything. She called the state college and enrolled. By fall she was immersed in a full-time graduate program. It was all just a memory.

A happy ending. For Helen, yes. But not for Dave. What neither of them knew at the time is that parasites like giardia are transmitted on human hands and in water and food. Whenever she cooked for Dave and handled the food, the bug could be passed along to him. Dave didn't get diarrhea, but he did get the infection. And in the end he came out worse than Helen. As the doctor says, "When it comes to parasites, don't pussyfoot around. Get tested and get treated."

ARE PARASITES A PROBLEM?

Timothy Kuss, Ph.D.

Worldwide more than one billion people are infected with parasites. The United States is now seeing an increasing prevalence of parasite-related problems. Research by the Centers for Disease Control (CDC) shows that far more than 90 percent of the parasites found in U.S. lab tests are microscopic—invisible to the naked eye and difficult to detect in the lab without special expertise. In Milwaukee in 1993, more than 40,000 people were sickened by the microscopic parasite cryptosporidium. Of these more than 4,000 were hospitalized and at least 100 died.

In a national survey about one in seven people were found to have parasites. The review was conducted in 1976 by the Centers for Disease Control. Almost half a million samples (450,000) were reviewed. If the survey had been conducted today the figures would probably be quite a bit higher—maybe twice as high, about one person in three—due to more advanced lab techniques and increased incidence.

Parasitic disease is on the rise due to many factors, including:

- Increased international travel
- Immigration
- The manufacturing and shipping of food internationally
- Worldwide urban crowding
- Restaurant food handlers as a major source of parasite dissemination

These trends are occurring on a massive scale that makes monitoring difficult. World travel, migration, transport, and trade occurs on a level unheard of at any earlier point in history. People, animals, food, even ships are all potential mediums for the transport of microbes. As the CDC points out, disease is only a plane flight away from anywhere in the world. Ships that discharge ballast can transmit an entire microbial population, which then infects the shellfish and sea life in that area, spreading contamination such as cholera.

People may be unknowing carriers. In tropical regions people inherit immunity developed over generations of adaptation to the microbes of that particular area. They themselves may be free of symptoms, but they may transmit the disease through personal contact or food handling to others who have not developed these immune protections.

Common Symptoms

Typical symptoms of an acute parasitic infection (in the early stages) include recurrent diarrhea, alternating diarrhea and constipation, constipation alone, bloating and gas, abdominal pain or cramps, nausea, loss of appetite, or food cravings. These are often accompanied by poor digestion and poor absorption. General weakness or fatigue, which no amount of rest relieves, may be a sign.

Note that these symptoms are typical of a recently contracted infection. Once a parasitic infection becomes deep-seated and chronic, some of the more severe GI symptoms may subside. At this point the infection may cause other types of chronic illness, which can be quite serious. New symptoms may emerge in different parts of the body such as the skin, respiratory tract, or joints.

System-Wide Effects—Omar Amin, Ph.D.

Parasites can cause illness anywhere in the body. In a survey of people found to have parasites in their stool, the Parasitology Center, Inc., found they also had a variety of associated conditions.

- *Entamoeba histolytica* (amoebas)—fatigue, nausea, allergies, pain, weight loss, insomnia
- *Blastocystis hominis*—fatigue, nervous disorders, pain, skin conditions, nausea, allergies, muscle problems
- *E. coli* (*Entamoeba coli,* the parasite rather than the bacteria)—fatigue, allergies, headache, nausea, depression/lack of concentration, irritability, joint/back pain, skin problems
- *Entamoeba hartmanii*—nervous system, respiratory, and skin disorders; allergies; pain; nausea
- *Cyclospora*—fatigue, itching, nausea, anemia, headache, muscle aches, depression

Microscopic Parasites—Trent W. Nichols, M.D.

- *Amoebic dysentery* is an acute and chronic disease caused by the organism *Entamoeba histolytica,* which can affect the colon, the liver, and other organs. Symptoms may include diarrhea or constipation, cramps, or gas and bloating. An estimated 5 percent of the U.S. population is infected by amoebas. It tends to be even more prevalent in South America and Mexico, and is more frequently diagnosed in people who are traveling from tropical regions.

  Occasionally this pathogen can cause amoebic abscess of the liver. The sufferer will be extremely ill and typically have a history of travel to a tropical country, symptoms of bloody diarrhea, extreme discomfort, distention, and pain over the upper right abdominal area. Liver involvement or the presence of a cyst in the liver would be diagnosed by a CT scan.

- Giardia *(Giardia lamblia)* can cause diarrhea, cramps, and bloating, and is seen in patients with a history of drinking untreated water from camp sites, lakes, or rivers. Giardia is difficult to diagnose because of its variable life cycle; evaluation is usually done through stool testing or biopsy, but it may require several tests before a positive diagnosis is made. Giardia may also be diagnosed through antibody testing in blood, but the organism doesn't always match the antibody profile and may even be missed in this subtle testing. *Doctor's note:* Giardia is the parasite treated most frequently in my practice here in Pennsylvania. It is pandemic worldwide because water supplies frequently contain giardia, particular those in wilderness areas.

- *Cryptosporidia* is becoming much more prevalent in the United States. It has only been recognized since 1976 as a cause of diarrheal disease in humans; before that, it was thought to only infect animals such as pigs, calves, and mice. Cryptosporidium is transmitted through water and animal hosts including reptiles and birds. Both cryptosporidium and microsporidia are frequently contracted by AIDS patients.

- *Blastocystis hominis* is an intestinal protozoa that is becoming increasingly prevalent. Patients who test positive for blastocystus do not always have symptoms. Symptoms may include diarrhea or severe constipation, weight loss, cramping, flatulence, or bloating. In the recent past this microbe was considered to be nonpathogenic (an organism not causing symptoms). However, microbiologists have found that there are two different strains of blastocystus. One is believed to be tropical and quite virulent; some reports indicate that about a fourth of the people with blastocystus have this condition as a long-term chronic disease.

- *Microsporidia* is another pathogen observed in AIDS and immunodeficient patients, with symptoms of malabsorption, weight loss, and severe watery, nonbloody diarrhea.

A number of other parasites have been recognized or reclassified as "emerging pathogens" in the recent past. This indicates either a change in the virulence of the microbe (its strength and ability to cause harm) or a change in our assessment of it as a potential medical problem. Other pathogenic parasites include *Dientamoeba fragilis,* cyclospora, and *E. hartmanii.*

Parasitic Infection: How Do You Know You Have a Problem?
—*Jerry Stine*

- Parasites can be extremely difficult to detect.
- It's very common to get a report with no findings (a false negative) when there actually are parasites present.

- It is usually not adequate to trust a negative diagnosis on the basis of just one stool test. Labs will typically request two or three samples.
- There must be multiple stool collections.
- When checking the levels of friendly flora on lab tests such as the CDSA, an absence of *E. coli* suggests the presence of a parasite.
- If the person has been sick for a long time and nothing shows on the stool testing, it's worth doing additional testing for the chemical markers of parasites or bacteria. Antibody testing can also be quite helpful. Never lose sight of the fact that the symptoms and history may tell you as much as the lab work.

Lab Testing

In the case of parasites, lab work can be very constructive. Testing for parasites rarely finds parasites that aren't actually present (a false positive); this is almost unheard of. The following are the most common tests and where they may be obtained. Refer to Laboratory Testing in the Resources chapter for lab contact information.

- Antibody testing—Immunosciences Laboratory and Diagnos-Techs
- Markers of inflammation—Diagnos-Techs, Great Smokies Diagnostic Laboratory, and Immunosciences Laboratory
- Stool testing—Parasitology Center, Inc., Diagnos-Techs, Doctor's Data, and university labs nationwide

CANDIDA

OMAR AMIN, PH.D.

The overgrowth of *Candida albicans* is well known to practitioners of nutritional medicine. What is less well known is the fact that candida infections often accompany parasitic infections. The energy drain on the system by the parasite tends to provide an opportunity for the candida.

An overgrowth of candida can cause physical symptoms. It can also decrease the beneficial bacteria. Researchers have found a definite relationship between the higher levels of fungal spores and lower levels of the desirable bacteria. This means that the microorganisms are competing for the same limited space and finite supply of nourishment, in the closed ecosystem of the digestive tract. If there are factors that promote the growth of candida, it consumes the resources and the space that would have originally been allotted to the beneficial bacteria (lactobacillus and bifidus). These flora then decrease, limiting their positive role in the digestive process. Lab testing frequently demonstrates this change in balance.

Which came first—the decrease in the friendly flora or the overgrowth of candida? Stable flora are observed in very young children, and it is true that candida is normally present in the gut of most people as a harmless coexisting organism (a commensal). However, if yeast becomes the dominant gut flora, it can become a destructive pathogen and take over in the digestive ecosystem. If the population of candida becomes too large and its strength and virulence increases, candida can cause considerable damage, especially in immune-compromised patients. The yeast can migrate to other tissues and become systemic. Once candida becomes blood born and systemic, then every organ system is at risk. Systemic candidiasis can cause serious damage, particularly to the reproductive system in females once it develops as a chronic urogenital infection.

When candida is present at low levels, especially if there are no symptoms, the patient is not treated. However, when a parasite is present (for example, an amoeba such as *E. histolytica*), even a low-level yeast overgrowth is to be taken much more seriously, since it could become a moderate overgrowth or worse within a brief period of time.

Candida is sometimes a factor in ADD and autism. Overgrowth of candida and other species of yeast, particularly in children, due to overuse of antibiotics and sugar in their diet, can lead to the formation in the gut of abnormal organic acids, which are neurotoxic and have been associated with both attention deficit disorders and autism.

BACTERIAL OVERGROWTH

Anaerobic Bacteria—W. A. Shrader, Jr., M.D.

In the treatment of allergies and digestive illness, when the therapy is not effective, it is often because of overgrowth or infection—dysbiosis. People who have very complex problems may have undiagnosed dysbiosis. Often their symptoms are simply chronic fatigue.

We've found that a useful approach to gastrointestinal problems is to first treat with antibiotics and other therapies for pathogenic organisms and then provide allergy treatment. Almost all the gastrointestinal problems we've been seeing seem to respond to this approach. Our treatments have addressed bacteria such as klebsiella and proteus.

We found that in certain cases, patients had an overgrowth of bacteria that wasn't showing up on lab tests. With some patients the bacteria turn out to be anaerobes—microbes that live in the digestive tract without oxygen, such as bacteroides and *Clostridium difficile*. Although anaerobes make up more than 90 percent of the flora in the colon, they are not directly detectable in lab tests.

IBS and Bacterial Overgrowth

A recent report in the *Journal of the American Medical Association* proposed that in some cases irritable bowel syndrome (IBS) may be caused by the overgrowth of bacteria. IBS affects more than 35 million Americans—and 40 percent of all people with GI problems. IBS has been considered a stress-related disorder, just as ulcers were until the discovery of *H. pylori* bacteria.

IBS is characterized by diarrhea or constipation (altered motility), and increased immune activity, as well as discomfort and bloating associated with meals. Many people with these symptoms also report difficulty with concentration or mental tasks and higher stress levels. Research indicates that 92% of IBS patients share the symptom of bloating, regardless of their primary complaint. Among these patients, 84% of those tested for bacterial overgrowth had positive tests results on a lactulose breath test. Of IBS patients who were treated for small intestine bacterial overgrowth, 75% show improvement.

Like ulcers, these are conditions that tend to become chronic and persist, year in, year out. Many people will be interested to know that IBS can be caused by bacterial overgrowth, which can be treated with medication or with medication and herbs in combination, and resolved relatively quickly. (Reference: H.C. Lin, MD. Small intestinal bacterial overgrowth: a framework for understanding irritable bowel syndrome." *Journal of the American Medical Association* 2004; vol. 292: page 773.)

Testing Indirectly for Anaerobes

To date, there are only indirect ways to identify anaerobes by testing for the metabolic by-products of the bacteria. We use these tests as the basis for drug and allergy therapy, and typically see significant improvement.

There are currently a number of ways to indirectly gain information on anaerobes:

- Antibody testing—Immunosciences Laboratory.
- Organic acids testing—Metametrix and Great Plains Lab.
- Monitoring metabolic by-products—A comprehensive digestive analysis measures various biochemicals in the stool that reflect the health of the digestive tract and possible bacterial overgrowth. These evaluations are available from Great Smokies Diagnostic Laboratory (the CDSA), Doctor's Data, and Meridian Laboratory. Useful information can also be obtained through the tests of Vitamin Diagnostics. (See the Resources for information on all of these labs.)
- This area of testing is still under development and will continue to be refined in the coming years. Currently we use it to obtain indirect information on anaerobic bacteria.

MICROFLORA COMPOSITION IN THE COLON

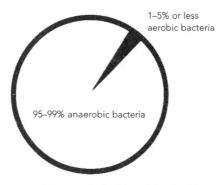

1–5% or less
aerobic bacteria

95–99% anaerobic bacteria

SOURCE: Diagnos-Techs, Kent, WA, © 1995

CHRONIC VIRAL INFECTION

There is evidence that some viruses and even certain viral vaccines are now thought to damage GI lining cells, leading to eventual inflammatory and degenerative diseases of the gut. Many viruses that enter the body through the GI tract can cause systemic disease or disease in other organs. If the GI flora, digestion, or physiology are disrupted, this can lead to impaired gut function and allow viruses easier access to the body. (See chapter 22 for more information on GI viral infections.)

INTEGRATIVE TREATMENT

Treatment involves destroying and clearing harmful bacteria or parasites. If the problem is due to yeast or bacterial overgrowth, treatment may mean minimizing the overgrowth of a microbe that is normally harmless (a commensal yeast or bacteria). These commensals can take over the ecosystem of the digestive tract and crowd out beneficial bacteria. (Also see the information on candida in part V.)

The most destructive of the pathogens are generally the parasites, usually single-celled protozoa such as amoebas. In other cases, overgrowths can involve potentially aggressive species of bacteria, including clostridium, bacterioides, or other anaerobes that are not directly detectable on lab tests. In the stomach, *H. pylori* bacteria has been identified as a causal factor in gastric ulcers. (For more information, see the entry under ulcers in part V.) When these infections or overgrowths persist, they can have major consequences to health.

Treatment Steps

Lab Testing

Drug therapies are designed to target specific organisms—whether they are bacteria, parasites, or yeast—so it is important to have the most complete, accurate laboratory evaluation(s) available. When there are digestive or GI symptoms but the cause is unknown, consider antibody testing (Immunosciences Laboratory) as well as stool testing. There is also value in a comprehensive digestive analysis (Great Smokies Diagnostic Laboratories, Doctor's Data) or other types of testing that include markers for various types of dysfunction (Diagnos-Techs, Great Plains Laboratory). The longer the condition has persisted, the more important it is to get the most definitive lab testing possible.

Preparing for Treatment

Someone weakened by chronic illness may need a period of strengthening before taking medication. Preparing for treatment involves enhanced nutrition and possibly an alternative liver evaluation to be sure the liver can handle the medication. (Consider either genetic testing or a functional liver evaluation, both available from Great Smokies Diagnostic Laboratories.)

Treatment

Your doctor may prescribe antibiotics to combat a bacterial infection, antifungals to reduce candida, or other specific medications against various types of parasites. The objective of treatment is to kill off the targeted microorganisms as completely as possible. Some drugs that are widely used against parasites, such as metronidazole, appear to be losing their effectiveness. This drug-resistance is due to a number of causes, but one thing you can do to assure more effective treatment is to complete the full course of medication. Bacteria and parasites that survive the drug are stronger than those killed off in the first days, so it is essential to be thorough and resolute in treatment. It can also be helpful to follow the medication with a course of herbs. This approach is used by many integrative physicians.

Dosage

The appropriate dosage is important: Microdosages may be helpful in the early stage of treatment. Begin by increasing the dose gradually in order to prevent uncomfortable die-off (see page 183). Then proceed to the full dose for the entire duration. Low dosages have the potential to create a generation of microbes that are drug resistant, having survived the initial dose.

Dosage must also be determined in part by body type and by body weight. A. S. Wheelwright, a famous herbalist, suggested that people tend to have either robust or sensitive body types. The robust types are large-boned and hearty, often have large livers, and are rarely sick. However, because they do not experience low-grade symptoms, they may develop cumulative illnesses. Sensitive body types are more delicate and tend to be more prone to chronic illness.

Die-Off

The die-off reaction typically occurs when you're killing off microorganisms (yeast, fungus, protozoa) at a pace quicker than the eliminative organs (the liver and the GI tract) can competently handle. This can occur when taking drugs or potent botanicals and can be disruptive to the entire body because the eliminative resources must be utilized to minimize the ill effects of the microbes.

The toxic by-products of the microbes can circulate and recirculate through the blood and lymphatics, causing possible symptoms of die-off such as fatigue, achiness, fever, and difficulty with concentration, sometimes resembling a mild case of the flu.

Avoiding Reinfection

It is important to observe the best possible personal hygiene. Effective resolution of these problems often require treating family members or a partner to be sure the microbe in not simply being passed back and forth through food handling, intimate contact, or exposure in the household environment.

Avoiding Overgrowth

In the case of candida and some of the other organisms that tend to overgrow, we have a different situation. It's not that difficult to get rid of candida, but keeping it from overgrowing again can be a problem. It is important to remember that improving GI immune function is the real key when it comes to the overgrowth of organisms like candida. It also involves looking at some of the other steps in the digestive repair process. See chapter 25 on restoring and repairing the GI tract as well as the suggestions on the next several pages.

Parasites, Bacteria, and Candida—Sample Program

JERRY STINE

HISTORY

- The Health Profile (score of 50 or above is significant)
- GI, skin, or upper respiratory symptoms are key (need not be acute)
- Emotional or mental complaints
    - Anxiety or depression
    - Spacey, foggy-headed, poor memory
- Possible factors
    - Exposure to contaminated drinking water, lakes, rivers
    - Exposure to infected family member
    - Dining out at restaurants frequently
    - Extensive antibiotic treatment
    - Travel to third world countries (exposure to parasites)

LAB WORK

- Testing for markers of inflammation, protective antibodies—Immunosciences Lab
- Stool culture—Parasitology Center or Diagnos-Techs

STAGE 1. NUTRITION/LIFESTYLE

- Improve nutrition, decrease starchy diet, moderate carbohydrates (see *40-30-30 Fat Burning Nutrition*, *The South Beach Diet*, and *Atkins for Life*)
- Supplements—individual
- Reduce toxins in personal environment
- Duration—until improvement is seen
- Walking or other exercise
- Meditation or relaxation

STAGE 2. TREATMENT

- Drugs as prescribed by a physician
- Recommended herbs during and after treatment

FOLLOW-UP

- Rehab program—see chapter 25

OTHER TREATMENT OPTIONS

Herbs

Using Drugs and Herbs in Combination—Timothy Kuss, Ph.D.

In an integrative approach, medication and herbs may be prescribed together as two components of a specific program. Additionally, herbs are often used in follow-up to drug therapy. As important as medications are in the treatment of GI infections or overgrowth, they cannot be taken indefinitely. Some are too harsh for the lining of the GI tract or cause nausea unless taken with food. Others may result in certain side effects.

Herbs with General Antimicrobial Properties
(can be used to follow drug therapy; see chapter 37)

Botanical Supplements*

Artemisia	Grapefruit seed extract (NutriBiotic)
Berberine (goldenseal extract)	Olive leaf
Cat's claw	Oregano oil capsules
Garlic or garlic oil capsules	Pau d'arco
Ginger	Tannic acid (Tanalbit)

Mineral-Based Supplements*

Bismuth tablets (Pepto-Bismol)	Elemental iodine (Paracidin)
Colloidal Silver (Allergy Research Group and others)	MSM (sulfur-based formulas of methyl sulfonyl methane)

Antiparasitic Formulas

Artemisinin (Allergy Research Group)	Systemic Formulas
Family Clear (Awareness)	VRM 1 (tapeworms)
Tricycline (Allergy Research Group)	VRM 2 (roundworms)
Para-Relief (Prevail)	VRM 3 (microscopic protozoa)
Parex Intensive Care (Metagenics, available through physicians)	VRM 4 (flukes)

General Antimicrobial Formulas

Biocidin (Biological Research)	DE-P Formula (Osage)
Combat Acute (following antibiotic therapy; helpful against viruses and bacteria)	Grapefruit seed extract
	WO Oil (Systemic Formulas)

*Green herbs can be alternated weekly with mineral-based supplements or bitter herbs.
SOURCE: Timothy Kuss, Ph.D., Infinity Health; Jerry Stine, Lifespan Institute; Omar Amin, Ph.D., Parasitology Center, Inc.

Maintaining Inner Balance with Herbs

Once a course of medication has been completed, it can be helpful to take herbs—which are milder—to prevent reinfection and keep any residual candida overgrowth under control. Although the herbs are natural substances, they too function as antimicrobials to some degree and therefore must be treated with respect just as a drug would be.

If well tolerated, herbs can be taken with every meal to minimize discomfort or bloating after eating. Ideally a different herb is used each week; the botanicals can also be rotated every three days if that is more beneficial. Herbs found effective in improving digestion (especially when there is dysbiosis or overgrowth) include garlic or garlic oil capsules, oregano oil capsules, ginger, and grapefruit seed extract. For example, you may want to begin the first week with garlic, the second week use oil of oregano caps, and the third week take ginger. (See the table on page 185 for additional options.) This type of rotation tends to minimize any reaction due to the overuse of a particular botanical.

Individualizing Your Use of Herbs

Herbs are best begun gradually. To test your tolerance to a particular herb, take one capsule the first day, preferably in the morning and preferably on a weekend. Begin on a day when you will be home for several hours so if a sudden bowel movement or diarrhea develops, you can adjust the dosage or stop the herb. Maintain this low dosage for another day or two and then gradually increase it, building up to four a day—one twenty minutes before each meal and one at bedtime.

If the dosage is too strong, a headache may occur—frequently a sign of toxicity. Occasionally this type of symptom may accompany a healing crisis, but it could also indicate that the herb is not compatible. In that case, stop the herb and retry it in a week. (For additional strategies, see chapter 37 on herbs.)

Nutrition

Diet

Doctors and nutritionists have observed that those who do everything else but do not lower their intake of carbohydrates tend to have greater difficulty restoring inner balance. Minimize or moderate intake of sweet and starchy foods, which are high in carbohydrates. Eat fruits and complex carbohydrates in moderation. Remember that each individual is unique and the ideal diet will vary from person to person. If additional advice is needed, see an integrative physician or a nutritionist.

Digestants

Digestants are the natural substances the body produces to promote good digestion, such as hydrochloric acid and digestive enzymes. The production of these factors may be low in some people due to heredity or can be compromised by GI infection. For those who are low in these factors, supplements can be taken.

If you normally experience discomfort *during a meal*, try betaine hydrochloride and one of the herbs with meals. If you are more likely to experience discomfort *following a meal*, try taking an enzyme product with the herbs.

- *Betaine hydrochloride.* Some people with bacterial or parasitic infections do not have enough hydrochloric acid, which makes them more vulnerable to invading pathogens. This acid is also essential to complete digestion. Hydrochloric acid (HCl) is available in the form of betaine hydrochloride, an extract from beets. Betaine hydrochloride should be taken at the beginning of a meal (see box on page 27 for more information).
- *Pancreatin (pancreatic digestive enzymes).* If the body's enzyme production becomes compromised as a result of infection enzymes may need to be supplemented to maintain digestion. Digestive enzymes come in a variety of forms, including pancreatic enzymes (from an animal source, usually bovine) and vegetarian enzymes. (For additional information on using digestants see chapter 24. For background information see chapter 3.)
  - Enzymes taken *with* meals. If adverse symptoms occur as a result of eating, you will want to explore the use of a good enzyme product. These supplements are taken with a meal to promote more thorough digestion and minimize the sense of bloating or indigestion.
  - Enzymes taken *between* meals. Another complementary strategy is to take enzymes between meals to lower inflammation and minimize microbial overgrowth. Enzymes used for this purpose must be enteric-coated, which enables them to survive the stomach acid.

Nutrition—Len Saputo, M.D.

The health of the mucosal lining of the gut is important in maintaining our resistance, and immune resistance is a powerful determinant controlling which microflora can survive. It is easy to understand that nutritional support for the cells of the gut mucosa is necessary to maintain our most effective defense mechanisms. Some important nutrients that are often used to support gut nutrition and repair include:

- A good multivitamin with minerals
- Vitamin A, 10,000–25,000 IU per day (not for premenopausal women)

- Special nutrients like L-glutamine, phosphatidyl choline, essential fatty acids, magnesium
- Antioxidant support with vitamin C, CoQ$_{10}$, lipoic acid, glutathione, ginkgo biloba, grapeseed extract, vitamin E, betacarotene
- Epidermal growth factor
- Bioflavonoids like quercitin
- Immune stimulants such as deglycyrrhizinated licorice, *Saccharomyces boulardii,* beta glucans, inositol hexaphosphate, echinacea, astragalus, and thymus extract
- Consider juicing with vegetables (one to two quarts per day of fresh veggies)

WHAT IF YOU DON'T GET WELL?

If the problems are caught early enough and the treatment is resolute enough, this may be enough to restore the person to his or her normal way of life, and this entire experience becomes just a memory, something like a bad dream. However, some people find that testing does not provide a definitive diagnosis or that they do not recover after the very first round of antibiotics. In this situation there is value in considering:

1. Treatment to support the whole body and the immune system.
2. A major therapy such as acupuncture, once a month or once a week, as affordable.
3. Additional testing for antibodies (Immunosciences) or for markers of infection (comprehensive digestive analysis). Multiple GI infections could be present. In other cases the infection may be resolved, but function is still compromised as in post-infectious IBS.
4. A lab analysis of general nutrient levels, since the deficiency of one or more essential nutrients has been found to compromise healing. This has been reported in the medical literature in thousands of studies.
5. Other systemic therapy, such as treatment with thymus extract or intravenous vitamin therapy to boost the immune response.
6. Removing other drains on the immune system, such as food allergies (see chapter 20) and environmental toxins (see chapter 23).
7. Rebalancing lifestyle and including walking or gentle exercise.
8. Increased attention to self-nurturance to reduce stress (see especially chapters 44 and 47). However, we now know that conditions such as IBS (like ulcers) can be caused by bacteria or food allergies rather than just stress. Maintain a meaningful life while you and your doctor, working together, sort through the options to find the right combination that heals you.

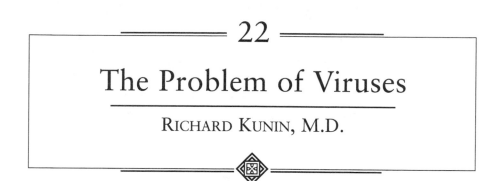

22

The Problem of Viruses

RICHARD KUNIN, M.D.

Whenever possible, use preventive strategies to avoid viral infection. Removing a virus is extremely difficult. We have fewer treatments for viruses, and among the microbes, viruses tend to be some of the most pathogenic and virulent. Our main strategies against viruses at this point are primarily avoidance, and maintenance of strong immunity. Since most viruses are transmitted by contact, personal hygiene is ultimately the best defense.

Viruses are mysterious infective agents. They are capable of passing through filters that retain most bacteria (such as your water filter). They are usually not visible through the light microscope, which meant that for years we were missing them in the lab until the electron microscope was invented. Viruses contain only DNA or RNA, but not both, which is why they are incapable of growth or reproduction apart from living cells. So they must seek out a host in order to grow and multiply. They have a protein coat, which is what our immune antibodies identify in order to detect them.

When it comes to the digestive tract, we often think of the bacteria that cause food poisoning, such as salmonella or *E. coli*. But we should also be taking viruses seriously. When we have the flu we remember all over again how formidable viruses can be. They are also an ongoing problem because they mutate and new strains emerge. This should motivate us to sustain our nutrient levels, preserve our immunity, and maintain basic hygiene.

FOCAL AREA OF SYMPTOMS

Mouth

Cold sores (herpes and aphthous stomatitis) are usually caused by the herpes virus. Lowered immune resistance is a big factor. Treatment with a liquid sodium selenite gargle three times per day for five days can be soothing. Vitamin C gargle has also been helpful. The amino acid lysine has been found effective in the case of herpes mouth ulcers, and along with vitamins A, B complex, and E and the mineral zinc tends to be generally preventive of cold sores.

The lymphoid tissue in the tonsils and adenoids (also known as Waldeyer's ring) is a common site of viral and bacterial invasion and combat. Most sore throats are relieved by the local application of vitamin E. The synthetic d-alpha-tocopherol is better tasting, though recent evidence suggests gamma-tocopherol may be a stronger antioxidant. The low 100 IU dose is usually appreciated for its soothing qualities and anti-inflammatory effect. General immune enhancers include echinacea, goldenseal, vitamin C, garlic, and pau d'arco.

Stomach and Upper GI Tract

Inflammation in the upper intestine by viruses and other microbes usually sends a signal to the lower tract via the nerve networks of the bowel. This can promote bloating and disturb motility along the length of the gut.

Intestinal viruses (enteroviruses) often cause intestinal complaints, even though they are especially identified with respiratory tract symptoms. In fact, they can also cause neurological symptoms.

Paralysis is associated with several of the enteroviruses: Coxsackie A7, echovirus 4,6, enterovirus 71, and polio viruses 1–3. The Coxsackie virus group B is also known to cause inflammation of the brain, heart, lungs, and pancreas, leaving some infected children with Type I diabetes. Herpangina syndrome is a painful rash on the palate and pharynx in children, and is caused by the Coxsackie virus. Persistence of Coxsackie viral infections is known to occur and may be a cause of chronic fibromyalgia and chronic fatigue syndromes. One clue is that such infections induce interferon alpha and beta production in the infected cells, which can be measured by blood tests.

Epidemic intestinal viruses, such as rotavirus, Norwalk virus, astrovirus, and adenovirus 40 and 41 that cause gastroenteritis typically travel in epidemics. This makes diagnosis a bit easier. Adenovirus usually expresses itself as pneumonia, with diarrhea as a frequent accompaniment. Poliomyelitis begins with nausea and diarrhea and can be mistaken for flu. Paralysis occurs in only a small number of cases, so misdiagnosis is common.

Measles in the GI tract is important because it can persist and cause reinfection, even years or decades later. It has been reported in the dendritic immune cells of the intestine, but this finding remains controversial. However, it is known that the measles virus binds to receptors on T cell lymphocytes (the CD46 receptors). Binding to the receptor inactivates the T cell and also appears to suppress transmembrane signaling by the lymphocytes, inhibiting the activation of nearby immune cells.

This causes localized immune deficiency and would explain some cases of chronic inflammatory bowel disease in which measles appears to cause inflammation indirectly, by creating vulnerability to secondary infection. Such infections might involve microbes that are normally noninvasive, but which cause symptoms due to the local immune suppression induced by the latent measles virus. Because the secondary infection can be caused by any of a great number of microbes (yeast, bacteria, or parasite species), the syndrome is extremely individual and the diagnosis elusive.

It is helpful to know that the invasiveness (virulence) of measles is reduced by vitamin A (retinol) supplements. By that token it makes sense to measure vitamin A levels and treat bowel disease with vitamin A at restorative doses. Of course vitamin A is essential for immune response in general, and as an integral part of cellular healing. In addition the use of Monolaurin, which contains lauric acid, a fatty acid that binds to the fatty coat of the measles virus, is also worthy of consideration in treating dysbiosis of the intestine.

Lower Small Intestine (Ileum) and Colon

There remains a surprising amount of confusion over the role of viral infection in chronic bowel disease. From my own clinical observation and experience, I am inclined to consider the herpes virus as an additional inflammatory factor, especially since this family of viruses is notorious for reinfection under conditions of stress or tissue inflammation from other, unrelated causes. Herpes I and II both thrive when the host's defenses are down and serve to amplify inflammation and aggravate the damage to the bowel lining at such times. There is undoubtedly interaction between food allergy and viral infection—both ways.

The Liver

Inflammation of the pancreas and liver are common in viral illness. Hepatitis virus A, B, and C and hepatitis due to the Epstein-Barr virus (the cause of mononucleosis) can all cause loss of appetite, nausea, vomiting, bile retention, and impaired digestive function that can go on for weeks, months, or years. The use of N-acetyl-cysteine 500 mg, milk thistle 300 mg, lipoic acid 100 mg, and ascorbic acid 1000 mg—all taken three times per day for a couple of weeks—has been associated with remarkable recoveries. These viruses can often be measured in blood by testing for antibody levels (titer) for IgG antibodies (gradual onset) and IgM antibodies (acute episode).

Anal and Perineal Area

Venereal warts are caused by viral activity in the anal area and are becoming more and more common. They can be difficult to eradicate. When the venereal warts become enlarged and covered by a fibrous coat, they are best removed by a CO_2 laser. (Preventive measures: Sexual contact is the means by which this infection is acquired and spread to others. Condoms tend to be generally preventive.)

Herpes viruses are especially common in the anal canal and associated with hemorrhoids, rectal prolapse, and perineal blisters. Treatment with Monolaurin capsules taken orally and local salve or cream are a safe adjunct in quelling herpes infections and deserves a trial for at least a week. Doses up to five capsules three times per day have been helpful in my experience. Local application of skin cream containing lemon balm (melissa), lysine, or lithium have all claimed success. Of course if herpes antibody tests are positive, the use of antiviral agents such as acyclovir (Zovirax) is standard. I prefer Monolaurin, however, due to its safety, its lack of adverse effects, and its broad spectrum of activity against lipid-coated viruses.

Richard Kunin, M.D., is founder and president of the Society for Orthomolecular Health-Medicine, and he has been active in private practice in nutritional medicine and psychiatry since 1963. He took his medical degree at the University of Minnesota and was an NIH Special Fellow in neurophysiology at the Stanford University. Dr. Kunin is a diplomate in psychiatry and has served as an instructor at Cornell University School of Medicine and the College of Osteopathic Medicine of the Pacific, and was consultant to the state of California in mental health research. He is the author of the best-sellers *MegaNutrition* and *MegaNutrition for Women,* and he has given more than sixty presentations worldwide on a wide variety of topics in nutrition. Dr. Kunin has a private medical practice in orthomolecular health-medicine in San Francisco and can be reached at (415) 346-2500.

The Society of Orthomolecular Health-Medicine can be contacted at 2698 Pacific Avenue, San Francisco, CA 94115, or by calling (415) 922-6462.

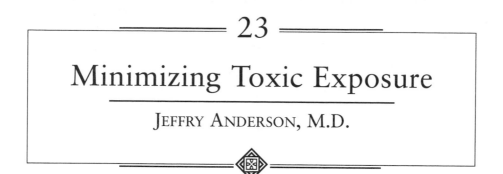

23

Minimizing Toxic Exposure

Jeffry Anderson, M.D.

For the average American, toxic exposure is subtle and yet ever present. To minimize ongoing exposure, it's important to think about the source of your water, the safety of your food, chemicals in everyday products, and other exposures in your environment. The primary concept of environmental medicine is to diminish the load—the burden on your body—and to stop further exposure. Some people tend to be more sensitive to toxins than others. Both low-level exposure through water, food, cosmetic products, our homes and gardens, and even the mercury filllings in our teeth and intense exposure from industrial environments, toxic buildings, and other occupational hazards can cause a wide variety of symptoms in the GI tract and throughout the body.

MINIMIZING LOW-LEVEL EXPOSURE

Chemicals in Water

As many as 45 million Americans are supplied with tap water that fails to meet basic health standards. This was the finding of the Environmental Working Group (EWG) in a review of federal and state records for 1994 to 1995. Updated studies indicate that our water continues to be contaminated from multiple sources. Here's what the EWG found: More than 25 million people used water contaminated by bacteria, with more than 12,000 system violations! Another 5 million had lead levels above standard, meriting more than 3,500 violations. Inadequate treatment was a problem for 20 million consumers.

Federal and state sources also reflect contamination with chemicals and pesticides in the water of a million people. But a separate EWG study, focused just on agricultural states, found that more than 14 million people used tap water routinely contaminated with five major herbicides.

The Centers for Disease Control and the U.S. Environmental Protection Agency have advised anyone with a compromised immune system to consult a physician before drinking ordinary tap water. The American Water Works Association, a trade group for water utilities, advises all individuals with the HIV virus to boil tap water before drinking it.

Worth the Effort

Sarah had been sick for about 14 years. She knew she was getting better a little bit at a time, but the source of her GI inflammation remained an unknown to both Sarah and her doctors. When she began reading up on pesticides, the size and extent of the problem overwhelmed her and she decided to eat more organics. Since her menu was quite restricted, it wasn't hard to switch over, so she began buying everything organic—just as an experiment. She was astonished to realize that her symptoms were better! Clearly not the whole answer, but eating food free of chemicals seemed to reduce the inflammation—perhaps 10 or 15 percent.

She was so encouraged that when she learned fluoride can also be an irritant, she switched toothpastes as well and began using baking soda and hydrogen peroxide. To her amazement, more improvement! And the improvement has lasted. Definitely worth doing.

Sources of exposure: Water often contains fluoride (added for the prevention of cavities) and chlorine; by-products of chlorine interaction (THMs); pesticides, herbicides, and inorganic fertilizer chemicals such as nitrates; heavy metals, including lead; petrochemical derivatives, PCBs, and dioxins; and radioactive compounds such as radium, radon, and uranium, as well as organic matter and bacteria.

Solutions: Clearly this is a complex subject. One ideal water source is bottled mountain spring water tested for purity and rich trace mineral content, stored in glass; ask the vendor to send you a copy of the results on its water testing. If you decide to buy a water filter or filtration system, you'll probably want to do some reading and talk with more than one vendor. If you have specific requirements or well water, have your water tested before you select the filter. Each system offers benefits and has drawbacks. Reverse osmosis (RO) filters remove more contaminants from the water than any other system. Ceramic and carbon block filters are both respected as decent filters. Microwater units that alkalinize water appear to be useful in reducing an acid state in the body.

Information on Municipal and County Water

Call your county water system.

Environmental Defense Fund, www.scorecard.org. Reports on water quality by state and county.

Environmental Working Group, www.ewg.org. Reports on water quality by state and county.

EPA's Safe Drinking Water Hotline. (800) 426-4791, www.epa.gov/water

Information on Bottled Water

International Bottled Water Association, IBEW in Virginia, (800) 928-3711, www.bottledwater.org. Bottlers of water need to meet certain standards to be members of the IBEW.

Bottled Water Web, www.bottledwaterweb.com/links.html; useful links on the topic of bottled water.

Before purchasing home delivery of bottled water, you may want to request testing information directly from the vendor.

Testing Your Tap or Well Water

Internet resources can be accessed under *water testing* or specific topics such as *lead testing*. You can also find extensive entries under *water filters* and *water filtration*.

You may also want to check your local yellow pages, under headings such as *water testing*, *environmental and ecological services*, and *laboratories, analytical*.

Information on Sources of Clean Water

A'o, Lono Kahuna Kupa. *Don't Drink the Water*. Lotus Press, 2004.

Consumer Reports, January 2003.

Stauffer, Julie. *The Water You Drink: Safe or Suspect?* New Society Publishers, 2004.

Environmental Advocates

Environmental Working Group (EWG), Washington, D.C., (202) 667-6982, www.ewg.org

Clean Water Action, Washington, D.C., (202) 895-0420, www.cleanwateraction.org

World Water Council, Marseille, France, www.worldwatercouncil.org

Chemicals in Our Food

Sources of exposure: The United States uses a fifth of the world's pesticides—more than 4.5 billion pounds a year, all sources totaled. Specific pesticide use in the United States has averaged from 1.2 to 1.5 billion pounds a year, yearly for the past twenty years. In developing nations many pesticides banned here and in Europe are in common use. Worldwide use of specific pesticides is 6 billion pounds every year.

Minimizing Toxins in Your Water

Source or Filter	Advantages	Disadvantages
Tap water Call your water district and check www.ewg.org	Inexpensive, available, may be good; boil for fifteen to twenty minutes to remove chlorine, bacteria, some parasites	Chlorine, fluoride, heavy metals, THMs; can contain cryptosporidium, giardia, and other parasites and their cysts
Bottled water Request testing information from vendor before ordering water service; sources of water include natural spring, distilled, or filtered municipal water; check label	Usually tested and prefiltered; spring water may be a good natural source of minerals	Soft and even hard plastic containers off gas toxic compounds, including plasticizers (phthalates), vinyl chloride, bisphenol-A (an endocrine disrupter); glass is still best
Ceramic carbon filters Two-step filtration— compacted activated carbon and porous ceramic	Removes most bacteria and parasites, cysts, sediment, chlorine, some radioactive pollutants, most solvents, pesticides, and chemicals, some heavy metals	Doesn't remove fluoride or certain heavy metals, viruses, or very small microbes
Carbon block, **activated carbon** Check manufacturer's specifications	Removes chlorine, solvents, and pesticides, some radioactive contaminants	Doesn't remove bacteria, heavy metals, some radioactive compounds, asbestos, or fluoride
Mechanical filters, some impregnated with silver compounds	Filters out debris, bacteria, large parasites, and cysts down to 1 or .5 microns; bacteriostatic also kills some bacteria	Does not remove chlorine, fluoride, asbestos, THMs, most volatile chemicals, including solvents or pesticides, or heavy metals
Reverse osmosis filters	Removes almost everything, except radon, pesticides, and volatile organic chemicals; to compensate, many systems come with add- on carbon filtration units	Also removes good minerals and makes water "lifeless"; may supplement with unit to add minerals back in; requires periodic filter change or back-flushing with chlorine; can out- gas plastic compounds into water, requiring additional filtration step

Source or Filter	Advantages	Disadvantages
Granulated, activated charcoal, typically in small portable filters and some prefilters (best is a unit that filters to 1 micron absolute)	Better than no filtration; removes THMs, chlorine, mercury, some chemicals, large parasites, particulates	Doesn't remove bacteria or protozoa under 4 microns, asbestos, most radioactive compounds, some heavy metals, or fluoride
Alkaline water, with granulated activated charcoal prefilter, impregnated with silver; can be linked to carbon block for additional filtration	Can restore normal acid-base balance in the body and aid detoxification; may be linked with another filtration system as a prefilter	Same limitations as other granulated charcoal filters; best in combination with a prefilter; misses viruses, fluoride, chemicals, and heavy metals
Shower filters	Removes some chlorine that off-gases while you shower	

About half of our produce and a third of our grains are reported by the FDA to have pesticides residues. However, by their own report, 90 percent of wheat samples tested contain residues. And the Environmental Working Group found that illegal pesticide levels on imported produce tended to be about twice as high as those reported—averaging 7 percent on some, but contaminating as much as 50 percent of the crop in other cases (in 1992 to 1993 records).

Meat, dairy products, and poultry may have traces of pesticides, hormones, antibiotics, tranquilizers, steroids, or other drugs. Fish and shellfish may contain mercury, lead, arsenic, cadmium, chromium, and chemicals such as dioxins and PCBs.

Least expensive strategy: Residues on some vegetables can be minimized by peeling. Buy produce in season as possible, since imported produce tends to have higher levels of residues and more illegal residues (since pesticide laws in some countries are less strict than ours). Some fruits and vegetables have been found to be typically low in residues when tested. Others consistently test high, sometimes because of the way they must be grown or stored. These are to be minimized or bought organically.

Most thorough strategy: If you have access to certified organic produce and products, that's definitely the best option. You will taste the difference and you may even notice a difference in your health. In part this is because truly organic products are not only free of pesticide residues, but are also raised in soil that is more nutrient rich. Testing has shown increased nutrients in organically raised vegetables from 50 to 200 percent! Although organics tend to be a little more expensive, you may come out ahead because of reduced health care costs.

Helpful Publications

Cummins, Ronnie, and Ben Lilliston. *Genetically Engineered Food: A Self-Defense Guide for Consumers.* Marlowe & Company, 2004.

E Magazine, Marion, Ohio, subscription number: (800) 967-6572

Haas, Elson, M.D. *The Staying Healthy Shopper's Guide.* Celestial Arts, 1999.

Hart, Kathleen. *Eating in the Dark: America's Experiment with Genetically Engineered Food.* Pantheon, 2002.

Harte, John, and others. *Toxins A to Z: A Guide to Everyday Pollution Hazards.* University of California Press, 1991.

Lyman, Howard, and Glen Merzer. *Mad Cowboy: Plain Truth from the Cattle Rancher Who Won't Eat Meat.* Scribner, 1998.

Rifkin, Jeremy. *Beyond Beef.* Plume Books, 1993.

Robbins, John, and Dean Ornish, M.D. *Food Revolution: How Your Diet Can Help Save Your Life and Our World.* Conari, 2001.

Organizations

Environmental Working Group (EWG), Washington, D.C., (202) 667-6982, www.ewg.org

Mothers for Natural Law, www.safe-food.org. Information on genetically modified food

National Coalition against the Misuse of Pesticides (NCAMP), www.beyondpesticides.org

National Resources Defense Council (NRDC), Washington, D.C., (202) 289-6868, or San Francisco, (415) 777-0220, www.nrdc.org

Pesticide Action Network of North America (PANNA), www.panna.org

Safe Tables Our Priority (STOP), www.safetables.org. Information and advocacy on the issue of foodborne illness, including microbial food contamination.

Toxins in the Home and Garden

Sources of exposure: Solvents such as turpentine, paint and paint thinner, paint and wax strippers, spot removers, degreasers, gasoline. Pesticides in home and garden bug sprays, pet sprays, flea collars, and pest strips have been consistently linked to higher rates of cancer.

When Organic Food Isn't Available

Strategy	Specifics
Wash vegetables thoroughly.	Vegetable washes (usually based on coconut oil) appear to be helpful; dish detergent got mixed reviews as a vegetable wash.
Peel fruits and vegetables.	High residues on skin or outer leaves can be reduced by peeling. Fruits: apples, bananas, grapefruit, oranges, pears. Vegetables: lettuce, corn (mixed reviews).
Buy in season.	Imported vegetables have higher residues in testing and more violations, since some chemicals allowed are illegal in the United States.
Avoid foods that test very high for residues of known or illegal toxins.	Fruits: strawberries, peaches and other stone fruits, grapes. Vegetables: celery, bell peppers, green beans, spinach, leafy greens, cucumbers. Staples: wheat (90%), rice.
Avoid produce frequently treated with systemic toxins.	Systemic toxins are absorbed and can't be washed off. Toxins in animal products are systemic by nature. In plants, they're found in produce such as broccoli, cabbage, celery, cauliflower, cucumbers, green beans, lettuce, potatoes and other root vegetables, spinach, tomatoes. Fruits: grapes, cantaloupe, watermelon, peaches and other stone fruits, strawberries.
Know the source of seafood.	Buy your seafood from a source you trust; inquire; keep up with current information to see what's safe.
Shop wisely.	Buy grains in bulk; support your local cooperatives and buying clubs.
Shop selectively.	Buy the most important foods organic—baby food, dairy products, meats, staple grains such as rice and wheat.

Solutions: If your exposure is from the home or garden, it may mean changing the products you use and shifting to organic gardening and nontoxic solutions to household maintenance. A number of excellent resource books can guide you in solutions. Some of the books, for example, offer simple, nontoxic alternatives to household cleaning products. Others provide solutions to complex problems, such as building materials or furnishings. Mail-order catalogs can be useful when purchasing specialty products.

• Reframe your expectations. If you and your family want to be safe from toxic exposure, you may not be able to have an effortless, picture-perfect lawn with no crabgrass. On the other hand, consider the possibilities. Minimizing the use of toxins on your lawn may mean planting hardy weed-resistant species of grass, or going for a more natural look by putting in a rock garden, or planting part of your yard in wildflowers or ivy.

- You can have a wonderful garden using the clever techniques of integrated pest management. These strategies minimize the use of toxins and also nurture the land and the environment. Plant flowers and crops that repel pests, develop healthy soil, mulch for weeds, alternate your crops (intercropping) and rotate them, water your garden deeply and frequently, and encourage natural predators (a ladybug farm).

Helpful Reading

Berthold-Bond, Annie. *Better Basics for the Home: Simple Solutions for Less Toxic Living*. Three Rivers Press, 1999.

Berthold-Bond, Annie. *Clean and Green*. Ceres Press, 1994.

Garrett, Howard, and Malcolm Beck. *The Organic Manual*. Tapestry Press, 2002.

Moses, Marien. *Designer Poisons*. San Francisco: Pesticide Education Center, 1995. An in-depth review of the research on toxins in our foods and homes, including the dangers they pose to children. For more information, see www.pesticides.org.

Organic Gardening, Rodale Press, Emmaus, PA, (800) 763-2531; a magazine and books.

Wolverton, B. C. *How to Grow Fresh Air: 50 Houseplants that Purify Your Home or Office*. Penguin, 1997.

Resources

The Bio-Integral Resource Center (BIRC), www.birc.org.

Co-op America, Washington, D.C., (202) 872-5307, www.coopamerica.org. Publishes the *National Green Pages*.

Ecomall. A virtual environmental shopping center at www.ecomall.com.

Real Goods. Products for an ecologically sustainable future at www.realgoods.com.

Chemicals in Cosmetic Products

Sources of exposure: Many everyday personal products contain additives that can be harmful to the GI tract, including fluoride (in most toothpastes) and toothpaste additives—propylene glycol (major constituent of antifreeze!), sodium lauryl sulfate, DEA (di-ethanolamine). People who are highly sensitive will find that inhaled substances from fabric softeners, colognes, and even scented laundry detergents may make their GI symptoms worse. Some familiar products are actually quite toxic: for example, lindane is still widely used as a treatment by prescription for lice in children, despite its known neurotoxicity and bioaccumulation!

Become informed about which additives are toxic and then read labels avidly. Consider shifting to simpler products—those without coloring, scents, or complex chemicals. Most health food stores carry a line of safe, nontoxic toothpastes, shampoos, deodorants, and cosmetics. Even there it is important to read labels; for example, some brands of toothpaste in the health food store now contain fluoride. When you note the caution on toothpaste labels, you'll notice that the toothpaste manufacturers label fluoride as a toxin and caution not to allow children to swallow it! Since these products are widespread, a realistic goal is not total avoidance but minimizing exposure.

Helpful Reading

Steinham, David. *The Safe Shopper's Bible: A Consumer's Guide to Nontoxic Household Products, Cosmetics, and Food.* John Wiley & Sons, 1995.

Winter, Ruth. *A Consumer's Dictionary of Food Additives, 5th ed.* Three Rivers Press, 1999.

Resources

American Environmental Health Foundation, Dallas, (214) 361-9515, www.aehf.com. Catalog of environmentally safe products and books on related topics.

Effects of Mercury Amalgam Fillings

Mercury (along with silver and tin) are found in dental fillings (mercury-silver amalgams). These metals may promote antibiotic-resistant gut bacteria and cause harmful overgrowth (dysbiosis); species include klebsiella, citrobacter, and proteus. Mercury is released from dental fillings continuously in very small amounts, but can accumulate in the body in dangerous amounts. Mercury-silver amalgams have been outlawed in Europe and Scandinavia for several decades.

Symptoms: People with long-standing multiple mercury-silver fillings (dental amalgams) often suffer diverse generalized problems associated with chronic low-level toxicity from mercury and tin (another component of amalgam). Typical symptoms include problems with the nervous or immune systems, metabolic disorders, and GI dysfunction.

Solutions: Consider having your amalgams removed and replaced if possible.

Referral Sources

Environmental Dental Association, (800) 388-8124. For book orders call EDA at (619) 586-7626. To receive a list of alternative dentists, send a self-addressed stamped envelope with $5.60 postage to EDA, P.O. Box 2184, Rancho Santa Fe, CA 92067.

For additional dental health resources see www.holisticmed.com/dental/dental.res

LONG-TERM OR HIGH-INTENSITY EXPOSURE

Sick Building Syndrome

These exposures are frequent or long-term, such as one might get on the job, and are characterized by poor ventilation and a high level of synthetic materials, such as certain paints, some synthetic carpets and underpadding, adhesives, formaldehyde, sealers, waxes, disinfectants, cleaning agents, photocopier solution and toner, pesticide applications, and PCBs (from older electrical equipment, fluorescent light transformers) in tightly insulated buildings that lack adequate ventilation and outdoor air exchange. Environmental testing can be obtained for some of the potential allergens and toxins in the home. This may include testing indoor air for formaldehyde and other toxins out-gassed from various materials such as Sheetrock, particle board, insulation, and synthetic carpeting.

For example, the pesticide of choice for termite control was traditionally chlordane (an organochloride) until it was banned because of its extreme toxicity. Many homes were treated with chlordane for decades, from the 1950s through the 1970s. It was often injected into the soil under the house. Like DDT, it persists, and since it has a half-life of centuries, it continues to be released. Chlordane causes low-level chlordane toxicity, contaminating the breathable air inside the treated house. So if you live in a house built before 1980, check any records on termite treatment. It can also be detected by testing the soil under the house.

Helpful Reading

Alvord, Kate. *Divorce Your Car!* New Society Publishers, 2000.

Chrias, Daniel. *The Natural House.* Chelsea Green Publishing Co., 2000.

Dadd, Debra. *Home Safe Home.* Tarcher/Putnam, 1997. Resources for a safer home environment

Pearson, David. *The New Natural House Book.* Fireside Books, 1998.

Rogers, Sherry. *Chemical Sensitivity.* McGraw-Hill/Contemporary Books, 1998. A good brief review of the health effects of toxic exposure.

Other Resources

American Environmental Health Foundation, Dallas, (214) 361-9515, www.aehf.com. An online catalog of environmentally safe products, books, and videos.

The Cutting Edge, Southampton, N.Y., (800) 497-9516, www.cutcat.com. Another good online product catalog.

Occupational and Industrial Exposures

Exposures: These concerns are often associated with the use of chemicals on the job, such as pesticides (agricultural and pest-control workers and landscapers); solvents (building trades); PCBs, dioxins, and hundreds of thousands of other chemicals (heavy industry, chemical manufacturing); and petroleum and its by-products (the petrochemical industry).

Acute, intense exposure from a single incident: An intense occupational exposure, an industrial accident, or a spill can involve solvents, pesticides, agricultural activities such as crop dusting and aerial spraying, petroleum spills, and other sources of exposure.

Helpful Reading

These books, written for health care professionals, provide a wealth of information for both professionals and consumers. They are most often available through medical libraries, environmental groups, or the publishers.

Hayes, W., and E. Laws, eds. *Handbook of Pesticide Toxicology.* Academic Press, 1991. A foundational text, out of print but available.

Keifer, M.C., ed. *Human Health Effects of Pesticides.* Hanley & Belfus, Inc., 1997. One of the most important books written on this topic, it offers compelling evidence on the risks of pesticide exposure.

Rea, William. *Chemical Sensitivity.* Lewis Publishers Inc., 1995. Another essential text.

DIAGNOSING TOXIC EXPOSURE

There are a number of tests available to detect the presence of toxins in the body or assess their effects. These tests apply to health conditions that result from long-term exposure, whether low level, moderate, or of high intensity. Some of the tests may also apply to acute, short-term exposures.

Assessing environmental factors in illness: There are objective lab tests that can be very useful in diagnosing both digestive and systemic illness with an environmental component. A detailed history of environmental exposure is key to determining the probable sources. Remember, many toxins and pollutants accumulate over a lifetime (stored in body tissues), and can have both additive and synergistic effects (one magnifying another). Certain chemicals can accumulate in what is known as the total load, or the total body burden of toxins. Therefore it's important to begin assessing and minimizing all your exposures. Once you begin to think in this way, you'll also want to use this approach to protect your children, by avoiding exposures from birth (or even before!).

Testing GI Consequences

There are a limited number of tests of the gastrointestinal system that provide objective markers of gut damage. Unfortunately there are no available practical affordable tests for heavy metals specifically in the gut.

- Secretory IgA in mucus, stool, or saliva
- Intestinal permeability, which tests for leaky gut syndrome
- Digestive stool analysis (CDSA) to measure digestion and absorption
- Measures of liver function—the functional detox panel (Great Smokies Diagnostic Lab)
- Testing for parasites and candida or other microbes, which tend to occur more often when the integrity of digestion has been stressed and challenged by toxins

These tests are all discussed in greater detail in the testing section, chapters 14 through 18. If the GI testing identifies a problem area and you have evidence for the presence of toxicity, there is a strong possibility that the exposure to toxins has compromised your digestive function. This provides the basis for developing a strategy. When there is a high likelihood that environmental influences are contributing to your illness, seriously consider seeing a good environmental physician. Check with the American Academy of Environmental Medicine, a source for referrals at (316) 684-5500, www.aaem.com.

HEAVY METAL EXPOSURE

The metals involved are mercury (Hg), lead (Pb), cadmium (Cd), chromium (Cr), nickel (Ni), tin (Sn), arsenic (As).

Sources of Exposure

- *Devices or materials placed in your body:* mercury/silver dental amalgams (mercury, tin), remnants of orthopedic surgical procedures (stainless steel screws, pins, plates, nails, wires—nickel).

- *Residential/commercial:* paints (old lead paint, marine and masonry paint); rodenticides, fungicides, pesticides (mercury, arsenic, thallium), old plumbing, with brass fittings or soldered lead joints.
- *Industrial/occupational/hobbies:* soldering, welding, foundry work, jewelry making, artist's materials, especially paints (cadmium); multiple industries.

Testing: Toxicological Assays

- *Hair analysis (quantitative):* Inexpensive, but not always accurate or reliable.
- *24-hour urine:* Measures actual content of body (quantitative) by output of toxic metal(s). More expensive, but very accurate and reliable. This assessment can be enhanced by administering a pharmaceutical *chelating agent* (such as DMSA, DMPS, or penicillamine) by injection or by mouth that "pulls out" heavy metals bound in tissue, acting as a specialized molecular magnet. This is called a chelation challenge.
- *Blood testing:* Most appropriate for acute or high-intensity occupational or industrial exposures. Not applicable to long-term low-level or midlevel exposures.
- *Biological marker assay:* Measures key metabolic products in blood, urine, or stool of hemoglobin synthesis and breakdown (called porphyrins) and associated enzymes, often abnormal in type or amount due to heavy metal toxic damage, and can produce serious neurological, dermatological (skin), and metabolic symptoms.

PESTICIDE EXPOSURE

Due to the extremely wide use of many diverse types of pesticides, these chemicals are virtually impossible to avoid (they include insecticides, fungicides, herbicides, rodenticides, agricultural fumigants, and structural fumigants/wood preservatives). Although pesticides are composed of a wide range of chemical types and molecular structures, almost all share similar toxic effects on tissues and organs. Many classes of these chemicals are designed to be toxic to the nervous systems of insects, and are toxic to the human nervous system as well. They can also cause problems to our gastrointestinal and respiratory systems; many of these chemicals are clearly toxic to the immune system, others are documented to be harmful to bone marrow, and many are cancer promoting.

Organophosphates and Carbamates

The combination of heavy metals (particularly mercury) and pesticides (such as organophosphates and carbonates) can have devastating effects on GI health. These toxins can injure the nerve and muscle function of the GI tract. In particular they can affect the visceral nerves that innervate the GI tract, creating a type of impairment comparable to neuropathy. Toxic effects can also damage the muscle cells. These injuries have the potential to cause motility problems in GI disorders such as irritable bowel syndrome, resulting in spasms or cramping.

Inflammation is another consequence that occurs through a different mechanism, as a "side effect" of the immune response. Inflammation can also impair normal nerve and muscle function and even more profoundly affect the lining of the digestive tract.

These chemicals, most frequently used as agricultural and residential insecticides, degrade rapidly in the soil, where they're broken down by microorganisms, but can persist for weeks on "inert" surfaces such as wood, metal, stone, or concrete. They are very difficult to measure directly in the tissue or blood. These classes of pesticides include malathion, parathion, chlorpyrifos, Diazinon, aldicarb, and carbaryl.

How they harm: They can damage the body by inhibiting an enzyme that is essential to the function of the entire nervous system (acetylcholinesterase, or AChE).

Testing: Markers in the body chemistry for AChE are relevant to both acute and long-term exposure. They can be measured through a blood test in plasma (less expensive but less accurate) or red blood cells (more expensive and highly accurate). In acute and chronic exposures significant depression of AChE can occur.

Organochlorines

Organochlorines include DDT and chlordane, which have been illegal for a number of years but are still found in abnormal levels in most individuals tested, due to slow breakdown. For this reason high levels of DDT and chlordane can still be found in a large percentage of the population. Common organochlorines currently in use include lindane, dieldrin, and hexachlorobenzene, among others.

These widely used pesticides are characterized by slow breakdown and long persistence in the environment and the body (years or decades). Exposure can occur through water, food, air, or skin absorption. Although we don't yet know all the mechanisms by which they work, we do know for certain they are endocrine disrupters, even in minute exposures. These toxins have the greatest impact on fetal development, growing children, and adolescents. Organochlorides are also known to be carcinogens. They are all neurotoxins, and the organs most vulnerable to this damage are the brain, liver, kidneys, heart, and reproductive tissue. Organochlorides have been found to inhibit essential energy-dependent functions in the cell.

Other classes of chemicals characterized by relatively slow breakdown include herbicides, chlorphenoxy acids (such as 2,4-D and 2,4,5-T) and nitro-phenolics (including DNOC and DNBP). Other classes of chemicals that share certain characteristics with organochlorines include industrial chemicals such as PCBs and dioxins. These chemicals also tend to persist in the environment, are highly toxic to the nervous system, and are known as endocrine disrupters. They are actively used in manufacturing and continue to be released into our environment as contaminants.

General assessment includes measurement of organ/tissue damage or dysfunction. Markers for toxics can be measured in blood or in fat, which provides direct measurement of chemical or by-products of breakdown (metabolites). A fat biopsy is especially important in accessing chronic exposure.

SOLVENTS

Solvent exposure is common in the household and in certain occupations, especially for painters and artists, people working in the field of electronics, in the petroleum industry or gas stations, and in gardening or landscaping.

Testing involves direct measure in urine or blood, or through a biopsy of fat tissue. This is particularly important for both solvents and organochloride pesticides.

- Biological markers, which measure damage done by toxins
- Measures of the integrity of the immune system—levels of antibodies and T and B cells
- Specific tests to measure neurological function—brain scans, PET scans, EEGs, neuropsychological performance tests

You may find you have underlying damage from long-term low-level exposures, as inflammation and dysfunction can continue even after the day-to-day exposure has been eliminated. Although the day-to-day exposures may be eliminated, you may still have the toxins in your body, stored in fat and tissue (chemicals and pesticides) or in bone (heavy metals). Until you completely detoxify you will probably continue to have problems.

So eliminating the external sources of exposure is important, and you may feel better rather quickly. But to get totally well you may need to go through a more long-term detox to get rid of what has already accumulated in your body. The goals are to eliminate the toxins you may already have accumulated, which are already doing damage, and to lighten any additional burden from your current environment. Toxins stored in the body can continue to challenge digestion and overload the liver. If you have developed chronic degenerative diseases in addition to the GI problems, it is essential that you absolutely eliminate toxic exposure. Otherwise it becomes extremely difficult to overcome these problems.

Resources

Chemical Injury Information Network, (406) 547-2255, www.ciin.org. The Network provides a newsletter, bibliography, and a research service on chemical injury.

American Environmental Health Foundation, Dallas, (800) 428-2343 or (214) 361-9515, www.aehf.com. Extensive catalog of environmentally safe products, including those for the home and garden and for personal care, as well as furnishings, building products, water filters, and books.

Additional Helpful Reading

Brown, Lester, et al. *The Earth Policy Reader*. W. W. Norton & Company, 2002.

Hill, Julia Butterfly. *One Makes the Difference: Inspiring Actions That Change Our World*. HarperSanFrancisco, 2002. Inspirational stories, practical actions steps, and resources.

Suzuki, David, and Holly Dussel. *Good News for a Change: How Everyday People Are Helping the Planet*. Vancouver: Greystone Books, 2002.

Biographical information for **Jeffry Anderson, M.D.,** appears on page 86.

24

Replacing Digestants and Restoring Flora

THE TEAM

In this chapter we'll look briefly at each of the major elements of digestion—enzymes, hydrochloric acid, bicarbonate, and friendly flora. Why are they important and what can we do to replace and restore them?

It's essential that we digest our food thoroughly. If food goes through the digestive tract partially digested and leaky gut occurs, the leakage of these by-products makes the body a little more toxic and reactive to sensitivities. We also want to avoid the fermentation or putrefaction that can occur if food isn't fully digested.

STOMACH ACID, ENZYMES, AND BICARB

Starch digestion begins in the mouth, through enzymes in saliva. Chewing well enables the food to mix with saliva and be broken down small enough to be well digested. The first step in proper digestion is to slow down and savor your food.

Stomach acid (hydrochloric acid, or HCl for short) protects us from bad bugs before they become a problem. Stomach acid begins the process of protein digestion and is one of the signals to the pancreas for enzymes and bicarbonate. The pancreas secretes our basic enzymes: lipase (fats), protease (proteins), amylase (starches), and others with specialized functions. The pancreas also provides the bicarbonate that neutralizes stomach acid, as well as insulin, which is released directly into the blood stream to regulate blood sugar.

Strategies to Provide Digestants
1. Testing is available to evaluate how your body is functioning.
2. Hydrochloric acid can be supplemented—with great care—using a product from the health food store. If used carefully this can help in the short term, but is not always a long-term solution. Both enzymes and bicarbonate can also be supplemented.

3. The function of your pancreas can be supported with glandular supplements.

4. You can also improve pancreatic function by moderating sweets and starches in your diet (see chapter 31).

Testing
Conventional Methods

- Hydrochloric acid (HCl) production can be measured as part of an endoscopic exam, by drawing a sample of gastric juices. This test can also be performed with a hormone stimulus, pentagastrin.
- HCl production can also be tested using a Heidelberg capsule; in this test, the patient swallows a capsule that sends signals back via radiotelemetry to detect low output of hydrochloric acid.
- The pancreatic secretion of bicarbonate is evaluated by giving secretin, a synthetic hormone, intravenously and measuring bicarbonate output over a 60-minute period.
- A 72-hour fecal fat analysis tells how well the pancreas is supplying the enzyme lipase to digest fats. This test can be performed by any major lab.

Alternative Testing

- *The Comprehensive Digestive Stool Analysis* (CDSA) is another practical test for measuring acidity and other aspects of digestive function.
- *Testing for overgrowth in the small intestine* (the CDSA, a candida evaluation from Diagnostic Labs, or other testing). An overgrowth may mean the pancreas is not totally doing its job.
- *Testing for a marker for inflammation in the small intestine.* Calprotectin is now available as a marker for bowel inflammation as part of the CDSA. Very low or high levels of this marker may reflect low enzyme production.

Supplements
Hydrochloric Acid

- Hydrochloric acid is available as betaine hydrochloride in most health food stores. In some cases that addition helps digestive problems. We encourage you to add betaine hydrochloride under the supervision of your doctor, because if you take too much it will cause heartburn.
- When you begin any new supplement be sure that is the only addition to your diet for at least one to two weeks so you can more easily identify unwanted effects.
- If you take only one capsule and that causes heartburn, it may mean you already produce too much acid. Take no more, and check with your doctor.

- The labels recommend a dose of 1 to 2 capsules with meals. Remember that we're all different—the nutritional requirements of a 100-pound woman are quite different than those of a man who weighs 200 pounds.
- Any time you get heartburn following the use of betaine hydrochloride, it usually means you are taking more than you need. Check with your doctor and be sure to cut back the dose.

Pancreas Glandulars

If your pancreas is struggling, taking betaine hydrochloride may be only a short-term solution. Some people feel better in the beginning, because they finally have enough stomach acid for digestion, but less well later on because the pancreas is still struggling. Another solution favored by complementary practitioners is to take a good-quality product that supports the healing of the pancreas. These are extracts called glandulars and are available from vitamin companies in health food stores and from reputable mail-order companies. Reliable suppliers of glandulars include Allergy Research Group and Standard Process.

TAKING GOOD CARE OF YOUR PANCREAS

The pancreas produces enzymes, bicarb, and insulin. Knowing how essential these functions are, please be sure to take the best possible care of your precious pancreas. The easiest way is to cut down on sweets and refined starches.

Our ancestors ate whole food. The hunters ate meat and plants, and the farmers that followed them ate whole grains as well. So the body did not evolve to handle sweets and simple starches. When we eat that kind of food, it's a shock to the pancreas and requires a huge blast of insulin. If we eat too many sweets too often, we can actually cause diabetes—what the old-timers called sugar diabetes.

The solution is to eat foods that don't trigger insulin, that are low on the glycemic index. (See Joyce Daoust's *40-30-30 Fat Burning Nutrition* or *The Zone* by Barry Sears.)

Low Levels of Digestive Enzymes

An infection by microbes is known to actually suppress enzyme production. This is a survival strategy on the part of the microbe. In addition our modern diet tends to be very stressful to the pancreas. This is unfortunate, because the pancreas has a major role in both digestion and the regulation of blood sugar. Without enough enzymes you can't fully digest your food.

Enzyme Supplements

Some practitioners use the results from the CDSA to tailor enzyme supplements to the needs of the patient. Enzyme products favored by practitioners include Protozyme, a German enzyme product from MarcoPharma (available by mail order from Smart Basics); Creon (an entera-coated product) or Ness (both available only through doctor's offices); or N-Zymes 10, a multiple vegetarian enzyme product available from the health food store.

The question of which type and brand of enzymes to purchase is a huge one. There are vegetarian enzymes and those extracted from animal sources (pancreatin). Some vegetarian enzymes are produced by a mold-growing process, so for mold-sensitive people, this is not the answer. Pancreatin, a frequently used animal-based multiple enzyme product, is generally extracted from animals in the slaughterhouse, and some individuals report the development of spots of pigmentation following heavy use of pancreatin. If you favor vegetarian enzymes, ask about the manufacturing process or consider ordering Protozyme, a product known for low reactivity. If you want to use pancreatin, spend the extra money and buy a top-quality brand. The same quality issues apply to glandulars.

The Use of Bitters to Stimulate Digestion

There are a wide variety of digestants on the market. A traditional strategy is the use of gentian to stimulate our own hydrochloric acid secretion. Gentian is available in bitters, a liqueur that has been made in Europe for centuries. Angostura Bitters can be purchased in many liquor stores. Health food stores also carry European bitters. Gentian root can also be purchased in bulk, ground, and put in capsules, and taken twenty minutes before meals to promote digestion.

Bicarbonate

Another strategy to encourage digestion is taking bicarbonate after a meal (Alka-Seltzer Gold, which is bicarbonate without aspirin). This can sometimes dispel the symptoms completely within five minutes. When you add extra digestive enzymes and some bicarbonate, the theory is that the food will be broken down more thoroughly. This approach is most helpful in someone whose body doesn't produce enough enzymes or enough bicarb.

BENEFICIAL FLORA

Beneficial flora turns out to be so significant, it is even proving useful in the management of HIV. Research on AIDS has found a link between those who remain in remission and those who supplement their friendly flora. It may be that keeping down pathogenic bacteria in the gut frees up the immune system to deal with other issues.

However, out of more than 1,400 articles over the course of fifteen years on the nature of probiotics and their safe and beneficial uses, there are at least two dozen reports of lactobacillus causing serious infection, including a few by acidophilus. The majority of these cases have been identified in transplant patients (more than twenty patients, mainly liver), recent surgery (fourteen), cancer (six patients), diabetes mellitus (four), and ostomy (one). Researchers indicate that this is a very uncommon condition. Balance this against the knowledge that there are literally tens of thousands of people who have been monitored in research studies and found to have specific benefits with no problems.

As with any supplement, food, or other substance you take into your body, make the addition of a probiotic product or yogurt the only major change for that week. If you are scheduled for surgery you may wish to cut back on your supplement or at the very least discuss your use of probiotics with your doctor.

Testing for Flora

There are several ways to test for flora.

- *Measure flora levels directly* with a test such as the Comprehensive Diagnostic Stool Analysis (Great Smokies Diagnostic Lab).
- *Check for an overgrowth of yeast (candida), bacteria, or parasites.* Whenever there is an overgrowth or parasitic infection, you know that the levels of flora are depressed.

The status of the flora can be an indicator of how severe the overgrowth is when the problem is due to anerobic bacteria, which are not usually measured directly, or caused by a parasite that isn't showing up on the tests. The lactobacillus are the most vulnerable and are generally destroyed first, then the bifidus, and then *E. coli* (the benign forms). If the *E. coli* are gone you have real problems and can assume there is a serious disruption in digestive function. The loss of beneficial flora can be caused by the use of medications or by the presence of a parasite. A parasitic infection that significant must be treated. If the bifidus is gone but the *E. coli* have survived, the problems tend to be more moderate.

Disruptions in gut flora patterns are very individual and can vary greatly. Some people are deficient in certain species of lactobacilli, others in bifidobacteria or beneficial *E. coli*. The only way to know for sure is to have the flora levels checked through stool cultures, ordered by your health care practitioner. Once flora levels are established it is easier to know what kind of probiotic cultures to take to rebuild your flora.

SUPPLEMENTING FLORA

Although there are currently more than 1,400 studies on *Lactobacillus aci-dophilus* alone, we still don't have all the information on the best way to supplement flora. Still, we do know that replenishing the good bacteria helps most people become better able to resist illness. There is very extensive research on the beneficial effects of supplementing with lactobacillus, particularly *Lactobacillus acidophilus* and *Lactobacillus plantarum*, as well as the yeast *Sacchromyces boulardii*.

Yogurt

It appears that yogurt can provide a dietary supplement of flora. Although current research suggests that it's only a temporary replacement, we know that people from cultures in which yogurt is a staple often have a history of being long-lived. We do know flora tend to diminish in yogurt due to storage and refrigeration. The best products are fresh yogurt made locally or home-made, as well as supplements.

The first consideration with yogurt is to be sure you don't have a dairy allergy (IgE) or a delayed allergy or sensitivity. In some intermittent allergies, yogurt can be tolerated every fourth or every seventh day. People who cannot tolerate cow's milk yogurt may want to try goat's milk yogurt. Tolerances are always totally individual.

Certain brands agree better with specific individuals. Some people, for example, find excellent results with yogurts that are also high in bifidobacteria, such as Brown Cow yogurt, available nationwide. Be sure to read labels and track your responses.

If you are dairy intolerant, excellent yogurt can be made at home with your favorite soy milk.

Yogurt can be useful following antibiotic therapy, illness, digestive upsets, in response to stress, and before and during long-distance travel. *Lactobacillus acidophilus* is the culture found in most yogurts. Others also contain bifidobacteria, another major resident of the GI tract. *The other bacteria that are found in yogurt can be indirectly beneficial but are not primary residents of the GI tract. Streptococcus thermophilus* and *Lactobacillus bulgaricus* exist only briefly in the human digestive tract after being consumed. However, they do produce lactic acid, which encourages the growth of other friendly bacteria.

Complementary Nutrients

Colostrum (freeze-dried from goat's or cow's milk) is a rich source of secretory IgA and other immunoglobulins to replace deficient gut immunity. It is also available with added lactoferrin.

A strategy that clinicians are finding helpful is to take colostrum in combination with a probiotic. Since colostrum can cause symptoms in dairy-intolerant people, if you are sensitive try half a capsule only with your probiotic. Watch for new colostrum products coming out in the future.

Lactoferrin is one of the primary components of colostrum and the second most abundant protein in colostrum. It stimulates the immune system, is antiviral and antibacterial, and has been found to selectively block the absorption of iron by tumor tissue while releasing iron to the body.

NAC (n-acetyl cysteine) is also important in reestablishing normal flora because it helps decrease the toxicity of abnormal bacteria while rebuilding beneficial flora.

Researchers recommend adding a complex carbohydrate called FOS (fructo-oligo-saccharides), which tends to support the growth of certain beneficial flora, although people who are carbohydrate intolerant may experience gas and bloating.

Products that Help to Restore Beneficial Flora

	Product	Source
Probiotics	Megadophilus (DDS strain)	Natren (health food stores)
	Repleniss (powder and capsules)	Lifespan Institute (LifespanProducts.com)
	Primal Defense	Garden of Life (health food stores)
	All-Flora	New Chapter (health food stores)
	Ultra Dophilus, Ultra Bifidus, Ultraflora Plus (with colostrum)	Metagenics (from physicians only)
Immunoglobulins that promote healing	New Life Colostrum	Health food stores
	Bioplex	Metagenics (from physicians only)
	Transfer Factor	4-Life (available through the Web and distributors)

Research on Supplementing with Probiotics

- In a small study at the University of Bologna, ulcerative colitis was treated using eight different strains of acidophilus and bifidobacteria, causing long-term remission of symptoms in twelve of fifteen patients.
- A four-year review of the safety of lactobacilli among people in southern Finland of more than 3,300 blood culture isolates found no case in which lactobacilli appeared to be the cause of infection.

Lactobacillus DDS is one of the most well-studied acidophilus strains and is available nationwide in health food stores. It has been documented to survive storage in dry form in the capsule, to produce viable cultures in the gastrointestinal tract, and to boost GI immunity.

Bifidobacteria is one of three major beneficial bacteria in the digestive tract. Some people find them quite health promoting. Clearly the last word is not yet in on the optimal ratio of any of the flora. Bifidus is contained in some fresh yogurt cultures, such as Brown Cow.

Sacchromyces boulardii, a naturally occurring yeast that is a close relative of the yeast used in baking, is another frequently recommended supplement. It stimulates the production of secretory IgA by the gut lining. There is a tremendous amount of research indicating that this yeast in supplement form can improve the course of GI illness:

- Traveler's diarrhea was effectively treated with *S. boulardii* in a group of 95 German patients. Of these 67 percent had failed to respond to previous antidiarrheal or antibiotic drugs.
- Colitis associated with *Clostridium difficile* responded well to the use of *S. boulardii,* which was used in conjunction with the antibiotics vancomycin and metronidazole in a study at the University of West Virginia.
- *S. boulardii* was found to prevent diarrhea in critically ill tube-fed patients in a French study.

Soil-based bacteria are gaining attention as viable GI flora. They are also known as homeostatic soil organisms (HSO). See, for example, *Beyond Probiotics* by Ann Louise Gittleman (Keats, 1998). HSO are an addition to the usual probiotic agents such as lactobacillus and bifidobacteria. Some people find they make a moderate difference. In other cases they may be quite important and anecdotal success has even been reported in a patient with Crohn's disease, after the patient had tried virtually every treatment program and many supplements.

HSO produce superoxide dismutase, a free radical quencher, and stimulate the production of alpha-interferon, a key immune system regulator. They also stimulate the production of human lactoferrin, which helps absorb iron and interferes with pathogenic bacteria. The theory is that in times past, vegetables and plants from the soil were less sanitized and people regularly took in soil-based organisms clinging to their food. An interesting study in England found that when people began buying their vegetables in supermarkets, health declined somewhat. The researchers suggested that the removal of all traces of soil-based organisms could be a factor. You will continue to hear more about this in the future. Note that some products contain an extract of wheat grass, so if you have any suspicion of celiac disease or wheat intolerance, these particular products are to be avoided.

Lactobacillus plantarum is another beneficial strain that has produced good outcomes in research studies. Children with recurrent abdominal pain took *Lactobacillus plantarum* 299V; of these 60 percent experienced a decrease in pain over the four-week period, in a study at the University of Nebraska. Irritable bowel syndrome treated with *L. plantarum* found rates of improvement of 67 percent to 90 percent, in a study conducted in a Polish hospital. Those who used drug therapy instead improved by 30 percent, and those who took the placebo showed no improvement.

In general research does show that probiotics can boost gastrointestinal immunity. Recent studies have found major benefit in the use of flora supplements to treat GI conditions. Although there are studies that have reported no benefit, there appear to be many more studies that have found probiotics to be a safe and effective therapy or supplement to treatment. Be sure to ask your health care provider about how to best explore this underappreciated supplement. Always remember that your body's requirements for specific probiotics and your response are totally individual.

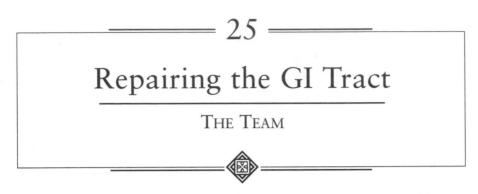

25

Repairing the GI Tract

The Team

How can we restore beneficial microflora and repair the gut lining? How do we support healing in the GI tract after an event or an illness in which the gastrointestinal environment has been disrupted? This disruption can include routine antibiotic therapy. How can we strengthen the entire system when there has been a chronic GI problem? And how do we heal the leaky gut, to increase the integrity of the GI tract and decrease allergies?

THE STRATEGY: GI REPAIR

JERRY STINE

A rehab program is used after antimicrobial therapy, particularly after very aggressive attempts to clear out parasites. It could also apply after being hospitalized for surgery. Most often it's used when there has been a heavy program of antibiotics or other medication that may have disrupted the GI environment and the flora.

There are several objectives under rehabilitation. One goal is to restore the beneficial microorganisms, the normal microflora of the GI tract. Another objective is to facilitate and support the healing of the gastric mucosa, to support the growth of new lining cells. A third goal is to normalize the function of the gastrointestinal immune system.

The duration and intensity of the GI problems will define the extent of repair efforts. A mild example is seen in a relatively healthy person with no history of chronic illness who has had an episode of antibiotic treatment. A relatively mild and simple rehab program that may take only three or four weeks would be very adequate here. At the other end of the spectrum is the person who has had many years of chronic illness involving major problems with digestive malfunction or dysbiosis. In someone with health issues of this intensity, the rehab program may take several months, perhaps six to nine months in really advanced cases. It depends on the original stresses on the GI tract and how long-term the condition has been.

The areas addressed in any of these rehab cases are:

- *Test for allergies* to make sure there is rotation or complete elimination of trigger foods from the diet.
- *Effective replacement of microflora* is more effective when accompanied by immunoglobulin supplements. Adding immunoglobulins to the flora usually substantially improves results.
- *Include nutrients that encourage the healing of the cells of the GI tract,* or that protect those cells, or both, such as N-acetyl-glucosamine, L-glutamine, slippery elm.
- *Slow or shut off inflammation,* particularly inflammation of the gut but also hypersensitivity, generally speaking.
- *Deal with long-term malabsorption and any actual malnutrition* that has occurred as a result.

We are looking at supplements that promote repair—vitamins, minerals, amino acids, and fatty acids. All of these features are components of the rehab protocol. Keep in mind that these protocols often follow an eradication protocol. Eradication is treatment to minimize an overgrowth of yeast or bacteria, or to remove invasive parasites. Although this type of treatment is necessary in many cases because of some kind of parasite or overgrowth, it can actually add metabolic damage. This is because antimicrobial drugs tend to be indiscriminant, knocking out both the harmful pathogens and the beneficial flora. In addition medications may aggravate sensitivity in the gut lining.

The repair phase must be worked out carefully on a case-by-case basis. And the rehab phase is the most lengthy, the most complicated, and the most important stage in returning the person to normal health, or achieving as healthy a balance as possible. Many of us take an antibiotic for a bug and consider the job done. That is really just the first step. Like strip mining, the gastrointestinal ecology must be restored or it will remain a barren interior environment, unable to provide nourishment for the other areas of the body.

Here is a list of nutrients and their use in decreasing intestinal permeability. This treatment for intestinal permeability is somewhat nonspecific. This simple kind of protocol is used while we are waiting for the results from the lab work to be returned.

- *Fiber.* Permavite contains an insoluble fiber, cellulose, which seems to decrease and clear toxins. In powder form it mixes well with water and has a mild flavor. The general recommendation is to use this prior to two meals a day.

It is specifically formulated for intestinal permeability, based on observations made by Dr. Leo Galland that different kinds of fiber affect intestinal permeability. He found that insoluble fibers reduce intestinal permeability and that soluble fibers tend to increase it. So this formula is based on insoluble cellulose and has other components in it to soothe and heal the GI tract. Cellulose products available in drugstores include Citracel and Fiber-Con. Permavite contains specific added nutrients, and is available from Allergy Research Group.

- *Quercetin* is a bioflavonoid that is very useful in some kinds of food allergy sensitivities. This can be a helpful component in dealing with intestinal permeability.
- *Enzymes and enzyme stimulants* provide digestive support using either digestive enzymes to promote thorough digestion or glandular products to stimulate the body's own enzyme production. Related but stronger products are Wobenzyme and Marcozyme, excellent quality digestive enzymes from Germany (available through Lifespan). There are vegetarian equivalents to these products; Interplexus has such a product, which is called Polyzyme. Since many of these plant-based products are made from mold fermentation, it's important to monitor your response.
- *Bioflavonoids* aid in strengthening the gastric mucosa and also help settle or reduce liver reactivity due to allergies.
- *N-acetyl cysteine* (NAG) is also important in reestablishing normal flora because it helps decrease the toxicity of abnormal bacteria while the person is rebuilding normal flora.

Reducing Inflammation

This part of the protocol adds components that may help with inflammatory tendencies. These nutrients may have a beneficial impact on inflammation at sites remote from the GI tract.

Inflammation can show up in a couple of ways. One is the actual perception and symptoms of inflammation, such as burning and irritation. There are many other conditions that do not produce a strong sense of inflammation but still involve reactions—diarrhea or cramping, gas and bloating, or spasms (as in irritable bowel syndrome). Inflammation can also take a form called subclinical inflammation, which doesn't show up on testing or even on an endoscopic exam, but which produces symptoms, for example, in response to certain foods.

- *Peptide products* can have a settling effect on inflammatory processes. Seacure is a specially processed fish protein, rich in nourishing peptides.

- *Magnesium* is available in a number of different forms. There are some kinds of lab work that can delineate specific magnesium compounds appropriate for each person's individual chemistry. Two labs highly respected for their metabolic profiles include Vitamin Diagnostics and Body-Bio Corporation. Some of the more easily assimilated forms of magnesium are magnesium citrate, magnesium glycinate, magnesium fumerate, magnesium aspartate, and magnesium malate. These are usually well tolerated and well absorbed.
- *MSM, a therapeutic form of sulfur,* is a way to deliver sulfur to the system in a soluble form. Methyl-sulfonyl-methane is now widely available. It is sometimes used to supplement treatment for *H. pylori* and many practitioners in the field of nutritional medicine have specific regimens for its use.
- *Digestive enzymes* often minimize inflammation, but if the gut is inflamed they occasionally worsen the condition. The most trouble-free brands that I have seen are the German products such as Marcozyme and Wobenzyme, available from Lifespan. Also check with your compounding pharmacy.

Essential Fatty Acids

These essential (in other words, necessary) fats have been found to decrease gut inflammation and leaky gut (hyperpermeability). Essential fatty acids are very powerful regulators of our chemistry, toning down inflammatory processes in the body triggered by the prostaglandins. This means that having sufficient levels of the right essential fatty acids may moderate inflammation. When you are supplementing with these nutrients, consider these factors:

- *Individual variations are the rule and not the exception.* The guidelines and suggestions here are extremely general. To ensure that you are getting the right combination you might invest in testing, such as the red blood cell membrane fatty acid test offered through BodyBio Corporation in New Jersey. This type of testing tells exactly which nutrients are and which are not there and allows extremely precise fatty acid supplementation.
- *Absorption and digestion of the essential fatty acids is often complicated by damage to the GI tract.* The villi, the fingerlike structures of the small intestine, have the job of absorbing fatty acids. If there have been long-term GI problems, the villi are often damaged. For instance, a gluten sensitivity that has gone undiagnosed and unchecked can destroy so many of the villi that a person may be operating with only 10 percent of the total

villi. The impact of this damage on their capacity to assimilate fatty acids, especially the long-chain fatty acids, may be 10 percent or less. In that case taking supplements may provide very little benefit, in spite of a great nutritional need for them.

- *Fatty acids most often supplemented are the omega-3s and the omega-6s.* The omega-3s are extracted from cold-water fish and dark green plants (the foods of our ancestors). They are also available in soy, walnuts, and flaxseed oil. Many people tend to be low in the omega-3s. Omega-3s are known to have a beneficial effect on the brain and the nervous system, and deficiencies are characterized by excessively dry skin. Cod-liver oil is the traditional supplementary source of omega-3s.

   Omega-6 fatty acids are found in vegetable oils such as corn and safflower oil (as well as flaxseed oil), so most Americans get enough omega-6s. But about 15 percent of the population is unable to fully break down omega-6s, perhaps due to a genetic defect. These people benefit from supplements rich in omega-6 that are already partially metabolized, such as evening primrose oil, which supply fatty acids called GLA (gamma linolic acid).

There are two tricky aspects to these supplements that makes nutritional testing the most ideal way to supplement them. First, they compete with each other. Dr. Leo Galland points out that feeding fish oil to a person who needs GLA may actually increase their omega-6 deficit (*Power Healing,* Random House, 1998). People whose dryness does not respond to omega-3s may have a need for omega-6s.

Omega-6 fatty acids are important in toning down inflammation, so this supplement is very relevant to many people with GI conditions. But too much omega-6s can cause inflammation through the buildup of arachidonic acid in the body. So be sure to moderate your intake of simple carbohydrates as well as red meat, dairy products, egg yolks, and shellfish if you are taking an omega-6 supplement.

There is believed to be an optimum ratio between the two oils, which is usually one part omega-3 to four parts of omega-6. This is the baseline. Flaxseed oil happens to contain that ratio inherently, which is one of the things that is so attractive about it. You are just taking one product. On the other hand, if you are one of the people with a need for the GLA form of omega-6, you will need borage or primrose oil and may find that your health improves significantly with this addition. There is no way to be certain which will work best on a case-by-case basis prior to using them. Body Bio Laboratory provides special testing of individual requirements for fatty acids.

STRENGTHENING THE BODY

JERRY STINE

This is a more intensive rebuilding program for people who have had long-term chronic conditions or strong indications of environmental illness. It is aimed at improving overall strength and reducing some of the gastrointestinal-based metabolic stresses for those with GI conditions or illnesses that result from hyperpermeability, such as asthma, allergies, chronic fatigue, or joint problems.

This protocol is to strengthen people who have a sense of feeling debilitated or physically stressed. It is an important preparation for an aggressive eradication program, particularly in the treatment of parasites. That is the major point of strengthening.

Objectives

The primary goals of the strengthening program are to reduce stress on the GI tract and on the liver. Stress can be reduced by cutting exposure to food allergens and dealing gently with overgrowths of candida or whatever kind of overgrowth shows up in testing. When we talk about gently, we mean *not* using harsh or fast-acting substances. We are also talking about supporting the liver detoxification systems as completely as possible. But all of this is done very carefully. There is always the slow buildup of each nutrient used and very careful attention to the diet in terms of any food that could be problematic because of allergies or because of starch/carbohydrate or wheat/gluten sensitivities.

When to Use this Approach

Use this program if you are frequently fatigued, highly stressed, sensitive, or feeling brittle; this protocol can be helpful if you have multiple symptoms in multiple areas. A good way to screen for this is to note the scores on your metabolic screening questionnaire (see chapter 1); any indication of sensitivity to perfumes and chemicals or strong reactions to foods and drugs is a sign to proceed carefully.

Promote change gradually. Protocols should not be too complicated. Supplements must be introduced at very low doses and built up gradually to the optimal doses. The main consideration here is attention to detail and taking the time to work through this. A strengthening protocol can take a month to arrive at full doses of all the products. That is not at all unusual. Then it is usually maintained for at least another month to make sure that the body has "cooled off" as much as it can from whatever stresses are coming from the GI tract.

What to Eat

In these kinds of protocols the choice of foods in the program is absolutely critical. I strongly encourage testing to determine allergies. Foods can be problematic in a number of ways.

With an overgrowth of bacteria or yeast, avoid diets high in sweet and starchy foods (carbohydrates) because they tend to encourage the "bad bugs" and people notice that they feel worse after eating these foods. Some parasites also thrive on simple carbohydrates, and you can help to minimize your condition by carefully selecting what you eat. That means getting a book that gives the carbohydrate content of foods, becoming an avid label reader, and monitoring your reactions to what you eat. Helpful books include *40-30-30 Fat Burning Nutrition* by Joyce Daoust and *The Zone* by Barry Sears.

There are other kinds of sensitivities that accompany inflammation or ulcers, which may mean that foods with lots of fiber may cause pain or spasms. Each person and each response to every food is individual. And it often changes from day to day as well.

Allergies can have disastrous effects on the gut and be significant factors in conditions as serious as Crohn's disease. A respected nutrition journal published photos of the inside of the digestive tract during the intake of milk by an allergic person: The image was like a tiny little explosion inside the gut.

Foods that show up as allergenic in testing or that are a problem in any way should be carefully avoided for at least a month. It is sometimes viewed as a hardship, but this is absolutely essential at this stage. This stress on the body from allergenic or high-carbohydrate foods (which might stimulate yeast or some bacterial overgrowth) must be really avoided. You need to be supported in sticking to this—enlist the help of those you love, and avoid those who sabotage your efforts to get well.

SUPPLEMENTS TO HEAL LEAKY GUT

Jeffry Anderson, M.D., and Michael Rosenbaum, M.D.

When the integrity of the GI lining is impaired, undigested food particles and toxins can be absorbed much more easily.

Major nutrients that can be useful in healing leaky gut include:

Immune Support
- *Colostrum* (freeze-dried from goat's or cow's milk) is a rich source of secretory IgA and other immuno-globulins to replace deficient gut immunity.

- *Lactoferrin* is an immune complex derived from molecules found in the milk of lactating mammals: Both colostrum and lactoferrin act as major immune barriers against the invasion of pathogenic bacteria, viruses, and parasites. Lactoferrin is a potent natural antibiotic.
- *Thymus extracts* stimulate and enhance the immune response both in the gut lining as well as generally throughout the body. One is Thymic Longevity Compound from Econugenics. Probably the strongest (and most expensive) is Nat Cell Thymus from Allergy Research Group. This contains frozen liquid thymic growth peptides from fetal and juvenile bovine thymus.

Nutrients from Protein

- *L-glutamine (amino acid)* is the preferred fuel of the cells lining the mucosa of the small intestine. It's an important building block for the production of normal intestinal mucus, and it's required for adequate production of SIgA and to maintain normal intestinal permeability following injury or infection. Lining cells in the small intestines (enterocytes) need to be fed with glutamine and the large intestine lining cells (colonocytes) require butyrate, which is metabolized by beneficial flora in the gut.
- *NAC.* In addition to its benefits as a natural chelator and potent antioxidant, NAC (N-acetyl cysteine) is also a potent detoxifier and enhances the detoxification of toxins produced by pathogenic bacteria. It rebuilds immune function by stimulating cellular immunity in the gut lining and directly increases macrophage and lymphocyte or white blood cell function in the gut lining. NAC also helps replenish intracellular glutathione. Again NAG is important in reestablishing normal flora because it helps decrease the toxicity of abnormal bacteria while the normal flora is being reestablished.
- *Seacure* is composed of peptides, which are the building blocks of protein, extracted from predigested whitefish. Many of the small peptides contained appear to duplicate growth factors. So the effect that you get on the GI tract far exceeds the six small capsules a day. You don't get that much protein—only three grams of protein a day—but the effect on conditions like irritable bowel syndrome can sometimes be very profound. These particular peptides appear to act as growth factors to help to heal the lining of the GI tract.

Protective and Soothing Nutrients

- *Vitamin A* is essential for production of protective antibodies (secretory IgA) and to maintain the integrity of the GI mucosa.

- *Zinc* is necessary for growth and wound healing, and it's rapidly depleted in the body. It is much more necessary in cells that have a rapid turnover. Zinc is especially relevant for the lining cells of the GI tract, which are replaced about every four days. So zinc is critical when it comes to the lining of the GI tract.

  Among its many functions, zinc also increases the release of vitamin A from the liver. If you are zinc deficient you may actually have enough vitamin A in the liver and be unable to make use of it. Vitamin A is responsible for the integrity of the cells lining all the mucosal surfaces of the body, including the entire respiratory tract and the entire digestive tract.
- *MSM, a form of the mineral sulfur,* enhances the body chemistry probably by raising glutathione levels in all the cells. This helps to prevent oxidative stress throughout the GI tract. It is supposed to prevent pathogens—bacteria, yeast, and parasites—from adhering to the bowel wall, so that the body can flush them out much more easily.
- *N-acetyl-glucosamine (NAG)* is essential for the secretion of the protective mucous lining of the gut (the glycocalyx).
- *Quercetin* is one of the bioflavonoids, which are especially helpful in food allergy/sensitivity and leaky gut, as well as inflammatory processes in the gut lining.
- *Epithelial growth factors* can be particularly helpful in healing the GI lining cells. They are found in several widely different sources: peptides (from protein), glandular extracts, deglycerated licorice, and in stevia, the natural sweetener. They have been used to treat all kinds of intestinal disorders, including colitis, Crohn's disease, and irritable bowel syndrome.

Vitamin B Complex

Phosphatidal choline supports normal barrier functions by repairing and maintaining the integrity of cell membranes and tight junctions, which helps to diminish leaky gut and sustain normal permeability.

Fatty Acids

The butyrates are short-chain fatty acids that are important for the lower portion of the intestinal tract, particularly the colon. The major role of the colon is to reabsorb water and maintain electrolyte balance in the body. Butyrates are the preferred food of the colon-lining cells. Our primary source is from the beneficial bacteria, so when there is an overgrowth and dysbiosis, butyrate levels drop. Butyrates are available as a supplement from a number of manufacturers.

Healing Herbs

These herbs are specific for healing leaky gut and damaged gut mucosa. Some of these botanicals also enhance detoxification. Part of the process of rebuilding the lining is the ability to repair.

- *Olive extract* is a natural antibiotic that tends to have antibacterial, antifungal, and antiparasitic effects on undesirable flora; the active constituent is oleuropein.
- *Silymarin* is an exceptionally healing herb extracted from the milk thistle weed and has a potent anti-inflammatory effect on the GI lining. It also has a direct antioxidant effect.
- *Ginkgo biloba extract,* which we usually consider a mild mental stimulant, has also been found to protect cell membranes from free radical damage. It has an anti-inflammatory effect as well.
- *Licorice root* (whole licorice root) is a herb that has profound anti-inflammatory effects on the gut lining.
- *Deglycerated licorice* has had the glycerin removed. So it is called deglycyrrhizinated licorice, or DGL. That form of licorice is also very soothing to the upper GI tract and may help to promote healing and get rid of leaky gut. It's useful in decreasing inflammation related to gut permeability and therefore stabilizing to the gut-barrier function.
- *Slippery elm* has a soothing effect on inflamed gastrointestinal lining.
- *Stinging nettle* has an antihistamine, anti-inflammatory effect that tends to reduce allergic inflammation.

Comment on Supplements

All of these supplements may have bearing on healing. It depends on the particular case—each person has his or her own individual issues. There are other considerations here that we have not discussed, including the possibility of trace element imbalances or the presence of toxic metals like lead and mercury. Those possibilities have to be explored. This is part of the history-taking process—to identify all of the issues that must be dealt with to help people increase their metabolic resilience and to decrease their metabolic stress.

A REVIEW OF TREATMENT STRATEGIES

LEN SAPUTO, M.D.

1. Correct, or at least improve, the underlying disease condition whenever possible.

2. Eliminate the known triggers of leaky gut: NSAIDs (nonsteroidal anti-inflammatories), alcohol overconsumption, infections, parasites, malabsorption, malnutrition, and allergic triggers.
3. Provide nutritional support.
4. Avoid or minimize toxic exposures.
5. Provide liver support based on the status of liver function and detoxification.
6. Supplement with "permeability factor" nutrients (the combination of L-glutamine, glucosamine, GLA, gamma oryzanol, phosphatidal choline).
7. Support with the four Rs: remove, replace, restore, repair—based on the protocol of Dr. Jeffrey Bland, a respected biochemical researcher who has provided much of the groundbreaking analysis in this field.
8. Insure adequate exercise; rest; stress reduction; and balance of body, mind, and spirit.
9. Be very careful about antibiotic usage.
10. It's important to assess GI function in order to manage GI conditions.
11. Whenever we detect leaky gut syndrome, we must also assess and manage the liver, beginning with a liver detoxification profile as the basis for understanding the situation.
12. Enhancing immune function is vital.
13. Screening with stool and intestinal permeability testing is a reasonable step in assessing chronic conditions and is essential in the seriously ill.
14. Ideal nutrition is critically important, but unless the GI tract is functioning ideally, much of this value is lost.

See the pages listed below for biographical information on the following authors.

Jerry Stine, page 12.

Jeffry Anderson, M.D., page 86.

Michael Rosenbaum, M.D., page 41.

Len Saputo, M.D., page 56.

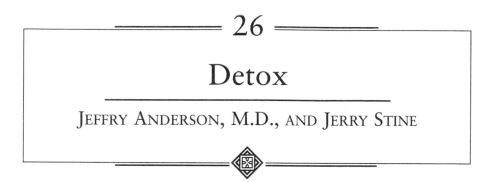

26

Detox

JEFFRY ANDERSON, M.D., AND JERRY STINE

Stored toxins can continue to cause damage to cells, tissues, and organs, creating inflammation and dysfunction even after the day-to-day exposures are eliminated. Although the external sources may be removed, the toxins remain in the body until they are cleared. To fully detox it's essential to support two specific processes:

- *Detoxication,* the internal processes of the liver by which toxins are eliminated from the body
- *Detoxification,* enhancing the release of toxins from the tissue through the use of specific therapies, including sauna, exercise, and nutrient support

SOURCES OF TOXINS

The gut is the source of much of the toxicity in the body because a good deal of what goes through the gut is absorbed, whether by design, accident, or pathology. Leaky gut can cause absorption of material that clearly should not be absorbed.

1. *The first category of toxins are actually produced within the body (endotoxins).* These toxins can occur in the gut due to impaired digestion and abnormal bacteria or yeast overgrowth, which leads to:

   - Fermentation and putrefaction by-products from yeast overgrowth and poorly digested food
   - The presence of parasites and their toxic by-products
   - Constipation

   These processes lead to a certain amount of internally generated toxins, which will be absorbed by the body before they are eliminated and will eventually be stored in tissues and cells.

2. *The second category of toxins are accidentally ingested from contaminated food or water.* This category includes food additives, pesticides, agricultural contaminants in meats and dairy products, and heavy metals in fish. Water may contain chemicals and their by-products, pesticides, and heavy metals as well.

3. *A third category are the toxins recycling through the body.* Toxins intended for discharge may accidentally be released back into the body. When the process works as it is meant to, toxins are bound to special transport molecules (conjugates) in the liver as part of detoxification. Conjugated toxins are then secreted into the bile and on to the GI tract, where they are further bound to the stool for final disposal from the body.

   Certain harmful bacteria secrete an enzyme that unbinds toxins and chemicals from the stool, and they are reabsorbed again. Some of the toxins will be disassociated from the binding site, rereleased into the system, and reabsorbed back into the liver and general circulation.

AVERTING A TOXIC DOMINO EFFECT

The starting point is the gut: If the gut is toxic and toxins are absorbed, they all go through the liver. Ideally the liver will be able to detoxify them or at least diminish their toxicity by changing them into less toxic substances, to be excreted in urine or feces. Toxins absorbed on the skin or through the lungs can also damage the GI tract and contaminate the cells and tissues.

If the liver is overburdened due to a chronic or persistent toxic overload, then a bottleneck effect can occur that may eventually reach a level beyond the capacity of the liver to handle. The liver detox machinery can become stressed and compromised. The overburdened liver will make every effort to do its job but may actually create an additional toxic load—more free radicals and even more toxic intermediate metabolites. If they can't be excreted, the body must store them. Internally generated toxins and especially ingested chemicals and pesticides will be stored in fat. Heavy metals will be stored in protein tissue such as muscle, bone, and cartilage.

The increasing accumulation can cause widespread cellular damage. You must begin detoxing by starting with first things first, which is the gut. Make sure that you are not constipated, that you don't have putrefaction, and that you don't have an overgrowth of yeast or bacteria and their toxic by-products. Clean out. Get rid of bad bugs and put in the beneficial flora by taking probiotics (acidophilus and bifidus). Once you have begun to clear the GI tract, you can start addressing the liver and body detox issues.

When you improve the GI tract environment, you take the stress off the liver because the burden of toxins is decreased. And there is less stress on the immune structures in the gut (the lymph tissue) as putrefaction drops and overgrowths decrease. Then there is less need for a constant high-level defense effort, and everything in the body just starts to work better. But the essential point is this: You can't deal with the downstream problems (symptoms in the body) until you have treated the upstream problem (malfunctions in the gut).

LIVER SUPPORT

Liver support refers to the general activity of supporting detoxification mechanisms within the liver, and reducing detoxification stress. There are several key issues here: facilitating the detoxification mechanisms, encouraging recovery and healing in the liver, and reducing stress in the liver.

Reducing Toxic Burden

Reducing liver stress means reducing intestinal permeability and minimizing the intake of any substance that will be a toxic burden on the liver. The objective of enhancing detoxification chemistry in the liver is to supply those nutrients or herbal products that seem to reinforce the liver detoxification mechanisms. The goal is to help the liver regenerate and rebuild, and that involves supplying nutrients essential to that process. Luckily the liver has rather phenomenal regeneration capabilities.

This program is potentially useful to anyone who has a chemical sensitivity, a food allergy, or chronic GI problems. Checking with the doctor is the first step, as with any illness. These situations and quite a number of others, especially chronic degenerative conditions, will benefit from the liver protocol support.

Supplying Key Nutrients

Another major component of detox is to supply the specialized nutrients for the GI tract and the liver—those specifically necessary for healing the digestive tract, and other nutrients specifically useful for facilitating liver function and recovery. Improving the liver's ability to detoxify both toxins generated in the body (endotoxins absorbed from the gut, from metabolic processes) and those from external sources is crucial.

Avoiding Detox Overload

Overloading the detoxification mechanisms in the liver is of concern for several reasons, because it also causes changes in the internal metabolic environment of the liver and interferes with the liver's role in key metabolic processes, including regulation of fat, carbohydrate, and protein metabolism.

At this point the body begins to deplete key nutrients, including vitamin C and the amino acid glutathione. If we don't have vitamin C, we can't recycle glutathione. Glutathione is extremely important. When the liver is under stress, we use glutathione in lavish amounts. So the body may be using up precious key nutrients. And this can create a kind of a deficiency condition in the body.

If first-pass detoxification fails, metabolic junk begins to circulate throughout the system, some of which activates the immune response. Allergies and autoimmunity can develop. Direct toxicity can occur from some of the chemicals in foods (both natural and manmade chemicals).

During Phase 1 liver detox, biotransformation of the toxins occurs, transforming them into chemical forms that may be even more highly toxic. The only way to deal with the toxicity is to give the body tremendous support with antioxidant factors to compensate for the overstimulation of Phase 1, which typically occurs in anyone experiencing toxic overload. These factors include: glutathione, NAC, and alpha-lipoic acid, as well as vitamin E (preferably mixed tocopherols) and the anthocyanins (a family of antioxidants from plant sources).

Specific Nutrients for Detoxification

Support for Phase 1 detoxication: Antioxidants tend to be protective against damage from an overstressed Phase 1 detox pathway, which generates a large number of free radicals.

Antioxidant support includes glutathione, NAC (N-acetyl-cysteine), alpha lipoic acid, selenium, alpha- and beta-carotene, vitamins B_2, C, and E, anthocyanins, and riboflavin.

Support for Phase 2 detoxication: This includes glutathione, NAC, alpha-lipoic acid, glycine, L-glutamine, L-taurine, L-cysteine, glutamic acid, aspartic acid, and a form of organic sulfur—MSM (methyl-sulfonyl-methane).

Both Phase 1 and 2 processes depend on a number of critical enzymes. Various B vitamins and minerals are required as essential catalysts for these enzymes to function. These include manganese, zinc, copper, B_3 (niacin), B_5, and folic acid. Broad-based nutritional supplementation is recommended. Required doses of the nutrients are quite varied from one individual to another. Working with exposures requires assessing individual needs on a case-by-case basis.

DETOXIFYING CHEMICALS AND HEAVY METALS

The elimination of toxins involves stimulating the release of fat and toxins stored in the fat cells. Most chemical toxins and pollutants like pesticides and solvents are stored in body fat (as opposed to heavy metals, which are not). Removing these toxins involves mobilizing them out of body fat to make them available for excretion.

This is done through a combination of therapies, by raising the body temperature through saunas (depuration therapy) and/or sustained aerobic exercise. These mechanisms gradually cause the body to break down fat and release the chemicals into the circulation so they can be detoxified and eliminated. This can be compared to melting lard under low heat in a saucepan. Basically you are melting solid fat to make it liquid. The stored chemicals are bound to fat, and to a degree can be driven out of fat by increasing the temperature. This is analogous to increasing the evaporation of alcohol if you heat it. The chemicals tend to be volatile, which means that they change from a liquid to a gaseous state through the application of temperature. If the body temperature is raised in a sustained way, the fat cells tend to break down, discharge the fat, and so release the chemicals.

Heavy metals are not stored in fat, so they are not amenable to elimination by this method. They must be pulled out of the body by molecular magnets. This is called chelating. Heavy metals are bound to protein complexes of the body, such as muscles, tendons, and bone. To encourage the release of heavy metals, you can use chelating agents such as vitamins and also specific chelating drugs. The majority of chemical toxins are solvents and pesticides and are basically bound to body fat.

Detoxification is a complex and challenging procedure that should be carried out under medical supervision. Everything we have listed here has potential problems. Aerobic exercise challenges the cardiovascular system. The use of saunas raises the body temperature and can cause dehydration if done incorrectly. It can also cause the loss of body fluids and electrolytes. None of these therapies should be done without medical supervision. This is extremely important because if the chemicals are being released into the body, you don't want them to cause further injury. You don't want them to recirculate and cause additional secondary damage.

Detoxing Cells and Tissues: Sauna Therapy

Sauna therapy is highly useful to bake toxins out of the body because they're stored in fat. The object is to burn fat—that is, break down fat cells, as discussed above. So the toxins stored in the fat are released and mobilized for elimination through liver detoxification as well as directly through the lungs and skin. This can be accomplished with aerobic exercise, saunas, or a low-carbohydrate diet, or a combination of these strategies. (See also chapter 31 on personalizing a diet low in starches and sugars.)

- You may want to join a health club with a sauna or build one yourself.
- If you have chronic fatigue and are unable to exercise, use the sauna longer.

The protocol usually involves twenty minutes of mild aerobic exercise, a dose of niacin, and then a sauna. The process quite naturally encourages the body to expel the toxins from the fat cells. The ideal temperature is 140 to 150°F. It's important to start slowly—as little as five to ten minutes each day or every other day. The time is gradually increased as tolerated.

Niacin (vitamin B_3) should be started in small amounts of 50 to 100 mg per dose (one to three doses a day) and gradually increased to a maximum of 1,500 mg total. Niacin (B_3) flush can be eliminated by taking one baby aspirin twice a day, for those who tolerate aspirin. This eliminates the flush completely.

Some people experience liver inflammation from higher doses of niacin (B_3), and many people can experience worsening of their condition if detoxification is too aggressive. Toxins can be mobilized more rapidly than the liver can handle, stimulated by too much sauna, too much exercise, or too restrictive a diet. For this reason medical monitoring is rigorously advised!

Nutritional Supplements To Be Used with Sauna Therapy

- *B vitamins,* especially niacin—up to 1,000 to 1,500 mg per day can be used. Medical monitoring is required. This would be taken two hours before entering the sauna.
- *Minerals:* potassium, magnesium, and a mixture of trace minerals, including copper, zinc, selenium, manganese, chromium, iodine, and boron.
- *Salts that make the body more alkaline:* sodium bicarbonate, potassium bicarbonate, calcium carbonate; 1 to 3 grams are generally taken one to two hours before or after the sauna depending on the individual's needs.

Miscellaneous Nutrients

- *Alpha-keto-glutarate,* 75 mg three times a day. This helps the detoxification pathways to operate more efficiently.
- *Activated charcoal,* 1 to 3 teaspoons a day for no more than three days per week.
- *Bentonite clay in colloidal suspension,* 1 to 3 tablespoons a day for not more than three days a week. Both bentonite and activated charcoal bind

toxins to be eliminated in stool. However, they also bind essential nutrients and must be restricted.

- *Polyunsaturated vegetable oils,* including olive, saffron, safflower, corn, walnut, or avocado oils, or a mixture of these oils. The polyunsaturated vegetable oils help prevent the recirculation or reabsorption of fat-bound chemicals in the GI tract. They also serve to replace the eliminated chemically contaminated fat in the body that has resulted from the sauna therapy.
- *Herbs:* Botanicals can be used to support the liver's detoxification pathways and protect the liver from damage during detox and the breakdown and release of toxins. Useful herbal remedies include milk thistle seed extract (silymarin), red clover, dandelion, goldenseal root or Oregon grape root, curcumin extract from turmeric, and ginger.

Detoxing Cells and Tissues: Aerobic Exercises

Aerobic exercise can be highly beneficial. Even walking is helpful—just do what you can do. (Also see chapter 43 on gentle exercise.)

Foods That Heal

Antioxidant-rich foods tend to protect all organs and tissues as well as the GI tract. These factors buffer cells against oxygen or free radical damage generated by pollutants. Antioxidants also aid the cell in repairing damaged structures such as cell membranes, and restoring cellular function, including detoxification. These nutrients include the carotenoids and vitamins A, C, and E. Antioxidants come in many different molecular or chemical forms and are present in extremely diverse sources of plants or foods. They are far too numerous to list. The most common ones are the ones we have suggested.

Vegetables

- *Green leafy vegetables:* Rich in vitamin A, carotenoids including alpha- and beta-carotene, lycopenes, and lutein. Kale, collard greens, dandelion greens, chard, beet greens.
- *Yellow-orange vegetables:* Also high in carotenoids and other plant-based nutrient factors (therefore called phytonutrients). Carrots, yams, squash.
- *Cruciferous vegetables:* Red cabbage, broccoli, Brussels sprouts.
- *Tomatoes (cooked) and beets:* Rich in lycopenes and anthocyanins, which are both types of nutrients with a protective antioxidant effect.

A liquid diet can be used for a short period to give the gut a rest. Another helpful strategy during detox is to simplify the diet, which reduces the GI load.

The Benefits of Raw Foods

It's become apparent that eating a variety of raw foods can be of great value. In essence, raw foods are beneficial because they contain "live" enzymes that have not been damaged by cooking. These natural enzymes aid in digestion, contributing significantly to the digestion of the foods in which they are contained.

After a plant has been picked, while it is still raw the enzymes remain active. When you eat raw fruits or vegetables, the enzymes take part in the digestive process in breaking down that fruit or vegetable. This "pre-digestion" takes a major burden off the pancreatic enzymes and the digestive tract.

The body must expend a great deal of energy to produce pancreatic enzymes for digestion. (The actual energy output consumed in a day is quite amazing.) This means that whenever we eat a meal consisting entirely of cooked food, this requires a huge amount of work on the part of the digestive tract and the pancreas. You've probably noticed the drop in energy that occurs after eating a large cooked meal—and the energizing effect of eating a fresh salad.

When we include raw foods in our diet, the digestive processes are able to cut back on enzyme production over time, conserving energy for other tasks. This is one of the reasons why people who are put on raw food diets start to heal and we sometimes see real improvement in chronic conditions. This seems to occur for at least two reasons: The first is that cooked food in the GI tract tends to promote more putrefaction, and as a result more toxins are produced. In contrast, raw food in the diet results in fewer toxins. And second, since much less energy is required to digest the food, that energy can be applied to cellular maintenance and repair (this seems to be borne out in the research).

Although a raw food diet is not always practical for people with digestive disorders, the higher the percentage of raw or organic food, the better.

It can be important to moderate the consumption of high-carbohydrate root vegetables such as carrots and beets. The majority of people do better on vegetables and fruits that are lower in natural sugars and lower in carbohydrates.

For those who do not have inflammation, the fiber content is one of the benefits of raw foods. On the other hand, fiber is a mechanical irritant. Consequently for people who have inflammation or sensitivity we usually recommend a low-fiber diet.

Those with sensitivities often do quite well with raw vegetable juices. When you use a juice extractor the fiber is eliminated. What you are really getting is the essence—simply the enzymes and the nutrients.

Fruits

Each antioxidant has a subtly different biochemistry. For example, vitamin C is a pure water-soluble antioxidant that protects certain tissues and structures vulnerable to oxidative damage, whereas other antioxidants are fat-soluble and protect structures like the fatty layer of the cell membrane against oxidative damage. These include vitamin E and glycolic acid, which is found in citrus fruits, grapes, plums, red currants, blueberries, and raisins.

Antioxidant Supplements

People with high susceptibility to toxic damage probably require supplements of antioxidants and cellular protective agents in addition to food sources. Antioxidants work much more efficiently if they are taken in combination, and they seem to be more effective when they are present with other factors in fresh foods that may act as synergists or enhancers of the antioxidant function. This is why it is important to get at least a large part of your cellular protection and antioxidant factors from fresh foods—vitamins (including antioxidants), minerals, and other nutrients.

Protein and Amino Acids

It is also important to have a balance of amino acids in your diet from a wide variety of protein foods, including nuts, seeds, legumes, dairy products, eggs, fish, and meats and poultry, depending on your diet. Obviously some of those things do not apply for vegetarians. But the wider the variety of protein foods you consume, the more balanced your amino acid pool will be for the body to use for cellular repair and protection. Many of the most important chelating and antioxidant amino acids (for example, glutathione and NAC) are found in both vegetable and animal protein foods.

People also need digestive enzymes that can help break down the protein into amino acids (protolytic enzymes) as well as peptides for absorption. People with a significant problem probably need amino acid supplements. The first step is a supplement that has all the essential and nonessential amino acids in balance (basically determined by measuring normal people's amino acid profiles). This will include all the amino acids we are talking about in the list, which are antioxidant, cellular protective, or chelating. These often provide some benefit.

Amino acid supplements can be tailored in a much more individualized program, but that requires professional testing and guidance. The simplest way to do this without having to test is to get health food store supplements that have 25 to 30 amino acids in them. They will contain the most important ones listed. One good basic amino acid supplement is Amino Caps 1 by Intensive Nutrition Incorporated (www.intensivenutrition.com), which is patterned after the amino acid content of human breast milk. Another very good amino acid formula is All Basic by Montiff (www.healingedge.net).

Nutritional Supplements

These individual nutrients are generally available in most health food shelves:

- *Amino acids:* N-acetyl-cystine, glutathione, methionine, taurine (all act as both natural chelators, as well as antioxidants)
- *Vitamins:* alpha-lipoic acid, vitamin B complex, vitamins C and E, mixed carotenoids, anthocyanins and pro-anthocyanins (which are powerful antioxidants)
- *Fatty acids:* omega-3, omega-6, and omega-9 oils, all essential fatty acids (found in primrose, flax, and fish oils)

Chelators

Foods with a high chelating value will help to draw heavy metals from the body. These include eggs, beans, and other legumes and the herb cilantro. Amino acid supplements that act as natural chelators include alpha-lipoic acid, N-acetyl-cysteine, glutathione, methionine, and taurine (they are also antioxidants).

A clear-cut problem with heavy metal toxicity or pollutant damage often requires laboratory work and individualized supplement programs. The more complex the problems of pollutant damage and gastrointestinal dysfunction, the more complex the treatment. There are nutritionally based physicians who have many tools to help individuals find the right solutions. But if you want to get started on something on your own without doing any damage or missing too many factors, you can eat a balanced diet consisting of a wide variety of good-quality organic-food protein sources, preferably from vegetables and animals, and take enzymes to help with the breakdown and assimilation.

Pharmaceutical Chelators

If the heavy metal toxicity is serious an environmental physician should be consulted. Such a physician may consider treating with a pharmaceutical heavy metal chelating drug, such as DMSA, DMPS, or penicillamine.

For biographical information for **Jeffry Anderson, M.D.,** see page 86 and for **Jerry Stine** see page 12.

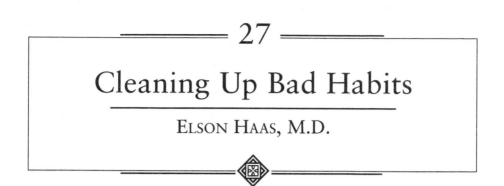

27

Cleaning Up Bad Habits

Elson Haas, M.D.

If you have digestive illness, you'll want to pay particular attention to toxins that may irritate or upset your digestive tract from the regular use of sugar, nicotine, alcohol, caffeine, or chemicals—what I call SNACCs. There is value in taking breaks from these kinds of habits to reassess your health and how you feel. You can't truly tell what effect these SNACCs are having until you take a little vacation from them. Research shows that all these substances can upset the digestive tract, and I have observed that in my patients. Digestion almost always improves when they let go of damaging habits.

These habits can initiate or aggravate many digestive problems:

- *Sugar* supports the infestation and overgrowth of the bad bugs—yeast, certain bacteria, and parasites.
- *Nicotine* can cause increased acid production, exposing the body to adverse effects.
- *Alcohol* is a direct irritant to the gastrointestinal mucosa. It commonly causes gastritis, liver damage, and all kinds of inflammatory problems in the GI tract.
- *Caffeine* also increases acid production. It is an irritant and can cause gastritis and ulcers.
- *Chemicals* include a wide variety of food additives and pesticides that can act as irritants to the gut. Over-the-counter medications, especially NSAIDs, are direct irritants to the gastrointestinal mucosa. Unfortunately NSAIDs can also promote gastritis and ulcers.

If you have any of these habits, you don't want them to become burdensome or addictive. You want to occasionally take a breath, take a break, take a vacation so you can clearly assess whether these are adverse influences in your life. And the only way to do that is to not do them. That means avoiding them. All of these substance abuses, so common in modern-day cultures, can act as insidious poisons when used consistently over the years. The incidence of chronic, debilitating disease is steadily growing, often linked to these long-term habits. They are also prime contributors to poor health in our aging years.

Clearing substance abuse is the first step to restoring health. If you have a problem in your body, correcting your lifestyle may significantly cut your exposure or eliminate the cause. This is an integrated approach to medicine. Another important aspect of integrated medicine involves the way we look at problems. From the Western point of view, problems of the body become "What can I take to make this go away?" But we need to ask basic questions about our health: Why is this present in my body? Are there things that I can change? Are there things that I can do or not do that will relieve me of this problem? Then we have a better understanding of the major influences on our health. One of my patients confided in me that when he stopped smoking and drinking coffee, he no longer had acid reflux.

There's a great quote: "There are no diseases, only mistakes in living." That is the core of this philosophy. I address each of these substances fully with ways to clear them in my books *The Detox Diet: How-to and When-to Guide for Cleansing the Body of Toxic Substances, Updated* and *The New Detox Diet: The Complete Guide to Lifelong Vitality.*

SUGAR

There are many problems associated with sugar abuse:

- *Allergies and sensitivities* may be increased by high sugar intake.
- *Diabetes* is the end result of insulin burnout and a depleted pancreas, which alters sugar metabolism.
- *Low blood sugar (hypoglycemia)* is associated with excessive sugar intake and linked to chronic fatigue, mood changes, and depression.
- *Obesity* can occur due to too much insulin or its effects on other hormones; this is discussed in books such as *The Zone.*
- *Altered immune responses*—sugar may trigger inflammation in the gut or immune suppression, as well as a temporary drop in the level of our white blood cells.
- *An overgrowth of yeasts, certain bacteria, or parasites,* the fermentation of food, and infection by any of these microbes; sugar is one of the favored foods of yeasts and some bacteria.

Often people have the strongest emotional resistance to the idea of getting off sugar. But physically it's probably the easiest! In the beginning it may be hard just to take the first step, mostly because of the emotional and mental attachment that people have to sugar. Sweets may serve as a comfort to us, linked to feelings such as "I want my sweets. Mama, tell me everything is going to be okay." What I find working with people to get rid of their habits is this: Once they get through their first few days, they come to realize that they are no longer subject to those cravings and begin to feel clearer and more alive. Some people go through a couple of days of irritability and lost sleep, but they typically steady out quite soon. Then they find they are not so run by sugar. It's almost like a bad relationship, when they are finally free of it and begin to feel better. Often a week or two later, they say that their moods are steadier, their energy is better, and they don't have those disturbing highs and lows. So people can see the actual difference as they progress from week to week.

What Drives Cravings for Sweets?

A couple of other important factors contribute to sugar cravings. Imbalances in flora and the overgrowth of yeast or parasites need to be addressed because they seem to drive people's cravings for sugar. Yeasts and many bacteria thrive on sugar and they also ferment sugars and starches, which generate gas, bloating, and other toxins. These toxic by-products may be absorbed into the bloodstream and affect mood, energy, and physical symptoms. Not enough protein in the diet can also cause sugar cravings. People typically have a diet that is too high in starches and sugars, especially refined carbohydrates. By improving protein quality and by creating a more alkaline diet, sugar cravings begin to decline. Eating more greens, grains, and proteins (both animal and beans), with less refined flour, cheese, and heavier food, they start to feel more balanced.

Key Nutrients

There are probably three or four key nutritional supplements that can help us with sugar cravings and addictions. One is chromium, which is the important mineral for glucose metabolism, as part of glucose tolerance factor, and it helps the body handle sugars better. L-glutamine seems to support the brain and to reduce cravings for sugar and alcohol. Vitamin B complex and vitamin C minimize the stress from the body's transition. Drinking lots of water to stay hydrated usually reduces cravings. Treat yourself to spring water or imported mineral water, lemon water (hot or cold), or herb tea (hot or iced).

NICOTINE

There are many problems associated with nicotine abuse. Nicotine is known to be an irritant, and has been found to inflame or aggravate existing inflammation of the delicate stomach lining—the gastric mucosa. Most of the research on nicotine has looked at smoking in general. A research review by the State University of New York found smokers are more likely to develop:

- *Reflux conditions* due to reduced saliva production and loss of muscle tone at the gastroesophageal sphincter.
- *Gastric and duodenal ulcers* that have a slower rate of healing, with a higher rate of relapse. Other research shows smoking to be one of three major risk factors for ulcers. A Norwegian study found the risk of perforated ulcers among smokers to be ten times normal.
- *H. pylori* infection and its complications, namely gastritis and ulcers.
- *Impaired stomach functions*—decreased blood flow and mucus and bicarb secretions.
- *More free radical production,* which leads to inflammation and disease.
- *Less responsiveness to medication.*

Nicotine also increases cancer risk. Numerous kinds of cancer are linked with smoking, as we see in the media. Lung cancer is of course the most common. However, gastrointestinal cancers may also be increased in smokers and tobacco chewers. These cancers include:

- *Stomach cancer.* Smokers have more than double the incidence over non-smokers (International Agency for Research on Cancer, Lyon).
- *Colorectal cancer.* Risk can be doubled for men over 50 who smoke (Finnish study).

The most promising information came out of the Finnish study of more than 56,000 people. Researchers found that men over 50 who quit for ten years reduced their cancer risk to that of nonsmokers! So that tells us that it's never too late to lower your disease risks by making healthy changes.

Smoking is one of the most difficult habits to stop. It's hard because it's so deeply addictive and tied into other lifestyle habits—drinking coffee or alcohol, talking on the phone, or a variety of work activities. It even becomes associated with our breathing; to keep breathing without nicotine is like being in a constant state of withdrawal for days or, weeks. For the average person, it takes about a week to begin feeling better. Nicotine patches help, but mindset is still the key. You have to be really determined to quit.

The research shows some benefit from nicotine patches or gum, although some nicotine continues to circulate in the body. Still, the nicotine in a patch is less than you would get from smoking, and many patches are designed to be used in stages, decreasing the nicotine as the body becomes more accustomed to doing without it.

Many of the serious problems from nicotine take twenty, thirty, or forty years to develop. Although it can take as long as a year to overcome the addiction to nicotine, the benefits to digestion and health are clear. The body is relatively forgiving of these addictive substances day to day, but on a long-term basis, there is often a big price to pay in health and life.

ALCOHOL

The continued use of alcohol over the years is very destructive to most of the components of the digestive tract. Alcohol can cause major gastrointestinal problems, including varicose veins in the esophagus (called esophageal varices); gastritis and ulcers; inflammation all the way through the digestive tract; cirrhosis and liver damage; and compromise of the pancreas's insulin production. So alcohol is a really important issue for anyone with gastrointestinal problems. Most people who are habitual drinkers eventually develop GI problems over time. Alcohol is likely the most damaging irritant of the common addictive substances.

Most people who just have a drink or two a day usually have no problem stopping. They may go through a mini-withdrawal for a day or two, and then usually they're fine.

Casual alcohol use commonly serves as a transition from daytime and work into the evening's relaxation. People want to loosen up. However, there are many better ways to accomplish this: exercising after work, doing yoga, taking a hot shower or a soak in the tub, or going for a walk. Most of these activities can help make that transition to a more relaxed state. The solution doesn't need to be an artificial substance to relax you.

People with GI symptoms should more seriously consider giving up that drink or two a day. If you have digestive illness, try taking a break from alcohol for two or three weeks to see if it makes a difference in how you feel. The whole point of removing irritants such as alcohol is to see if it helps you feel better. Some people will need a few weeks to see any significant results. They might see some change right away, but other benefits may take longer to experience.

Many of the changes in lifestyle habits we make require us to notice how we feel from week to week, rather than from hour to hour or day to day. If we give something up for three weeks we'll notice benefits that we don't usually see in just three days. And in three months we should see even greater improvement. Changes can be progressive. If someone diets and loses 10 pounds in two weeks, then resumes their old diet and gains it back, that makes no sense—it doesn't really help them. But a person who stays on that diet could lose 30 pounds over 60 days. Giving up alcohol is a good beginning for any lifestyle improvement. It can help us begin to lose extra weight, lower the stress and irritation on the digestive tract, and allow us to be more connected and genuine with our true feelings.

CAFFEINE

The research on caffeine and digestive problems is sparse. However, caffeine does seem to be connected with a number of GI conditions, including indigestion, stomach ulcers, and cancer. In general caffeine's adverse effects on the body are from its actions as:

- *An irritant.* One of the problems is that the acids in coffee are irritating. And research has confirmed that patients with indigestion were more likely to experience their symptoms after drinking coffee. There are links with stomach ulcers as well, and clearly it aggravates gastritis and ulcer conditions and the pain from them.
- *An intensifier.* A number of studies have found that caffeine intensified the effects of medications or other chemical habits, perhaps by its effects on body chemistry and the liver's many functions. Researchers noticed this relationship in a study that found caffeine worsened gastric ulcers when used in combination with nicotine.
- *A carcinogen.* Studies have linked high levels of coffee consumption to increased incidence of pancreas and bladder cancer.
- *Acidic.* Coffee can tend to make the body more acidic and stimulate acid secretions. Because it's a diuretic, it causes the loss of calcium, magnesium, and potassium, which are more alkaline. As we lose more of the minerals, our body chemistry shifts toward acidity, and this makes us more prone to inflammatory conditions.

At this point in time we don't know that coffee per se is a carcinogen, and the research does not offer a clear indication one way or the other. Whether this is a factor of too many chemicals used in coffee production, or the effects of the coffee bean itself, remains to be seen. The greater carcinogenic risk may be due to the chemical used in coffee growing, packaging, and processing. Might organic coffee use reduce this risk?

Caffeine tends to promote headaches, irritability, and ultimately fatigue. It makes people more tense, so there is increased tension throughout the system, including the GI tract. People tend to skip meals and replace them with coffee (and a pastry or a cigarette) to boost their energy. For example, a lot of people don't eat breakfast and then drink a couple of cups of coffee throughout the morning. This can have an adverse effect on the gut because we're taking in irritants, but we don't have any food or much digestive juice to dilute the coffee and make it less toxic to protect the stomach.

To break the coffee habit most people just need to go through a brief period with a headache and some irritability, and that can generally be handled quite well. Usually by the third day they are pretty clear and their energy begins to feel more balanced.

The detox process can be smoothed with a little aspirin or ibuprofen for the headache. Then the challenge is to get our own natural energy cycles back in sync. Coffee gives us a boost when we need it, as if by magic. But here too there's a price. This energy comes from the release of our deep stores of glycogen from the liver and the stimulation of adrenal and liver function.

If we become fatigued a little, this is an opportunity to find other ways to support our energy with herbal teas, the blue-green algaes, or a wholesome snack, such as almonds or sunflower seeds. Many people have better energy if they make a fruit smoothie with some protein powder. Then they get some carbohydrate and a few fructose calories, as well as the protein nourishment. Adrenal function is also important. The adrenals are key for sugar metabolism and for dealing with stress.

One of the primary questions is this: Wouldn't it be nice to feel what your own natural energy and natural cycles are? People who take in caffeine daily and then use relaxants later in the day to slow them down don't really know. what their own rhythm and potential are. This awareness becomes healing.

CHEMICALS AND DRUGS

Chemicals come in a wide variety of forms. There are chemicals in food (such as additives and pesticides), over the counter medications, and prescription drugs, not to mention street or recreational drugs. Many drugs have damaging effects and side effects, including problems related to digestive health, because chemicals tend to:

- *Act as irritants and carcinogens, especially additives and pesticides.* Pesticide residues on food can be irritants; some pesticides and food additives also have carcinogenic potential, such as the by-products of nitrates (the nitrosamines). Consuming the cleanest possible water and food, organic whenever possible, will minimize these irritants.

- *Cause leaky gut syndrome.* NSAIDs (nonsteroidal anti-inflammatory drugs) are well-documented irritants and triggers of leaky gut syndrome, a problem that leads to malabsorption.

Since there are tens of thousands of drugs, both over-the-counter and prescription, you can imagine the possibilities for gastrointestinal complications from drug use, overuse, and abuse. Check with your doctor and/or your pharmacist to be sure the medication you are taking or are considering doesn't have harmful side effects for your GI tract.

The medical literature shows that damage to the GI tract can also result from recreational drug use, primarily from crack cocaine, but occasionally from overuse of other street drugs as well. A couple major concerns include:

- *Stomach and intestinal ulcers as related to smoking crack cocaine.* This link was reported in many studies, from hospitals in Los Angeles, Brooklyn, and the Bronx.
- *Ischemic colitis and GI hemorrhaging* were seen in hospitals in the Bronx and London, as well as Michigan and Ontario.

The liver is important because it must detoxify most of the chemical substances we take in from our environment, our food, and our medication choices. And irritation can be caused in the gastrointestinal tract directly from the drugs.

When we make good choices in what we eat and minimize harmful habits, we give our digestive system the best chance for optimum health. Ideally as natural medicine comes more into mainstream thinking and practice, it will increase the use of reliable substitutes and natural therapeutics that have less potential for damage to our inner health.

Elson Haas, M.D., is the founder (1984) and medical director of the Preventive Medical Center of Mann, an integrated health care facility, in San Rafael, CA. A graduate of the University of Michigan Medical School, Dr. Haas has practiced medicine in a variety of clinical and hospital settings in the San Francisco Bay Area. He is the author of a number of highly successful books: *Staying Healthy with Nutrition* (a 1,200-page resource book on nutrition), *A Cookbook for All Seasons, The New Detox Diet,* and *The Staying Healthy Shopper's Guide* (all from Celestial Arts). Other books by Dr. Haas include *The False Fat Diet* (Ballantine Books, 2000), *Vitamins for Dummies* (IDG Books, 1999), and *Staying Healthy with the Seasons* (Celestial Arts, 1981; new edition, 2003).

Dr. Haas provides specialized health programs incorporating lifestyle counseling and natural therapies within his family practice. In conjunction with his work as an author and speaker, he gives workshops and presentations on integrated medicine, nutrition, and detoxification. He can be reached through the Preventive Medical Center at (415) 472-2343 or through his Web site www.elsonhaas.com.

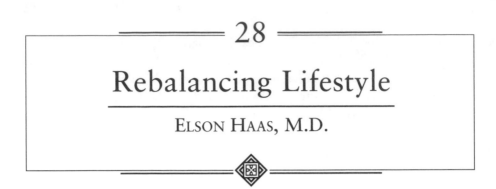

28

Rebalancing Lifestyle

ELSON HAAS, M.D.

Our health is a by-product of our lives—our genetics and constitutional state, our upbringing and the habits we develop, our diets, our stresses and how we deal with them, our illnesses and how we treat them. All of this and more affects our level of health.

How we live—our lifestyle choices—is the key to long-term health, quality of life, and vitality in our later years. The five keys to good health and disease prevention are:

1. *Diet*—eating wholesome foods and avoiding as much junk food as possible
2. *Exercise*—stretching and working the body regularly to keep it flexible and strong
3. *Sleep*—adequate rest and sleep (and dream time) for each of us, crucial to recharging our batteries, healing many problems, keeping our moods balanced, and staying healthy
4. *Stress management*—learning to deal with life's ups and downs, emotions, and frustrations
5. *Attitude*—keeping a positive outlook so that we treat ourselves and others with the life-supporting respect and care we deserve

NOURISHING YOUR BODY

Eat whole, natural foods. My nutritional message in my personal life, my practice, and my books has been to turn back to a nature-based diet for greater vitality and health. Eat closer to the earth's food sources—from the gardens, orchards, and farmer's markets. Move away from the boxed and canned foods and the refined and chemicalized cuisine. Focus on fresh fruits and vegetables, whole grains and legumes, nuts and seeds. Limit animal-based foods and refined/processed foods. This basic approach, emphasizing grains and vegetables, can greatly improve health, both in our immediate future and over the years.

Avoid toxicity and deficiency. Another key understanding about nutrition is the concept of toxicity versus deficiency. The basic premise is that when we get out of balance from a nutritional point of view, we have, on the one hand, toxicity, which means we have too much coming in that we can't handle. Toxic congestion can lead to all the chronic inflammatory degenerative problems. They're caused by too much intake of the things that the body doesn't process well—overconsumption of animal fat, excess chemicals, too many SNACCs—sugar, nicotine, alcohol, caffeine, and chemicals. We need periods of cleansing and letting go of these abusive habits to improve our health. These temptations/habits are potentially harmful to us. On the other hand, deficiency or depletion can occur when we are not getting enough of the things that we need. In this case what is called for is improved nourishment to rebalance the body.

Minimize processed foods. So when we eat a diet that is high in processed foods and low in all the fresh things and whole grains, we're getting toxins. But we're not getting enough nutrients. So we may have a chronic problem of imbalance, as a result of both excess toxins and not enough nutrients. That can result in what I call obese malnutrition, which is common in our culture. Our bodies are craving nutrients, but as long as we're eating out of habit we're not really meeting the basic needs of our bodies. If we just have steak and potatoes or coffee and doughnuts when we're hungry, we aren't really providing what our bodies are calling for, which is nutrient-rich food. One of the ways that you lighten up and become healthier and more vital is to get rid of foods that are high in calories and low in nutrients, and to begin consuming foods that are high in nutrients and low in calories, such as fruits and vegetables, whole grains, beans, fish, and poultry, which are basically healthier source foods.

EXERCISE

Exercise frequently. Our exercise program must be frequent (at least three to four times a week), consistent over the years, and balanced, which is very important. A balanced exercise program should include regular stretching for flexibility, weight work for building tone and strength, and aerobics for endurance and stamina. Exercising regularly will improve body function and health as well as attitude. It is one of our best stress managers, relaxers, and mood elevators.

Build strength gradually. We should exercise realistically at our current level of physical strength and endurance so that we can progress consistently and avoid injury. If we are just beginning and not in great shape, we can start slowly and build as our stamina and strength improve. If we have been working out regularly and are already fit, then it is beneficial to periodically evaluate our state and progress and make appropriate changes to exercise at our full potential, whatever that might be. If you have days when you don't feel well enough to walk in the hills or ride a bicycle, there are also quiet healing exercises you can do.

SLEEP

Get enough deep sleep. Sleep offers life's balance for all of our activity, on the physical, mental, and emotional levels. Like breathing fresh air, drinking good-quality water, and eating a nourishing diet, our nightly quality sleep is crucial to our well-being. There are many stages of sleep important to our body's recharging process, and although we all do not regularly recollect our dreams, we need to sleep deeply enough to go into that theta wave, REM (rapid eye movement), dream sleep. If we are not sleeping well, apply the other principles of preventive medicine, such as eating well and avoiding stimulants, exercising regularly earlier in the day, and managing stress. And we don't have to turn to medications for sleep because there are many natural remedies that can help, such as calcium and magnesium, 1-tryptophan (back again), and herbal relaxers, including valerian root and kava kava.

Get quality sleep. Sometimes when we don't sleep well enough, it may be that we can't digest well—both food and life experiences. In terms of sleep, we're just not current. We may have too many things we are thinking about, too many things we should have done, too many things we want to do. Then there are frustrations with our jobs, with relationships, or with money. All these things are stressors, which can also interfere with the quality of our sleep.

Change your environment. If you sense that you're not getting enough sleep, consider all possible factors: Is your bedroom too stuffy or cold? Is your bed too hard or too soft? Do you have allergies that would be improved by hypoallergenic bedding or pillows? Are you using an electric or synthetic blanket that overstimulates you? Are there pleasing routines that would enhance your sleep, such as meditation, warm milk before bed (if you tolerate dairy), or reading something relaxing before you fall asleep?

Relax and Recharge

BREATHING EASY

When you wake up in the morning, there are two simple exercises you can do. First, take five to ten minutes to lie on your back, close your eyes, place either hand just below your navel on your lower abdomen and the other hand over your heart. And as you breathe in slowly, bring your breath down into your lower hand and slowly let it fill your abdomen and then your chest. And then as you breathe out, go in reverse and end by contracting your lower abdomen.

This is a way that you can start to exercise with your abdominal muscles and intestinal tract. As you breathe in you say in your mind that you are breathing in relaxation, healing, and energy—whatever you wish.

LETTING GO

As you breathe out, you tell yourself you are releasing worries, fears, disease, or whatever you want to say. And at the same time you are just letting your body relax on the bed or floor and you are taking time to relax and recharge your body. Also let your mind relax, just breathing in this and breathing out that. Don't think about anything that may be troubling to you.

Some people report that the deep abdominal breathing can almost immediately create a positive shift in how they feel, in the quality of their consciousness and attitude. Relaxed deep breathing seems to make a fundamental and instant difference in the way they experience things.

GENTLE MASSAGE

After you do some relaxed breathing, start some gentle awakening in your digestive tract through a little self-massage. Start in the area around your navel. Slowly massage your colon. Work all the way around the outside of your abdomen. If you are looking down, it would be clockwise. You slowly massage the tissue. If it doesn't hurt, press a bit more firmly. Do that half a dozen to a dozen times. Breathe in between each time you go around. Go a little deeper with your massage as you breathe out. If you feel a tight area in your colon, you can massage that a little more. Self-massage is a way to support peristaltic activity. A lot of people with chronic digestive problems, especially those with a sluggish digestive tract, just don't have good peristaltic activity. You can stimulate that a little bit. Many people find that they can then get up and use the bathroom.

Change your patterns. Do you sense that you need more sleep? Try a variety of sleeping patterns. You can do this spontaneously, using your intuition to guide you. You can also explore your sleep habits systematically. For a week try going to bed half an hour earlier each day. If this is helpful, of course continue. Or you may find that you're still not getting enough rest. Healing chronic illness places a tremendous demand on the body, a requirement sometimes best met by extra sleep. If this is the case, for the second week add an additional half hour. Continue this pattern weekly in increments until you find yourself waking naturally, without an alarm clock, well rested and refreshed.

COPING WITH STRESS

We have known for some time that worry and stress can affect the health of the digestive tract. Managing stress is a key element in minimizing health risk and enjoying life. Stresses are our body/mind responses to our personal experiences, and we are individual in the issues to which we respond and react. There are so many illnesses and diseases that are generated or worsened by stress that it is imperative that each of us develop skills to deal with mental and physical demands and emotional challenges. Managing stress is important because it encourages a more relaxed and healthier mind and body. If you look at stress in terms of lifestyle, we don't grow up in a society that supports or educates us on dealing with the typical stresses that we have.

Exercise, sports, outdoor activities, and especially internal disciplines like yoga or tai chi are all extremely valuable in dealing with both daily and long-term stress.

Simple relaxation techniques. We are so oriented toward action that we probably don't put enough emphasis on learning how to just be. We're not really trained in relaxation exercises and meditation and doing stretching, breathing, and other things that unwind the body so we can let go of the mind-body stresses we tend to perpetuate.

Meditation is another very effective way to clear our minds of chatter and restore inner balance. Daily meditation can gradually shift our self-image and quiet some of the harsh inner voices we carry with us from our childhood.

Body work and massage therapy. When we're exposed to a conflict or challenging situation, we tend to internalize a lot of emotional baggage. When we have little episodes that we didn't fully resolve, they get stored in our minds as images and thoughts, but they are also stored in our bodies. Frustrations or anxieties that aren't completely resolved or healed can cause tension, muscle tightness, and even pain. Body work and massage therapy can help.

Water-therapy baths and showers, saunas, and swimming. Water is therapeutic. It is so cleansing, flowing, relaxing, and supporting. We are mostly water, so in a sense we are connecting with our dominant element. Hot water has the added benefit of soothing and relaxing tight tissues and muscles.

Coping skills. There is value in having a whole repertoire of constructive ways to cope with stressful situations. This involves refining our abilities in conflict resolution and good communication, and being able to read ourselves and others.

Emotional and spiritual nourishment. We may also crave nourishment on a more fundamental human level—the need for affection, intimacy, giving to others, and spiritual experience.

Spending time in nature is a wonderful stress reducer.

I believe that one of the greatest problems of modern-day life is the indigestion of life. Most of us do not have enough personal time to digest and assimilate our daily experiences—work, relationships, and food—that we consume in rapid-fire fashion throughout our day-to-day existence. This leads to the implosion of energy and the suppression and potential explosion of emotions or bodily symptoms. These are the body's attempt to convey the messages that we don't have time to receive and incorporate. It can be helpful if we take time to quiet ourselves, to breathe and listen, to experience and enjoy. The concept is to take the time to relax and assimilate our experiences, just as we would an excellent meal. To become current with our lives makes us ready for new creativity and experiences. This can lead us to more optimal health.

ATTITUDE

- Staying positive and motivated to experience life, unafraid to handle challenges or deal with uncomfortable emotions, is also crucial to health.
- Begin with a personal assessment. Our personal well-being is ultimately up to each of us. We can begin by assessing our health and lifestyle. We want to make changes that matter: changes that will provide more energy, improve our overall health, and increase longevity. Lifestyle medicine is the highest art of healing for each of us.

- Use supportive self-talk to maintain a positive inner dialogue. The way we talk to ourselves can make a difference in the decisions we make. If we use positive self-talk every time we start to have a negative thought, we can begin to shift our habits. Learning to think positively about the self is often a first step in loving ourselves and making healthy lifestyle changes to improve our overall well-being.
- We may need therapy to help us cope in some situations. We can't just change overnight by using positive self-talk alone. Sometimes these problems are more deep-seated and need to be addressed in therapy or with a counselor who can help uproot the psychological weeds that may be undermining personal habits.

As a doctor, I believe that the most important thing I can do is encourage my patients and readers to make personal changes in their lifestyle—diet, exercise, proper sleep, stress management, and attitude. Attitude underlies the whole pattern of how we take care of ourselves. I feel I have accomplished something useful if I can get people to change their attitudes and encourage them to care for the only body they have. The essence of this approach is to care for yourself with love.

My goal is to remind you that you hold much of the power over your health. What really matters is how you live—what you do, what you eat, and what you think and feel. Do what you can to be vital and healthy. It is really worth it! Be well.

Biographical information for **Elson Haas, M.D.,** appears on page 246.

29

Renewing Immunity— A Checklist

Michael Rosenbaum, M.D.

❖

KEY INFLUENCES ON YOUR IMMUNE SYSTEM

- Genetics in general
- Inherited allergies
- Nutrition
- Stress
- Age
- Health of the microflora
- The integrity of the gut lining
- The presence of infection in the gut or anywhere in the body

SUPPORT YOUR IMMUNE SYSTEM

- *Any kind of infection, even the flu, can lower your stores of antibodies* (our precious secretory IgA). An infection anywhere in the body, even a tooth abscess, can affect the gut by increasing stress and reducing the SIgA.
- *Stress reduces antibody levels.* Any kind of stress can do this. Two German studies indicate that mental relaxation procedures, such as meditation or biofeedback, can lead to increased secretion of SIgA, in comparison with a vigilant task. To promote this positive effect, stress reduction; moderate exercise such as yoga, tai chi, or Qigong; meditation; or any kind of mental relaxation are very important for a healthy digestive tract.
- *Poor diet and low nutrient levels generally also lower immune protection.* It's been shown that children in third world countries who have protein calorie malnutrition (PCM) have lower antibody levels and therefore frequently get diarrhea conditions because they're lacking the SIgA to protect

them against diarrhea. Once you get diarrhea you lose even more lining in the gut, and it becomes a vicious cycle.

- *Antibody levels decrease with age.* It seems that there are many more things that reduce secretory IgA than easily increase it, so you really have to be on guard. Research has found that nutrition can actually affect the way your genetic makeup is expressed. Good nutrition can tip the balance toward health.

- *Vitamin A in particular is critical in replenishing the lining of the gut* and maintaining the integrity of the mucosa. Unfortunately lack of vitamin A happens to be the most common vitamin deficiency in the entire world. Other nutrients that increase SIgA include zinc taken with vitamin A, colostrum (for people who are not dairy intolerant), and probably L-glutamine.

Biographical information for **Michael Rosenbaum, M.D.,** appears on page 41.

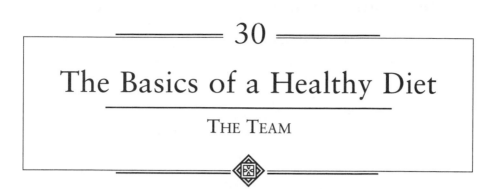

30

The Basics of a Healthy Diet

THE TEAM

Food needs and tolerances are very individual. Here are some foods known to be good for your health, and special concerns that may come up for people with digestive illness. The strategy is simple:

- Choose foods close to their natural state, source, and season
- Select foods that are free of additives and pollutants
- Whenever possible, use organically grown fruits and vegetables
- Plan meals around freshly cooked and, if tolerated, raw foods
- Minimize your use of packaged, boxed, and canned products

FOODS AND FLUIDS

Water

Benefits: Spring water is the best. Other good sources include bottled water that's well filtered, using a method such as carbon-block filter. Use bottled or filtered water in cooking, to make herb teas, and to dilute fresh fruit or vegetable juices (about half and half).

Concerns: Never drink tap water unless you know it's from a top quality source. Tap water is considered a major source of parasitic infection, according to doctors and the news media!

Vegetables

Benefits: Vegetables are the basic staple of this diet. Eat all the raw watery vegetables or juices your body can handle. Heavier vegetables such as broccoli and peas (if well tolerated) are best steamed or stir-fried in very little cooking oil. They can also be taken raw if you can handle them. Starchy vegetables (yams, parsnips, turnips, and other root vegetables) should be baked or steamed until soft. (Monitor for tolerance to starches.) Cruciferous vegetables (broccoli, cabbage, cauliflower, and Brussels sprouts) can be very health promoting. Sea vegetables (like those used as side dishes in traditional Japanese cooking) include dulse, hijiki, wakame, and nori. They are excellent sources of minerals.

Concerns: Some people with inflammatory conditions find that they can't handle the fiber of raw foods or salads, and in some cases, even cooked vegetables. In these situations experiment to find what you can tolerate by trying juiced raw vegetables or soft or pureed cooked vegetables. One of the benefits of vegetables is their alkalinity. If you find you must limit vegetables, supplement with liquid chlorophyll such as DeSoussa's or with a green food product such as Nutricology's ProGreens.

Whole Grains

Benefits: A secondary staple of this diet, grains provide valuable starch, fiber, minerals, and vitamins. Use whole grains only and flours made from whole grains. Brown rice, cracked wheat, buckwheat, barley, and oats are just a few of the many grains available from your natural food supplier. These can be prepared plain, baked into breads of many kinds, or made into different kinds of pastas.

Concerns: Whole grains are usually an excellent staple. But some people with digestive disorders can't tolerate grains, especially wheat and other grains containing gluten. Others can't tolerate starches or sweeteners (carbohydrates). This is especially true of those who have GI infections or bacterial overgrowth.

Legumes

Benefits: Legumes are another secondary staple. Beans and peas are excellent sources of protein, complex carbohydrate, and fiber. They can be eaten as a main course in various modifications of traditional beans-and-rice dishes. Soybean tofu is an excellent and versatile source of protein. Beans are also good chelators, substances that help to clear the body of toxins.

Concerns: Beans and soy products tend to be harder to digest and are known to cause flatulence in some, but all recommendations are individual. The product Beano is helpful to some people. Beans are also high in starch, so they don't work for people who are carbohydrate-intolerant because of overgrowth.

Lean Meats

Benefits: Another secondary staple, lean meats can supplement protein in the diet. In any case, they should be lean. The best are fish or fowl rather than beef or pork, which tend to be higher in fat. Roast, broil, or bake. Take care not to brown. Remove the skin from fowl, because it's very high in fat. Those who choose to be vegetarian can do fine with added legumes and other vegetable sources of protein.

Concerns: Meats are best obtained from organic suppliers. It is important that food preparers, especially at home, learn to protect food from prolonged exposure to temperatures that permit bacterial overgrowth. Keep foods cold until you cook them, then hot until they're eaten.

Eggs

Benefits: Eggs should be restricted to those from free-ranging birds fed organic foods. They are best soft-boiled or poached because frying will increase detrimental oxidation of fats. The best eggs are those from clean environments, as free of salmonella as possible. Eggs are high in lecithin (a precursor of cell membranes), and contain beta-carotene, the entire B complex, essential amino acids, and minerals such as sulfur and chromium.

Concerns: It is probably best to limit their use to several times a week. Be sure they're well cooked to avoid problems from salmonella.

Fruits

Benefits: Fresh, seasonal, and unprocessed are best. Take in limited quantity. They tend to promote good regularity. Best taken without other foods, in the morning as breakfast or as a midmorning or midafternoon snack. That is, when you eat fruit, eat just fruit. This is because fruits are digested more quickly than meat or grains and they move through the digestive tract more rapidly. If fruits are eaten alone, it will minimize fermentation due to slow motility.

Concerns: Dried fruits should be used only occasionally and with caution because they are very concentrated sweets and are often chemically treated, typically with sulfur, which tends to promote allergies. People who are carbohydrate intolerant due to GI overgrowth may crave fruits and sweets, and find they are gas producing. In that case, it's best to leave them alone or minimize them.

Nuts and Seeds

Benefits: Whole, untreated, good-quality nuts and seeds can be a great snack or even part of a substantial quick meal. They can be added to various vegetable and grain dishes for flavor and added protein. They are high in fat, however, so use nuts and nut butters in moderation. Keep nuts and nut butters in the refrigerator after opening.

Concerns: Watch out for rancidity. When nuts and seeds are hulled (especially if they are broken), they become more susceptible to oxidation, which is what makes them rancid. If there's any hint of a funny taste, discard them, because rancid fats are a major source of free radicals. If you're concerned about heart disease, you might want to use peanut butter sparingly. It seems to have an unidentified substance that contributes to heart disease. Peanuts often contain a low level of mold called aflatoxin, known to cause cancer; the amount of aflatoxins allowed is regulated by the government, but this is still a reason to monitor your response and moderate your intake.

Oils
Benefits: These are an important part of the diet. The body needs about two tablespoons a day of a good-quality oil rich in the essential fatty acids. The best oil to use on a daily basis is canola oil or olive oil (rich in monounsaturated fats) as a condiment and in salad dressings. Fresh flaxseed oil is a superb source of essential fatty acids. One tablespoon can be taken as a daily supplement. Additional vitamin E should be taken with it—about 400 IUs a day. Don't cut out fats altogether—your body needs fats to make hormones, cell walls, and the myelin that coats and protects your nerves.

Concerns: Purchase natural oils rather than hydrogenated ones. For the same reason, it's best to use natural butter rather than margarine products. The basic rule, however, is that the diet should be low in fat overall. Aim for about 20 percent of total calories.

Fermented Foods
Benefits: These are an excellent source of trace nutrients and friendly bacteria for some. They include modest amounts of good-quality live-culture low-fat yogurt, miso paste for broths, and health food store sauerkraut.

Concerns: Like everything else, response is individual. People with candida overgrowth or GI infection tend to have more problems tolerating fermented products.

Sweeteners
Benefits: These are best used very sparingly. Raw honey, real maple syrup, and stevia are probably the best.

Concerns: For people with carbohydrate intolerance, stevia maybe the only option. Any sweetener, no matter how pure, provides food for bad bugs. Monitor your response.

Salt

Benefits: Requirements are highly individual. Vegetarians have a higher requirement because they naturally get less salt in their diet. Best used very sparingly. Good sources include sea salt, sesame salt (a mix of sea salt and sesame seeds), Bragg's Liquid Aminos, and natural soy sauce. Some of the low-salt products and salt substitutes are quite decent, such as Vege-Sal, Spike, and Mrs. Dash.

Concerns: Many people are virtually addicted to large amounts of salt and salty foods. This can contribute to high blood pressure and may be a factor in other degenerative conditions. Moderation in all things—base your use on your health needs.

Spices

There are almost countless herbs and spices that can be used to add flavor and medicinal effects to our foods. Choose nonirritating, natural, and organic herbs and spices whenever possible. Some spices probably have antimicrobial benefits. But for people with inflammation strong spices must be moderated or avoided.

Vitamin and Mineral Supplements

Best to use natural sources rather than synthetic. A plan for your optimal supplements can be worked out with your nutritionally oriented practitioner. In addition seek advice on specific health conditions, but continue to monitor your reactions to what you eat, since no one can totally predict your own unique responses.

Beneficial Flora

The first consideration is to be sure one is not dairy intolerant. In some intermittent allergies, yogurt can be tolerated every fourth or every seventh day. If not supplements are available containing *L. acidophilus* and bifidobacteria without any added components of milk.

These foods and products can be quite helpful:

- Following antibiotic therapy
- Following illness

- Following digestive upsets
- In response to stress
- Before and during long-distance travel

WHAT TO AVOID OR MINIMIZE

Canned or Bottled Drinks and Sodas

Apart from mineral waters, these drinks tend to be high in sugar and low in nutrients. Carbonated beverages are high in phosphoric acid, which contributes to the demineralization of bone (osteoporosis). Alcoholic beverages are to be avoided, except for those who want to add one or two glasses of wine to their daily health regimen. The research on this is still mixed, so use moderation.

Even bottled fruit juices have been processed in bottling and are nowhere near as nutritious as fresh fruits. In addition juices are too sweet for your body—they require a blast of insulin to metabolize, which puts a real stress on your pancreas. A good way to deal with this is to eat fruit rather than drink juice. A pint of orange juice, for example, contains the juice of ten oranges. We would almost never sit down and eat ten oranges, but we think nothing of drinking a pint of juice.

Better options: Spring or mineral water, fruit juice cut half and half with water, lemon water (hot or cold), or herb tea (hot or iced).

Sugar and Other Sweets

Humans naturally like sweets. But in nature, sugar is present in small quantities in various foods, mainly fruits. Concentrated sweets imbalance the metabolism, accelerate aging, contribute to atherosclerosis, and can hasten the onset of diabetes. They also encourage the overgrowth of bad bugs.

Better options: Sweets also seem to drive a craving for more sweets. You can cut those cravings by drinking more water and other wholesome liquids. Cravings can also be minimized by taking a little extra vitamin C or an anti-candida herb such as Nutribiotic (grapefruit seed extract with artemisia).

Hydrogenated Fats

These altered fats can have damaging effects on the body and are best avoided. They're found in soft margarines; many other processed foods contain them because they are inexpensive and have a long shelf life. However, this is another good reason to avoid processed foods.

Better options: Monounsaturated oils such as canola or olive oil (try Bertolli Light), and for some people butter (such as sweet butter) or ghee (clarified butter, used in East Indian cooking).

Caffeine

Minimize coffee. Decaf may be acceptable in small amounts, although there is some evidence that even decaffeinated coffee may be bad for your health. Also minimize black tea, caffeinated soft drinks, chocolate, and over-the-counter medicines like No-Doz, which are the major sources of caffeine. It is best to get your energy by other means. Try a grain-based coffee substitute like Caffix or Pero, but don't expect them to taste like your normal cup of java.

Better options: Consider how you use coffee. If you use it for a morning pick-me-up, consider adding some form of protein to your breakfast, perhaps a smoothie with protein powder. Carry snacks with a little protein (like nuts) for later in the day. If it's just a beverage, try switching over to spring or mineral waters. If it's social, go out for tea (herb or green teas).

Canned Foods

With the exception of quality tomato products that can be used in moderation, canned foods are to be generally avoided. They have been heat treated and tend to be low in nutrients. Furthermore, they often contain trace contaminants from processing. Commercial canned foods are also typically very high in salt. Like everything else, practice moderation.

Better options: Develop a routine that allows you the few minutes to quickly cook fresh vegetables (steamed or sautéed in the wok). Most vegetables take less than ten minutes. Consider investing in a mini–food processor to cut prep time.

White Flour Products

These include breads, pastries, and pastas. White flour, even when "fortified," is low in nutrients and thus provides only empty calories. The high starch content of the flour tends to promote yeast and bacterial overgrowth.

Better options: Whole-grain breads, especially low-yeast breads such as whole-wheat pita bread and whole-grain tortillas.

Processed and Luncheon Meats

These often have many additives, altered fats, and high salt content. The preservatives nitrate and nitrite are of special concern because in the body they may become nitrosamines, known to cause cancer.

Better options: Read labels. Some deli meats are nitrate free.

Fried Foods

Frying uses heat levels that damage many nutrients and changes the structure of the fats, making them unhealthy for the heart. It is best to avoid fried foods altogether.

Better options: Try oven-baked potatoes! They're astonishingly good. Stir-frying vegetables in a small amount of a good-quality oil and water is okay because they will cook at temperatures that are more like steaming.

Browned Foods

Avoid all browning of foods. Browned proteins are aged protein. The brown stuff contains toxic and carcinogenic compounds created by the process of browning. This is true of meats, vegetables, and starches.

Dairy Products

There seem to be several issues with dairy products. Sort through the concerns and see if any affect you. Some people lack the enzyme lactase and therefore can't handle lactose, the natural sugar in milk sugar. For these people supplementing the enzyme or using acidophilus milk products may solve the problem. Others are sensitive to milk protein (especially casein), and that can be more difficult to overcome. Nonorganic dairy products may also contain pesticide residues from feeds, drugs given to the cows (such as hormones), and bacterial and chemical contaminants from processing.

Better options: Organic whole milk is now more readily available, and for those who tolerate dairy can be a decent food. Of these, plain yogurt, plain kefir, and butter can provide significant nutrients. As always, tolerance is totally individual. Calcium is the only nutrient you are likely to miss if you find you must cut out dairy products.

Low-fat cheeses such as Swiss, sharp cheddar, Edam, and Jarlsberg are lactose free, and used in moderation are a good source of protein. Goat cheese can also be a quality food. Blood type and heredity are important factors in dairy tolerance. Check *Eat Right 4 Your Type* (D'Adamo. G. P. Putnam, 1996) for information on the genetic aspect of your food tolerances.

Fast Foods

There is a huge industry producing fast and convenience foods that are typically highly processed, devitalized, and calorie-rich goodies. Avoid these foods or keep them to a bare minimum. We now believe they contribute to the huge problem of obesity in the United States.

Better options: If you're on the road and don't have many choices, remember that some of the major fast food chains now offer salads with grilled chicken or feta cheese, pita pockets, and even decent vegetarian burgers.

Junk Foods

These are another side of the fast food category, especially sweet and salty munchies. They add empty calories, altered fats, and sometimes harmful additives to the diet. Since many of them are sweet or starchy, they tend to encourage the bad bugs. Cut your cravings with the strategies listed under "Sugar and Other Sweets" above.

Preservatives: These chemicals add shelf life to packaged convenience products. They are added to virtually all processed foods and are another reason to avoid packaged, bottled, and canned processed foods. There's a lot of research available about the concerns. For more information browse Ruth Winter's book *Food Additives* (Three Rivers Press, 1994).

Alcoholic Beverages

Extreme moderation is needed. It depends on your genetic heritage. If you come from a teetotaling family alcohol may not be for you; some people just can't metabolize alcohol. But the research shows that for others alcohol in moderation can be beneficial. For example, the Mediterranean tradition of red wine turns out to offer benefit for the heart, not only because of the helpful bioflavonoids, but also because it contains anthocyanins, the red-pigmented nutrients.

HOW TO ADAPT TO A HEALTHIER DIET

Take it in stages. It will depend on where your diet is now and how fast you want to move. It is best to expect that it may take you quite some time to make all of these changes you want in your diet. And generally make one change at a time so you can tell what's working and what isn't.

Cut out the elements worst for your health first.

1. Cut out tobacco, sugar, and junk foods. Sometimes that's all you have to do. You may find you don't need other changes.
2. After getting used to that, check your response to dairy and wheat. These are the two foods most likely to cause digestive allergies. In addition check for sensitivity to corn and citrus.
3. Begin phasing out processed foods and white flour products.
4. Work to refine your program to fit to the needs of your own unique body and chemistry.

The Glycemic Index

Foods that are low on the Glycemic Index tend to cause lower insulin production. Oatmeal, for example, is relatively low on the index. Wheat triggers more insulin than rice or oatmeal. Potatoes, starchy breads, and sweets all require a huge output of insulin. Over time this type of stress can lead to weight gain and even diabetes. The Glycemic Index is a great resource for anyone who wonders what to eat to stay healthy. The key is to select foods that are low on the index—the foods that also happen to be your favorites. (See Glycemic Index on page 274.)

What to Do When Eating Out

Simply choose menu items you know you can tolerate. Don't worry about blowing it once in a while. It isn't what you do now and then that counts, as much as what you do day in and day out. What if you get serious cravings? Don't try to bully yourself into accepting this way of eating.

Reason with yourself. Give yourself a vacation meal now and then (say, every Saturday night at first) when you can eat anything your little heart desires for that one meal. Call it your freak-out dinner. After a while, as your body adapts to eating well, you'll find that you don't really need such meals that often. But even then an occasional freak out will help you be less obnoxious to your friends and family.

Food Combining

The basic idea here is that every food has a specific condition for optimal digestion. For example, fruits need very little digestion in the stomach and can pass through quickly. On the other hand, proteins require a more prolonged time in the acid environment of the stomach for best digestion. Starches are mostly digested in the small intestine.

- Fruits are best eaten alone—that is, without any other food in the stomach.
- Proteins or starches are combined with vegetables. Using this system a meal would not typically contain both a large amount of starch and a large amount of meat. For example, fish might be served with a big salad. Rice would be served with cooked vegetables. An Oriental dish might contain meat in small quantities with the rice, but not a large portion.
- Try this system and see if you find your meals more digestible. If so it becomes quite easy to integrate into meal preparation and actually seems to make planning a little easier.

Staying Attuned to Your Biorhythm

The body has many natural rhythms. They range from long cycles like yearly hormone production peaks to the very rapid cycles of the brain waves. In terms of food consumption, the most important rhythm is the daily cycle.

Another natural rhythm to keep in mind is the breath cycle. You will get the most out of what you eat if you breathe well. Make sure to stop to breathe between bites. Don't be in a big rush to finish your meal. If you are in a hurry or under time pressure, take juice rather than solid food: You'll find it more digestible.

A final natural rhythm to tune in to is the annual cycle. Many foods have a season when they are available fresh locally. The body tends naturally to eat more heavily in the winter and more lightly in the summer. You may also want to consider engaging in an annual cleansing diet or brief juice fast to help rebalance the excesses of your preceding year. This can contribute greatly to your health.

Eat Right for Your Type

Consider your genetics, the physical heritage from your ancestors. We can't change genetics overnight. The implications are that it can be helpful to eat as our ancestors did. This approach also makes an argument for eating whole foods rather than refined, since that's what our ancestors ate. Check out Dr. Peter D'Adamo's book *Eat Right 4 Your Type* (G. P. Putnam, 1996).

Acid-Alkaline Balance

Excessive acidic waste in our body can stimulate a variety of problems, including chronic infections, difficulties with incomplete digestion, and allergies. One way to counter that is to make your diet more alkaline. The Japanese, for example, have structured their diet to be alkaline. They also drink alkaline water to overcome other sources of acidity. One helpful approach is to shift our habits by finding more alkaline substitutes for foods we enjoy.

Benefits: Not overconsuming pasta and bread can be helpful in this regard. Rice, millet, and tofu are much more alkaline than wheat. We may choose to eat more rice and less pasta. We may want to change to green teas and herb teas. Bitter greens tend to be very healthy for the gallbladder and pancreas.

Concerns: Meat, tomatoes, and wheat are more acidic. Coffee and black tea are also acid producing. There are so many variables in our diets that push us toward acidity that we almost have to do something every day as a counterbalance. The key here, as in most things, is balance.

Easy Ways to Eat an Alkaline Diet: Consider adding a green salad at least once a day and also at least one cooked green vegetable a day. In addition try a tablespoon of liquid chlorophyll a day, choosing one of the tasty brands such as DeSoussa's or World Organics. These three simple additions will help to keep your system more alkaline over the course of the day. This can encourage good digestion and minimize toxicity.

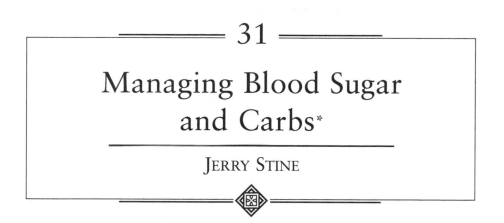

31

Managing Blood Sugar and Carbs*

JERRY STINE

One of the most important influences on our health, minute to minute, is the stability of our blood sugar. When we refer to blood sugar, we are referring to the level of glucose in the blood. Glucose is one of the primary sources of fuel and energy for the body. Most of us are all too familiar with the feeling we get when we skip a meal and our blood sugar falls too low. At times like this our energy usually drops as well. Some people are also prone to anger or irritability, and others tend toward depression. Some experience a loss of concentration, a state that isn't alleviated until they eat something.

BLOOD SUGAR AND THE IMMUNE SYSTEM

Most of us don't think of our blood sugar as a powerful regulator of immune function. But blood sugar can affect immunity in a number of important ways:

- Lower levels of white blood cells have been associated with a diet high in sugar.
- The overgrowth of yeast or bacteria can also result from eating too many starches and sweets, since carbohydrates are the preferred food of many microbes.
- Impaired immune function can result from internal chain reactions that involve insulin and other hormones. This stress can inhibit antibody production.

*Excerpted from *Boosting Immunity: Creating Wellness Naturally* edited by Len Saputo, M.D., and Nancy Faass (Novato, Calif.: New World Library, 2002). Reprinted with permission of New World Library at www.newworldlibrary.com.

Jim was a competitive marathon runner. At 35 he was also a busy professional with a wife and young children. In preparing for races he found that if he trained thoroughly enough to be competitive, he caught every cold or flu his children brought home from school, causing him to miss work. When he didn't train that hard, he wasn't as susceptible but then he wasn't well prepared for the race. He was anxious to resolve this dilemma—running was important to him, and he was one of the top fifty runners in the state.

Like many of us, he had never paid much attention to his diet or eating on a schedule. In our nutritional counseling sessions, we focused on improving both athletic function and immune response, so that Jim could train to his competitive level and stay healthy. His choice of foods was an issue, because as a runner, he believed he had to eat a diet high in carbohydrates. It took a while for him to become convinced that "carbo loading" was not always the best strategy, particularly in his case.

Through experience he found that when he reduced his carbohydrate intake, he stopped getting sick. He made it a point to include reasonable levels of protein and fat in his diet and to eat at regular intervals. He was surprised and pleased to find that his immune function improved, and so did his running.

The stability of our blood sugar has a wide range of effects on:

- Moods
- Mental clarity
- Energy
- Allergic sensitivities
- Metabolism
- Weight
- Potential for diabetes
- Heart health

Maintaining stable blood sugar (glucose) is simpler than you would think. It involves just three steps:

1. Eating the right foods. Foods that release glucose slowly don't cause drastic highs and lows in blood sugar level.
2. Finding food options you really enjoy that are also good for you.
3. Ideally having a regular eating schedule, eating every four or five hours. That may mean just a piece of fruit and some nuts or a protein shake. The idea is to provide the body with a consistent supply of nutrients.

THE BENEFITS OF STABLE BLOOD SUGAR

Blood sugar (glucose) is one of our primary sources of fuel. Most people find that their performance and sense of well-being are improved by having a steady source of energy—stable blood sugar. But many of us tend to eat too many sweet and starchy foods—simple carbohydrates. This has resulted from the modern lifestyle centered on junk food, fast food, and low-fat diets. High-carbohydrate diets can cause health problems, because it's more difficult to maintain consistent blood sugar and energy with a diet that's heavy in simple starches.

Major research has found that diet and poor blood sugar regulation are important risk factors for adult-onset diabetes, Type 2 diabetes. This condition currently affects more than 15 million Americans. A diet low in sugars and starches can often help to prevent the onset of diabetes and is also appropriate for those who are already diabetic. Research also links high-carbohydrate intake with conditions such as obesity, high cholesterol and triglycerides, and heart disease. This is a little confusing, because we tend to think of high cholesterol and heart disease as the result of a high-fat diet. But the carbohydrate connection to these diseases has been confirmed in some of the most extensive research ever conducted. On the other hand, a low-starch diet has been found beneficial in:

- *Lowering stress on the body.* Rapid changes in blood sugar are a major stress on many crucial systems. Maintaining stable blood sugar can minimize this stress.
- *Improving health and chronic conditions.* Drastic highs and lows in blood sugar can cause immediate problems, including fatigue, mood swings, difficulty concentrating, or insomnia. Over time it can be a major factor in weight gain, digestive disorders, or chronic depression.
- *Cutting the risk of disease.* Over a lifetime poor regulation of blood sugar has been linked to obesity, cholesterol problems, heart disease and stroke, diabetes, and the serious disorders that can result from diabetes.
- *Avoiding weight gain.* Since obesity has been linked to both diabetes and heart disease, it is an important health issue. It's much easier to maintain the weight we would like with this style of eating. It is a highly effective tool for natural weight loss.
- *Supporting healing.* Ensuring a steady, reliable source of energy can support the healing process. Correcting this issue in our diet is one of the most important things we can do.
- *Promoting greater alertness and energy.* It's especially important that the brain have a steady supply of glucose.
- *Improving athletic performance.* If you have an athletic interest, this style of eating substantially improves endurance and recovery from intense physical activity.

REGULATING BLOOD SUGAR

We can avoid dramatic highs and lows in our energy and mood by choosing foods that encourage stable blood sugar. The key is to eat slow-burning carbohydrates, foods that are broken down gradually to provide the body with a steady source of nourishment. This means foods such as nuts, popcorn, oatmeal, or sweet potatoes. In contrast, refined sugars and starches are processed too rapidly in the body because they are already partially broken down due to manufacturing. Soon after we eat them, they are quickly absorbed into the bloodstream. As a result they raise our blood sugar too quickly. This is not only true of foods containing sugar and sweeteners but also of foods made with refined flour, such as breads or pastries.

Refined sugars and simple starches are so common in our modern diet that many people experience blood sugar highs and lows every day. When blood sugar (glucoses) is elevated too high, the body is forced to bring the levels down. To cope with high blood sugar, the body releases excessive amounts of insulin, a natural hormone. This brings the blood sugar black to normal levels, but at a price. The body must dispose of it. So some of the blood sugar is expended as energy—remember that energy rush you get right after you eat sugar? And some is stored or converted into fat.

Research has shown that this process is one of the primary causes of excess weight gain. This is also a form of metabolic stress. If we can avoid these rapid increases in blood sugar (and insulin) we can eliminate a major source of stress on the body.

EATING BY THE GLYCEMIC INDEX

One of the easiest ways to eat healthy is to select foods based on their rating on the Glycemic Index (see page 274). Most people are pleasantly surprised to learn which of their favorite foods are also good for them. You can copy the Pocket Index reference chart on the facing page and carry it in your wallet or purse.

The Glycemic Index is based on scientific research. It's the diet that provides the basis for the following four diet books: *The Zone, Sugar Busters!, Eating Well for Optimum Health,* and *The Formula.* Maintaining stable blood sugar is also described as glycemic control—referring to glucose (blood sugar). The index is simply a way of rating foods, based on how much they increase blood sugar and how rapidly it increases. Foods that have a high number on the Glycemic Index (55 to 150) tend to cause very rapid increases in blood sugar. This happens with foods that are very sweet, like desserts, or very starchy, like baked potatoes. Foods with a high number on the index also include those made from refined grains, like white bread or breakfast cereal, that metabolize quickly into glucose. It's helpful to read the Glycemic Index, because some foods are more problematic than we realize. Surprisingly, rice cakes, for example, are high on the index.

Foods that break down into glucose more slowly have a lower rating on the Glycemic Index. Those at 55 or below are either metabolized slower or contain fewer natural sugars. That avoids stressful, drastic changes in blood sugar levels.

The Pocket Index

Fresh Fruit

Berries like blueberries, strawberries, blackberries, and raspberries

Stone fruits, such as peaches, plums, and cherries

Apples and pears

Citrus fruits, such as oranges and grapefruit

Mangos, kiwi fruit, and grapes

(Juices tend to be too sweet because they are so concentrated. Minimize tropical fruits, such as bananas.)

Hardy Starches

Nuts (fresh or roasted)

Popcorn (yes, butter is usually fine)

Whole-wheat pita bread

Oatmeal, brown rice, and wild rice

Sweet potatoes and yams

Pinto and lima beans

Black, kidney, and butter beans

(Minimize white rice, white bread, corn, and potatoes.)

Vegetables

Lettuces, spinach, cilantro, and parsleys

Tomatoes

Cucumbers

Leafy green vegetables for cooking: dandelion, chard, collards, and kale

Celery, cabbage, and bok choy

Peas, green beans, and peppers

Asparagus, broccoli, and Brussels sprouts

Eggplant

Summer squashes, including zucchini and yellow squash

Quality Protein

Protein tends not to trigger insulin production

Unsweetened or lightly sweetened dairy products as tolerated—yogurt, kefir, cheeses, creamed cheese, and cottage cheese

Soy and tofu products

Nuts of all kinds

Eggs

Nutrition bars and protein powders, if they are low in carbohydrates and contain protein

Meat

Poultry, fish, and shellfish

The Glycemic Index

Foods that are rated at 55 or below are easier for your body to handle. Minimize those above 55 because they trigger insulin.

Foods That Trigger Insulin

Grains, Breads, Cereals, and Vegetables		*Sweeteners, Fruits, and Dairy Products*	
White bread and baked potatoes	95	Maltose	105 to 150
Instant rice	90	Glucose	100
Cooked carrots	85	Raisins	95
French fries, pretzels, rice cakes	80	Honey, refined sugar	75
Corn flakes, corn on the cob	75	Watermelon, dried apricots	70
Frozen or canned corn	75	Pineapple	65
Plain bagels	75	Ice cream, ripe bananas	60
Crackers, graham crackers	75		
White flour products, puffed wheat	75		
Sweetened cereals	75		
White rice, taco shells, beets	70		
Spaghetti	60		

Foods That Don't Trigger Insulin

Starches and Vegetables		*Fruit and Dairy Products*	
Oatmeal, brown rice, wild rice	55	Mango, kiwi	50
Sweet potatoes, popcorn, whole-wheat pita bread	55	Pears	45
Yams	50	Peaches, plums, apples, oranges	40
Green beans, green peas	45	Yogurt, with fruit	35+
Pinto and lima beans	40	Milk, whole	30+
Black, kidney, and butter beans	30	Milk, skim	30
Nuts	30 to 15	Cherries, grapefruit	25
Artichokes	25	Yogurt, plain, no sweetener	15
Asparagus	20		
Tomatoes	15		
Green vegetables	15		

Applying the Index

Using the Glycemic Index involves just three steps:

1. Getting to know the Index
2. Using it to plan your meals and grocery list
3. Developing a schedule, so you don't go too long without something to eat

When we get hungry, that means we've waited too long to eat and our blood sugar is already beginning to drop. We don't have to eat very much to keep blood sugar steady—in fact, it's not desirable to eat large meals. For people who tend to become hypoglycemic, it is especially important to have three meals a day and two snacks between meals.

For those of us who are rushed in the morning, breakfast need not involve cooking at all. It could just mean having a protein shake, fruit and cheese, a tuna fish sandwich, or unsweetened yogurt. In general you don't want to go more than four or five hours without eating. Snacks may be eaten an hour or two before meals—this is another way to prevent overeating at mealtime.

- *Individualizing your diet.* The Glycemic Index is easy for most people to learn. It may take a month or two to become accustomed to this style of eating. Give yourself permission to adapt gradually. Remember, one of the keys is substitution—replacing foods high on the index with favorite foods that are low on the index. For example, have cherries or a peach instead of a banana or raisins.
- *Cut cravings.* Using the Glycemic Index successfully often involves finding ways to decrease cravings for sweets or starches. See *The Zone* and *The Diet Cure* for additional suggestions. Some of the most effective approaches include:
  - Increasing your water intake (see chapter 4)
  - Eating half an apple for dessert
  - Using the French approach for dessert: serve cheeses, salads, or nuts and wine (like Gorgonzola and walnuts with port)
  - Taking extra vitamin C, the buffered form
  - Taking chromium, a mineral supplement, one dose (200 mcg) on an empty stomach, first thing in the morning (usually well tolerated)

BALANCED MEALS

The ratio of nutrients in a healthy diet is typically 40-30-30: 40 percent carbohydrates, 30 percent protein, and 30 percent fats. This is the same ratio used in *The Zone* diet and in *The Formula*. In these diets every meal is built around low-starch vegetables and high-quality protein. A balanced diet consists of:

- *40 percent carbohydrates,* chosen from fruits and vegetables on the index that are rated at 55 or below. Portion size: about one to two cups of vegetables. You usually don't have to measure out portions as carefully as you would if you were on a diet, because these foods don't tend to cause weight gain. If you want to include starches high on the index, they should not make up more than one-fourth of your carbohydrates at any given meal.
- *30 percent proteins,* that is, three to five ounces of quality protein, depending on your body size and how active you are. The choice of protein varies from one person to another and can be adapted to a vegetarian diet (including dairy and eggs) or vegan diet (nuts, tofu, and soy).

  Quality proteins include:

Dairy	Soy and tofu
Eggs	Poultry and fish
Nuts	Meat
Protein powders and bars	

- *30 percent fat.* Good sources of fat include cold-pressed flaxseed oil, olive oil, safflower oil, and sunflower oil. Typical servings are $1/2$ to 1 teaspoon of oil per meal, which can be taken as salad dressing.

Dining Out

Restaurant meals typically consist of a lot of protein and a lot of starch—for example, a baked potato and a basket of rolls, or pasta and French bread, or a large serving of white rice. The vegetables are often served in small amounts. Keeping blood sugar steady can be achieved by reversing these proportions. Emphasize the vegetables, and just eat a smaller portion of the starch. Say "No, thank you" to at least one of the starches in advance, to avoid temptation and waste. If your willpower is stretched thin, dish up what you want before the meal begins and send back the rest so you won't be tempted to overeat.

To find food that adapts well to this style of eating, plan ahead and make conscious choices when you dine out. Some cuisines work well with this diet:

- Chinese or Thai cooking often offers a good balance with lots of vegetables and moderate protein. Cut down significantly on the rice or noodles, and avoid sweet-and-sour sauces.
- Green salads with grilled chicken are widely available.
- Fish with a salad or vegetables is a good choice.
- Specialty dishes, such as fajitas or antipasto, that are mainly vegetables and protein are also a good choice.
- Burritos or tacos work well, if you go easy on the beans and rice.
- Nouvelle or Continental cuisine frequently includes great vegetable dishes (be intelligent about the dessert course).

When you're cooking at home, plan ahead so you have leftovers for breakfast and lunch the next day, which really simplifies your routine.

Cheating on the Diet

What can we do about dessert; that special wedding cake; or the sweets served at birthdays, holidays, picnics, and other celebrations? When we indulge we may find ourselves bounced around emotionally—hyper, then depressed, and eventually feeling shaky. It's okay to indulge occasionally, as long as you don't do it too frequently and your reactions aren't too severe. You can avoid a low drop in blood sugar by eating a balanced snack about forty-five minutes to an hour after you eat something really sweet. The snack should include protein, which usually stabilizes blood sugar, and carbohydrates low on the Glycemic Index. The slower-burning nourishment of the protein tends to sustain the blood sugar, avoiding that blood sugar roller coaster that can be so depressing.

When Bob was first cleaning up his diet, one thing he didn't have the willpower to give up was root beer. He thought about it all the time and craved it, and it became one of the few items that was really a problem for him. This was odd, because beforehand he wouldn't have thought of root beer as a favorite beverage. It just surfaced as something he craved. So he let himself have it once a week. His reaction was so dramatic (and so negative) that eventually he stopped wanting it, because every time he indulged it made him sick. Finally he stopped craving it altogether. Note: This approach only works if your diet is really clean. Otherwise the symptoms won't show up in the midst of many dietary transgressions.

MORE BENEFITS OF USING THE INDEX

Following the Glycemic Index can help you reap many significant health benefits.

- *Better digestion.* Eating foods that aren't too sweet or starchy leads to improved digestive health. It also automatically addresses the issues important in food combining. One of the main issues in food combining is that too much sugar or sweet food causes the stomach to empty into the small intestine too soon. When this happens it means that the first important step of digestion has been completely omitted. This can cause the sense of bloating or indigestion and eventually contribute to allergies or overgrowth.

- *Fewer allergies.* When food passes through the GI tract undigested, it sets the stage for allergies. It can trigger a condition called leaky gut syndrome, in which large food molecules pass into the bloodstream. This puts a burden on the liver. It also encourages overgrowth and food sensitivities or intolerances, because these undigested food molecules may be viewed by the immune system as foreign substances. The response might be experienced as anything from very subtle symptoms to severe reactions.

- *Ability to identify hidden food allergies.* As you become skilled at using the diet, these stresses on your body will be reduced. At this point allergies or food sensitivities may become more apparent as other symptoms begin to decrease. You'll be able to see how different foods affect you, so you can individualize your diet, adapted from the suggestions on the Glycemic Index.

- *Protecting beneficial flora.* Sweets and starches create an environment that tends to encourage the overgrowth of microbes. When there is an overgrowth of yeast such as candida or harmful bacteria the good flora can be crowded out. Eating a diet moderate in carbohydrates encourages healthy flora. (See chapter 7 for more information about flora and digestion.)

- *Cutting the risk of diabetes.* Once we begin eating a glycemic-controlled diet, a massive stress is removed from the body. This type of diet is called "insulin sparing," because foods rated at 55 and below on the index do not call up as much insulin. When you eat a meal low in starches and sugars, your pancreas does not need to produce as much insulin. However, if the liver and the pancreas lose their ability to regulate insulin, diabetes results.

- *Inner balance.* The tendency toward inflammation is also minimized. When blood sugar levels get too high, a whole series of defenses in the immune system are called into play, which can result in inflammation. Keep in mind that blood sugar doesn't just affect one system. All systems of the body are affected by blood sugar and insulin levels, and there is an interrelationship between systems, including the nervous system, the hormones, and immune function.

Martha came to me with a variety of complaints, including poor energy and some memory loss. However, the main thing that motivated her to seek nutritional counseling was that she was getting sick too often. She had a cold or the flu almost every month. Even worse, the illnesses were quite severe; when she got sick she had a very tangible sense of vulnerability. Although she was in her midsixties she had never experienced anything like that before, and it frightened her.

Once she began a diet that was moderate in starches and low in sugars, her susceptibility to colds and flu declined dramatically. We stayed in contact over the course of a year, and during that time she was sick only once.

Eating Well to Strengthen Immunity

This type of approach provides a sound basis for good immune function. Glycemic control is one of the few things that is usually within our reach. We can't control our genetics. Many exposures to environmental toxins and stress are unavoidable. But most of us have the opportunity to choose the foods we eat. The Glycemic Index applies to anyone who wants to maintain or improve his or her health. It is also relevant to those with a health issue, whether it is fatigue, sleep problems, mood swings, difficulty with concentration, allergies, digestive disorders, stress, or any type of immune dysfunction. The most important thing I can tell you about diet is to learn how to use the Glycemic Index to maintain stable blood sugar. You'll find that using this approach in your day-to-day life will provide you with a steady supply of nourishment and energy.

Supplements that Cut Carb Cravings

- Chromium is the primary nutrient in the body that regulates blood sugar. When we don't have enough chromium, the body can't move glucose out of the blood and into the cells. This is probably the most essential nutrient to take to keep blood sugar levels even.
- Tryptophan is the raw material the body uses to make serotonin, a key neurotransmitter. Serotonin levels can be raised naturally by assuring enough of this essential amino acid. Having adequate levels of serotonin has been found to reduce carbohydrate cravings and improve mood.
- Glutamine can be effective in supporting blood sugar if you've missed a meal or have consumed too many carbs. When taken in powdered form, this nutrient is fast acting. Glutamine can also be effective in cases of food poisoning and for general digestive health.
- Amino acid supplement. At least nine of the amino acids found in protein are absolutely essential to the body for repair and healing. If we don't get enough, we can develop a constant sense of hunger. Difficulty in breaking down protein is a common digestive problem and a good supplement insures a supply of essential and critical amino acids.
- Fish oil. We now know that healthy fats are also essential and that fats play a major role in satiety—our sense of having eaten enough. Fish oil is the premier healthy fat and can be taken in supplemental form. Omega-3 fatty acids in fish oil can help reduce excessive cravings for sugar.
- Digestive enzymes. One of the causes of food cravings is incomplete digestion, reflected in a constant state of hunger if we're not being adequately nourished. When this is the case, a digestive enzyme can make a real difference. Taking a good enzyme supplement supports more complete breakdown of food and absorption of nutrients.

Courtesy of Jerry Stine, Lifespan Institute.

Biographical information for **Jerry Stine** appears on page 12.

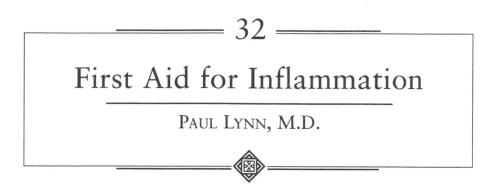

32

First Aid for Inflammation

Paul Lynn, M.D.

Nutrients can be used to soothe and heal inflammation. Suppose you have a case of immediate severe stomach distress. For these situations there are a number of simple but potent healers that include slippery elm, flaxseed, L-glutamine, and protein peptides (Seacure). These four nutrients can be used in a variety of combinations, based on your general symptoms. This approach can be helpful for a variety of conditions:

- Flu (a viral influenza)
- An acute food poisoning from a pathogen such as salmonella or shigella bacteria
- Food irritation or sensitivity that causes diarrhea (without any obvious pathogens)

If there's a fever, it is usually an infection that is bacterial or viral. Bacterial infections can also develop without a high fever.

- *See the doctor.* In all these cases, the first important thing to do is to make an appointment to see the doctor as soon as possible. If you are very ill go to an emergency room or acute-care medical center. While you are waiting to be seen, you can also take the L-glutamine and Seacure. They will not interfere with the medications, but they will make the work of the antibiotics or the antiparasitic therapies easier. The L-glutamine does not compete with medication; it is one of the building blocks of protein, which your body uses to repair tissue. For this kind of intense episode, consider taking 1,000 mg of L-glutamine and one capsule of Seacure every hour until the doctor is seen, and keep taking the preparations at a lower dose even after beginning the medication. Once the symptoms of diarrhea recede, cut down on the L-glutamine. When there is no inflammation present, L-glutamine can be constipating. So discontinue the L-glutamine once the diarrhea has stopped.

- *Guarding against infection.* Strong and healthy cell walls shield against the invasion of pathogens. If you have an infection (whether it be viral, bacterial, or parasitic) and you take preparations like L-glutamine, that can help repair the intestinal lining so it is less susceptible to future infections. This means the organisms will not present as much of a problem, even in parasitic infections. Research has found that when there is exposure to pathogens, the chances of getting sick are related to our tissue resistance to infections as much as to the degree of exposure.
- *For chronic, long-term conditions.* Where there is pain, diarrhea, or cramping, consider taking one L-glutamine and one Seacure twice a day, on an ongoing basis. That would keep an inflammatory diarrhea-like syndrome under control until there is a more definitive way to address it. Just that much will strengthen the lining and tissue of the intestinal tract, making it a less welcoming host to either allergenic or chronic infectious problems.
- *For chronic inflammation and constipation.* Consider taking the Seacure but not the L-glutamine. But in addition try taking flaxseed on a daily basis. It's the seeds, whole or powdered, that have a beneficial effect; flaxseed oil is not really that useful as an anti-inflammatory for the intestinal tract. If flaxseed causes a problem, try capsules of slippery elm. These plants reduce inflammation through a mucouslike quality they develop when they're combined with liquid.

  The flaxseeds act as a poultice to draw out inflammation and provide very gentle roughage that will allow more regular bowel movements. Typical doses would be two tablespoons of flaxseed a day. Slippery elm does the same thing, but it may be just a little less potent. One could take a few more capsules of slippery elm—anywhere from 500 mg a day to 3,000 mg a day (one to six capsules a day), or four to six capsules of Seacure. Always begin with one capsule per day and build up gradually by adding one capsule each day.

  Chronic constipation and inflammation do not constitute an immediate, medically acute situation, but it is essential to address this type of condition. If you have chronic constipation, seek medical help even if you are using the nutrients. Many doctors will prescribe the use of a stool softener. If someone with this condition does not seek medical care, the risk here is that constipation could develop into fecal impaction. This might require seeing a doctor in the emergency room to have the impacted material in the lower colon removed manually.
- *Integrative treatment.* Don't neglect your body while waiting for the nutrients to work. If a condition of chronic constipation has been going on for more than two weeks, it is essential to seek medical care to address the

underlying condition, regardless of taking nutrients. These techniques should not be used as a way to avoid the doctor. We say this as both a disclaimer and to inform you of the importance of tending to either extreme diarrhea or constipation. These suggestions on first aid are meant to be just that—first aid, and not a substitute for medical care.

FLAXSEED

Use the whole seed, taking a typical dose of two tablespoons a day. There are several easy ways to prepare it, depending on your needs. If your inflammation is mild, just use two tablespoons a day sprinkled over foods to provide a tasty nutlike flavor. The seeds will become a gel as you digest them, creating a soothing effect in the digestive tract. Another good way to take flax is to prepare the seeds as a cereal by simply pouring an equal amount of boiling water over 2 to 4 tablespoons of the seeds and letting them stand, covered, for five minutes. This produces a pleasantly flavored dish with the consistency of cooked cereal.

Flaxseeds provide fiber and essential fatty acids. People who find they are still sensitive to the seeds will want to try them ground as a complement to other foods, over salads or cooked rice, or added to their morning smoothie. This can be an effective remedy for constipation and some kinds of inflammation. Flaxseed can also be used to counter the effects of drugs or nutrients that tend to be constipating. For example, some people tend to get constipated when they take L-glutamine. If this happens the flaxseeds can be taken as a complement to the L-glutamine.

L-GLUTAMINE

This amino acid (from protein) works in a different way by strengthening the muscular and mucosal part of the intestinal lining. If you have a mild ongoing chronic inflammatory disease or condition, then taking low doses of L-glutamine (500 mg twice a day) may be sufficient to control the inflammation and clear that vague sense of intestinal ache. L-glutamine can also be specifically useful for leaky gut syndrome. L-glutamine and Seacure can be used together or separately. I usually use them together in the beginning. The Seacure and the L-glutamine are then taken in combination until you become stabilized. Then see if you can get by with just L-glutamine.

- *Repairing the GI tract.* L-glutamine helps to repair the mucosal lining and restore muscular function while discouraging diarrhea. It can be exceptionally useful in cases of food poisoning or infection through its action to slow diarrhea. In general it slows down transit time by restoring mucosal function. Most people tolerate and need high doses when having food poisoning or infections. However, remember there are always rare individual sensitivities. Monitor your own unique response whenever you take any substance. When food poisoning occurs, such an acute situation calls for L-glutamine, taken every two hours until the problem is corrected. It even helps both with viral stomach flu and dysentery caused by bacteria. L-glutamine is also a good nutrient for the nervous system. It is relaxing because it produces glycine, so it is a useful antistress nutrient.

- *The role of L-glutamine during infection.* If you have an acute inflammatory reaction or infection anywhere in the body, your system will draw L-glutamine out of the muscles and put it into the blood so it can be used for repair. That's what makes you feel as if your muscles are weak during a fever or acute illness. When you take the L-glutamine by mouth, your body doesn't have to pull this nutrient out of the muscle tissue. So taking L-glutamine can help you retain a certain sense of muscular stability during the intense acute phase of a cold or flu, which makes you feel stronger and better. It minimizes that sick feeling. L-glutamine also has a multifaceted action when addressing the inflammatory processes of the GI tract.

In modern medicine L-glutamine is given intravenously after intestinal surgery in order to quickly repair the tissue. In most cases any condition that tends to tear up the delicate lining of the GI tract will probably benefit from L-glutamine.

PEPTIDES

Peptides are the building blocks that make up protein, composed of specific combinations of amino acids. There is a product now available that is a combination of peptides and individual amino acids; it's called Seacure. It can be used for conditions of irritable bowel syndrome when no infection is present or detectable. When there's infection I rely more on high doses of L-glutamine along with Seacure. The combination works very well. Seacure's mechanism is to speed up repair of the mucosal lining that has been damaged through irritation or infection. It helps heal very quickly. You can take from three to twelve capsules a day, but typically six to eight capsules a day is the dose.

Doctors report that Seacure is quite useful for the treatment of irritable bowel and leaky gut syndromes. People with leaky gut syndrome may have any of a number of symptoms. Leaky gut can be viewed as an early stage or low-grade level irritable bowel syndrome. These conditions often lead to a susceptibility to food sensitivities. There may be bloating, gas, and pain, or sometimes just pain in the digestive tract without bloating or gas. Other people may have susceptibility to candida and other pathogens, which can be accompanied by fuzzy-headedness or drowsiness after eating.

These conditions also sometimes cause susceptibility to constipation or loose stools. Flaxseed can be used when there is constipation, and L-glutamine can be used for diarrhea. Seacure can be used when there is an acute circumstance of inflammation without infection. Using L-glutamine and Seacure can often allow you to regain control very quickly. In some cases just taking one of each twice a day, ongoing, may be enough to manage irritable bowel and leaky gut syndromes. Many people are maintained quite well on two to four L-glutamine and Seacure per day. It doesn't take a lot to support the body's ongoing maintenance.

CHLOROPHYLL

The other component of this anti-inflammatory program is to include the daily use of liquid chlorophyll to detoxify the GI tract and restore normal acid-alkaline balance. Chlorella, a freshwater algae, also works quite well, but it causes diarrhea in a few people. I never get a complaint about liquid chlorophyll, and it's a day-to-day detoxifying agent that is pleasant tasting. Using liquid chlorophyll on a daily basis can reduce everything from rectal burning or itching to skin rashes and general complaints related to toxicity. Two popular brands are DeSoussa's and World Organics. Use either one ounce of liquid chlorophyll or 1,000 mg of chlorella every day to keep your body more alkaline.

Minimizing toxins in the body. The nutrients that tend to reduce toxicity in the body are liquid chlorophyll, chlorella, and flaxseeds. Flaxseeds can draw inflammation and toxicity out of the body. In herbal medicine flaxseed is often used as a poultice on the skin, for example, to draw out a boil. If you use it on a sprained ankle, it will draw out the inflammation. Similarly in the digestive tract, another valuable part of anti-inflammatory treatment is reducing toxicity on a day-today basis. It's hard for some people to find a diet that won't cause some level of sensitivity or toxicity.

SLIPPERY ELM

This is an herb you can buy at the health food store. It's another alternative to flaxseed. Some people just don't like taking the seeds. You can buy slippery elm in 500 mg capsules, and typical use is one to four per day. Slippery elm reduces inflammation and irritation just about equally to flaxseed in the small and large intestines. But it doesn't help constipation the way flaxseeds do, nor does it provide the nourishing omega-3 fatty acids. It does provide fiber, and it's a strong anti-inflammatory herb. Slippery elm works quite well for people with loose stools or inflammatory stomach (in contrast to conditions that only involve the intestines). This can be helpful because many forms of fiber, such as wheat bran, have a tendency to be harsh. For highly sensitive people, even psyllium is too irritating.

Slippery elm has even less potential to irritate than flaxseed, which is fairly mild. Slippery elm can relieve the irritability related to the gastritis. (Flaxseed tends to work better farther down the intestine.) In contrast, flaxseed doesn't work particularly well for the stomach if there is gastritis. Chlorophyll is also reported to benefit gastritis.

MSM

Another nutrient that is beneficial for stomach inflammation is MSM. If it's clear that food sensitivities are a major part of the problem, try using 1,000 mg of MSM twice a day. Some people use up to two grams twice a day for food sensitivities. Continue it for up to about a month to see if it is working. MSM can also relieve gastritis and stomach ulcers quite dramatically and sometimes very quickly. I'd say that probably 75 percent of my patients who have taken MSM four times a day get a remission and a healing of their symptoms, with the ability to come off medications over time. Don't stop your prescription medication for ulcers or irritable bowel syndrome without consulting with the doctor who wrote them! Let them know of your improvement, and then work together on a plan to gradually end them.

EFFECTS OF ALLERGIES

If you have an obvious problem with intestines or intestinal health, you should eliminate dairy, wheat, and of course sugar. I'm not even saying all gluten—just wheat, dairy, and sugar. These three foods tend to be the three excesses in our diet that generate disease in our intestinal tract: They account for many digestive problems. Eliminating these foods alone can potentially remove the stress from the GI tract.

Wheat and dairy can be reintroduced after one to three weeks and monitored to note any sensitivity. I find that more people can tolerate grains such as oatmeal and rye. Perhaps this is because they don't eat these as much, and gluten in small amounts doesn't cause problems as often.

- However, people with conditions such as celiac disease may be totally gluten intolerant. For them it is essential to absolutely avoid all foods and products containing gluten. Gluten sensitivity can be confirmed through testing.
- Butter is often an exception to a diet with no dairy. Some people can eat butter, which seems to be more digestible than milk or cream. Others are totally dairy-intolerant.
- Sugar is another story. It typically causes fermentation.

If people can eliminate the foods that trigger sensitivities and keep their GI tracts tuned with the key supplements we have discussed, this can resolve a lot of problems with inflammation.

Paul Lynn, M.D., is director of the San Francisco Preventive Medical Center and has been involved in integrative medicine since 1971. A graduate of Louisiana State School of Medicine, he trained at Charity Hospital in New Orleans. He spent several years in Europe and India immersed in the study of natural medicine, and has also studied natural therapy under the pioneers Drs. John Christopher and Bernard Jensen. His work includes a focus on healing through diet, nutrients such as amino acids and peptides, and immune enhancement. Dr. Lynn's current contributions include innovative work in the use of low-dose natural hormone therapy.

Dr. Lynn is available for consultation at the San Francisco Preventive Medical Center, (415) 566-1000.

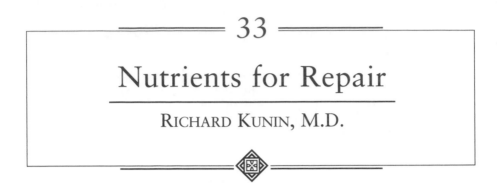

33

Nutrients for Repair

RICHARD KUNIN, M.D.

There are simple rules. You've got to eat—that's the first rule. But you'd like to eat healthy, and that's the second rule. The third rule is to eat in balance with the needs of your own body. That's a high goal. That's what orthomolecular medicine—also called nutritional medicine—is all about. If you ask for it, physicians will soon be providing it. The technology and the knowledge are here. But there is a need for more doctors trained in this field, in response to growing public interest.

HEALTHY OR NOT SO HEALTHY

In health, there is always a genetic component and an environmental component. The environmental component consists of the good things that nourish us (air, water, and nutrients) and the bad things we all must deal with (pollutants and other physical and mental stressors). We accept the need and value of adapting to stressors, but we would rather avoid and remove pollution. As a rule, stressors are inevitable, whereas pollution is largely unnecessary.

When all is well, we are hardly aware of the body and least of all the digestive system, except for the pleasures of taste, texture, and the fulfillment of appetite. The rest is automatic until something goes wrong.

When things go wrong, it's useful to focus on the key nutrients. Nutrients are the raw materials used in the thousands of manufacturing processes of your body; they're an integral part of this big complex system. They're key because if they're depleted nothing works right. If you look at the things that go wrong most often, you get some idea of why things can malfunction in the digestive machinery—the intestinal tract—and fail to heal. Repair is actually quite rapid in the gastrointestinal environment, which regenerates every five days or so. This suggests the possibility of rapid healing if all the right raw materials are in place. So theoretically an insult could begin to heal itself in less than a week if the right nutrients are available to the system.

For example, vitamin E serves as a vital backup if protective antioxidant levels in the cells are reduced, which is likely to happen whenever you have any illness at all. These deficiencies may not look so obvious under everyday conditions, but they really matter when you're sick. If you have chronic illness every one of these nutrients probably should be reviewed. This is key.

When you are chronically ill, a lack of any one of these nutrients could be the cause. In fact, we're saying that these factors should all be considered because they work in an interrelated way. Many have essential functions throughout the body and turn up in the most surprising places. If any one component is missing, it may short-circuit an entire process.

NUTRITION AND DIGESTION

In discussing optimal nutrients for intestinal health, we must think about the health of the entire body first and then the specific organs of the intestinal system. The functioning of each organ in our digestive tract provides evidence of the health condition within.

How do we determine our needs? First there is the old-fashioned way, the art of medicine based on the doctor's knowledge and acumen. Physical examination provides valuable clues. But equally important, we now have specific laboratory tests that identify the blood levels and tissue levels of vitamins, minerals, and other nutrients. And it's now easier to find a doctor who is familiar with these tests and employs them in orthomolecular or nutritional medicine.

ORAL SYMPTOMS

The Gums

The gums, teeth, and mucous membranes all reflect nutritional status. When your gums are bleeding you've got trouble. And that trouble is likely to affect your entire digestive tract because it means your connective tissues are weakened. So if you see bleeding gums think folic acid. Not unimportant because folic acid deficiency also implies the accumulation of homocysteine, a natural biochemical by-product in the body that can become toxic when the levels are too high. This in turn suggests an increased risk of heart attacks and strokes, and bleeding gums are a known predictor of coronary risk. Of course vitamin C is also important for healthy gums, but folic acid is the more common, chronic deficiency.

The Tongue and Mouth

Dental and periodontal infections can cause trouble. They are quite serious because they can become a reservoir of pathogenic bacteria or organisms that can (1) cause secondary abscesses throughout the body, particularly in the brain, kidneys, or heart valves, (2) act as a constant drain on your immune reserves, and (3) wear out the jawbones, which causes tooth loss. Folic acid is also one of the important nutrients here.

The condition of the tongue is a clue to vitamin deficiencies, sinus infections, and immune status (a coated tongue can be caused by yeast overgrowth). Yeast/fungi and other organisms can move up the esophagus from the stomach, gallbladder, and bile ducts, especially if there is weak stomach acid. The first sign of AIDS is often thrush, a yeast overgrowth on the tongue, due to immune suppression. This can also occur in pregnancy, because of the immune-suppressing effect of the pregnancy hormone progesterone. Diabetics are susceptible to thrush, perhaps as a result of high sugar levels, and probably immune suppression as well. Generally the most common cause of inflamed gums is the presence of resistant bacteria, often induced by mercury in dental amalgams. Other oral symptoms that reflect nutritional status:

- Vitamin B_2 deficiency: magenta tongue
- Vitamin B_3 deficiency: cracked lips, pigmented hands, diarrhea, mental confusion
- B_{12} deficiency: smooth tongue, beet red

Mucous Membranes in the Nose, Throat, Esophagus, and Intestinal Lining

Vitamin A deficiency can complicate inflammation and make it more difficult to heal any mucous membrane area, including the lining of the GI tract. In order to have normal production of mucus, there must be sufficient vitamin A. The active form of vitamin A is called retinol. This is not the same as carotene, but under healthy conditions carotene can be oxidized into vitamin A, and therein lies some confusion. The conversion is often very inefficient, particularly in people coping with illness, the very ones who need it most. In this case the solution is to provide vitamin A directly through a vitamin pill or cod-liver oil.

The Esophagus

Constriction of the lower esophagus (achalasia) often seems to cause regurgitation, burning under the breastbone, and a lump in the throat. Most often associated with deficient folic acid, but also B_6, magnesium, and vitamin A deficiencies.

THE STOMACH

Symptoms

Indigestion (dyspepsia, belching, bloating), nausea, and pain in the upper area of the abdomen, especially on the right, are common. (Left-side pain is associated with the colon.) When we eat, the stomach responds immediately, secreting acid even before we begin chewing or swallowing. It tells us right away what's going on in our body. Most people don't attend much to their body's messages. I encourage you to increase your mindfulness of how your body is working and the things you do that make it work better.

Heartburn is one of the key symptoms of the stomach. What does heartburn mean? Hyperacidity, but also that the tissue defenses aren't working so well. Why aren't they working well? There is often a diet connection—for example, a *selenium* deficiency. It is believed that the incidence of gastric cancer in the United States has dropped about 80 percent in this century since Dr. Kellogg invented whole-grain breakfast cereals in about 1910. By eating these regularly people have been getting better-quality grains, not just white bread. That little extra selenium in whole-grain cereal is enough to lower the rate of stomach cancer. And there is *copper*. Copper deficiency is associated with hyperacidity. Why? Because copper is necessary to the cell hormones that regulate acidity (called prostaglandins). Vitamin A is another important nutrient in the stomach, key in the production of protective mucus.

When the Stomach Won't Empty

Delayed emptying often involves the function of the pylorus, the muscular ring that holds the contents of the stomach until food is sufficiently digested to be moved on to the duodenum. The pylorus opens when acidity declines to the quality of vinegar, about pH 4. Hyperacidity delays emptying. When that occurs the stomach can become locked up and may hold the food for as long as three hours after eating—it's semidisabling to have this experience.

The first thing you can try is buffered vitamin C (calcium-magnesium ascorbate). The classic treatment is Alka-Seltzer Gold, which is sodium bicarbonate without aspirin. The other is Pepto-Bismol—essentially the mineral bismuth. Pepto-Bismol is especially indicated if there's an ulcer infection, caused by the bacteria *H. pylori*. Omega-6 fatty acids such as those contained in cod-liver oil are another dietary factor in some cases.

Eating too many sweets also affects the production of mucus by binding copper, which increases gastric acid and decreases the formation of protective mucus in the stomach, setting the stage for gastritis or ulcers.

Deficiencies that Affect the Stomach

- Copper deficiency: hyperacidity, indigestion/dyspepsia
- Zinc excess: stimulates hyperacidity and often provokes indigestion/dyspepsia
- Selenium deficiency: chronic indigestion, increased risk of gastric cancer
- Taurine deficiency (usually secondary to homocysteine excess): gallstones, pain in the abdomen, intolerance of fat

THE PANCREAS

Pancreatitis can cause abdominal and back pain and is associated with poor digestion as well. Antioxidant supplements are protective.

Water is important. Do you know how much in the way of pancreatic secretions you produce in a day? More than two quarts! So if you don't drink two quarts, how much pancreatic juice can you make? How much saliva? It's true that some liquids are reabsorbed and recycled in our system, in the colon, for example. But suppose you've got diarrhea. What happens to the level of liquids in your body? Clearly the body is at risk for dehydration when pancreatitis occurs, especially if diarrhea prevents the reabsorption of water.

Vitamin D is an endocrine activator. Since the glands of the pancreas must produce digestive enzymes, and these pancreatic secretions depend on vitamin D, you can see how important it is. In addition when there's a prediabetic state, there's an increased vulnerability to infection. Diabetes is also a vitamin D–related condition, in another aspect of its functions. So a strong case can be made for the importance of vitamin D.

THE SMALL INTESTINE

If you're looking for a symptom reflecting the condition of the small intestine, watch for abdominal bloating after meals, about 30 minutes to an hour later. Stomach symptoms are fairly immediate, and that makes diagnosing the upper intestine a bit easier. In contrast, second-guessing the colon is more complicated. Sometimes the peristaltic rush after meals focuses attention on large bowel irritation, spasm, or gassiness. But identifying the cause of these symptoms is challenging; colonic gas is a remnant of food eaten hours or days before.

Simple sugars and sweets are hard on the gut because they are a readily available food for opportunistic flora, especially yeasts, fungi, bacteria, and certain invasive parasites. A broad variety of sweeteners are added to most commercial processed and restaurant food, including corn sweetener, fructose corn syrup, cane sugar, brown sugar, honey, molasses, turbinado sugar, fruit juices, fruit concentrates such as apple or pear, as well as highly sweet dried fruits—raisins, dates, apricots, banana chips, and prunes. Minimize sweets to maintain a GI environment hospitable to beneficial flora, rather than encouraging the "bad bugs."

Vitamin A

The gut is the barrier between your precious self and the rest of the universe out there that wants to destroy you, wants to turn you back into a pile of molecules. And between your cells and the sanctuary that your body must defend daily (your digestive tract) lies a miracle substance called mucus. Mucus is the barrier. It's antioxidant, antibacterial, and a decoy all at once. It acts like fly-paper, catching the bacteria and carrying them out of your digestive tract in stools. The protective effect of this intestinal barrier is limited by the quality of your mucus and of your defending antibodies—secretory IgA. Both require vitamin A.

Yet vitamin A is deficient in one of five people to begin with. And if you don't eat the right foods or you don't make enough vitamin A from carotene, you can predict the outcome: trouble. Again here's where a single multivitamin or a daily teaspoon of cod-liver oil makes a big difference—by producing extra retinol, or vitamin A.

Maintaining the gut is a big job. No question about it. You have both a big surface and a high metabolic rate in the intestinal tract. Vitamin A is used in proportion to the surface involved and the metabolic rate. Vitamin A is a major factor in the growth and healing process of the GI tract—especially because the gut is constantly regenerating its lining, a two-to-four-day process (judging by serial biopsies during fasting). This puts a huge demand on certain nutrients that have to do with DNA synthesis. One of the premier nutrients is vitamin A, with folic acid and vitamin B_{12} close behind.

There are three major sources of vitamin A in nature and they are: butter, eggs, and liver. I often recommend cod-liver oil, which contains 1,250 IU per gram or 5,000 IU per teaspoon. Make sure you get good-quality fish oil that's been assayed for pesticides and peroxides. Vegetables do not produce vitamin A. Rather they produce carotene, which is a source of vitamin A, but not always a reliable one. In the case of intestinal disease, diabetes, hypothyroidism, or the presence of toxic metals or chemicals (which inactivate important enzymes), the metabolism of carotene into retinol is likely to be weakened. Exposure to toxins increases the need for vitamin A, but at the same time it decreases our ability to process it. One research study found that exposure to the highly toxic chemical dioxin caused a decrease in liver stores of vitamin A by 50 percent in just one hour!

Vitamin A also stands out because of its role in detoxification. Infections and pollutants take their toll on vitamin A, and when it's depleted nothing heals well. Your whole healing apparatus starts to malfunction. This is a practical thing. When disease lingers or is chronic, consider that problems occur not only from how bad the disease is, but also how insidious the depletion of nutrients is, and the general state of your immunity.

Vitamin A is a little essay all by itself, because of its interactions. For example, if you have inadequate protein you run into the problem of insufficient transport proteins for vitamin A. If vitamin A lacks the binding protein, it doesn't get to the tissues where it is supposed to go. But for the transport protein to work, you must have zinc. Vitamin A also requires thyroid, but thyroid itself requires selenium, and so forth. These are all depletable factors. That's why these nutrients are so important. You are not as likely to recover unless you also replenish your deficient nutrients.

The Vitamin B Complex

All the B vitamins have to do with the bowel because the gut is essentially a gigantic energy machine. Most of the micronutrients are actively transported into the bloodstream, which requires energy. It takes energy to make energy. The amino acid carnitine guarantees that this process will happen, so the energy will get to where it can be used. Once it is there the B vitamins are important in the activity of the engine of the cell, the mitochondria.

Niacin, for example: One of the cardinal symptoms of niacin deficiency is chronic diarrhea.

Pantothenic acid (B_5) deficiency also results in sluggish motility and gas. This nutrient is so important for motility, it is used after abdominal surgery to get the bowel moving again.

Folic acid is of major importance because it is involved at every level in dental, liver, and intestinal aspects. Folic acid is protective when yeast and parasites are present. And it's important for healing as well as resistance. When there's irritation of the upper duodenum due to wheat/gluten sensitivity or microscopic parasites such as giardia, folic acid isn't well digested. This is important. In these cases we do best to supplement with folic acid. The folic acid in vitamins is actually better absorbed than the folic acid in food, which has to be digested. This is an important consideration and explains why nutrients in vitamin form can be so important for people with digestive illness. But the point is that without the folic acid the healing mechanism is hampered and the process of inflammation can become chronic.

In order for your body to use folic acid, it requires T3, activated thyroid. Selenium and trace minerals are essential to this process. Thus supplemental selenium helps to correct the folic acid problem and improves immune resistance and healing of all kinds of GI problems.

Vitamin B_{12} is basically the same except B_{12} is absorbed in the terminal ileum (very farthest end of the small intestine, where it joins the large intestine), whereas folic acid absorption is mostly in the duodenum (the first portion of the small intestine, adjoining the stomach). B_{12}, folic acid, and vitamin A are particularly important to the healing of the GI tract and digestive enzyme production. Nutritional status can be seriously compromised if they are deficient.

When the cecum—colon valve—leaks back into the small bowel, bad bugs can migrate back up into the small intestine, which inevitably means an alteration of the transport proteins for B_{12}. So a B_{12} deficiency can occur not only at the stomach end of the small intestine, but at the ileum. Ileitis or ileocolitis leads to B_{12} problems, and the undigested food now goes on into the colon.

Vitamin B_{12} and Folic Acid

Because two B vitamins, B_{12} and folic acid, can be so beneficial in healing the digestive tract, we shall discuss them in greater detail here. Once deficiencies of these nutrients are restored, intestinal problems may improve substantially. In some cases these two nutrients turn out to be the most important factors in recovery. Since they work hand in hand, it is important to use them in combination.

How do these deficiencies occur? Leaky gut syndrome is a common aspect of many intestinal problems. Once leaky gut occurs the result is malabsorption. This means that the body is continually deprived of the necessary nutrition, with the potential for significant deficiencies. A number of other important causes and effects have been linked to deficiencies of B_{12} and folic acid.

Symptoms of B_{12} deficiencies: When B_{12} deficiencies persist they can result in pernicious anemia, a form of anemia that affects the gastrointestinal tract and the nervous system. People with pernicious anemia also seem to have a greater chance of developing other conditions, including autoimmune disorders—particularly those affecting the thyroid gland, parathyroid, and adrenals. Symptoms of B_{12} deficiency include fatigue or weakness, loss of appetite or nausea, bloating, diarrhea, anemia and palor, sore mouth and tongue, numbness and tingling of hands and feet, and premature aging.

Causes: B_{12} is generally stored in the body, so deficiencies occur slowly over a period of years. Common causes include:

- Digestive disorders
- Peptic ulcers, and high or low stomach acid

Symptoms of B$_{12}$ Deficiencies

- Fatigue or weakness
- Loss of appetite or nausea
- Bloating
- Diarrhea
- Anemia and palor
- Sore mouth and tongue
- Numbness and tingling of hands and feet
- Premature aging

Symptoms of Folic Acid Deficiencies

- Weakness or fatigue
- Depression
- Lack of appetite and weight loss
- Lightheadedness
- Forgetfulness
- Irritability
- Anemia and pale appearance
- Sinusitis and frequent colds
- Sore red tongue

Everyone knows that these nutrients are essential. Yet the importance of B$_{12}$ and folic acid is still not fully appreciated. What tends to be overlooked is the link between digestive disorders and deficiencies of both B$_{12}$ and folic acid.

It is vital to correct the damage of B$_{12}$ deficiency as quickly as possible because it can also cause irreversible dementia, similar to Alzheimer's disease.

- Celiac disease
- Bacterial and parasitic infections, such as giardia
- Chronic IBS (irritable bowel syndrome), Crohn's disease, and celiac disease
- Genetic deficiency of intrinsic factor (that enables the stomach to produce hydrochloric acid) and other transport proteins
- A strict vegan diet

Symptoms of folic acid deficiencies: Folic acid is used up relatively quickly unless it is replenished at least weekly. The half-life of folic acid is about 5 days, so deficiencies can occur in a few months. As with B$_{12}$, folic acid deficiency can result in a type of anemia. The symptoms can include weakness or fatigue, depression, lack of appetite and weight loss, lightheadedness, forgetfulness, irritability, anemia and pale appearance, sinusitis and frequent colds, and a sore red tongue

Causes: Digestive disorders can cause folic acid deficiencies. A number of factors related to diet can also play a role:

- Diet, due to a lack of fresh fruits and vegetables (this applies to more than half of Americans)
- Genetic disorders
- Malabsorption due to the same types of disorders that cause B_{12} deficiencies, including almost any digestive disorder, particularly celiac disease (gluten intolerance), giardia infections, irritable bowel syndrome, ileocolitis, Crohn's disease, and chronic diarrhea.

Bacterial overgrowth: Many chronic digestive disorders are characterized by bacterial overgrowth and dysbiosis. As dysbiosis worsens, this causes a chain reaction that can result in leaky gut and poor absorption, causing chronic nutritional deficiencies, including folic acid. (See chapter 6.)

Malabsorption: Folic acid deficiencies are aggravated by malabsorption and can result in immune deficiencies. Folic acid is required for the production of thymidine (a nucelic acid), which regulates T cells, our primary defenders against viruses.

When the intake of folic acid is sufficient, there is also the question of absorption. Folic acid must also be digested by enzymes in the duodenum to be absorbed in the liver and metabolized (reduced) in the cells. At various stages in the process folic acid can become depleted. In some cases this may be due to a genetic error that interferes with the ability to absorb the folic acid into the cells.

Reversing the damage: The chain of events that leads to deficiencies can be reversed. Key strategies include:

- Supplementing healthy bacteria
- Restoring nutrient levels with supplements that lead to better absorption
- The addition of folic acid to support immune function

Restoring folic acid levels: Supplements of folic acid are now available in sublingual form, which can be taken orally—dissolved under the tongue—in an activated form as folinic acid, which is better utilized by the cells. If this is not working, it is important to provide injectable folate.

Adding this essential nutrient can work wonders. I've had patients whose chronic hemorrhoids simply disappeared after the first week of folic acid supplementation, following years of discomfort.

Remember that B_{12} and folic acid must be supplemented at the same time. Otherwise providing one without the other could bring out a hidden deficiency in the other nutrient, with potentially severe symptoms.

Restoring B_{12}: Initially B_{12} can be given in sublingual tablets, containing hydroxy-cobalamin (rather than methyl-cobalamin or cyano-cobalamin). If patients do not respond within a month to oral supplements, it is important to provide injections. Since B_{12} deficiency (even without accompanying anemia) can cause permanent damage to the nervous system, it is vital to reverse the damage as quickly as possible, because it can cause irreversible dementia similar to Alzheimer's disease.

There are other ways to enhance the activity of the B_{12} and folic acid system. Nutrients that act in concert include serine, riboflavin, zinc, vitamin C, and niacin. The effectiveness of this approach has been well documented in the research literature, which shows that restoring nutrients also restores function. This logic underlies the most effective treatment strategies in nutrition and orthomolecular medicine.

Vitamins C, D, and E

Vitamin C is important for controlling inflammation and for immune resistance. Without vitamin C you encounter immune suppression. The intestinal tract is not only a digestive organ, but also an immune organ. It must resist the onslaught of infectious agents in food at every meal. The first thing that goes wrong when there's a deficiency of vitamin C is the possibility of a chronic infection in the gut wall. It doesn't always show up as diarrhea, but if you are deficient in vitamin C, the local immune cells in the gut are hampered too. The results are a digestive tract that is leaky, bloated, sore, malabsorbing, toxic, and digesting poorly.

We take vitamin C for granted because it has become so available in this country, but this kind of depletion still needs to be considered. Especially since people who are sick use up their vitamin C and B complex, so they need even more than usual amounts.

Vitamin D works at the intestinal level for the absorption of calcium. A vicious cycle can occur. Without adequate vitamin D, calcium is not absorbed, and then the function of all the glands of the body are diminished and the whole digestive process is ultimately compromised. This causes poor blood sugar regulation. So the lack of digestive abilities makes you more vulnerable to malabsorption, and then the body operates at a sub optimal level.

And then there's vitamin E. Antioxidant support is strongly dependent on vitamin E as a backup when the cellular antioxidants are compromised, which is likely to happen whenever you have an inflammatory condition. The antioxidants inside the cells are proteins. They are made by the cells, but they require amino acids (cysteine especially) and minerals (selenium, zinc, copper, manganese), all of which are often deficient.

Essential Fatty Acids

Essential fatty acids ensure that there's the right amount of moisture in the cell by regulating hydration. You don't want your cells to become shrunken or dehydrated, nor do you want them to be swollen with edema. The essential fatty acids also regulate calcium metabolism and the calcium traffic of the cell wall. They turn on inflammatory and anti-inflammatory defenses at the cell level (through prostaglandins and their products).

Because fatty acids are part of all cell membranes, they affect all cell activities. Deficiencies can cause almost any symptom: If you run short, the skin gets dry, the bladder cannot hold urine, bowels become irregular, hair falls out, skin itches, nerves get raw, and so forth. So the fatty acids are extremely important but confusing, in that deficiency can cause constipation on the one hand and diarrhea on the other. It is a paradox.

There are omega-3 fatty acids (such as flaxseed oil) and the omega-6s (like fish oil). Both classes are important. By and large, the omega-6s build up your resistance to infection. The omega-3 pathway provides anti-inflammatory nutrients (EPA and DHA), but at the expense of decreased resistance to infection. If you don't get enough omega-3s, the body can become pro-inflammatory.

Symptoms of an omega-6 fatty acid deficiency includes thinning of hair, dry skin, and increased susceptibility to infection. In mild cases you may see only the dandruff or eczema as it spreads across the face and the neck. Some people have claimed that fatty liver and anemia go with it too. An omega-3 deficiency, on the other hand, is more often associated with neurological problems, increased allergies, and inflammatory symptoms.

Other Nutrients

Glutamine and carnitine are amino acids specifically beneficial to the lining of the gut. Glutamine is an amino acid. Carnitine is a specialized amino product. It is a potential factor in support for the engine of the cell (the mitochondria), which converts fats into energy. To get the full energy out of any cell, particularly the high-energy cells of the gut that make all these secretions, you must have every cell working. Carnitine and glutamine nourish the digestive tract, so it can enhance nourishment of the rest of your system.

In summary the most important factors include vitamin A, short-chain fatty acids, carnitine, glutamine (the amino acid most prevalent in the digestive tract), and nucleic acid precursors, such as glycine (the metabolic by-product of glutamine in most people), and folic acid.

Of the nutrients that promote the production of antibody defenses (SIgA), vitamin A and zinc are most essential. B_{12}, folic acid, B_6, and the amino acids are all source materials required for competent GI defenses.

Glucosamine and other sugar aminos are found in aloe, a favorite treatment for digestive disorders. (Sugar aminos are also called glycoproteins or lectins.) They bind and dispose of undesirable microbes that otherwise bind to *you*. This is how aloe enhances your body defenses.

THE COLON

Food for Flora—FOS (fructo-oligosaccharides) are nonabsorbable carbohydrates often added to probiotic supplements of acidophilus and bifidus to support the growth of the friendly flora. There are pros and cons to this approach. The good news is that some of its sugars will break down into nutrients that both nourish the gut and feed the flora; these are acetate and especially butyrate. However, some sugars also ferment to lactic acid, which is an irritant in the colon. So for people who are lactose intolerant or especially sensitive, it is probably a better idea to get probiotics without the FOS. On the other hand, for those who have headache and lethargy, signs of ammonia intoxication, FOS can help promote fermentation—which uses up excess ammonia and thus cures headache and fatigue in some people. Monitor your response.

Short-chain fatty acids, such as butyrate, are the preferred fuel for cells in the lining of the colon. People who are depleted in butyrates have higher risk for chronic colitis and eventually cancer. You've read that butyrates are actually made by the friendly flora. While this is true, the friendly flora must have the raw materials to work with. Both starches and proteins are the source from which fatty acids are made by the flora. If these are not sufficient there are straightforward ways of getting them from fats: They're found in butter and cream. Some cases of bowel irregularity or diarrhea resolve quickly by simply increasing fat intake. For those who are totally dairy intolerant, butyrates are now also available in supplement form.

Bleeding from hemorrhoids, indicated by red blood passing with stools, is usually a sign of inflammation of the colon or rectum, and the most common causes are lactose intolerance and food allergy. Deficiency of vitamin B$_6$ has also been implicated. These symptoms need to be related to the doctor in order to make the necessary corrections.

Nutritional Deficiencies That Relate to the Colon

- All the B vitamins working together, and particularly
  - Vitamin B$_1$ deficiency: constipation, flatulence
  - Vitamin B$_6$ (pantothenic acid): flatulence, sluggish motility
  - Vitamin B$_6$ deficiency: irritable bowel, prediabetic conditions, high blood sugar
- Thyroid deficiency: constipation, irregularity, excess gas
- Carnitine deficiency: gas, chronic bowel irregularity, fatigue
- Glutamine: gas, chronic bowel irregularity, fatigue
- Excess lactose (milk sugar): gas, constipation, narrow stools, hemorrhoids.
- Excess fruit sugars (disaccharides): gas, constipation, narrow stools
- Calcium deficiency: unformed stools, increased risk of colon cancer
- Iron excess: constipation, abdominal cramps, black stools

THE LIVER

The liver is the chemical factory and detoxifier of the body. Large meals, especially those with a high intake of animal protein, can overload the liver. The liver is the most vulnerable organ in the body to damage by homocysteine, a metabolic by-product that can increase just from too much animal protein in a meal. Although homocysteine occurs naturally in the body, high levels also put us at risk for heart attack and stroke. The most protective nutrients in this cycle are folic acid, B$_{12}$, B$_6$, choline, and betaine (TMG). These nutrients are crucial in protecting the liver from homocysteine. Fortunately this nutritional protection is afforded by nutrients in diets adequate in fruits and vegetables (sources of folic acid, antioxidants, choline, betaine) and animal protein (B$_{12}$, choline). The liver also stores vitamin B$_{12}$, usually enough for a few years, so it is almost always available unless you happen to be on a strict vegetarian diet. If so be sure to have your levels checked and take a B$_{12}$ supplement, preferably the sublingual form.

In addition to the dangers of high homocysteine, there are many toxic substances and free radicals. Inflammation and toxic products from dysbiosis often produce free radicals that can reach the heart and cause inflammation there. Glutathione, a nutrient that acts as cellular defense, is a peptide manufactured by the cell from glycine (a form of glutamine), glutamic acid, and cysteine. To supply the cell with these raw materials, be sure to get enough of the sulfurous vegetables such as the mustard family: cauliflower, broccoli, Brussels sprouts; or animal proteins, such as fish, fowl, meat, milk, and eggs. These are the best sources of methionine, from which cysteine is derived.

Methionine is also reused for a number of other essential functions involving protein synthesis and methylation. Without it your body cannot produce choline, carnitine, creatine, adrenaline, or inactive histamine. However, every time you eat animal protein, you dump a load of methionine on the liver and the liver converts some of it into homocysteine, which is toxic, especially in the case of deficient folic acid, B_{12}, B_6, and betaine; if these vitamins are deficient, then liver damage is more likely to occur.

Betaine (TMG) is especially protective. If everything else fails, your body can use the supplemented betaine to rescue you from high homocysteine, recycling it into methionine before it can do any damage.

Vegetarians are less susceptible to this problem than those who eat high-protein animal foods because vegetables do not overload the methionine pathways. But vegetarians have their own nutritional challenges. They are at risk for B_{12} deficiency, since only meat has B_{12}. On the other hand, fruits and vegetables are rich in folic acid, antioxidants, choline, and betaine. Of course the liver also stores vitamin B_{12} in large amounts, so that it's almost always available for the first few years on a meatless diet. This fools some people, who don't run into problems until they've been on a meatless diet for several years.

OTHER NUTRITIONAL FACTORS

Fiber is important. Our food often lacks protective fiber. The right kinds of fiber can nourish friendly flora. Fiber also provides a biochemical (phytate) that binds and inactivates excess iron. Some sources of fiber appear to be easier to tolerate than others, particularly for people with GI conditions. Two excellent sources are flaxseed (whole or ground) and rice bran (as part of the grain or as a supplement in foods). Plant-based sources, depending on your tolerance, includes fibrous vegetables such as celery. Wheat and oat bran must be monitored for sensitivity and particularly for delayed reactions to gluten, which is an inseparable part of all the grains in the wheat family.

One way to be sure you get good fiber is to start making your own bread. The dangerous iron and trans-fats would be avoided. However, it's important to minimize fresh yeast in the diet, through a balanced emphasis on grains, beans, nuts, and seeds.

Trans-fats (otherwise known as saturated and partially hydrogenated oils) actually interfere with the cell energy required to produce enzymes, transport food molecules across membranes, and accomplish digestion and absorption. For example, although margarine appears to be a natural oil, the hydrogenation process makes it full of unnatural trans-fats. Research studies show that the energetics of the cell are weakened by 10 percent due to trans-fats. These fats get into the cell membrane and take twice as long to metabolize as normal fat cells. Once in place they slow down the cell activity, so that the energy of the cell is less efficient.

Vegetable oils also have a big effect on intestinal function. The polyunsaturates include almond, canola, corn, cottonseed, safflower, and sunflower seed oils (most of the sources of oil in the vegetable kingdom except for peanut and olive oils). But there is a surprise. Most vegetable oils turn out to be vulnerable to processing. Extracting with heat or chemicals can cancel out the very health benefits for which they've been touted. The highly processed vegetable oils are subject to oxidative damage, which affects human health by promoting damage to the cell wall (the membrane). Fortunately these vegetable oils are more stable if they are cold pressed or expeller pressed. So be sure to get good brands of naturally processed oils, store them in the refrigerator, and use them up within about six weeks.

The drawbacks of processed fats. Background: The U.S. Navy has long had a port of call at Hong Kong. An increase in intestinal complaints, particularly ulcers, has been observed when ships docked there. By contrast, when the same ships and crews docked in Singapore the intestinal complaints dramatically declined. Medical research revealed the reason. When the ships put into Hong Kong the food was cooked with polyunsaturated fatty acids. When they put into Singapore they used stable, saturated fats, from coconut oil and palm oil.

The polyunsaturates, when processed, are subject to rancidity and may cause irritation on contact, particularly upper-intestinal problems and ulcers. The tropical oils, coconut and palm oils, on the contrary, seem to have a healing and protective effect. Research on tropical oils indicates that although they are saturated fats and some do raise cholesterol, there is no associated increase in adverse health effects. You'll be hearing more about these oils in the future, as new research findings expand the dialogue on good and bad cholesterol and its function in human health.

Flaxseed oil. Protective processing is also important for the ultrapolyunsaturated omega-3 oils such as flaxseed, which are even more vulnerable than omega-6 oils. They need to be processed and stored in the dark. Reliable brands of flaxseed oil include Spectrum, Flora, Omega Nutrition, and Barlean's.

Blood type can be relevant. Recent research indicates your blood type can actually provide clues to detecting food sensitivities. Your blood type is based on chemical markers called antigens. The immune system tolerates the antigens of your blood type in order to avoid a self-destructive autoimmune condition. Your body also tolerates antigens from outside sources that resemble the constituents of your blood type.

All foods contain antigens (elements that trigger our antibodies), and since we best tolerate foods with antigens compatible to our blood type, this approach can provide valuable clues to overcoming food sensitivity. For some people, it doesn't matter if they eat a food that is different from their own type, particularly if it's taken in moderation. But if your body is combating any kind of illness, you don't want to waste precious immune energy.

The most important thing is to deal with the major factors. Learn to read food labels, avoid the foods that don't really nourish you, and change the other aspects of your situation that you can correct. You can't fix it all, but if you make good choices about the things within your control, you will most likely begin to see encouraging improvement.

Biographical information for **Richard Kunin, M.D.,** appears on page 192.

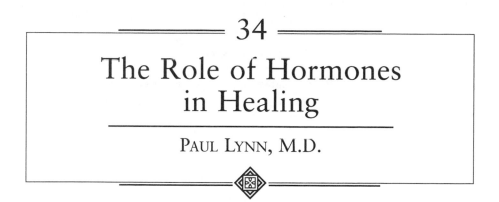

34

The Role of Hormones in Healing

PAUL LYNN, M.D.

Digestive problems are often accompanied by allergies and fatigue. People with these concerns say they're tired quite a bit, they have allergies more than average, and they have achy muscles. Some of these symptoms may relate to an underlying medical problem. Your doctor might call it adrenal insufficiency syndrome or subclinical adrenal hypocorticoidism. Basically the problem could be low-level exhaustion—the exhaustion of the adrenal glands from continually battling problems in the digestive tract and other physical and mental stresses.

Supplementing low hormone levels can definitely be worth while. Doctors who use hormone therapy report that even low dose supplements of specific hormones can improve blood levels of these hormones and translate directly into improved adrenal function.

HORMONE LEVELS

When medical labs report the results for hormone levels, there is a very wide range that is considered normal. The labs determine their normal range through statistics, rather than by comparing hormone levels with actual patient symptoms in a medical setting. Should low or low normal hormone levels be supplemented? One key factor is whether a chronic health condition is also present. Long-term illness can challenge adrenal function and may persist longer if the adrenals are compromised. In many cases these situations can be improved through the use of hormone supplements.

It's also important to consider individual response in evaluating the lab results. In addition to the issue of what constitutes a normal test result, there is the consideration of biochemical individuality. It's a fact that we're all a little unique in every aspect of our functioning. For example, think about the size and shape of the hands of everyone in your family; usually there is an enormous range in size, shape, structure, strength, and dexterity. In the same way, we each have patterns in our body chemistry that are a little unique. So levels that are perfectly normal for one person may not be for another.

Hormone Levels

Hormone	Normal Range (statistically determined by medical labs)	Adequate Range (observed in medical practice by doctors)
DHEA	90 to 430	Higher than 175
Cortisone	4 to 12	Higher than 6
Progesterone	1 to 25	Higher than 5

DHEA AND HEALING

If your adrenal hormones are low your immune system will not be able to function at full capacity and you may find you're more susceptible to certain conditions such as food allergies, for example. There are several ways in which a hormone such as DHEA (dehydroepiandrosterone, a steroid hormone made from cholesterol by the adrenal glands) can affect your ability to heal from a chronic illness.

When the Complaint Is Fatigue and the Lab Test Comes Back Normal

Do you have just enough energy to make it through the day? It could be a case of adrenal exhaustion. This problem is often not picked up in blood tests!

When doctors check the status of the adrenal glands, many people test in the normal range. The natural cortisone level (also called cortisol) wouldn't necessarily be low in terms of the standards given by the labs. Part of the confusion comes in because people with adrenal insufficiency often test in the low-to-normal range.

For example, the normal range for DHEA is 90 to 430. If someone tests with a DHEA level of 125, the lab report would indicate normal. And their doctor would probably say, "The test came back normal." But the person being tested may be struggling and exhausted most of the time.

Using DHEA to Improve General Functioning

Raising hormone levels closer to the middle of the normal range has been found to improve overall functioning. It can alleviate the sense of physical exhaustion. A greater tolerance for exercise often occurs, which in turn improves muscle tone and function. There also tend to be improvements in the pain in the knees and lower back that are associated with lower adrenal function. As these improvements progress, the overall functioning of the body is enhanced and you will find yourself more resistant to allergies and common infections.

Promoting Repair

The second way DHEA supports the immune system is by promoting quicker repair. DHEA is a hormone that promotes cell growth. It's an anabolic hormone (one that handles repair and rebuilding), so it also helps the body heal injured tissue. In the intestinal tract allergies or pathogens can cause major inflammation because the intestinal mucosa is very sensitive. The mucosa is much less durable and resistant than our skin. Whenever there is inflammation or damage from an allergy or an infection, you want it to be healed as quickly as possible so it doesn't become a chronic condition. DHEA helps speed up the repair necessary to make the mucosal tissues in your GI tract whole again. That's a second way in which DHEA can be beneficial to people with the syndromes of poor digestion.

Treating Autoimmune Conditions

DHEA is closely linked to the functioning of the immune system and has been used to treat autoimmune disorders. Stanford and other universities have done quite a bit of clinical testing of DHEA in high doses for people with rheumatoid arthritis and lupus. Much of the research has been done on lupus, an autoimmune disease believed to have similar features (in terms of the immune system) to irritable bowel syndrome. In both conditions it is the abnormal overstimulated response by our body that causes most of the injury. It is possible that DHEA can be beneficial in other comparable immune-related conditions.

Supporting the Immune System

Restoring DHEA levels also restores some of the functions of the immune system. It enhances the ability to create white cells to fight infection by bacteria or parasites. It also helps maintain the levels of antibodies such as secretory IgA that protect against invaders and allergens. So DHEA directly supports immune activity.

Providing Energy for Coping

Supplementing DHEA can also improve a person's psychological outlook, especially if hormone levels are really low. By the time I see patients they have often had these problems for years and they are understandably frustrated and discouraged. They may be coping with chronic indigestion and abdominal pain, or alternating diarrhea and constipation. Chronic conditions of this type can depress our hormone function in a number of ways.

If the adrenal hormones are burdened too much for too long, adrenal exhaustion can result. That has been known since the original studies on the stress syndrome by Hans Selye in the 1930s. With chronic illness, we're looking at a situation that may compromise function without bringing on total exhaustion. In these situations, when we test for adrenal hormone levels the results will often be in the low-normal range, as I suggested earlier. But despite hormone levels that look normal, actual adrenal function can still be very depressed and the person may really be struggling to maintain.

Brightening Mental Outlook

In some cases of adrenal depression, people feel so discouraged that they do not want to take the steps that would probably help them. They may have made many false attempts at improvements over the years. Although they're not so discouraged that they don't come into the office, they feel too discouraged to trying anything new. Part of this pattern of thinking is typically related to low adrenal function. A person may feel overwhelmed all the time as a state of being. That in itself makes immune function worse. That is another indirect but important way that DHEA can promote the healing process.

In these situations DHEA can help to brighten the outlook. People are then in a better position to look for new therapies that would benefit them. They have the mental energy to try new approaches. When DHEA levels rise the psychological outlook gets brighter, probably through improved supply of the neurotransmitters, and the person is more willing to take on a therapy program to help himself.

LOW DOSE CORTISONE THERAPY

Cortisone's main functions are antiviral and anti-inflammatory. Synthetic cortisone is given routinely by doctors as a medication under the generic name prednisone. It is important for people to know that when doctors say cortisone, they usually mean prednisone. They have begun to use those words synonymously, but they are very different compounds. I use only cortisone, since it is identical to what the body produces. Prednisone is not.

When you measure the cortisone level in the blood, the labs will label it cortisol. It is the same substance.

Using Cortisone to Address Inflammation and Viral Conditions

I have used cortisone as a compound for people with irritable bowel syndrome with good effect in some cases. It doesn't always help, but often it does. It usually helps people who have a low or low-normal level of cortisone, as I have mentioned before. In this case the cortisone certainly works as an anti-inflammatory in the intestinal tract, and cortisone itself shows the qualities of improving viral conditions quite effectively as well. It probably helps address some of the viral components of the immune suppression. The book *Safe Uses of Cortisone* by William McKinley Jeffries, M.D., is a helpful reference on the use of cortisone as an antiviral. It helps reduce inflammation from both infections and allergies. Cortisone also contributes to adrenal function.

Low Doses Can Make a Difference

Unusually low doses can provide these benefits. That's an important consideration. The doses for cortisone would be less than 9 mg of hydrocortisone a day. For example, 3 mg might be given once, twice, or three times a day. That is the most you would have to give. Most endocrinologists would consider that such a low dose that it would be considered insignificant, but it's not really. As patients and doctors try it, they will find it very beneficial for conditions such as irritable bowel syndrome.

In conventional therapy the normal dose for cortisone for someone with arthritis would be between 75 and 150 mg a day. The book *Safe Uses of Cortisone* recommends using up to 20 mg a day. Dr. Jeffries does not give 20 mg a day to everybody, but he considers that to be a safe dose in the low range. In my own medical practice I have found that people respond well to even lower doses, and usually doses as high as 20 mg a day are not really necessary. I give the 20 mg dose to people acutely ill with irritable bowel syndrome, but that is a very rare circumstance.

The cortisone typically doesn't have a positive effect unless a person's blood level is on the low side of normal. The usual low-dose treatment with 3 mg once, twice, or three times a day is an effective dose that is extremely safe. The use of low-dose hormone therapy opens up a whole exciting new arena in medical treatment.

My biggest challenge in getting people to try low-dose therapy is that they have the impression that such a low dose won't help, or they say, "I've come to a natural doctor and I don't want to take a steroid." But then I explain to them that they will be taking a substance in minute doses that is identical to what is in the body, and that makes people feel comfortable about taking it. Also I give them Dr. Jeffries' book as a reference.

NATURAL PROGESTERONE

The other hormone that is beneficial in healing is natural progesterone. It has frequently been helpful for women with digestive disorders. Gastroentero-logists or internists who specialize in digestive conditions typically get a higher number of women than men. In my practice it is probably a four-to-one ratio. In premenopausal women the hormone levels of progesterone should be checked only during the last week before the menstrual period. If a woman has symptoms of PMS or if her blood level of progesterone is below 5 at that time of the month, she would respond well to taking about 30 mg of natural progesterone from day 12 to the end of her cycle.

Using Progesterone to Deal with Inflammation and Stress

Progesterone is a hormone with both anti-inflammatory and antistress prop-erties. I do not know if it directly affects immune function the way DHEA does, although it has been suggested that it does. But it helps patients relax, as a natural kind of relaxant rather than being an antianxiety drug. It helps people sleep better and feel more balanced emotionally, in spite of their illness. Relaxation of the stress response is proven to be a strong enhancer of immune function. So that is the third hormone that should be measured in women.

The dosage of DHEA would typically be between 5 mg to 25 mg in men or women (which is very low). It would probably average about half that to get the blood level up sufficiently. People should take it at that level for a few months to see how their immune systems function, providing they have showed signs of low or low-normal levels in their initial blood tests.

Testing

I use laboratory testing on blood rather than saliva. At this time testing on blood tends to be more stable. Blood levels are more reliable. They tend to compare well with the changes observed in the body. I find that the changes in later blood levels reflect the treatment I've given.

Special Considerations about Progesterone

There are three forms of progesterone that I prescribe to my patients for everyday use:

- Skin cream
- Capsules in which the protesterone is contained in oil to protect it from being digested in the stomach
- Tablets that dissolve under the tongue (sublingual)

Unless the progesterone is in one of these three forms it probably won't be absorbed into the bloodstream for the body to use. Other oral forms are typically digested in the intestinal tract.

USING HORMONE SUPPLEMENTS

Natural vs. Synthetic

All these substances are molecularly identical in composition to the substances in the body. That is the key to their effectiveness in low doses.

Where to Get Hormone Supplements

DHEA is available in most health food stores. Progesterone as a cream is also available in health food stores. Progesterone in the oil-containing capsules or in sublingual tablets is available from specialized compounding pharmacies (see below and also Resources). Cortisone is available by prescription only.

Finding a Physician Who Uses Low-Dose Hormone Therapy

Check with organizations that provide practitioner referrals, such as the American College for the Advancement of Medicine (ACAM) at (800) 532-3688. To locate the nearest specialized compounding pharmacy near you, call the PCCA, Professional Compounding Centers of America, in Houston, Texas, at (800) 331-2498.

Biographical information for **Paul Lynn, M.D.,** appears on page 287.

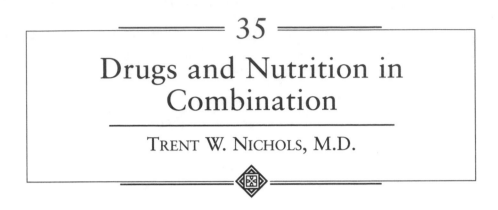

35

Drugs and Nutrition in Combination

TRENT W. NICHOLS, M.D.

It is important to tailor drug therapy to the needs of the individual to maximize healing. We each have a unique genetic inheritance and nutritional requirements. The stresses and toxic burden of our environment, coupled with our distinct patterns of liver detoxification, will also influence our response to various medications. In the context of these factors, medication and nutrition are currently being used together in highly successful treatment strategies.

THE ESOPHAGUS

Using Nutrients to Complement Drug Therapy

The esophagus is one of the places where drugs and nutrition in combination can be important in healing. Barrett's esophagitis is an inflammation of the esophagus known to be caused by chronic acid reflux. It predisposes people to esophageal cancer in somewhere between 3 and 17 percent of cases. The primary treatment is to block the stomach acid with a proton pump inhibitor. However, in this condition tissue repair is often overlooked.

Zinc and beta-carotene are typically depleted in such cases, and therefore supplements can make a difference in the course of the condition. Research has shown that 25 mg of beta-carotene, given in combination with the proton pump inhibitor, can increase tissue repair.

Nutritional Factors in the Esophagus
- Alcohol and caffeine should be restricted because they are potent stimulants of acid secretion and are also known to lower the pressure in the esophageal sphincter.
- Spicy foods tend to irritate the damaged lining of the esophagus.
- Fatty foods also can lower the pressure in the esophageal sphincter and should be avoided. These include fried foods, fatty meats, cream sauces, gravies, butter/margarine, oils, and salad dressings.

Using Nutrition to Save an Organ

George had reflux esophagitis. When we biopsied him the report came back with a diagnosis of Barrett's esophagitis, which meant his acid reflux condition was causing stomach tissue to grow into his lower esophagus. The report also indicated the presence of dysplasia, cells that are often precancerous. We knew we had to act quickly to prevent cancer.

He was put on Prilosec with a proton pump inhibitor to cut back the acid, but when he was endoscoped again, there was no change. At that time we added specific nutrients to his program—beta-carotene and zinc to assist with healing. We had him make some behavioral changes in his eating habits, making sure that he never ate before going to bed, having smaller meals throughout the day, and eating nothing after about five o'clock in the evening to diminish acid. After another five months, he was checked again by endoscope and we found that he was almost totally healed. There was no Barrett's esophagitis and no dysplasia.

The Other Side of the Story

In contrast, Andy didn't have such good luck with his esophagitis. We requested that he come back to be checked in three months, but he moved out of state and was lost to follow-up. I heard from him about a year later. He had developed cancer from the Barrett's esophagitis, which required that a large portion of his esophagus be removed. Unfortunately he now has chronic reflux all the time because he no longer has a true esophagus.

THE STOMACH

Using Nutrients in Combination with Medication

Gastritis with depressed acid production (atrophic gastritis) depletes intrinsic factor, a protein that is needed for the absorption of vitamin B_{12}. Sometimes in chronic gastritis acid production is decreased substantially. Since stomach acid performs part of the digestive process, in this condition it needs to be increased by supplementing with an over-the-counter preparation of betaine hydrochloride, usually sold in combination with the enzyme pepsin.

Infections due to *H. pylori* can cause stomach inflammation with or without ulcers. This bacteria has learned to live in the hostile environment of the stomach and to tolerate the hydrochloric acid by developing in a cocoon of ammonia. To get rid of the bugs you must first temporally get rid of the acid. When you reduce the acid level significantly in the stomach and create a nonacidic environment, the bacteria have trouble adhering to the wall of the stomach.

The mineral bismuth keeps them from adhering and thriving. After eradication of the bacteria, nutrients are needed to encourage mucus production and the growth of new lining cells. These include beta-carotene and vitamins C and E; the minerals zinc, copper, and manganese; and the amino acid N-acetyl cysteine. Gum mastic has been shown useful to treat *H. pylori* infections, in combination with olive leaf and colloidal silver.

Nutritional Factors in Ulcer Conditions

Why do some people get the adherent form of *H. pylori* and have recurrent ulcer disease, while others are cured after one course of therapy? In part it is due to genetics or because they lack the nutrients essential to repair. In other cases it is due to bacterial resistance to antibiotics.

In parts of Africa and Latin America almost everyone has *H. pylori* bacteria, but there is very little ulcer disease. Researchers believe this ability to tolerate the bacteria without developing symptoms is promoted by a diet of whole, fresh foods. However, when people with the bacteria immigrate to the United States and begin eating a diet of refined and junk food, they develop all the symptoms of ulcer disease. Refined foods that are high in white flour and sugar are actually lower in essential nutrients. On a diet that is deficient in basic nutrients and fiber (lost in refining), it is much more difficult for the body to repair damage.

When essential nutrients are increased, immunity and healing are improved. Traditional diets of grains, beans, fresh fruits, and vegetables provide enough nutrients to prevent the symptoms of the disease. Fiber is another factor. It's important for good motility. It's also essential because it nourishes the beneficial bacteria that manufacture the fatty acids (the butyrates) that nourish the digestive tract.

When symptoms of ulcer disease are present, it is rational to restrict alcohol and caffeine because they are potent stimulants of acid secretion. Spices such as black pepper and red pepper have also been found to impair ulcer healing.

THE GASTROINTESTINAL TRACT

Drugs and Nutrition in Combination to Save an Organ

Gastrointestinal surgery can sometimes be avoided by providing enteral feedings (via a nasogastric tube) or parenteral nutrition (via feedings through the

Saving an Organ: Ulcerative Colitis

Harry is a man with a high-stress job and ulcerative colitis. He owns a large landscaping business, travels throughout the state, and has a hectic life. He's had several severe episodes of ulcerative colitis. The first time this occurred we thought his entire colon would have to be removed, because he didn't respond to intravenous prednisone. It wasn't until we started him on intravenous nutrition and a liquid (elemental) diet that we got his albumen high enough to get the drug into his system and get the prednisone into the tissue. Soon he was able to leave the hospital by going home with a central intravenous unit.

In addition to the IV therapy, he continued to take Ensure. Initially he had it pumped in, and later when he could eat again, he used it in place of meals to rest the colon. He continued on oral prednisone for a time after he came off the IV steroids.

Now every time he starts getting into trouble, he knows just what to do. He starts by reducing the stress. He increases his intake of L-glutamine (to speed healing in the gut lining) and goes on UltraClear Sustain. He calls me and we increase his dose of Asacol, and he checks in for steroids, which aren't usually needed. He has also learned to increase his nutritional support early in the spring and fall to avoid the annual relapse that occurs for so many people with GI conditions.

veins) with high caloric content (protein, glucose, and fat). We have seen a number of successes with both methods to save the colon in patients with severe ulcerative colitis. In some cases nutritional therapy was successful even after the condition failed to respond to intravenous prednisone.

We've also had many patients with conditions of the small intestine, such as Crohn's disease, who have been able to avoid surgery. I can honestly say that all my patients who have been able to stop smoking and have followed a nutritional regimen have done very well.

Leaving the Hospital Early: Nutritional Therapy at Home

Patients who undergo surgery can sometimes leave the hospital sooner through the use of home nutritional therapy. Parenteral feeding can be given to provide intravenous fluids, using a small portable pump and a special catheter to prevent infection. However, total parenteral nutrition alone (providing nutrition entirely through the vein) can allow the gut to begin to atrophy. It is essential to put some nutrients into the small and large intestine to stimulate hormones such as growth hormone.

We now realize that if critically ill patients in the ICU or after surgery are left on sugar water, they heal much more slowly than if they are started right away on more nutrient-rich enteral nutrition. Parenteral nutrition is used if the gut is unable as yet to tolerate oral feedings.

Enteral nutrition (tube feeding) is provided with a portable pump and a nasogastric tube; this is typically used for inflammatory bowel conditions. In some cases, this type of nutrition is also enhanced with direct oral intake of a supplement such as Ensure FIN or Impact.

UltraClear Sustain is a hypoallergenic rice-based protein that contains essential nutrients to support the growth and repair of the gut lining. The formula is based on research that has identified the most essential nutrients in this rebuilding process, including L-glutamine to nourish the cells, fructo-oligo-saccharides and inulin to support the growth of new flora and decrease ammonia production, as well as probiotics.

Short-gut syndrome is known to occur after resection for Crohn's disease or a vascular accident. Short-gut syndrome occurs in patients who have had a significant portion of the small intestine removed and require continual par-enteral (IV) nutrition. We used to think that they would be on intravenous nutrition forever. We now know that there is a surprising degree of plasticity in the small intestine. As long as you keep feeding the digestive tract and giving it the right sort of stimuli, such as growth hormone, with large amounts of glutamine, the small intestine actually grows. This can be a long-term process. The Nutrition Restart Center in Hopkinton, Massachusetts, is currently treating patients with this technique.

Drugs and Nutrition to Treat Irritable Bowel Disease (IBD)

IBD tends to deplete vitamins and minerals due to the associated diarrhea and oxidative stress from inflammation. Zinc, copper, and manganese can stimulate the production of an enzyme vital to the protection of the energy unit of the cell. This powerful antioxidant enzyme, superoxide dismutase, is subject to oxidative stress when there is inflammation.

5-ASA drugs. One of the cornerstones of IBD drug therapy is the use of 5-ASA drugs. Azulfidine, Dipentum, Asacol, and Pentasa are able to squelch free radicals that occur as by-products of oxidative stress in inflammation.

Manganese deficiency was found to be frequently associated with IBD conditions, in association with the use of 5-ASA drugs, in a study by the author. We also noticed that low levels of manganese typically preceded a relapse. This suggests that replenishing manganese will probably benefit patients when they take 5-ASA medications.

Prednisone, another cornerstone of GI treatment, is used to keep excessive white cells from migrating from the blood into the tissue. These activated white blood cells, called macrophages, release toxic enzymes. The drug also decreases the production of antibodies and immune-messenger chemicals in order to minimize inflammation. However, the prednisone must be transported through the bloodstream into the tissue to do its job.

Albumin, a blood protein made by the liver, is needed to transport the prednisone. If malnutrition has depleted the levels of albumin in the body, the prednisone may never reach the tissue. Supplementing with protein is essential in cases of malnutrition, which deplete the production and stores of albumin.

The Importance of Nutrition in Coping with Diarrhea

Why do some people have a short-lived diarrhea due to a virus or bacteria from which they recover, and others don't? When the immune system is stimulated, many people are able to fight the virus, parasite, or bacteria. Two primary factors in the vitality of the immune system are the nutrients available and the level of stress draining the system.

When people are able to resist illness, it may be because they have replenished the good bacteria such as acidophilus and bifidobacteria and beneficial yeast such as *Saccharomyces boulardii.* These are the major beneficial bacteria in the GI tract.

Another aspect is the role of nutrients in repair. We need to repair the damaged villi (the fingerlike structures that line the small intestine and absorb nutrients from our food). Nutrients important in this repair include vitamins A, B complex, C, and E and minerals such as zinc, copper, and manganese.

NUTRIENTS FOR THE LIVER

Acute hepatitis and chronic liver disease are often accompanied by nausea, vomiting, and chronic malnutrition. When these symptoms occur it is essential to control the nausea and vomiting, using intravenous hydration. Secondary therapies that have been found helpful in our practice include the use of a liquid enteral diet with vitamin and mineral supplements. Therapeutic acupressure (Acu-Stim) is applied through a portable unit comparable to a TENs (using the P6 point).

Saving an Organ: The Liver

Sally and Rachel, two nurses, both looked like definite candidates for liver trans-plants, especially after we saw their biopsies, which came back as chronic bil-iary cirrhosis. But using nutrition with drug therapy, they were able to heal their livers to the point where the transplants were not necessary. They were on a protocol that included medications plus the herb silymarin, and amino acid sup-port such as NAC (N-acetyl cysteine).

The results have been very encouraging. These were women who had severe, liver biopsy–proven conditions. They have followed their diet, been very careful of what they eat, and avoided exposure to environmental toxins. They also take nutrients and probiotic support regularly, and they have been able to avoid transplantation. The combination of diet, herbs, and drugs has definitely been advantageous.

Reducing the Side Effects of Medications

Drug reactions occur more frequently when liver detoxification is compro-mised. This can happen if the nutrients necessary for Phase 1 and 2 process-ing in the liver are depleted. Phase 2 actually encompasses six different major detox pathways, each with specific requirements for essential nutrients.

Toxic hepatitis can result from the drug interaction between acetamino-phen (Tylenol) and alcohol when taken together by someone unable to perform phase 2 detoxification. Many drugs are broken down and metabolized in the liver through the same detox pathways, and therefore may deplete the enzymes essential to this process. When this occurs toxicity can result, because the liver can no longer perform at full capacity. What we call drug side effects can occur when this enzyme system is overextended. At last count research has identified thirty-five specific drugs that can deplete liver enzymes. The amino acid N-acetyl cysteine under the name Mucomyst is the emergency-room treatment for acetaminophen, which can cause death due to liver toxicity.

Gilbert's syndrome, which is rather common, is associated with an inher-ited defect in breaking down blood cells into bilirubin that can result in mild jaundice due to prolonged fasting or viral infections. It was recently discov-ered that this genetic uniqueness is linked to alterations of specific liver enzymes. Research shows that people with this genetic defect tend to be poor detoxifiers, based on functional liver challenges with small doses of Tylenol (acetaminophen). This suggests an unusual susceptibility to toxins. Another study providing nutrient supplements targeted at the flawed enzymes demon-strated improvement in symptoms.

By using supplements or eating certain foods, you can help to stimulate your own liver detoxification. Cruciferous vegetables, particularly broccoli and Brussels sprouts, can provide sulfur and other nutrients essential to liver detoxification.

Nutrients to Support Detoxification

UltraClear is a medical food designed to be used for liver detoxification. It comes in powdered form and contains vitamins, minerals, and amino acids tailored to the needs of liver detoxification. There is also a formula (UltraClear Plus) for people with slow detoxification. UltraClear is used whenever there is a liver detoxification problem, for both liver and nonliver conditions.

We know detoxification patterns are inherited. In addition many people now have a poor ability to break down toxins, due to the exposure to environmental pollutants. This is also occurring because people are living longer; most people who are older tend to have poor detoxification, just by virtue of a lifetime of requirements placed on the liver.

When multiple drugs are used, magnesium and vitamin B_6 are two of the nutrients that become depleted, affecting the capacity to detoxify and therefore the ability to tolerate medications. Two groups of people who often show these symptoms are those with diabetes and those who overconsume alcohol. These people have unusually high requirements for magnesium and B_6.

Whole foods are not always realistic if someone is severely depleted. Take, for example, sulfur. In someone who is ill the detoxification process uses up large amounts of sulfur. Sulfur is found in foods that can be fairly difficult to digest, especially during GI illness—vegetables such as onions, garlic, cabbage, Brussels sprouts, and turnips (and also eggs). This is the rationale behind supporting the liver's functions with nutritional supplements.

In some cases it's difficult to get as much of a particular nutrient as we need. Magnesium, for example, tends to be low in our diet. Our whole society seems to have a very high calcium intake because we eat a lot of dairy foods and many common products are supplemented with calcium. To get enough magnesium in order to create the right calcium-magnesium ratio would require eating about a bushel of spinach a day. Thus the value of supplements.

The Liver-Brain Connection

Ongoing research is being done in conjunction with Metagenics West (Gig Harbor, Washington) and the Institutes for the Achievement of Human Potential (Philadelphia). Work with brain-injured children is highlighting the

A Sample Protocol for Treating Chronic Liver Disease

DIET
- Often protein must be restricted. Nonmeat sources of protein, such as vegetable protein, contain lower amounts of mercaptan (an amino acid elevated in such cases) and ammonia.
- Salt (sodium) restriction is needed when edema and/or ascites (abdominal fluid) accumulate.
- Fluid restriction is also often necessary with edema and/or ascites.

MEDICATIONS
- Neomycin (an antibiotic) and/or beta-lactulose (a nonmetabolized sugar) can be given to reduce the ammonia production from bacteria in the gut.
- Spirolactone is a diuretic medication that is useful in treating ascites because it blocks the secretion of aldosterone, a hormone that is over produced in this condition.

NUTRIENTS TO SUPPLEMENT
- Water-soluble vitamins are needed to supplement the metabolism.
- Fat-soluble vitamin deficiency is very common in chronic liver disease, and water-soluble forms of these vitamins (Aquasol A or Aquasol E) should be used while monitoring blood levels to ensure adequate amounts.
- Calcium is often inadequate in these conditions, and dietary and/or supplemental calcium up to 1,500 mg per day should be encouraged in those at risk for osteoporosis.
- Zinc deficiency is common in many types of liver disease.
- Magnesium deficiency may occur due to malabsorption, small bowel disease, or pancreatic insufficiency.
- Specific branched-chain amino acid supplements also appear to be helpful.

NUTRIENTS TO BE RESTRICTED
- Iron supplementation is often to be avoided because of the dangers of iron overload or because of the Fenton reaction, in which iron can fuel oxidative stress.
- Copper and manganese should be restricted in causes of jaundice because excretion of these minerals is often impaired.

links between brain function, impaired liver detoxification, and GI integrity. This work builds on a decade of research on the effects of digestive toxins on the brain and nervous system. The research implicates a variety of subtle GI disorders in certain forms of learning disabilities, hyperactivity, and even autism.

Enhancing the Action of a Drug and Conserving Costly Medications

Transplant patients require cyclosporine, a drug that is very expensive. The effectiveness of the drug can be increased and the required dosage reduced by slowing liver metabolism through the use of grapefruit juice. An active ingredient in the juice, naringenin, blocks the activity of one of the liver enzymes, down-regulating liver activity. As a result less of the drug is needed. David Jones, M.D., a Linus Pauling Award recipient in 1997, makes similar use of grapefruit juice with patients to reduce the dose of Viagra, which is a very expensive medication used to treat impotence.

FUTURE DIRECTIONS

Nutrition for AIDS Patients

For AIDS patients proper nutrition is extremely important. Now that we have potent protease inhibitors for HIV and treatment for pneumocystis, what is most dangerous to AIDS patients is malnutrition. Mitchell Kaminski, M.D., and Jeffery Bland, Ph.D., have done research on the treatment of the AIDS wasting syndrome as a gastrointestinal disorder.

To restore the destruction from the wasting effects of AIDS, they recommend a nutrient-rich protocol including antioxidants such as vitamins C and E; amino acids such as N-acetyl cysteine and arginine; and minerals including selenium, manganese, zinc, and copper to reduce inflammation. Damage from overly reactive immune responses to inflammation is moderated with CoQ1O, essential fatty acids, and lipoic acid. Pepto-Bismol (containing the mineral bismuth) is given to decrease the adherence of cyclosporidia and microsporidia to the intestinal lining and decrease the diarrhea. UltraClear Sustain and extra L-glutamine are also provided as part of this extensive gut-repair program.

The Future of Nutritional Therapy

We predict that nutrition will become a tool that any physician or healer will use. Now we tend to think of food as just something that provides calories and satisfies our taste buds. However, we are seeing the distinction between nutrition and medicine blend. The use of specific, carefully chosen nutrients can provide many healing benefits and positive health outcomes, as the new science of nutritional medicine demonstrates. In the future with advances in genetics, clinical nutrition, and bioelectromagnetics, twenty-first-century health care will achieve what Thomas Edison predicted.

The Doctor of the future will give no medicines. But will interest his patients in the care of the human frame, in diet and in the causes of disease.

—THOMAS EDISON

Biographical information for **Trent W. Nichols, M.D.,** appears on page 104.

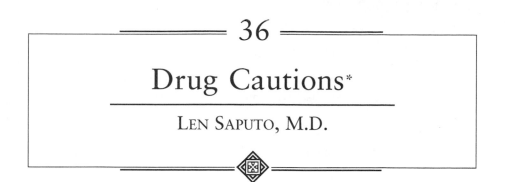

36

Drug Cautions*

LEN SAPUTO, M.D.

We all know that pharmaceutical drugs are an important aspect of medicine. They can improve symptoms—at times they reverse illness, and in some situations can be lifesaving. We value them highly and need them. It is also well known, as mentioned in a recent article in the *Journal of the American Medical Association,* that pharmaceutical drugs are the third leading cause of death in America and result in more than 5 million hospitalizations every year! Only heart disease and cancer result in more deaths.

This paradoxical situation emphasizes the importance of using pharmaceuticals only when the benefits of their use clearly outweigh their possible risks. This requires a value judgment. Often the assessment of a clinical situation and the decision to use or not to use a specific drug can be very difficult. We may not really know what to do. We may not really want to go through the process of exploring nonpharmaceutical alternatives, nor do we want to take responsibility for the downside of what can happen. We just want to get better and hope that the doctor knows best.

The cells of our body are highly complex, microscopic industrial plants. We know a lot about how they operate biochemically, but this knowledge represents only the tip of the iceberg. The synthetic drugs produced by science and manufacturing and then introduced into our bodies are a unique phenomenon in human history. Nothing quite like them has ever existed in the past. We don't understand fully how they operate and have no idea what they will do to some distant biochemical reaction until some time after they have been in use and a problem develops "out of the blue." This information is sometimes learned the hard way, and a drug is recalled from clinical practice because of serious complications or even death.

This same toxicity is not seen nearly as often when natural therapies (nutraceuticals) are used, such as vitamins, minerals, food extracts, and herbs. Despite the fact that nutraceuticals only occasionally cause serious problems,

---

How Things Go Wrong

Dan developed severe diarrhea at the age of 16, and he was hospitalized for the major dehydration that resulted from the 15 to 20 bowel movements he was having every day. Over the prior three months, he had lost more than 20 pounds, and at 5 feet 10 inches, he now weighed just 130 pounds. His physician did a colonoscopy with biopsies, which confirmed the diagnosis of ulcerative colitis.

Dan was treated with prednisone and Asacol, and his symptoms improved markedly. He began to feel good, gained back about ten pounds, and was having only two to three soft bowel movements a day. Unfortunately over the following several years, Dan would have a recurrence of the ulcerative colitis symptoms whenever the prednisone was decreased below 10 mg a day. So he and his doctor felt it was essential that he remain on the drug.

However, he began to develop signs of Cushing's disease associated with the overuse of steroids—overweight with a swollen abdomen, yet thin legs and wasting muscles, and weakness with a tendency to bruise easily and heal slowly. He also had chronic indigestion from the prednisone. His physician ordered antacids and Zantac, which controlled his indigestion, but the Cushing's-like side effects of the prednisone continued to develop. There was talk of doing a colectomy. Dan knew he was in trouble.

When Dan first came to me, he was depressed and worried that he might never get over his ulcerative colitis. He felt dependent on the drugs, and at the same time feared that they were causing problems that would eventually damage his body in a very serious way. He was right.

Rather than suppressing the symptoms of the ulcerative colitis, we elected to support his digestive tract with the best nutrition possible and to see if his body could heal itself. He began a program of supplements that included L-glutamine, friendly flora (probiotics), licorice extract, butyrate enemas, antiyeast herbs, essential fatty acids, antioxidants, and a diet high in nutrients and low in allergens. He was gradually able to decrease the drugs, and within four months he was off the drugs altogether. For the first time in years he was having normal bowel movements and yet was no longer on medication. Dan has gained back his confidence and his lost weight, and now has to "diet" to maintain a normal weight!

we read about them in the headlines whenever they do occur. They don't even begin to rival synthetic pharmaceuticals in their magnitude of danger. They are nowhere near the third leading cause of death in America.

One of the major conceptual differences between conventional and nutritional approaches in managing illness is that in mainstream medicine, the treatment is often based on suppressing the symptoms of a disease, and in nutritional medicine it is generally to support the defenses of the body to cure itself of the disease. Working in harmony with the body is much less intrusive to natural biochemical processes and is less likely to result in serious complications from therapy.

Many natural alternatives to synthetic pharmaceuticals are important to consider, especially in people who are ill. Some of the drugs that should be avoided in patients with gastrointestinal disease include NSAIDs, HZ blockers, prolonged antacid therapy, corticosteroid usage, antibiotics, drugs that affect intestinal peristalsis, and artificial fiber.

Nonsteroidal anti-inflammatory drugs (NSAIDs) should rarely, if ever, be used because they are so toxic. It is well documented in the medical literature that each year approximately 15,000 deaths and over 300,000 admissions to hospitals occur from the direct effects of these synthetic pharmaceuticals. Most problems are related to gastritis, ulcers, and gastrointestinal bleeding, though there are also serious kidney and liver abnormalities as well. In addition, there are profound changes in the permeability across the intestinal lining that result in toxic overload to the liver and to the immune system. It has been shown that intestinal bacteria can pass across the intestinal lining and invade the body as a consequence of this increased intestinal permeability. These changes in permeability have been documented to occur after even a single dose of NSAIDs.

H2 blockers such as cimetidine (Tagamet), ranitidine (Zantac), famotidine (Pepcid), and omeprazole (Prilosec) are powerful inhibitors of acid secretion into the stomach. They work wonderfully to relieve our symptoms of indigestion, but there is a price to pay. They all but abolish acid production, and consequently we don't have the necessary acid to digest protein properly or to absorb vitamin B_{12} or various minerals. These medications can also cause other changes that affect the composition of the intestinal microflora.

Deglycyrrhizinated licorice (DGL) has been shown to be equally effective to Tagamet and Zantac in clinical trials, and it has no effect in changing acid production. What it does do is strengthen the protective mucous layer that lines the stomach, increase the longevity of gastrointestinal cells, improve circulation to the intestinal mucosa, and stimulate the production of secretory antibodies that are shed into the gut. It may even help the body to rid itself of *Helicobacter pylori,* the bacteria thought to be responsible for some ulcer formation in the first place.

Sucralfate (Carafate) is a popular synthetic pharmaceutical that is believed to coat the stomach and form a protective layer that keeps stomach acid from access to the ulcerated tissues. Again it has been shown to be effective in healing stomach ulcers. However, it is full of aluminum, just like several antacids! It is well documented that aluminum is highly toxic to the nervous system, and it has been shown that there is a significant increase in both blood and urinary levels of aluminum after standard doses of these substances. Aluminum toxicity has been implicated in numerous studies on Alzheimer's disease. Why use something that is toxic when it is just as effective to use a natural remedy that is totally safe?

Corticosteroids (cortisone products) can be lifesaving in patients with certain gastrointestinal problems, and there is a clear place for their usage, especially in Crohn's disease and ulcerative colitis. However, they should be reserved as a last resort. Nutritional support of the gut can be vitally important in preventing the progression of these illnesses. Nutrients such as L-glutamine, probiotics, antioxidants, essential fatty acids, and butyrate frequently promote natural healing and obviate the need for even considering corticosteroids. The very serious effects of steroids can be devastating and have been linked to the development of ulcers, osteoporosis, psychosis, high blood pressure, fluid retention, potassium and magnesium depletion, and more.

Antibiotics similarly are often critical in the management of serious life-threatening bacterial infections. When used appropriately they are of clear value. However, whenever an antibiotic is taken there are potentially serious consequences. Maintaining a normal balance of the microflora of the gut is very important in sustaining good health. In the extreme situation a potentially life-threatening condition called pseudomembranous enterocolitis can develop. This is the result of using antibiotics that kill the normal intestinal microflora and allow the selective overgrowth of highly pathogenic bacteria *(Clostridium difficile)* to dominate. In addition antibiotics disturb other important aspects of nutrition and GI function.

Pharmaceuticals that "balance" intestinal motility may relieve our abdominal cramping, diarrhea, or dull aching pains, or speed up a sluggish gut, as in esophageal motility disorders. While the symptoms are often improved or relieved, nothing is accomplished regarding the causes of these disorders. In fact, this approach will actually mask the symptoms of the disorder, making us feel like the problem is no longer present. In addition potential complications may result from the unwanted side effects of the medication.

Occasionally these complications can be lethal, as in the case of a recently withdrawn drug, Posicor, a calcium-channel blocker for high blood pressure. When this medication is processed in the liver, it competes with other drugs that use the same two specific CP-450 enzymes; these medications have included Propulsid, Mevacor, Hismanal, erythromycin, and others. In some cases heart arrhythmias have developed, in a few cases fatal. Drug combinations have become more prolific and more problematic—one of the reasons pharmacists now use computerized drug-interaction databases.

Most patients with digestive disorders are labeled as having "irritable bowel syndrome" or "spastic colon." Nearly all of the associated problems can be managed successfully without the use of any synthetic pharmaceuticals, by correcting the ecological balance of the intestinal flora (dysbiosis), providing nutritional support for the gut, improving the diet, and eliminating food allergies or intolerances, like gluten sensitivity or lactose intolerance.

We are repeatedly told that we need more fiber in our diets. It is important in preventing constipation, in lowering cholesterol, in adding bulk to the stool, and in detoxification. It is also critically important as a nutrient for those friendly bacteria in our intestinal tracts, vital for the normal function of the digestive tract. So we should be eating fiber that is found in food.

When we eat artificial fiber, it may well provide some of the functions that we've discussed, but it cannot function as a nutrient for the bacteria in our intestinal tracts. And many of these artificial fiber products have other "inert" ingredients such as sodium lauryl sulfate, mineral oil, and povidone that are clearly unhealthy for our body chemistry.

So when we are looking for solutions to our health problems, while synthetic pharmaceuticals may save our lives in severe illnesses, because of their ever present inherent toxicity to the biochemistry of the body, we must beware. Medications have their place, but overuse can be dangerous because of the many potential drug-to-drug interactions and consequent side effects. Another issue is the increased demand drugs place on the liver for detoxification. It is not prudent to rely on these powerful drugs in situations where it is possible to use natural alternatives that have also been documented to be of equivalent value. We would be wise to use an integrated approach to solving our health care issues, one that offers safer alternatives when common sense (and our doctors!) tells us they are reasonable choices.

> *Greater than the tread of a mighty army is the power of an idea whose time has come.*
> —VICTOR HUGO

Biographical information for **Len Saputo, M.D.**, appears on page 56.

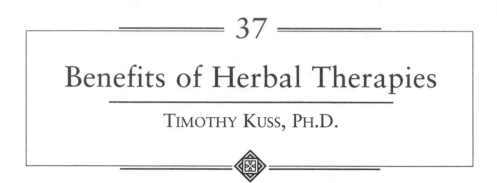

37

Benefits of Herbal Therapies

TIMOTHY KUSS, PH.D.

Since the dawn of time, herbs have been used for their potent healing and recuperative powers. Medicinal plants contain a multitude of active ingredients used by humanity for their healing properties. Aspirin, the most widely used drug in the world, is based on salicylic acid—naturally present in white willow bark.

Herbs can be used to renew the body, season by season. Their healing constituents supply important ingredients that can enhance immunity and optimize health. Medicinal plants have provided the foundation for the modem pharmaceutical industry. In turn modern science is now validating the efficacy of botanicals in a wide variety of health conditions.

Therapeutic herbs have many benefits. Their primary action is to stimulate (anabolic effect) or soothe (catabolic effect) a given organ or body system. For example, milk thistle stimulates the liver to release toxins and protects it against the potentially damaging effects of the toxins themselves. Herbs may also be used to cleanse, build, detoxify, promote tissue repair, improve digestion, stimulate bile flow, regulate hormonal activity and metabolism, fight infection, reduce fever or inflammation, and so forth. With a thorough knowledge of plants, the herbalist has an incredible array of strategies for healing.

Herbs, when used with prudence and good judgment, can assist greatly in correcting many symptoms and disorders. They must be used properly and with discretion. Choose the right herb for the right reason, at the right time, in the right combination, and for the right duration. A trained herbalist can be a major ally in the pursuit and maintenance of good health.

GENERAL GUIDELINES FOR USING HERBS

1. *Determining dosage.* The physical condition of each individual must be considered in regard to dosage. Age, body size, body strength, and gender should all be considered. A 40-year-old 225-pound man might take three capsules of a particular herb; a 110-pound woman only one.

2. *Sensitivity issues.* Sensitive individuals can experience reactions to certain herbs, especially if introduced at too high a dose. The key principle here is to begin an individual herb very slowly. Avoid making any other changes in supplements at that time. I recommend one dose a day for at least three days. Once you've found the herb is well tolerated, the dose can be gradually increased.

3. *Selecting the right form.* Botanicals are now available in capsules, tablets, powders, teas, liquid extracts, tinctures, and the whole form of the original plant itself. Preferences tend to be highly individual. Experiment for yourself, buying the smallest quantity possible until you become accustomed to what you like.

   For medicinal purposes your health practitioner may prefer that you take a particular form of a certain herb. For example, St. John's wort standardized extract in 300 mg capsule form offers the most dependable delivery of the active ingredient, hypericin at 0.3%. In comparison, St. John's wort in liquid extract form does not deliver the active hypericin as reliably.

4. *Using fresh herbs.* Select herbs in their freshest form possible. Freshly picked herbs are delightfully potent and carry the greatest life energy and a higher concentration of enzymes, vitamins, and volatile oils; they are generally more effective. In bottled herbs look for expiration dates, and select products from reputable companies.

5. *Strengthening the body, as the first step.* If you have chronic illness or don't feel well, it is important to initially emphasize herbs that are building and sustaining in nature. The body's energies and healing capacity must be increased before a cleansing, detoxification program is begun. Herbs such as fo ti (he shou wu), cayenne, ginger, green tea, and milk thistle help to nourish and revitalize the body's life force.

6. *Time for cleansing.* Once you feel stronger a cleansing program can be started. Then the life force is sufficient to allow detoxification without overstressing the eliminative organs. Liver, colon, and kidney cleanses, as well as parasite detox programs, may be undertaken directly. If a cleansing is undertaken before the body is ready, reactions or a healing crisis may occur.

7. *Acute conditions.* In acute conditions, such as an active bacterial or viral infection, herbs may be taken every three to four hours throughout the day as necessary.

8. *Bowel regularity.* It is vitally important to maintain bowel regularity. Toxins and wastes must be excreted daily to maintain good health. Mild laxative herbs such as aloe vera (capsules or inner leaf), cascara sagrada, or yellow dock may be used to promote a regular elimination pattern.

9. *Overcoming congestion.* In Oriental medicine there are thought to be two primary causes for most disease—congestion and depletion. When congestion or depletion occurs, or both, blood and lymphatic circulation are disturbed. Signs of congestion include mucus buildup, lymphatic tenderness or swelling, circulatory disorders, cold hands and feet, infection, and inflammation. To clear congestion it is important to increase circulation. Consider capsicum, cayenne, ginger, ginkgo biloba, ginseng, hawthorn, horse chestnut, rosemary, or watercress. In the beginning of your program use mild herbs, such as burdock, that have both strengthening and cleansing properties.

10. *When to take herbs.* In general for maximum effect, herbs are best taken between meals, on an empty stomach. However, most may be taken with food as required. In fact, the herbs fennel, ginger, and gentian promote optimal digestion when taken with food. Stimulants such as ginkgo biloba are best taken early in the day to avoid disrupting sleep patterns. Nervines, such as valerian and skullcap, are herbs that tend to relax the body temporarily, and are best taken before bed.

11. *How long is long enough?* Herbs can be used therapeutically or tonically. Therapeutic use is for short periods of one to four weeks at a time. For example, goldenseal and echinacea are used therapeutically, and it is important that they not be taken for more than three weeks at a time.

    Tonic herbs can be used for longer periods of time, typically two to six months or longer, to address deep-seated imbalances. Ginseng, milk thistle, and turmeric are often considered tonic herbs. Others such as aloe vera, garlic, and ginger can be taken either as tonics or therapeutic agents. The old rule of thumb is that herbs are used one month for every year the patient has had the condition. Rely on your herbalist or health practitioner for advice in this area.

12. *Rest cycles.* Give the body a rest from the use of a specific herb (or herbs) at certain intervals. In Chinese medicine herbal blends are used for one- to two-week periods and then usually stopped and alternated with other formulas. In contrast, when the same therapeutic herb is used for many weeks at a time, homeostasis can occur and the herb loses some of its beneficial impact on the body. In the case of antibacterial or antimicrobial herbs, changing the formula may prevent the microbes from becoming adapted to the anti-infective properties and overgrowing again. Tonic herbs such as milk thistle or dandelion are an exception to this rule and may be taken for many weeks at a time.

13. *Herbs and vitamins.* Herbal medicine is compatible with almost all other forms of treatment. In fact, herbs are usually synergistic with vitamins,

especially naturally derived nutrients. Check with your homeopath if you are taking a prescribed remedy.

14. *Herbs and prescription medicines.* Consult with your personal physician or pharmacist on questions of individual compatibility of herbs with prescription medicines. If your doctor has approved the use of an herb in tandem with a drug, whenever possible to minimize interactions, take the herb at a different time of day than the medication. Herbs can also be highly effective following a course of treatment, or alternated with drug protocols.

15. *The herbal advantage.* As natural plant-based medicines, herbs are usually quite compatible with the human body. Taken properly, side effects usually do not occur. Herbs can also be quite effective in dealing with the microbial kingdom. The herbal advantage is further magnified when a group of herbs are used together in a combination herbal remedy, and the effect of the active ingredients are exponentially greater.

16. *Gathering herbs.* All plants are best gathered when they are at their peak of growth, usually during the spring and early summer months. The best time to pick herbs is in the early morning hours, after the evaporation of dew and before the sun is high in the sky. The plant's aromatic oils are at their peak at this time. Select plants that are freshly in bloom and that have retained their natural color. Avoid plants sprayed with insecticides.

17. *Quality herbs.* Good choices typically include products labeled "organic" or "wild-crafted" (which means the plant was gathered in a natural environment and may be organic). Ask a well-informed staff person in the health food store which companies tend to have the freshest, highest quality herbs. If you use herbs frequently you may want to order directly from a company that is regarded as a supplier of superior botanical products.

18. *Storing herbs.* Botanicals are delicate and require attentive handling. Heat and direct sunlight quickly destroy the plant's value. Keep your herbs in sealed, clean, airtight, lightproof containers in a cool, dry, dark location. Store herbs away from microwave ovens, computers, televisions, and heat ducts. At airports, hand-check your herbs to avoid X-ray exposure.

19. *Making tea.* When leaves or flowers of a plant are used, pour a cup of boiling water over one teaspoon of the loose herb and let it steep for about ten to twelve minutes; then strain and drink. For roots, seeds, bark, or tough leaves, cover with cold water and bring just to a boil; then simmer for ten to twelve minutes and strain.

20. *Body type and dosage.* Different body types can be classified as sensitive or hearty. When a range of dosages are offered, the lower dose is usually appropriate for the sensitive body type, whereas the higher dose is for the more hearty body type.

HERBS TO PROMOTE DIGESTION

Cardamom (Elettaria cardamomum) makes a wonderful, warming, and soothing digestive toner. It is excellent as a tea for indigestion, gas, or colic or to stimulate the appetite.

Chamomile (Matricaria recutita) is so popular in Germany many call it "capable of anything." Chamomile is used for many mild gastrointestinal disturbances. It can have antispasmodic effects. It also possesses a powerful anti-inflammatory influence on the mucous membranes of the entire GI tract. Chamomile helps prevent and soothe gastritis and mild ulcerlike conditions and speed their healing. It is also used as a mild sedative to calm the nerves and relieve anxiety without impeding normal motor coordination. Chamomile is used for its calming and therapeutic effects.

Gentian (Gentiana lutea) is a highly useful bitter tonic herb. Germany's Commission E (scientists who evaluate the safety and effectiveness of herbs) reports that gentian stimulates the taste buds and appetite and increases the flow of saliva and both stomach and bile secretions. Improving these functions may be relevant in cases of dyspepsia, gastritis, heartburn, nausea, jaundice, or diarrhea. Gentian may be taken as a tea or in capsules. It is also available as a tincture (called bitters) sold in health food and liquor stores.

Ginger (Zingiber officinale) is known in Asia as the "universal medicine." Research published in *The Lancet* and other prestigious medical journals has validated many of ginger's traditional uses. For example, it was confirmed to be more effective than drugs in treating both motion sickness and nausea. The optimal delivery of active ingredients is best found in the liquid extract, such as New Chapter's Daily Ginger Extract. Ginger in tea form is second best.

Ginger has been found to calm the stomach, improve digestion, lower cholesterol, increase circulation, and enhance overall immune function. These improvements may benefit conditions such as colitis, constipation, irritable bowel, malabsorption, colds, flu, and many other digestive disorders. It tends to amplify the benefits of other herbs and nutrients taken with it. Consider ginger for almost any gastrointestinal complaint. For GI conditions use the tea or the liquid extract in a glass of pure water.

Fennel (Foeniculum vulgare): Hippocrates recommended it to treat infant colic in the third century B.C.E. Licorice-flavored fennel helps relieve stomachaches and cramps and also flatulence. Chew a few raw fennel seeds immediately following a meal to improve digestion and to reduce gas and bloating.

Neem leaf (Azadirachta indica) is a cooling and bitter herb used in Ayurvedic medicine. Neem has been found to improve digestion, has antifungal properties, and broad antimicrobial properties. This herb stimulates an immune response, which is helpful in treating ulcers and in detoxifying the liver. Neem is usually taken in capsule form or as tea.

Papaya leaf (Carica papaya) contains papain, a potent protein-digesting enzyme so effective it is the active ingredient in meat tenderizers. Take capsules or tablets or a slice of papaya fruit with or just after protein meals.

Peppermint (Mentha piperita) contains volatile oils and other compounds that may settle an upset stomach, absorb gas, improve digestion, and relieve heartburn and colic. Some people find it useful in controlling diarrhea or constipation. It is used in a wide variety of products, such as Tums.

Peppermint's essential oils can improve digestive activity by stimulating bile flow. In some, peppermint promotes muscular activity, reduces cramps, and helps relieve headaches caused by poor digestion. Research shows peppermint has anti-ulcer and anti-inflammatory properties. Peppermint also has antimicrobial characteristics inhibiting more than thirty different strains of bacteria, viruses, and yeast organisms. Peppermint may be taken in the form of a tea, in a concentrated oil, in tincture, or in enteric-coated capsules.

HERBS FOR INTESTINAL HEALING

Aloe (Aloe spp.) is one of nature's most incredible curative agents. Currently aloe is being effectively used in some hospitals to heal radiation and first- and second-degree burns. Since the skin and the gut lining have some of the same properties, it is understandable that aloe has been found to work wonders there as well.

Aloe helps soothe and heal the stomach and small intestine lining, which is useful when coping with myriad insults from allergic reactions, celiac disease, gastritis, or ulcers. It can promote bowel regularity as an excellent mild and soothing laxative, taken in capsule form at bedtime. To determine the right dose begin by monitoring your body's response at home on a day off from work. Fresh aloe is rich in mucilaginous polysaccharides, its active component, which can be depleted in processing. For best results use the fresh inner gel from a live plant. When using a leaf from your own plant, simply remove the firm outer leaf with a knife so all the toxins are eliminated. Even the gel of the plant near the skin is safe to use. Try one teaspoon of fresh gel in a blender drink. Excellent benefit can also be derived from commercial juice or gel, intended for internal use only. Avoid brands using the outer leaf, which is toxic. Aloe concentrated in capsules or tablets is also beneficial, but can be laxative, so time your use judiciously.

Buckthorn bark (Rhamnus catharticas) is quite popular in Europe as a laxative and has the same key constituents found in cascara sagrada, promoting peristaltic action and intestinal mucous secretions.

Cascara sagrada (Rhamnus purshianus) was called the "sacred bark" by the early Spanish explorers. Cascara is a safe laxative that promotes peristalsis and restores tone to the colon and liver. Begin with just one capsule and use just enough to produce the desired results. Decrease and discontinue dose as your GI function returns to normal. *Note:* Overdose can cause diarrhea or cramping. Not recommended for pregnant or lactating women or for ulcers, irritable bowel syndrome, or inflammatory conditions in general. *Important:* This herb can cause a sudden, unpredictable rapid cleansing, which may occur as much as six hours later. When you begin the herb try it at home on the weekend and monitor its effects on your system. For laxative use, if cascara is not the right choice for you, consider trying aloe vera in capsule form, taken at bedtime.

Cat's claw (Uncaria spp.) is an Amazonian immune-strengthening herb, and is beneficial to the digestive tract as well. It reputedly has the power to influence deep-seated pathology. Cat's claw is known as the "opener of the way" for its remarkable ability to cleanse the entire intestinal tract and help many different stomach and intestinal disorders. Cat's claw has been found to relieve swelling and inflammation relevant to the prevention and treatment of ulcers, colitis, irritable bowel, Crohn's disease, and chronic inflammation. Use only cat's claw concentrates for best results, in either liquid extract or capsules. *Caution:* The liquid is bitter.

Flaxseed is an excellent bulking agent and imparts a very mild laxative effect. Try one to two tablespoons of seeds whole or ground sprinkled into a cereal, soup, salad, yogurt, or smoothie. If you have no problems with inflammation, prepare the seeds as cereal by pouring ¼ cup of boiling water over ¼ cup seeds; cover and steep for five minutes.

Marshmallow root (Althaea officinalis): The Roman naturalist Pliny stated, "Whosoever shall take a spoonful of the mallows shall that day be free from all diseases." Marshmallow may be used as a tea, powder, tincture, or in capsules to soothe an upset stomach, ulcer, or any irritation of the GI tract. In lab studies it has demonstrated biological activity and stimulated macrophage activity. Marshmallow increases function in the GI tract as it nourishes and heals sensitive intestinal mucous membranes.

Slippery elm (Ulmus rubra) is a remarkably effective gastrointestinal soother, due to its unusual gelatinous, mucilaginous content. It heals sore and inflamed mucous membranes, including those of the digestive tract. Slippery elm has been used to address ulcers, diarrhea, and diverticulitis, and to increase stool motility. It may be taken in capsules or prepared like oatmeal, by adding hot water to the powdered bark to make a cereal.

Yellow dock root (Rumex crispus) is a nourishing and purifying herb often used in seasonal detoxification cleanses and as a general anti-inflammatory. It is high in organic iron and other minerals, so it has been used in the treatment of anemia. It also has a mildly laxative effect. Use for short periods of time, up to eight weeks, in capsules, tea, or liquid extracts.

LIVER-PROTECTIVE HERBS

Boldo leaf (Peumus boldo) is a South American herb and one of the world's foremost liver and kidney tonics. Boldo is an antioxidant that nourishes the liver, which nourishes the blood, to the benefit of the whole body. Boldo is applied in many liver and digestive disorders, including jaundice, constipation, poor digestion, and gas and bloating. The botanical literature contains references to the use of boldo in cases of hepatitis. The herb may be taken as a tea (one teaspoon per cup) or in capsule form. *Caution:* To be safe, pregnant women should avoid boldo.

Dandelion (Taraxacum officinale) has centuries of use as excellent nourishment for the liver. Dandelion stimulates bile flow and reduces bile duct inflammation, liver congestion, and gallstones. These improvements are relevant to the treatment of jaundice, mild hepatitis, and edema caused by liver toxicity.

The leaves may be eaten as a salad green or steamed like spinach, or a tea may be brewed from the roots. Dandelion can also be taken in capsule form.

Milk thistle (Silybum marianum) has more than 2,000 years of medicinal use and is the subject of over one hundred clinical trials. It contains three powerful liver-protective flavonoids known collectively as silymarin. Silymarin imparts potent therapeutic benefits as an antioxidant, by regenerating liver-cells (hepatocytes) and by inhibiting inflammatory enzymes. Research has found that silymarin neutralizes the toxic effects of a wide variety of poisons, including alcohol, excessive iron, industrial toxins such as carbon tetrachloride, acetaminophen (Tylenol) overdose, and the deathcap mushroom, *Amanita phalloides*.

Silymarin prevents the depletion of the key liver antioxidant glutathione. In fact, silymarin has been shown to increase liver levels of glutathione by up to 35 percent. The higher the glutathione levels, the greater the liver's ability to detoxify. Studies indicate that Silymarin has benefits in treatment regimens for liver disease, cirrhosis, hepatitis, jaundice, fatty degeneration of the liver, and indigestion. I predict silymarin will one day likely become standard preventive treatment taken with any liver-toxic drug.

Mountain mahogany (Cercocarpus spp.) is an herb growing on the lower slopes of the Rocky Mountains. Indians of the region customarily chewed the tender leaves for stamina during long treks through the mountains. It is quite supportive for the liver and overall endocrine system.

Phyllanthus (Phyllanthus amarus) is an ancient Ayurvedic herb known for its liver-strengthening abilities. Phyllanthus is a mild, slow-acting herb ideal for individuals who need to detoxify in a gradual manner. In other words, phyllanthus does not aggressively and hastily flush toxins out of the system, but does so in a gentle process that does not overwhelm the body. It is helpful for many liver conditions, as it protects the liver cells against damage and disease. Phyllanthus is available in capsule form. This botanical has a long history as a liver-supportive herb. However, the jury is still out on its specific therapeutic applications.

Schizandra (Schizandra chinensis) is one of the most beneficial of the Chinese herbs for the liver, containing a dozen active compounds that are liver protective. In Chinese medicine schizandra has many uses, including its role as a tonic for both men and women and for viral hepatitis. It may be taken in capsule form, or the dried berries can be found in herb shops. When taken for acute conditions the herb is divided into several doses throughout the day.

Turmeric (Curcuma longa) is honored in Ayurvedic medicine as one of the foremost digestive tonics and overall remedies. It quiets indigestion and helps to reduce gas, bloating, and inflammation. Turmeric lowers cholesterol and is a general antimicrobial agent. This herb stimulates bile flow, helping digest oils and fats. These benefits make it relevant to the treatment of hemorrhoids. Animal studies show that it protects and detoxifies the liver. Curcumin, an active compound in turmeric, is reported to directly inhibit carcinogens.

Curcumin suppresses prostaglandin synthesis, which reduces pain in a manner similar to aspirin or ibuprofen, only milder. At high doses curcumin stimulates the adrenal glands to release cortisone—the body's natural anti-inflammatory and pain management agent. If you consume alcohol, smoke, or take frequent doses of prescription drugs or Tylenol (acetaminophen), you may want to include turmeric or milk thistle in your daily regime. However, individuals suffering from gallstones or bile duct blockage do best to avoid turmeric and also curry powder, which is typically one-third turmeric. For sensitive types turmeric may be best tolerated in combination with a product by NOW called Silymarin (with turmeric included in the ingredients).

HERBS FOR ULCERS

Fresh raw cabbage (Brassica oleracea) juice contains two compounds that are used as anti-ulcer agents, the amino acids glutamine and S-methyl-methionine. In a recent study 92 percent of patients with ulcers showed a marked improvement within three weeks on a program of daily cabbage juice, compared with 32 percent drinking a look-alike placebo. Cabbage soup can also be helpful, especially with the addition of ginger, cloves, and just a hint of licorice. Typically two to four cups of the fresh cabbage juice are taken daily or eaten in soup form.

Ginger (Zingiber officinale) is reported to relieve inflammation and has the potential to protect the digestive system from ulcers. Ginger contains eleven different active constituents with proven anti-ulcer properties.

Licorice root (Glycyrrhiza glabra) is approved by German Commission E as an ulcer treatment. The preferred form is deglycyrrhizinated licorice root (DGL), which does not increase blood pressure rates. DGL promotes healing of the sensitive mucosal membranes of the GI tract. DGL is best taken in chewable tablets because the mixing of saliva with DGL activates the licorice's healing properties.

Meadowsweet (Filipendula ulmaria) is used extensively in Britain as an anti-ulcer agent. Meadowsweet contains tannins, which have been found to be antibacterial in research studies. Meadowsweet is a logical treatment for ulcers, since most are caused by a bacteria (*H. pylori*).

Neem (Azadirachta indica) is a highly useful bitter herb that can improve digestion. In India neem is used in cases of ulcers. It is also a respected immune stimulant and liver detoxifier, and helps diabetics lower their blood sugar levels.

Okra is a mucilaginous vegetable that is a potent gastrointestinal soother and healer. It is rich in chlorophyll and beta-carotene, and when eaten as a cooked vegetable assists in repairing the sensitive stomach and intestinal lining. The gelatinous quality of the vegetable tends to be quite healing.

Slippery elm (Ulmus rubra) also has an unusual gelatinous, mucilaginous content with traditional therapeutic use for ulcers, diverticulitis, ulcerative colitis, and Crohn's disease. It may be taken in capsules or prepared like oatmeal, adding hot water to the powdered bark to make a cereal.

Turmeric (Curcuma longa) is an excellent anti-inflammatory, anti-ulcer agent, and applied as a general healer for the GI tract in capsule or powder form.

ANTIMICROBIAL HERBS

All herbal roots and barks exert general antimicrobial properties. Otherwise they would succumb to the widespread presence of microbes in the soil. Certain herbs exert an even stronger antimicrobial effect than others. The most potent of these herbs will now be discussed.

Black walnut (Juglans nigra) has traditional uses in Asia and America for its antiparasitic properties. Black walnut also possesses potent antiyeast and mild antiviral properties. One study showed that fresh husks of the black walnut killed candida better than the commonly prescribed antifungal drug, without the side effects. In China it is used with good success to kill tapeworms. The black walnut's broad antimicrobial success is due to its high tannin content. The green hulls or the bark of the tree are used. Black walnut is usually effective in stopping diarrhea. It makes a good liver tonic and has been applied in cases of hemorrhoids and organ or tissue prolapse. Black walnut may be used in liquid extract form or in capsules.

Clove (Syzygium aromaticum) is the most stimulating and carminative of all aromatic spices (a carminative is an agent that dispels gas from the intestines). Clove possesses strong and proven general antimicrobial properties against fungus, bacteria, and parasites. Clove has a long tradition of use in China and in India, where cloves are used to stop diarrhea, gas, and bloating.

Clove acts as a restorative tonic to the digestive and circulatory systems. It is an excellent blood cleanser, relieves nausea and vomiting, and stimulates peristalsis. Often added to bitter herb-medicine preparations, clove tends to make them more palatable. Eating cloves is said to be an aphrodisiac. *Caution:* Do not use clove when pregnant, or for children under 2 years of age. Clove is generally taken in capsule form.

Echinacea (Echinacea spp.) has a great range of activity against viruses, bacteria, fungi, and protozoa. It contains an antibiotic compound (echinacoside) with broad-spectrum activity often compared to that of penicillin. Echinacea bolsters the immune defenses in various ways. (1) It strengthens the body's local defenses by use of a substance (echinacein) that deactivates germs' tissue-dissolving enzyme. This prevents germs from spreading and infecting other body tissues. (2) A study in *Infection and Immunology* showed that echinacea stimulated production of white blood cells and phagocytes and increased macrophage germ-killing activity. (3) A University of Munich study demonstrated that echinacea boosted production of infection-fighting T lymphocytes up to 30 percent more than standard immune-supportive drugs.

One study showed that echinacea has significant antiyeast qualities. In Germany echinacea is used in the treatment of flu, colds, bronchitis, tonsillitis, ear infections, whooping cough, psoriasis, wounds, and abscesses, and is even included as one aspect of treatment for meningitis and tuberculosis. The root of the plant offers the greatest healing potential. Root extracts of echinacea are believed to boost interferon levels, vital to the body's defenses. The German Commission E recommends echinacea to be used for short periods of time not to exceed eight successive weeks. It is best taken as liquid extract or in capsules.

Garlic (Allium sativum) is the botanical kingdom's best example of an herbal wonder drug for fighting infections. When the Russian army ran out of penicillin in World War II, garlic was their second choice, and they used it to treat typhus, dysentery, septic poisoning, and gangrene in battle wounds. Hence the nickname "Russian penicillin." Garlic contains several antimicrobial compounds, including allicin, one of nature's strongest broad-spectrum antibiotics. Research has found garlic to have antibacterial activity against bacillus, brucella, citrobacter, *E. coli,* hafnia, klebsiella, *Salmonella typhi,* shigella, *Vibrio cholerae,* and various forms of staph and strep.

At Benares Hindu University in India, one of garlic's constituents, ajoene, was found to be almost as effective against mildew fungus as pharmaceutical antifungals. In test tube studies garlic has demonstrated viricidal activity against many viruses, including rhino viruses and herpes simplex I and II. Garlic is often used in cases of food poisoning and GI tract infections. It exerts antiparasitic properties applied in treatment against pinworms, roundworms, and certain protozoa, including *Entamoeba histolytica.*

Garlic is also used to help relieve gas pains and as an antispasmodic. It is most active in raw form as a food or a fresh-pressed juice. A few cloves may be juiced along with carrots to make the medicine go down easy. Or it can be taken in gel capsules, two to three per day as prevention, or two to three, three times daily, in acute situations. *Note:* To help counter the powerful smell, chew one or more of the following herbal breath fresheners: parsley, fenugreek, or fennel.

Ginger (Zingiber officinale) has been found to possess inhibitory action against various pathogenic microorganisms, including the bacteria *E. coli,* salmonella, *Staphylococcus aureus,* and *Streptococcus viridans.* It also possesses anti-influenza, antiviral, antifungal and antiyeast activity. Studies show ginger is quite effective against numerous parasites, including various protozoa. Remarkably this versatile herb also acts as a probiotic, promoting growth of friendly flora species like *Lactobacillus acidophilus.*

Grapefruit seed extract (GSE) is a general antimicrobial agent with specific antibacterial, antifungal, antiviral, and antiparasitic properties. This bitter herb is known for its excellent application against *Candida albicans.* In lab testing, GSE has shown effectiveness against a long list of other microorganisms as well, including *Staphylococcus aureus, Salmonella typhi, E. coli, Proteus vulgaris, Pseudomonas aeruginosa, Aspergillus parasiticus, Entamoeba histolytica, Giardia lamblia,* herpes simplex type 1, and influenza A virus. Applications also include controlling diarrhea. It's especially helpful for infections of unknown cause, because it is nontoxic and its activity is so broad.

GSE offers a safe, simple way to disinfect drinking water when camping or traveling. Available water should first be filtered (at the least, let suspended water particles settle). Retain the clear water and add 10 drops GSE for each gallon of water. Shake vigorously and let stand for a few minutes before drinking.

GSE may be used in liquid concentrate form or in capsules. GSE may be taken internally, in minute doses such as 2 to 4 drops twice daily, diluted in at least 4 ounces carrot, orange, pineapple or grapefruit juice.

Licorice root (Glycyrrhiza glabra) helps prevent and remedy infections, fevers, and inflammation. It has broad antimicrobial activity against viruses, bacteria, yeast, and fungi. Licorice contains at least eight antiviral and twenty-five antifungal compounds. Licorice's active fungicidal constituents are greater than those of any other herb. It also possesses antiviral compounds that promote interferon release, part of our body's antiviral arsenal. A Japanese study showed licorice to be effective against *Staphylococcus aureus,* which was already resistant to penicillin and streptomycin. Furthermore, licorice remained just as effective against successive drug-resistant generations of the same staph.

In Chinese medicine licorice is called the great unifier. It is used in small amounts in numerous herbal formulas for its exceptional harmonizing and synergistic qualities. Licorice heightens the beneficial effects of other herbs it is used with.

By itself licorice is a dynamic herb and should only be used for short periods of time. Caution: Use only DGL (deglycyrrhizinated licorice) if you have high blood pressure. Avoid licorice altogether during pregnancy, or if you're diabetic or have glaucoma, water retention, heart disease, or a history of hypertension or stroke. Licorice has a naturally sweet taste and it may be taken as tea, liquid extract, or in capsules.

Additional Antimicrobials

Astragalus (Astragalus spp.) is a supremely versatile and potent immune strengthener. Astragalus builds up the body's vitality, prevents and hastens infection's exodus. Research in China shows *baikal skullcap (Scutellaria baicalensis)* has broad-spectrum antimicrobial activity, so it is associated with the treatment of pneumonia, flu, and other respiratory infections. It suppresses viruses and pneumonia causing fungi. *Cinchona bark (Cinchona* spp.) was the primary source for quinine until the drug was synthetically produced. Cinchona bark has more than twenty active compounds; in addition to quinine it has antiviral, antimalarial, antiprotozoal, and antiyeast properties. Use in capsule form.

Dandelion (Taraxacum officinale) is used against respiratory infections. It may be taken as a tea, in capsules, or the fresh greens as a salad. *Honeysuckle (Lonicera japonica)* is much used in China to treat bacterial and viral conditions. It is taken as a liquid from flower extracts or as a tea. *Olive leaf (Olea europaea)* has general antimicrobial properties, providing relief against bacteria, virus, fungi, and certain protozoa. For GI conditions its leaves contain a rich amount of FOS (fructo-oligo-saccharides), which nourish and promote the growth of good bacteria.

ANTIBACTERIAL HERBS

A number of outstanding bactericidal botanicals have just been discussed in the section on antimicrobials. Of these the most important include *echinacea, garlic, ginger,* and *grapefruit seed extract.* Also antibacterial but milder in their effects are clove, licorice, honeysuckle, and olive leaf. Additional outstanding antibacterial herbs follow.

Chaparral (Larrea divaricata) is a powerful antimicrobial herb. It can be effective against a broad spectrum of infectious agents, viruses, yeast, and bacteria. One compound in chaparral, nordihydroguarietic acid, is a viable antiseptic. Chaparral is one of nature's best blood cleansers and is quite immune supportive in general. The tea works well but tastes bad, so capsules are usually best.

Goldenseal (Hydrastis canadensis) is the antibacterial herb in greatest demand today. Due to this popularity it is greatly overharvested and nearing extinction in the wild. Goldenseal stimulates macrophage activity, the microscopic Pac-Men of our immune system that engulf and devour bacteria. Goldenseal contains the active compounds berberine and hydrastine, which are anti-inflammatory and antihistamine and stimulate bile flow.

Berberine is strongly antibacterial, amoebicidal, and somewhat antifungal and antiviral. It helps stop diarrhea. Berberine appears to work by staining microbes (to be targets for the macrophages) and by preventing the microbes from attaching to cells. *Note:* Other berberine-containing herbs are oregon grape root, barberry, and Chinese goldthread. Goldenseal has broad applications for the GI tract and liver and is a potent blood cleanser.

Goldenseal is too bitter as a tea, and the active ingredients may not translate into the liquid extract form. Thus capsules are preferred. Use goldenseal only for brief intervals of two to three weeks at a time. When used longer goldenseal is reported to deplete the body of B vitamins, and to a lesser extent vitamin C. Goldenseal can also be harsh on the kidneys and should be used judiciously. If the herb causes stomach discomfort, mouth irritation, or other symptoms, use less or stop using it altogether. Do not use it when pregnant.

Goldthread (Coptis chinensis) is from Asia and is sometimes called Chinese goldenseal. It offers an excellent substitute for American goldenseal, as its berberine content is twice as high. *Caution:* Do not confuse Chinese goldthread with American goldthread *(Coptis groenlandicum).*

ANTIVIRAL HERBS

In addition to the herbs listed here a number of outstanding viricidal botanicals were discussed earlier. Of these the most important are: *echinacea, garlic, licorice,* and *astragalus.* Also antiviral but milder in their effects are Baikal skullcap, cinchona bark, ginger, grapefruit seed extract, honeysuckle, and olive leaf. Other outstanding antiviral herbs include:.

Black elderberry (Sambucus nigra L.) has been used in cases of flu, coughs, colds, and upper respiratory infections for more than 2,500 years. Recent studies demonstrate black elderberry's effectiveness against all strains of influenza virus. An enzyme present in black elderberry (neuraminidase) has been found to inhibit the virus from piercing the cell membrane and entering. Black elderberry is most effective in either a syrup form or in lozenges.

Black-eyed Susan root (Rudbeckia spp.) is about to be discovered for its virus-fighting capabilities. A recent report showed black-eyed Susan to be a more potent immune system stimulator than echinacea.

Forsythia (Forsythia suspensa) is a traditional Chinese herb used when there are colds, flu, and other viruses. It is often mixed with honeysuckle *(Lonicera japonica)* and sometimes lemon balm and/or ginger as a tea.

Isatidis (Isatis tinctora) is one of the best-known Chinese antiviral herbs. Isatidis is an excellent remedy for any virus. Because it helps reduce both swelling and liver inflammation, it has been used against hepatitis. Isatidis is mild and can be used for children or those who don't tolerate heat well (described as pitta types in the Ayurvedic system). Less well known, isatidis is also a good antibacterial agent.

Leptotaenia (Lomatium dissecutim). Research in 1948 demonstrated leptotaenia inhibited the growth, with varying degrees of success, of all sixty-two strains of bacteria and fungi tested. An oil extract of leptotaenia was shown in a 1949 in vitro test to completely inhibit growth of ten microbes, equivalent to penicillin at the same strength. Leptotaenia is available in both capsules or liquid extract. Because of these properties it is applied in the treatment of a number of viral conditions, such as pneumonia, flu, colds, and bronchitis, as well as all viruses, including herpes simplex I and II and hepatitis C. Leptotaenia also possesses activity against many forms of yeast.

Schizandra (Schizandra chinensis) has uses in Chinese medicine as an antiviral herb, in cases of viral hepatitis. Schizandra may be taken in capsule form or the dried berries may be found in herb shops.

ANTIYEAST HERBS

A number of outstanding bactericidal botanicals were discussed in the antimicrobial section. Of these the most important antiyeast herbs are garlic, grapefruit seed extract, and licorice. Also antiyeast but milder in their effects are Baikal skullcap, black walnut, cinchona bark, clove, echinacea, ginger, and olive leaf. Additional antiyeast herbs include:

Celandine (Chelidonium majus) is a well-known herb with benefits to the liver and can help detoxify and eliminate the waste by-products from candida treatment. Celandine also possesses active antiyeast properties in its own right. It is usually taken in capsule form.

Cranberry (Vaccinium macrocarpon) contains the compound arbutin, which has antiyeast and anticandida properties, so it is used in fighting urinary tract infections. Use the unsweetened juice or capsule form.

Gentian (Gentiana officinalis) is a bitter herb that acts as a first line of defense against yeast overgrowth. Gentian stimulates gastric juice secretions. When our stomach acids are sufficient, microbes and yeasts are destroyed, "cooked" in the highly acid gastric medium. Gentian may be taken in capsules or liquid extract form.

Goldenrod (Solidago virgaurea) is approved by German Commission E for prevention and treatment of urogenital ailments, including yeast infections. Goldenrod contains a number of potent antiyeast compounds. Can be taken as a tea or in capsules or in drop form.

Licorice (Glycyrrhiza glabra) contains the largest number of antifungal compounds of any single herb. For these properties it may be taken in capsules, in liquid extract, or as a tea, but not as the supplement DGL.

Oregano oil (Origanum vulgare) is a potent antiseptic. Research shows this tasty spice packs a whale of a wallop against a wide range of fungi, yeasts, and bacteria, with some antiviral and antiparasitic properties as well. *Caution:* The vast majority of oregano oil is mislabeled, usually derived from thyme or marjoram, and not nearly as effective. Add a few drops of oregano oil into juice. Emulsified oil of oregano is now available in caplet form.

Pau d'arco (Tabebuia spp.) is a highly revered South American herb that excels in controlling candida and yeast overgrowth. It contains three antiyeast compounds—lapachol, beta-lapachone, and xyloidine—active against *Candida albicans* and other common fungi. Lapachol's antiyeast action alone has been found comparable to the drug Nizoral (ketaconazole). In Brazil pau d'arco is commonly used for a host of conditions, including constipation, colitis, ulcers, diabetes, arthritis, respiratory problems, and infections of all kinds. Pau d'arco exhibits antiviral and antibacterial properties. The herb is effective in tea, liquid extract, and capsule form. Start slowly with whichever form you use, to avoid strong die-off reactions.

Pseudowintera colorata is a New Zealand herb containing a powerful anti-fungal agent called polygodial. It has been found effective against *Candida albicans* and other fungi. When combined with anethole, the active constituent of aniseed *(Pimpinella anisum),* polygodial's effectiveness against *Candida albicans* was found to increase thirty-two times, as confirmed by studies at the University of California.

The combination of *Pseudowintera colorata* and aniseed work by damaging the cell membranes of *Candida albicans* and other yeasts. The yeast's cell division is thus significantly impeded. *Note: Pseudowintera colorata* and aniseed are found together in a product manufactured by Forest Herbs called Kolorex, typically taken at the end of a meal.

Spicebush (Lindera benzoin) is an Appalachian herb quite effective against *Candida albicans.*

Honorable mention herbs include *ivy (Hedera helix),* whose leaves inhibit candida and many bacteria as well. *Tea tree oil (Melaleuca* spp.) has a history of use against topical yeast problems, so it's applied in treating athlete's foot. Use cautiously to determine suitability for your skin type. *Uva-ursi (Arctostaphylos uva-ursi)* possesses antiyeast properties, and therefore is taken for urogenital disorders; take as a tea or liquid extract, or in capsules.

ANTIPARASITIC HERBS

A number of prominent antiparasitic botanicals were discussed in the section on antimicrobials. The most important are *black walnut, garlic,* and *grapefruit seed extract.* Also antiparasitic but milder in their effects are cinchona bark, clove, ginger, and olive leaf. Additional outstanding antiparasite herbs include:

Artemisia annua, derived from the Chinese herb Qing-Hao, is used in Chinese medicine in treating a variety of protozoan infections caused by amoebas (amebiasis), giardia (giardiasis), and other microbial agents. Also known as Sweet Annie, artemisia has also been found in research at the Walter Reed Army Research Institute in Washington, D.C., to be effective in fighting malaria. The organism that causes malaria is a species related to the amoeba. Artemisia is in the wormwood family of herbs, all of which are extremely bitter. They are used for indigestion, heartburn, flatulence, gastric pain, and jaundice, for general weakness, and in stimulating appetite. Wormwood also stimulates liver and bile flow, as well as general circulation.

Caution: One member of the wormwood family, *Artemisia absinthium,* has been declared unsafe by the U.S. Food and Drug Administration, and its use was outlawed in France in the nineteenth century because of its adverse effects on the nervous system.

Chaparro amargosa (Castela emoryi and *C. texana)* is used against some of the nastiest protozoa on the planet, including *Entamoeba histolytica* and giardia. Known in Spanish as bitter bush, *Chaparro amargosa* is also helpful in rebuilding the intestinal tract after antibiotic therapy or a bout of gastroenteritis. It is an excellent preventive to avoid diarrhea when traveling. *Chaparro amargosa* is usually taken in liquid tincture form, followed immediately with a more pleasant juice or tea to diminish the taste.

Kamala (Mallotus philippinensis) is used in India and elsewhere because of its antiparasitic properties. It is most effective when used as a part of an herbal combination remedy, usually in capsule form.

Quassia (Picraena excelsa) is a bitter herb with strong antiparasitic qualities. A tea is made from quassia wood chips. Historically it is used to kill roundworms (ascaris). Taken internally as an enema, it is used against pinworm.

Wormseed (Chenopodium ambrosioides) is one of the most highly respected antiparasitic remedies, known for its ease of use and low toxicity. Wormseed is believed to act as a direct poison to parasites. Traditionally wormseed oil has been used against roundworms and hookworms, paralyzing them and causing them to lose their grip on the intestines. A strong laxative administered shortly after wormseed is said to drive the parasites from the body. Wormseed is often found by the Spanish name epazote. Mexicans prize epazote for dispelling gas associated with bean consumption. The fresh or dried herb is added to bean and lentil dishes when they are almost done.

Caution: Wormseed is quite potent. An overdose of the oil can cause poisoning or even death. A one-year-old baby died after taking a dose of four drops three times a day for two days. Wormseed is not recommended for pregnant or lactating women or children under the age of six. Often a strong laxative is taken after the last dose of the oil. Wormseed is also available in capsule form. Consult your doctor for proper dosage, as each product is slightly different.

Special note: Eliminating parasites successfully can be tricky business. To minimize the challenge we strongly recommend consulting with an experienced health practitioner whose training includes herbology *and* a track record of success in treating parasites.

COMBINATION REMEDIES

Individual herbs may be all that you need. However, most herbalists will agree that combination herbal remedies are even more effective due to the combined synergy of benefits. The potency of a single herb can usually be significantly enhanced when correctly combined with other herbs. The overall results are greatly augmented. Traditional Chinese medicine and Ayurveda offer classic examples of herbs specifically combined for their distinct synergistic and therapeutic effects. Combination herbal remedies offer state-of-the-art clinical results and serve as the foundation of modern herbalism. Refer to the Resources for a list of professional companies that offer high quality, effective combination herbal remedies.

Timothy Kuss, Ph.D., is founder and director of Infinity Health Systems, a private nutritional practice consulting with both doctors and patients on the therapeutic use of nutrition. He holds a Ph.D. in nutrition and an N.D. in naturopathy, is a certified nutritional consultant, and studied with the respected biochemist and herbalist Stuart Wheelwright. He is cofounder of the Institute of Bio-Energetic Research, dedicated to nutritional research, and is nutrition director for Recovery Systems, a clinic that uses diet and nutrients to aid recovery from addictive lifestyles. Author of *A Guidebook to Clinical Nutrition for the Health Professional* and articles on a variety of health topics, he also formulates herbal and nutritional supplements. Timothy Kuss is available by phone for herbal and/or nutritional consultations at Infinity Health in the Denver area at (800) 733-9293.

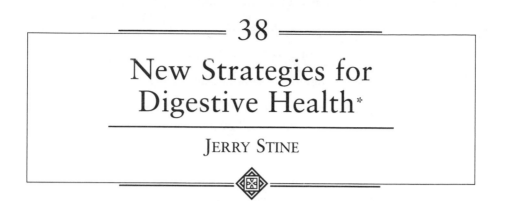

38

New Strategies for Digestive Health*

JERRY STINE

Nowhere is the phrase "Knowledge is power" more true than in health. Recent research is providing new ways of looking at dynamics in the body—dynamics that underlie a great many diseases. This chapter includes important information on:

- Microcirculation
- Homocysteine
- Low-carb/no-carb diets
- Insulin resistance
- Iodine deficiencies

MICROCIRCULATION

Breakthrough in Chronic Illness

Microcirculation problems may turn out to be one of the key factors in chronic illness and aging. The role of microcirculation in illness is a story that has only recently been brought to light. We now have a better understanding of how subtle changes in blood coagulation affect the course of many diseases. Adding microcirculation therapy to the treatment plan for many of these conditions is producing dramatic outcomes.

Microcirculation defined. When we talk about microcirculation, we're not referring to the larger blood vessels or arteries. It is the microcapillaries, microscopic blood vessels that are smaller than a red blood cell, that we are concerned with here. (These capillaries are so small that the red blood cells have to compress themselves into an oblong shape to fit through these tiny blood vessels.) They're found everywhere in the body, in every tissue, next to

---

*This chapter appears with permission of the author; © 2005, Jerry Stine, Lifespan Institute, LifespanProducts.com.

Losing Microcirculation

This condition can be an important factor in chronic illness.

1. The initial problem is inflammation of the lining of the capillaries. We know that this inflammation can be caused by many forms of stress:
   - Infections
   - Chronic illness
   - Surgery or physical trauma
   - Exposure to toxic metals or chemicals
   - Eating foods to which you're allergic
2. All these stresses cause irritation to the lining of the capillaries. The mechanisms may be different, but they all result in some degree of compromise and damage to this delicate lining (endothelial cells).
3. The next step is the thickening of the blood (hypercoagulation). Stress in any form activates blood-clotting mechanisms and thickens the blood. Whenever we're under intense physical stress, coagulation factors circulate in the blood so that clotting can occur more quickly. This is a normal aspect of the body's response to emergencies—the blood prepares to clot in case we're injured. In the short term this can be beneficial and protective. However, this situation sets the stage for potential problems.
4. Putting a Band-Aid on the problem. When the blood thickens under stress, the coagulation process is set to respond more rapidly. Once the blood detects capillary irritation it responds by laying down a thin coating of fibrin to heal the irritation. Fibrin is one of the materials the blood produces to coat injured tissue, a kind of internal Band-Aid. This is a perfectly normal response. The process of healing injuries to the capillary lining begins with this fibrin coating.
5. Healing enzymes. The next step of healing requires specific enzymes to dissolve the fibrin, removing that hindrance to circulation. In addition substances are released from the fibrin as it dissolves, which contribute to repair. As the fibrin is broken down there are a number of protective effects that result in clearing and healing the capillary.
6. Losing the battle with fibrin buildup. Over time if the fibrin isn't totally cleared, we can get into trouble. Circulation to the cells and tissues can be impaired if the fibrin isn't completely dissolved. Then the capillaries remain partially blocked (occluded) by this coating of fibrin. This is how the micro-capillaries lose their ability to deliver all the oxygen and nutrients our cells require.

almost every cell. This is the point of contact where blood flow nourishes each individual cell, delivering nutrients and oxygen.

What goes wrong. Impaired microcirculation interferes with the capillaries' ability to deliver nutrients and oxygen to the cells and carry away waste products and carbon dioxide. This impairment is caused by subtle damage to the capillaries that impedes blood flow.

Symptoms. The symptoms of microcirculation problems are widely diverse because it can affect *any* of the cells in the body. So this is a syndrome that often underlies other conditions. The "symptoms" are those of the presenting illness, whatever that happens to be. We are learning that microcirculation is one of the factors that sustains chronic illness—that makes chronic illness chronic.

The Digestion Connection

Microcirculation is an issue of incredible importance to people with digestive disorders. Here's why: The digestive tract is a surprisingly large organ—the largest in our body. It is essentially a long assembly line for processing food. The job here is the absorption of nutrients, which are then transported to the liver to be further metabolized. This absorption occurs along the entire length of the digestive tract and is carried out by the microcapillaries.

Miles of capillaries are required to transport the nutrients. Any type of recurring irritation in the GI tract will tend to promote fibrin coating in the gut capillaries. The irritation could be due to gluten sensitivity, a yeast overgrowth, a parasite infection, alcohol consumption, or food allergies. If these capillaries become damaged, it limits their ability to support and nourish the lining of the gastrointestinal tract. Consequently a wide range of digestive disorders appear to be associated with damage to the microcapillaries.

When People Don't Heal

We're now seeing that this is one of the issues that makes some people's GI problems so intractable, so resistant to treatment. Even when we think we understand the problem—when we have identified the bacteria, the right medication, and the right supplements—in some cases success still doesn't happen. We are now seeing that these problems with microcirculation are a major factor that underlies many chronic illnesses and can make them so resistant to treatment.

Testing and Treatment

Doctors who are now using this approach for patients with chronic illness report major breakthroughs in treatment. When they give patients products that dissolve the fibrin, an improvement in GI function often occurs, sometimes very dramatically.

Testing. Specialized blood tests from Hemex Laboratories (Phoenix, Arizona) are available to diagnose the extent of problems related to fibrin buildup. Other tests are available to identify individuals who have the genetic tendency to this problem.

Multistaged treatment. The first step in therapy is to improve circulation. The most commonly used medication for this is heparin. A number of herbal and botanical products are also highly useful in this regard, particularly nattokinase and lumbrokinase, which dissolve fibrin. There are also herbal formulas from Chinese medicine, based on their experience with blood chi stagnation—the inability of the blood to deliver energy. These products can help improve the health of the capillaries and the red blood cells. It is interesting to note that traditional Chinese medicine has recognized this phenomenon for centuries. This Chinese medicine concept fits the recent perception of impaired microcirculation to a T.

Low-dose heparin therapy. Many of our readers may have heard of the use of heparin for the treatment of blood clots and heart conditions. In the treatment of microcirculation, referred to as microheparin therapy, much lower dosages of heparin are used. The dosage is far below what would be used for serious blood clot conditions. Consequently the safety of low-dose heparin, even in long-term use, is good, and side effects are rare. The heparin can be given in small, very shallow injections under the skin (subcutaneously). It can also be given as a slow-dissolving lozenge (a trouche) or sublingually, squirted into the mouth under the tongue.

We want to emphasize that microcirculation problems can be a major factor in chronic illness. People who clear the fibrin efficiently tend to get over diseases more completely. For those who can't clear fibrin this low-dose therapy is now available. Doctors are reporting that a great many patients with long-term chronic illness see improvement with this approach.

HOMOCYSTEINE

Homocysteine has been in the news for the last few years because it is a major risk factor in heart disease and cancer. More recent research has also definitively linked it with memory loss, dementia, Alzheimer's disease, and osteoporosis.

Homocysteine defined. Homocysteine—a marker of impaired metabolism—is an amino acid compound normally produced through a type of detoxification called methylation. Methylation chemistry occurs in every cell in the body, particularly in the liver.

What goes wrong? Methylation relies on a number of B complex vitamins to do its job. When these raw materials are lacking, methylation can be impaired and homocysteine levels start to rise in the blood. This amino acid, in excess, is now recognized as a major factor in a range of disorders. These diseases tend to cluster in families, suggesting a possible genetic susceptibility to high homocysteine. Associated conditions include:

- Heart attacks and strokes
- Memory loss, dementia, and Alzheimer's disease
- Parkinson's disease
- Osteoporosis
- Rheumatoid arthritis
- Cervical cancer

Testing. There is a basic blood test that can be ordered by your doctor to check for elevated homocysteine levels. This test can be given again at a later time to measure the response to treatment. It is generally desirable to have your homocysteine level in the low end of the normal range.

What can be done about it? Fortunately this problem can be quite easily resolved by taking a few important nutrients, which are relatively inexpensive and quite effective.

Therapy. The key nutrient here is trimethylglycine (TMG). A number of vitamin products on the market include TMG and the related B vitamins necessary to support methylation and reduce homocysteine levels. Many doctors are reporting that this is a tremendously effective strategy. While homocysteine can be a serious problem, it can be easily detected and treated. Consider getting tested at your next doctor's visit. In the meantime an easy preventive measure would be to use one of the widely available nutritional products that prevent homocysteine buildup.

LOW-CARB/NO-CARB DIETS

Reading Between the Lines

Recently there's been an absolute storm in the popular media about the low-carb diet. What's unfortunate about the media's coverage on this topic is that they're only telling part of the story. What they're not talking about is the question of *what kind* of carbohydrates we should be eating.

The carb issue defined. The point is not just how many carbohydrates we're consuming; it's whether the carbs are refined or not. This determines how quickly the carbs are metabolized into sugar in the body. All carbs are broken down into sugar (glucose). It is how quickly that occurs that determines whether a carbohydrate is good or bad.

Low-Carb Diets

What goes wrong? There's more to this story. The low-carb diets tend to be high in protein, high in fat, and very low in carbohydrates. This diet can produce rapid weight loss, but there are serious concerns about the long-range effects of not eating enough vegetables.

What can be done about it? If you really want to try low-carb eating, you might want to pick up a copy of *Atkins for Life*. This book includes about 50 pages worth of menus. The meals are rated at different levels of carbohydrate, ranging from 20 to 100 grams of carbs. Once the reader has lost some initial weight, he can move out of that low-carb mode into a more moderate-carb diet that emphasizes plenty of veggies.

Which Carbs?

Refined carbohydrates are partially broken down, so they are quickly processed and metabolized. The sugar from a candy bar can be in your bloodstream in minutes. You feel great. But the stress on your body is tremendous. And there's a price to pay. In less than an hour blood sugar spikes and then starts to plummet. Soon you're out of energy and moving into a depressed funk. Your internal chemistry doesn't fare any better. Over time the up and down of the blood sugar exhausts crucial body systems, and they just wear out. This is type 2 diabetes.

Examples of foods that cause a rapid rise in blood sugar are white bread and baked potatoes. The strategy is simply to substitute foods that are broken down more slowly. Brown rice is a good choice. Almost any vegetable will work (except many root vegetables—they're too starchy). Most of the veggies that taste great in Chinese stir-fry are good choices, such as snow peas, onions, peppers. They offer two advantages: They break down more slowly, and they don't contain as many carbs to begin with.

The solution is quite simple. Find foods that you like that don't spike your blood sugar. The process is as simple as substituting a peach for a banana or stir-fry for spaghetti.

Learn to use the Glycemic Index. This is simply an easy-to-understand list of good and bad carbs (see page 274). There are a number of useful books on the subject. We especially like those by Joyce and Jim Daoust, including *The Formula* (Ballantine, 2001) and *40-30-30 Fat Burning Nutrition* (Wharton Publishing, 1996). Barry Sears's books are also classics on this topic, particularly *The Zone* (Regan Books, 1995).

INSULIN RESISTANCE

Insulin resistance defined. This condition is essentially the stage before diabetes, and the key issue in syndrome X or metabolic syndrome. In insulin resistance, insulin is not able to help the body maintain stable blood sugar.

What goes wrong? Insulin resistance involves difficulty with the metabolism of starches and sugars—carbohydrates. When this condition develops, insulin is no longer able to efficiently pull blood sugar (glucose) out of the blood and into the cells. Another undesirable aspect of this problem is that insulin levels in the blood are too high much of the time.

Conditions that can result. This is a growing problem that is almost population wide. It frequently occurs when there is obesity, which now affects 61 percent of the U.S. population. Symptoms include excessive weight gain and fatigue, but insulin resistance is the main metabolic defect in many other serious conditions:

- Obesity
- Hypoglycemia (low blood sugar)
- Diabetes
- Increased risk of heart disease and stroke
- Hypertension
- Rheumatoid arthritis and other inflammatory conditions

Insulin resistance adds a second level of complexity to these serious illnesses. We now see that the successful management of these common, life-threatening diseases must include the management of insulin resistance. Dealing with this problem later, when there are more complications, is more difficult than dealing with it in the early stages. The problem with subtle conditions like insulin resistance is that there are no immediate symptoms that let you know things are starting to go wrong. This is not something that you wait to find out about. We encourage you to take action now.

What can be done about it? The prevention or management of insulin resistance involves a few simple lifestyle issues. We need to eat quality food—we can't eat junk food, we can't eat refined carbohydrates in any quantity. That's the diet.

We encourage you to look at your lifestyle right now and assess it: Ask yourself if you're eating well (are you a carbohydrate junkie?). If you're not sure of what to eat, take a look at the chapters in this book on diet. The whole idea behind carb balance is not life on celery and carrot sticks—it's about finding great food that you like, that tastes good, and that keeps you healthy. Here are the main lifestyle issues that help prevent insulin resistance:

- It is important to eat modest amounts of quality protein and complex carbs—lots of vegetables. In fact, vegetables are more than a source of complex carbohydrates. They're also a great source of a wide range of vitamins, minerals, and phytonutrients.
- Regular exercise is absolutely essential.
- Sleep is crucial. Even getting 8 hours of sleep but getting it at the wrong time of day contributes to more rapid onset of insulin resistance. So sleeping at night and being awake during the day is vital.
- There are a few nutritional supplements that are extremely important. The mineral chromium is key in regulating blood sugar. Lipoic acid is another, because it helps insulin do its job.
- If you are at risk or have insulin resistance, it's vital to see a doctor or nutritionist who is quite familiar with this issue. Doctors who practice complementary and integrative medicine tend to be especially knowledgeable about this problem.

IODINE DEFICIENCIES

We've known about the importance of iodine for more than 100 years. Only recently has its broader impact on health and performance come to light. Recent research has challenged our previous picture of the amount of iodine required for good health. Over the past 50 years, it was believed that if we're getting enough iodine to prevent goiter (a disease of the thyroid gland) we're getting enough iodine to stay healthy. It is becoming apparent that appreciably higher levels of iodine are beneficial.

How much iodine is enough? Iodine levels that prevent goiter are considerably less than 1 mg per day. The question is whether that's enough to support optimal function. In the past we've never had a practical test for determining sufficiency. Now testing and research are changing our perspective on iodine.

A review of the evidence across large populations suggests that higher levels of iodine intake offer huge benefits in overall health and performance. Much of what we know comes from the data on the Japanese population, which has the best health of any industrialized country in the world. Their average level of iodine consumption is 10 to 30 mg a day. People who live in inland cities get more than 10 mg on average. In the coastal cities they take in over 30 mg a day. Almost all of this is coming from seaweed and sea vegetables, which are common foods in the daily Japanese diet. The benefits are particularly dramatic in Okinawa, where there is an unusually high number of people who are over 100 years old and copious amounts of sea vegetables are consumed daily. (The average American gets less than 1 mg of iodine a day.)

What can be done about it? Among the doctors who have been exploring the use of iodine supplements, one of the things that they're universally reporting is that their patients' ability to recover from infections has been tremendously improved. Anyone with any type of chronic infection or bacterial or yeast overgrowth might consider iodine testing and getting a consultation on iodine dosage.

Testing. Practical testing for iodine deficiencies is now available from FFP Laboratories at (828) 684-3233. It simply involves a 24-hour urine collection. One takes a dose of iodine and collects a urine sample for 24 hours. The lab measures how much is excreted into the urine over the 24 hours. If most of the iodine is excreted, then you don't need any more iodine. If your body saves it, conserves it, that is a sign that you need more.

Supplements. The new research suggests that iodine supplements need to be a mixture of iodine and iodide. In fact, there has been a very traditional iodine solution called Lugol's Solution, which was routinely used in medicine for more than 100 years. It tends to have a very strong flavor. The modern products are very similar in composition to Lugol's.

The supplements that have been developed by these researchers are available through integrative-medicine physicians. Kelp and other types of seaweed extracts are available in health food stores, although they are not nearly as concentrated. Lugol's Solution is available in drugstores.

All these concepts are relatively new but are vitally important to our health. We want to reemphasize that these dynamics underlie a great many diseases. It has been our experience that integrative doctors and nutritionists are particularly aware of these concerns and their treatment. If any of these issues sound relevant to you and you're interested in exploring them further, you'll want to begin by discussing them with your doctor. The more we know about how our bodies work, the more likely it is that we can get healthy and stay healthy.

Biographical information for **Jerry Stine** appears on page 12.

39

Medicine for the Future: Bioelectromagnetic Therapy

Trent W. Nichols, M.D.

MRI AND OTHER DIAGNOSTIC DEVICES

The use of magnetic and electromagnetic devices has many medical applications and has proven to be one of the safest, most effective means of diagnosing human diseases available. For example, MRI (magnetic resonance imaging) provides a highly accurate method of imaging that is replacing X-ray diagnosis because it does not involve radiation and yet is more detailed. As a result MRI technology is frequently used in place of earlier technology, such as the CT or CAT scan (computer axial tomography). Similar technology is also beginning to replace EEG as the preferred technique for recording brain activity.

Other familiar applications of electromagnetics in diagnosis include ECG (electrocardiography) to record the functioning of the heart, EEG (electroencephalography) for the electrical activity of the brain, EGG (electrogastrography) for the stomach, and EMG (electromyography) to evaluate muscle function. In sum, electromagnetic devices are now widely accepted as the primary technology for use in diagnosis.

THERAPEUTIC APPLICATIONS OF ELECTROMAGNETIC ENERGY

Eight major applications of electromagnetic energy in medicine were reviewed at a National Institutes of Health (NIH) Consensus Conference held in Virginia in 1992, on bioelectromagnetic therapy. It is worthy of note that a number of these areas are relevant to the healing of GI illness.

- Wound healing
- Tissue regeneration
- Immune system stimulation
- Neuroendrocrine modulations
- Treatment of osteoarthritis
- Bone repair
- Nerve stimulation
- Electroacupuncture

359

Sources of Magnetic Energy

Magnetism is one of the fundamental forces of nature and has been studied and used since antiquity. A magnetic field is defined as a field of magnetic force extending out from a permanent magnet or produced by moving electrical currents. Biomagnetism exists in all living organisms. The earth is surrounded by magnetic fields, generated from the massive molten iron core in the center of the planet, of such intensity that it radiates thousands of miles beyond the earth's surface. Incoming electromagnetic radiation from solar storms also has powerful magnetic effects on the earth.

On a human scale the body produces subtle electromagnetic fields that are generated by the chemical reactions within the body. This electromagnetic energy travels from the nerve cells of the brain (astrocytes) along the cells covering the nerves of the spinal cord (Schwann cells), out to organs and limbs. The energy is returned via the connective tissue. These routes of electromagnetic transmission in the body were first defined as meridians more than 2,000 years ago by Oriental medicine practitioners.

It has been long known that exposure to electromagnetic radiation (ionized energy comparable to the effects of X-ray) can cause extreme damage in living tissue. Only recently has it been discovered that electromagnetic fields (non-ionized) with low frequency can have a beneficial effect on biological tissues and thus can be therapeutic. Our systems appear to require a certain amount of low electromagnetic current, which the brain transmits every night in cycles to regenerate various organ tissues during sleep. (Researchers have actually measured this current and found it to be comparable to a DC current of about 2 to 8 Hertz.)

TREATMENT OF CHRONIC PAIN

Acupuncture

In 1997 the National Institutes of Health issued a *Consensus Statement* on acupuncture. The report included confirmation that acupuncture is considered appropriate for the treatment of chronic pain.

How does acupuncture work? Research indicates that acupuncture treatment raises the threshold of pain in the body. When acupuncture or electroacupuncture is performed, endorphins are released by the body, which significantly decrease the sensation of pain. This mechanism has been confirmed through more than a decade of studies by a team of researchers from St. Louis Medical University and Bejing Medical School.

Thousands of clinical trials have been conducted on acupuncture. More than 200 have focused specifically on the treatment of pain, confirming the effectiveness of acupuncture in pain relief. Findings of recent studies include:

- A French study of pain in cancer patients found that 36 percent given acupuncture experienced a decrease in pain intensity. Of those who received "sham" acupuncture (but were not actually treated), only 2 percent had less pain.
- An Italian study of acupuncture for lower back pain found that among patients who received five treatments, 68 percent obtained a good result. In those who received ten treatments, 86 percent experienced a good result, which was defined as having less than half the pain.
- A German study on rheumatoid arthritis and the associated pain used electromagnetic millimeter waves (MW) applied to acupuncture points. Patients in the treatment group reported such significant pain relief and reduced joint stiffness (during and after the course of therapy) that the research was halted so all the participants could receive this therapy.

TENS Units

In the United States, TENS units (providing Transcutaneous Electrical Nerve Stimulation) are now frequently prescribed by doctors for the control of pain in patient self-care. Handheld TENS units have a sensor enabling the treatment of acupuncture meridians and points. These units stimulate acupoints using low-intensity, low-frequency electrical current to affect small-muscle nerves, releasing the body's endorphins to moderate pain. Although these treatments are brief (approximately 30 minutes), the beneficial effects do not diminish over time. Research has confirmed the effectiveness of TENS in managing pain:

- A study at Peking University in Beijing evaluated the effect of using TENS on acupoints to treat pain. Researchers reported that TENS treatment reduced pain without blunting sensation.
- At the Department of Rehabilitative Services at Hong Kong Polytechnic University, researchers measured the response to both electroacupuncture and TENS in patients with painful osteoarthritic knees. The conclusion: "Both electro-acupuncture and TENS treatments were effective in reducing osteoarthritis-induced knee pain."
- Successful treatment using a TENS unit has been reported for achalasia, a disease of the esophagus (treating acupoint LI4, reported by Ann Ooyang, M.D., Penn State University).

- Clinicians report that pain relief can diminish over several months of continuous therapy with standard TENS devices. To overcome this limitation, newer TENS-like and electroacupuncture devices have been developed in both the East and West.

Other Electroacupuncture Devices

A variety of safe, low-frequency electroacupuncture units are widely available in the Orient and are used by both doctors and patients. These devices are used by the author in his practice and are found to be very effective in pain control. Patients are instructed in how to use the unit at home, which has made possible the successful elimination of narcotics for many patients with chronic pain.

- The author has treated many patients with nausea using a handheld electroacupuncture device applied to specific acupuncture points (the Acustim unit, particularly when applied to acupoint P6).
- Another small portable device that utilizes acupoints is designed to control symptoms of motion sickness. This device is available as a wristband that stimulates an acupuncture point on the wrist (acupoint P6), using a device developed by Dr. Kenneth Koch, Penn State University. This type of unit was utilized by astronaut John Glenn to control nausea during his historic reentry into space.
- A number of other promising applications of magnetic therapy in pain management are described by Drs. Paul Rosch and Ronald Lawrence in *Magnet Therapy, the Pain Cure Alternative*.

TISSUE REGENERATION

Low-Intensity Microwave Therapy

Microwave resonance therapy is being studied for bone repair in trials under way in the United States. This research was begun in Russia using low-intensity radiation (continuous or pulsed-modulated) to treat ulcers and esophagitis, chronic pain and arthritis, neurological disorders, and side effects of chemotherapy. Research on the mechanism of microwave indicates that there is an increase in immune system competence at very low intensities. Thousands of Russians have been treated by this therapy, which uses low-level microwaves applied at certain acupoints.

Pulsed Electromagnetic Fields

Restoration of nerve and bone tissue with pulsed electromagnetic fields (PEMF) was approved for the treatment of fractures in 1979 and has been given full FDA approval as a treatment device. Since that time success rates have averaged 80 percent (based on the research of Dr. Andrew Bassett and the electro-chemist Arthur Pilla, Columbia-Presbyterian Medical Center, New York). A detailed account of this research is described in the book by Dr. Robert Becker, *The Body Electric: Electromagnetism and the Foundation of Life.* In the early 1970s,

> Bassett and Pilla published empirical evidence that pulsed electromagnetic fields accelerated the healing of bone fractures. . . . Several experimenters, notably Stephen Smith, have now proven that the electrobiology bone-healing device . . . speeds up the division rate of cells that are already proliferating rapidly. Among normal cells, this includes skin, gut, and liver cells. In 1983, A. R. Liboff, a biophysicist at Oakland University in Rochester, Michigan reported on the effects of . . . magnetic fields [at specific frequencies], all enhanced the replication of DNA during the synthesis phase of mitosis [cell division] . . .
>
> It is important to bear in mind that, in stimulating DNA synthesis, a [pulsed] electromagnetic field does not distinguish between desirable and undesirable growth. It affects all cells in the same way, but cell systems that are already rapidly dividing are speeded up the most. . . . These susceptible processes include healing [cells], embryonic growth, and cancer.

In essence this pulsed energy can be very beneficial when focused on a specific area of the body, such as a fracture. However, if it is applied to the entire body and an undiagnosed tumor is present, it could stimulate the rate of cancer growth. For this reason other types of electromagnetic therapy, such as MME, are used when the goal of treatment is to stimulate the entire body or the immune system.

MME: Magnetic Molecular Energetics

Wound healing, tissue regeneration, and immune enhancement are all possible using MME (magnetic molecular energizing). MME is a therapeutic device developed by Dr. Dean Bonlie for the Advanced Magnetic Research Institute in Calgary, Alberta. MME consists of two strong DC, nonpulsed electromagnets, comparable to those used in MRI equipment. In MME technology the electromagnets create a therapeutic magnetic field. Because MME uses nonpulsed electromagnetism, the entire body can safely be treated. Of the 1,200 patients treated to date, the most serious problem that has occurred is one patient with a nosebleed.

This electromagnetic field leads to enhanced electron transfer, which is the basis of all chemical reactions in the body. We have direct evidence from our research that this therapy improves oxygen capacity (confirmed in measures of oxygen levels through ear oxymetry testing). It also enhances chemical processes, improving the assimilation of nutrients, removal of metabolic waste, reduction of free radicals, and increased manufacture of enzymes. These improvements in physiological functioning provide the basis for healing. (Another mechanism of healing is improved detoxification. This effect has been confirmed in the research of Jan Walleczek, using static magnetic fields. He documented a 35 percent increase in the activity of beneficial detoxification enzymes.)

MME technology is now being used in a six-site clinical trial approved by the FDA and the Central Institutional Review Board. Patients are receiving therapy for neurological conditions including spinal cord injury, brain injury, stroke impairment, multiple sclerosis, cerebral palsy, and Alzheimer's and Parkinson's diseases. In the trial orthopedic conditions involving bone and joint repair, such as sports injuries, are also being studied. Presentations of this research have been given at a number of international scientific conferences over the past five years. As mentioned, more than 1,200 patients in North America have been treated to date. (See www.amripa.com for abstracts of cases.)

Dr. Andrew Bassett made this prophetic statement in 1992:

In the decades to come, it is safe to predict bioelectromagnetics will assume a therapeutic importance equal to, or greater than, that of pharmacology and surgery today. With proper interdisciplinary effort, significant inroads can be made in controlling the ravages of cancer, some forms of heart disease, arthritis, hormonal disorders, and neurological scourges such as Alzheimer's disease, spinal cord injury, and multiple sclerosis.

This prediction is not pie-in-the-sky. Pilot studies, and biological mechanisms confirmed in basic research, form a rational basis for such a statement.

Biographical information for **Trent W. Nichols, M.D.,** appears on page 104.

The Advanced Magnetic Research Institutes (AMRI) provide treatment for neurological and degenerative disorders. The technique described above is now being researched in a six-site clinical trial approved by the FDA and the Central Institutional Review Board. Patients are receiving therapy for Alzheimer's disease, brain injury, multiple sclerosis, muscular dystrophy,

Parkinson's disease, spinal cord injury, and stroke impairment. Treatment is also provided for orthopedic conditions involving bone and joint repair, herniated discs, and sports injuries. For more details and appointment information contact Advanced Magnetic Research Institute of Pennsylvania, Eichelberger Professional Building, 195 Stock Street, Suite 211B, Hanover, PA 17331; (717) 632-0300; www.amripa.com.

Advanced Magnetic Research Institutes are also currently located at:

27652-B Camino Capistrano, Laguna Niguel, CA 92677; (949) 367-0877;
www.amri1.com
Dayspring Medical Center, 217 Dayspring Way, Mocksville, NC 27028;
(336) 492-2874; www.amri-nc.com
43393 Schoenherr Road, Sterling Heights, MI 48313; (586) 254-7711;
www.amri-mi.com
Tahoma Clinic, 801 SW 16th, Suite 121, Renton, WA 98055; (425) 264-0059
ext. 260

40

Improving Digestive Health with Chinese Medicine

EFREM KORNGOLD, O.M.D.

Chinese medicine is a complete medical system that has been practiced continuously throughout Asia for more than twenty-three centuries. Not only has it successfully treated and prevented illness among Asian people, but it has also become part of the health care of millions of Westerners in Europe and North and South America for more than one hundred years. Chinese medicine alleviates sickness while enhancing immunity and recuperative power—in other words, it promotes health.

It is the ability of the body to resist illness and disease, as well as to repair and regenerate itself, that enables it to remain adaptable and well. The capacity to recover balance or physiological homeostasis and to restore the body to a healthy condition is entirely dependent upon the quantity and quality of *Qi* (pronounced chee), often translated as "vital force" or "vital energy." Qi is the fundamental power that we are endowed with at birth and that we strive to maintain and increase by cultivating a healthy and satisfying lifestyle. All healing in Chinese medicine is directed toward conserving, protecting, restoring, and regulating Qi. And in the broadest sense Qi refers to all the substances, resources, and capacities within our bodies that we use to remain alive and well.

HOW THE BODY IS ORGANIZED

Chinese medicine maintains that preserving the strength and integrity of the body as a whole is the most important defense against disease. This means that while acupuncture, herbal medicine, appropriate diet, and exercise are used to relieve symptoms and heal sickness, an equal or greater emphasis is placed upon replenishing the body's natural substances or body constituents (called Shen, Qi, moisture, blood, and essence) and optimizing the function of the body's primary organ systems or networks (known as the liver, heart, spleen, lung, and kidney networks).

- Shen is our spirit or charisma, mirrored in our thoughts, feelings, sensations.
- Qi, our vital force, is observed in the body's warmth, movement, and metabolic activity.
- Moisture encompasses all of the fluids and internal secretions that lubricate the joints and form tears, saliva, urine, and cerebrospinal fluid.
- Blood contains all of the nutritive elements from which the body's tissues are made and provides the structural components that form skin, muscles, vessels, nerves, bones, and visceral organs.
- Essence is the basic *stuff* that enables us to maintain primary vital functions such as growth, repair, reproduction, metabolism, sensation, and imagination.

These five body constituents are managed or *organized* by the five organ networks:

- The heart network governs Shen, maintaining awareness and propelling the blood through the vessels.
- The lung network governs Qi, establishes the rhythm of breathing, and maintains the integrity of skin and mucous membranes.
- The spleen governs moisture, distributing fluids and nutrients and maintaining the integrity of muscle.
- The liver governs blood, regulating the smooth circulation of Qi and blood.
- The kidney network governs essence, providing the basic foundation for life in all of its aspects—physical, mental, emotional, and spiritual.

DISHARMONY: THE ROOT OF DISEASE

The colloquial use of the term *stress* actually suggests a state of distress—a sometimes vague, sometimes distinct sense of disquiet, discomfort, and disequilibrium that is often a prelude to the overt outbreak of an illness. The notion of stress is parallel in meaning to the classical Chinese medical concept of disharmony or imbalance. By the time stress is experienced as an impediment, a variety of symptoms may occur, depending upon the tissues and organ systems that are already weak or vulnerable.

Health is a result of the harmonious interaction of the five body constituents and the five organ networks. In contrast, illness is the result of a depletion, obstruction, or abnormal alteration of the five body constituents and a disturbance of the coordinated activity of the organ networks. Chinese medicine considers all sickness to be a consequence of the body's inability to preserve its own equilibrium in response to constant and inevitable changes, internally and externally—in other words, *stress,* the stress of living.

PRESERVING INTEGRITY, STABILITY, FLEXIBILITY, AND ADAPTABILITY

It is the central purpose of Chinese medicine to invigorate the individual's power to function in a natural and integrated way. This is facilitated through a number of methods:

- Acupuncture (the insertion of thin stainless steel needles at specific locations along the meridians that traverse the surface of the body in order to regulate the body's vital energy or Qi)
- Herbal medicine (natural plant, animal, and mineral substances combined into specific formulas that are taken in the form of teas, powders, pills, and tablets to strengthen the body and antidote the disease process)
- Diet therapy (the use of special combinations of foods and herbs to nourish and strengthen the body)

The practitioner of Chinese medicine seeks to enable the body to restore itself to a condition of stability, flexibility, and adaptability. And while a condition of perfect health is not always completely attainable, these gentle and noninvasive methods of treatment will almost always restore or enhance immunity, vigor, and functionality. In addition Chinese medicine can prevent or reverse many of the harmful effects of medical treatments that may be necessary to preserve and prolong life. In fact, using Chinese medicine in combination with Western medicine enables a person to better withstand the impact of aggressive medical interventions such as chemotherapy and surgery by building strength and accelerating the rate of recovery, maintaining the quality of life, and increasing the likelihood of long-term survival.

THE DIGESTIVE SYSTEM IS THE SOURCE OF QI

Each cell of our nervous and digestive systems must function appropriately every minute to ensure coordinated muscular movements of the gut and the proper secretion of enzymes, hormones, and mucus. Digestion is therefore a crucial aspect of our intelligence.

According to Chinese medicine, Qi is the intelligent power of the body. So if Qi is adequately distributed throughout the body, then the body will

Chinese Medicine in Action

In 1991 Elaine was diagnosed with proctitis, and in 1993 she was diagnosed with ulcerative colitis. After four years of treatment with prednisone, steroid enemas, Rowasa suppositories, Asacol, and mercaptopurine, she was told that she needed to undergo surgical removal of her colon. At this point she decided to try something different—Chinese medicine.

When she began treatment with acupuncture and Chinese herbal medicine in 1997, Elaine was experiencing constant abdominal bloating and gas, intestinal pain and sensitivity, urgency and frequent bowel movements, very low energy and stamina, depression, and anxiety. Not only was she not responding well to her medications, but she also was having trouble figuring out what to eat that didn't aggravate her condition.

After ten acupuncture treatments over a period of eleven months, along with dietary modification (basically elimination of all grains, starchy vegetables, and milk products) and herbal formulas in the form of pills and liquid extracts, she has improved enormously. She rarely has gas, bloating, urgency, or diarrhea, and she has no pain, intestinal bleeding, or mucus in her stool. She has reduced her medications considerably but still relies on a daily dose of mercaptopurine, which has been reduced from 75 to 50 mg, and Asacol, which has been reduced to once every four days.

More important, her energy, stamina, and sense of hopefulness and optimism have returned, enabling her to go back to work, expand her spiritual life, and think about changing her career. All of this has occurred without major surgery and with a decreasing need for medication. The longer she continues with acupuncture, herbal medicine, and an appropriate diet, the more functional she becomes and the stronger she feels.

know what to do in each of its parts all the time. Each of us has an operating system, an organizing power (Qi), that has much in common with other beings but is unique to each individual. Every moment that we are alive we're literally re-creating ourselves, and we do it a little differently every day—we don't remain exactly the same. Because our world is always changing we must continually adapt, so one of the indications of disease is the loss of adaptability—when we're no longer able to adjust comfortably and naturally to the shifting circumstances of our lives. The health of the digestive system is crucial to maintaining our ability to adapt and to be well, for a lifetime.

It is the spleen network that governs all digestive processes, including those of the mouth, esophagus, stomach, small intestine, large intestine, and pancreas. The spleen network is subdivided into two organ systems: the stomach, which regulates the digestion of food and fluids, and the spleen, which regulates the absorption of nutrients and their distribution within the body. It is the job of the spleen network to supply the body with the raw materials it needs on a daily basis to produce all the substances of the body, primarily Qi, moisture, and blood. So the digestive system is the source of all that we require for daily living, including the nutrients we need to grow and mature.

THE THREE PILLARS OF HEALTH

Because it supplies us with Qi the digestive system is one of the three pillars of health—what are known as the Three Treasures—the other two being Shen and essence. Shen is our spirit or charisma—what we experience as emotional warmth and presence of mind. Essence is the vital power and substance that we are endowed with at birth—what we "inherit" from our parents and from our mother while we're growing in her womb—and it enables us to have children, to be imaginative and creative, and to develop into mature and competent adults.

The signs of good digestion are:

- Feeling good in the belly. Your stomach and intestines, your upper and lower abdomen, feel comfortable, especially after eating or eliminating— so comfortable, in fact, they actually induce pleasurable sensations.
- Experiencing regular and distinct feelings of hunger. When you're hungry you have a clear sense of what it is that you want and need to eat. When you eat and drink what is appropriate and nourishing for you, you feel satisfied, better after eating than you did before. You become revitalized and happy, ready to work and play.
- Feeling good in the mouth. You have a pleasant taste in your mouth, it feels comfortably moist, and your breath smells good.

Frequently when people feel unwell, if there is no clear evidence of illness or disease from a conventional Western medical perspective, their distress may be viewed as if it were merely a psychosomatic problem. It can be distressing to experience poor digestion and not recognize the cause. In situations like these, in which there is no clear understanding or diagnosis, Chinese medicine can often be helpful. Vague complaints—the kind that mysteriously come and go or simply make us uncomfortable and discouraged—

are taken to heart by the practitioner because they're seen as the vanguard of what could develop into a more serious condition. The goal is to treat problems before they become severe. One of the strengths of Chinese medicine is that it can offer interventions at the early stages of nonspecific illness, whereas conventional Western medicine is geared more toward treating problems that are full-blown and therefore easier to identify with objective tests and diagnostic procedures.

TONGUE DIAGNOSIS: A SIMPLE WAY TO EVALUATE DIGESTIVE HEALTH

In Chinese medicine the tongue is perceived as a window through which the signs of health or sickness can be directly seen. The condition of the tongue and its coating—the tongue fur—indicates quite clearly whether or not the digestive system is functioning well. By carefully noting the shape, color, and moisture of the tongue and its fur, we can tell if there is a disorder of the stomach or the intestines. If there is congestion in the stomach due to a lack of digestive secretions, inhibited peristalsis, toxins in the food, poor-quality food, or food that is staying in the stomach or intestines too long and beginning to ferment or putrefy, it will appear as a change in the moisture, texture, thickness, and color of the fur.

A healthy tongue is a ruddy pink color, lays comfortably in the mouth (is neither too large or fat nor too small or thin), and has an even shape, a smooth texture, and a thin, moist, light white fur that covers its surface evenly from the back to the front. The appearance of coarse, thickened, wet, dry, absent, or discolored fur (translucent white changing to opaque white, gray, yellow, or brown) is an early sign of congestion in the stomach and of poor digestion. By examining the tongue fur each morning and evening, you will know whether your digestive health is improving or worsening. Usually if the tongue fur is becoming thicker and/or more yellow, it indicates either a disturbance of digestion and elimination, the development of an acute illness like stomach or intestinal flu, or both. If the fur is becoming progressively thinner, whiter, and clearer it represents a general improvement in the entire condition of the body as well as the digestive system. On the other hand, if the fur becomes very thin, patchy, or entirely absent, it represents a worsening of health in general, and a weakening of the Qi of the whole body.

Very often visible signs on the tongue are associated with a subjective experience of distress, generally as well as locally in the digestive organs. A sensation of bloating in the stomach or belly, belching or flatulence, irregular bowel movements, strong food aversions or cravings, irritability, and pain are symptoms of congestion, whereas feelings of fatigue and weakness, chilliness, melancholy and dull thinking, vague discomforts that can't be easily localized, slow or infrequent bowel movements, loose stools, and cravings that are difficult to describe or satisfy are symptoms of depletion. Another early warning of poor digestion is a sense of dissatisfaction, irritability, or malaise after eating—lingering hunger, queasiness, or feeling as if you ate something spoiled or improperly cooked.

The Appearance of the Tongue

The appearance of the tongue and its fur have specific meanings:

- A very red tongue indicates an excess of heat: systemic fever and/or inflammation.
- A very pale tongue indicates deficiency of Qi and blood: generalized weakness and/or anemia.
- An enlarged or swollen tongue with "tooth marks" indicates overall weakness of the digestive system, usually in a person who tends to be tired, lethargic, and unable to sustain a desirable level of physical and mental effort: deficiency of Qi, especially of the spleen network.
- A small or thin tongue indicates an insufficiency of moisture and blood, usually in a person who tends to be tense, nervous, and working beyond the limits of his or her true capacities.
- Yellow fur, especially in the central area of the tongue, indicates heat in the stomach: inflammation in the stomach and/or small intestine and/or large intestine.
- Very white (like paper) fur indicates excess of cold in the stomach and spleen: diminished metabolic and digestive activity leading to congestion of food and fluids in the stomach and/or small intestine.
- Very thick fur indicates a condition of Qi stagnation: congestion of food and fluids in the stomach and/or small intestine.
- Very thin fur indicates a condition of Qi depletion: weakness of the stomach and/or small intestine and a diminished capacity for absorbing nutrients.
- A very wet tongue or slimy-looking fur indicates an excess of moisture (also known as a condition of dampness): retention of fluids in the body as a whole (wet tongue) or in the digestive system (slimy fur).
- A very dry tongue or fur indicates a deficiency of moisture (also known as a condition of dryness): generalized dehydration (whole tongue) or a lack of fluid secretions in the digestive system (fur only).

HOW DIGESTIVE PROBLEMS BEGIN

From the point of view of Chinese medicine, disorders such as esophagitis, gastritis, ileitis, and colitis are all variations on a theme—the disordered function of the stomach and intestines (the spleen network). These organs can become disturbed for a multiplicity of reasons: poor diet; irregular eating habits; physical and mental strain; a viral, bacterial, fungal, or parasitic infection; allergies; toxicity; and harsh medications like antibiotics (tetracycline, metronidazole, Biaxin), anti-inflammatory drugs (aspirin, Motrin, Indocin, Asacol), steroids (prednisone, cortisone), chemotherapy drugs (methotrexate, cisplatin, 5-FU, Adriamycin). These influences can undermine the health of the digestive system in the short term—as in diarrhea and nausea caused by antibiotics or chemotherapy—and if present over a period of months or years, probably distort the normal gut ecology by encouraging local or systemic yeast (candidiasis) and bacterial overgrowth in the stomach and intestines, decreasing enzymatic functions (inhibiting fat, protein, and carbohydrate-digesting enzymes), and compromising gut immunity (decreasing immunoglobulins and increasing antibodies that cause allergic reactions to food and other substances). It's unusual for chronic problems to arise out of a single acute incident, although they may appear that way to the individual. Invariably there is a history of symptoms—minor but persistent or recurring problems that go unnoticed, ignored, or neglected, or that may even be considered normal—that actually may begin as early as infancy or childhood.

The first stage of diminishing digestive function is signaled by vague or generalized feelings of discomfort—a little indigestion or heartburn, queasiness once in a while, bad breath, slight bowel irregularity, and variable cravings or hunger. In Chinese medicine these initial signs reflect the disorganization of Qi. This means that the normal activity of the gut—the smooth, peristaltic waves that push food through the digestive tract—have become disrupted. When the gut ceases to function naturally, people begin experiencing gas in the intestines and stomach or a sensation that food is stuck in the throat, chest, stomach, or belly. This condition is called stagnation of Qi, and different manifestations mirror the same basic syndrome. Instead of food and fluids moving easily, sequentially, and comfortably in the right direction (from the top down, like squeezing toothpaste out of a tube), they get blocked or even go in reverse, which can cause nausea, regurgitation, heartburn, and belching.

This is the way that many digestive problems begin—as a condition of stagnation. In fact, many diseases begin in this way. After a long period of stagnation, the ability of the digestive system to extract nutrients becomes diminished, and the syndrome of stagnation eventually transforms into one of depletion, a weakness of the body as a whole. When that happens people no longer have the dependable resources they need in order to work, think, re-create, enjoy life, and cope with its challenges. When this feeling of inade-quacy is present there is the sense that there is not enough strength or endurance, people begin to compensate, usually unwittingly, by taking stimu-lants to squeeze more energy out of themselves, because they're not getting what they need from their food.

Additionally poor digestion can lead to lack of rest, due to disturbed sleep patterns. When your stomach is uncomfortable you don't sleep as well. Because of work schedules or long commutes, many people eat too late and too much before they go to bed, allowing excess food to remain in the stom-ach and intestines while sleeping. Ordinarily digestion is facilitated by getting up and moving around after eating, whereas eating just before going to sleep can interfere with this process.

SELF CARE

When And How To Eat
The Chinese medical model describes an optimum time for each organ system during the 24-hour cycle of day and night. Ideally soon after you awaken in the morning, you have a bowel movement. That way the gut is emptied and prepared to receive the first food of the new day. Between 7:00 and 9:00 A.M. is the optimum time to empty the bowels. The optimum time for eating and digesting is from midmorning to early afternoon, 9:00 A.M. to 3:00 P.M. This is the time of peak activity for the stomach and the small intestine. So from the point of view of the digestive organs, breakfast and lunch are the most important meals. The midday meal should be the largest, breakfast should be moderate, and dinner should be the lightest and easiest to digest.

Most of us eat breakfast fairly early, somewhere between seven and nine o'clock in the morning, when we're not yet ready physiologically for a large meal. We need to eat something nourishing and filling in the morning because we're empty and somewhat weak after sleeping for eight hours, but we should eat just enough to get the juices flowing. As a general principle you should eat a small meal for breakfast. On the other hand, it's important not to go with-out breakfast, because you'll be too hungry for lunch and end up overeating. The better you keep to a regular schedule of meals, the better you'll feel.

Another issue is how quickly we eat. Many people eat too fast—they're always in a hurry. The only time they're not rushing is late in the evening, when they're physically and mentally worn out from the day. Not only do you feel weary in the evening, but your digestive system is at a low ebb because its prime time is long past. Yet when the evening meal is delayed, you'll be even hungrier and more tempted to overeat. If you overload yourself with food at that time your body will perceive it as a burden, not as a pleasure.

Food Temperature and Good Digestion

Another habit that Americans indulge in that can have damaging effects on digestion is eating too much cold and raw food, especially in the beginning of the day—like reaching for the orange juice right out of the refrigerator first thing in the morning, or having cold yogurt or a piece of chilled fruit, or all three. Sometimes the cold and raw food is chased with a hot cup of coffee. And even though a cup of hot coffee warms things up, it's often so intensely hot that it is an insult to the stomach. Drinking something extremely hot right after eating something very cold is a little like running cold water over a very hot cast iron frying pan, which can sometimes crack under the strain. Such a sudden and extreme change can damage the stomach Qi and lead to Qi stagnation syndrome, causing chronic indigestion over the long term.

Raw foods, like refrigerated and frozen foods, are also considered to have a cooling influence on the body. A diet that consists primarily of raw and cold foods will often lead to persistent diarrhea with abdominal gas and bloating. Cooling or cold food may be appropriate when the body is overheated in hot weather or during an acute illness with a high fever. For example, eating watermelon on a hot day helps to cool us down, and watermelon juice can actually bring down a fever that comes as a result of being too long in the sun.

The inherent coldness of raw and refrigerated foods chills the stomach, and instead of helping to increase its blood supply for effective digestion and activate its digestive secretions, it causes the stomach to contract, to reduce its blood supply and inhibit its secretions. The mixing of hot and cold foods in quick succession can easily lead to Qi stagnation syndrome and may ultimately result in chronic indigestion.

A more healthful morning ritual would be to first drink something warm, even plain hot water. What this does is to prepare the stomach—it "wakes it up," just as a hot shower invigorates you and gets your blood moving. The hot shower invigorates you from the outside, and drinking something hot invigorates you on the inside. After drinking something hot, eat something else that's warm, like cooked cereal or steamed vegetables or even stewed fruit—something that you can digest easily and that provides more nutrients than a piece of toast or a muffin with a cup of coffee. Cooked foods have a warming influence that helps the stomach and intestines function more effectively. Then if you want to finish your morning meal with something fresh, like a piece of fruit or some yogurt, as long as it's at least room temperature, that's fine, because the digestive organs are already "warmed up." If you must eat something cold—because you're in a hurry or feeling hot or thirsty—always eat or drink something hot first.

Throughout Asia hot water is considered to be the universal remedy for any illness, as well as being a simple health tonic. Just sipping hot water (or hot lemon water, vegetable broth, diluted fruit juice, or even weak green tea) throughout the day is very good therapy for your digestion. The reason that the frequent ingestion of warm or hot (but not scalding) liquids is so beneficial is that it restores and maintains the natural condition of the digestive organs. For example, recall how you feel when you go into a cold environment and you're not dressed warmly enough: You become rapidly chilled and begin to feel lethargic or even sleepy, like you want to curl up in a ball in order to get warm and conserve your body heat. Exactly the same thing happens to the internal organs when they're subjected to cold influences.

When I was a child I loved ice cream, and I would always ask to have ice cream for dessert. I was a rather thin child, so when we would go to a restaurant my father would always say, "Now, if you get ice cream, you're going to feel really cold when you go outside." I would never believe him. And every time I'd walk outside and get really cold. The point is that eating cold things makes us cold. And naturally the body responds defensively: It contracts, the pulse slows down, and metabolic activity becomes depressed. The more the body slows down, the harder it is to eat, digest, assimilate, and transform the food nutrients into energy, blood, and tissue.

Factors in Good Digestion

The primary factors that promote good digestion include:

- Timing—when you eat
- Manner—how you eat
- Quantity—how much you eat
- Condition of the food—whether it's raw, cooked, warm, or cold
- Quality—whether the food is fresh, clean, and pure
- Appropriateness—whether the food is compatible with your digestive capacity and relevant to your nutritional requirements

The quality, quantity, condition, and appropriateness of your food are all important from the Chinese medicine point of view. But even more crucial are the conditions of eating—the manner in which you eat, how quickly you eat, whether you're standing or sitting or moving about, whether you're paying attention to your food or continuing to work. If you continue to work while you eat—to engage in intense problem-solving or read something that makes you tense—you are depriving the digestive system of the energy it needs to perform its function. If reading or conversing while you eat relaxes you, then it's good; if not then it's an unnecessary stress and potentially harmful.

If you're trying to work while you eat you're forcing the body to divide its resources between action or thinking and the work of digestion. This uses up the Qi instead of restoring it, so that you wind up competing with yourself. People who eat and run or who eat on the run will progressively begin to lose energy and digestive power. This is also true of those who eat without stopping or who eat and then immediately get up and go back to work, without allowing time for digestion. The consequence of this is an increased risk of diminished physical capacities and deteriorating health. Chronic health problems generally originate very early in life because that's when our habits around food and eating are established, like not chewing well and eating too fast.

In my family my father ate so fast that he was always finished before everybody else and couldn't tolerate leaving the food and dishes on the table. He immediately began to wash the dishes and put the leftovers away. So if I didn't finish quickly I wouldn't get to eat all of my food, and I was a dreamy child who ate particularly slowly. Eventually I learned to eat very quickly, and as a result I've had to learn to undo that conditioning in my adult life. Being tense and gulping your food leads to a lot of discomfort, especially for children, who often get stomachaches after eating too much and too quickly—often in response to messages like "You can't leave the table until you eat everything on your plate."

When There's No Time to Eat

If you're in a hurry, if you really don't have time to sit down, it is better to drink your food rather than eat it. Drink something warm, like soup or even plain broth. If you have to eat in a hurry, it's a lot easier to digest cooked vegetables than raw salads. Later, when you have time to sit, to calm down, and to chew thoroughly, then you can eat more dense, solid food—and you'll be able to digest it.

Even before you put something in your mouth, you should feel good in your belly. This good feeling comes as a sign that the body is getting ready for the food. When you begin to put the food in your mouth, chew, and swallow, you'll start to feel even better: As the food slides smoothly down the esophagus and into the stomach, it should induce pleasurable sensations all along the way. Then as you eat more, it gets pushed along and pushed along, and eventually you say to yourself, "That's it, I'm finished. I'm not hungry anymore."

RESTORING VITALITY, RESTORING QI

People with digestive disorders often miss the pleasurable experience of eating, but they certainly want to regain it. The purpose of acupuncture, herbal medicine, and dietary modification is to restore the normal activity of the Qi, to relieve stagnation—to promote the normal secretions and peristalsis of the digestive tract. This is essential to good health.

To restore the Qi means to restore the normal pattern of movement: the movement of blood and fluids and the activity of the organs themselves. One of the early signs of poor digestion is reflux, which means that food, air, and fluid are reversing their normal direction, going up instead of down. This is what causes problems such as esophageal irritation and spasm. On the other hand, when the gut is hyperactive food and liquid are passing through too quickly to be properly transformed and absorbed. This is also abnormal movement. Gut hyperactivity can be a manifestation of irritability and anxiety; and under these conditions, food is experienced as an irritant and the body tries to get rid of it as quickly as possible, resulting in urgency and diarrhea.

The Body's Communication System

In Chinese medicine the body is conceived of as a microcosm of society in which the organ systems interact like the members of a family. In order for the family to work together harmoniously there must be cooperation, coordination, and accommodation. The basis of this is communication.

Adequate circulation plays an essential role in healing, because circulation is an important form of interbody communication. Candace Pert, a respected NIH researcher, discovered that there are chemical messengers called peptides that circulate in the blood. Every tissue makes these same chemical messengers. So the blood is not only a vehicle for transporting nutrients, it's also a medium for delivering information. Every cell is constantly sending messages to every other part of the organism.

If circulation to a certain part of the body is reduced, then there will be a breakdown in the information network. As a consequence a process of isolation due to a loss of contact begins to occur that can eventually develop into a condition of confusion and conflict within the body. Disease is a breakdown in the process of coordination that binds the organism together. The body should function as if it were a unified entity, and when it begins to function as if it weren't, the process of disease begins.

The Importance of Immunity

The gut is not only a digestive organ, it is also an essential component of the immune system. It functions as a boundary, a permeable membrane, just like the skin, except it's on the inside of the body instead of the outside. In fact, the lining of the gut—its surface area—is much greater than that of the skin. If you were to lay out the entire gut it would fill up the area of a tennis court. In comparison the skin would only cover a desktop. So even though the gut is considered to be an internal organ, it is exposed to the external environment by direct contact with the gases, liquids, and solids that enter the digestive tract. Thus the gut is the body's first line of defense against multitudes of invading pathogenic organisms, including viruses, bacteria, fungi, and parasites. And since the gut functions as an immunological boundary, it's normal for there to be bacteria in the mouth, the throat, the stomach, and the intestines. But these organisms should remain on the surface, outside the digestive barrier, not inside it. And if the lining of the gut is in some way compromised, our resistance is diminished and we become subject to infection and the toxic metabolic by-products of those same microorganisms.

There are many factors that can lower our resistance or diminish the integrity of our boundaries—illness, improper diet, stress, exposure to damaging toxins (poisons in the food or bad medicine), or a combination of these things. Take, for example, a sunburn. Once the skin becomes damaged by exposure, some people become more prone to herpes or vulnerable to other kinds of problems like warts, fungi, or bacterial infection. Similarly damage to the lining of the digestive tract can make us more vulnerable to other conditions.

Because everything in the body is interconnected, what happens to the body that's good benefits the whole body, and what happens to the body that's bad ultimately harms the whole body. When one aspect of function is impaired the others are also diminished. You can't separate them: Poor digestion also weakens immunity. Compromise of the immune function of the membrane of the gut eventually leads to disturbed digestion and absorption. From the Chinese medicine point of view, resistance—the ability to defend oneself against what is "not me"—is completely dependent on the quality of Qi, and the quality of Qi is completely dependent on digestion, which is its source.

Managing Stress

It's not just what you do specifically to improve your health that's important, it's everything you do. You're not healthy just because you're taking digestive enzymes or beneficial intestinal bacteria or herbs to improve digestion and elimination. These may all be very good for you, but they're just parts of the picture, not the whole view. That is the typical approach of Western medicine and even some forms of alternative medicine—a tendency to be simplistic or reductionistic, being more concerned with the parts rather than the whole.

How you take care of yourself, how you manage yourself physically from day to day, is as important to your health as any medicine or therapy. For example, some people with Crohn's and colitis know that their condition is aggravated by mental, emotional, and physical stress. Yet a lot of people with these problems lead very strenuous lives. In spite of their illness, they continue to push themselves, to overextend themselves, and to put themselves in situations which make them feel inadequate.

It may be that the vast majority of people have these same habits, but not everybody has inflammatory bowel disease. Other people get problems that may be just as serious, but they arise elsewhere in the body. And so the issues of stress and lifestyle are ever present factors that are always influencing our health.

Wherever your weakness lies, that's where the greatest distress is going to appear. This means that conducting your life so that you are not overextending and weakening yourself is fundamental to successfully managing these kinds of illnesses. Success doesn't mean achieving a complete cure, but it does mean enabling people to be functional. The goal is to become competent to the degree that the illness is no longer a disability. After all, nobody's perfect and very few of us are going to get through life without some kind of injury or insult.

Part of the problem in our culture is that we're always looking for a total cure—it's all or nothing. Yet a complete cure may be an unrealistic expectation for many people with chronic illness. People need to learn how to cope with their impairments realistically and not feel defeated by them. The goal is to increase our capacity to the point where our limitations will not prevent us from fulfilling our purposes in life.

THE BENEFITS OF CHINESE MEDICINE

In Chinese medicine Qi is the vital force that heals us, and Qi is also a kind of intelligence. It is the mind or consciousness. It's the body being aware of itself. You're able to be self-aware because all the parts of you are linked together by Qi, the dynamic intelligence of the organism. Qi is everywhere, all the time, as it flows with the blood through a special system of channels or meridians.

Immunity is an important aspect of that intelligence, which is able to distinguish between what is you and what is not you, what is of benefit to you and what harms you. Acupuncture restores the circulation of Qi, which in turn renews the integrity of mind, self, and body, invigorates immunity, and enables healing to occur.

Illness is a consequence of the disorganization of Qi—a kind of disintegration. Acupuncture can often reorganize the Qi and reestablish bodily unity.

The more consistently a person receives acupuncture, the more long lasting the effects. The experience of well-being that follows an acupuncture treatment is the renewed feeling of being integrated, as if your body has been reunited, rather than continuing to be an assemblage of conflicting and competing parts.

When a part of the body is in pain or inflamed—like a shoulder with bursitis or an irritable colon—then it becomes our whole world, taking over a large portion of our waking life. A process of self-alienation begins in which there is a desire to disassociate from the offending bodily part; it becomes like an adversary that we begin to resent for the discomfort it creates. In fact, the shoulder and the stomach are still part of us, but there's been a breakdown in the sense of unity between the self and the body. What acupuncture works to restore is coordination and communication within the body, brain, and mind. Once that begins to happen, the natural mechanisms for repair, recovery, and regeneration are permitted to function again.

Efrem Korngold, O.M.D., has been practicing Chinese traditional medicine since 1973 at his clinic, Chinese Medicine Works, in San Francisco. He received his early training in the United Kingdom and has twice traveled to China for advanced studies. A diplomate in acupuncture and a doctor of Oriental medicine, he has contributed his expertise as an examination consultant to the National Commission for Certification in Acupuncture and Oriental Medicine. He is coauthor with Harriet Beinfield, L.Ac., of the book *Between Heaven and Earth: A Guide to Chinese Medicine* (Ballantine, 1991) and the herbal guide *Chinese Modular Solutions Handbook for Health Professionals* (available through K'AN Herb Company). Dr. Korngold is currently on the faculty of the American College of Traditional Chinese Medicine in San Francisco and is a peer reviewer for the journal *Integrative Medicine,* edited by Dr. Andrew Weil.

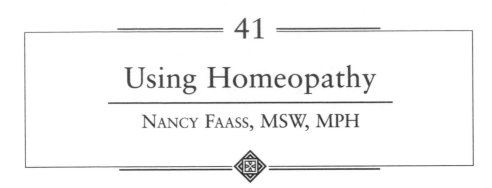

41

Using Homeopathy

Nancy Faass, MSW, MPH

Imagine a highly effective type of medicine that has no side effects—one that works when nothing else does. Doctors and patients can see the healing benefits, but researchers are unable to define exactly how it works.

This is homeopathy, a subtle method of healing based on the use of exceptionally small doses of medication. Since the doses are microscopic, the remedies are extremely safe. Given this safety, homeopathic treatment is a practical approach for self-treating stomach upsets, diarrhea, flu, mild food poisoning, and other types of everyday concerns.

A PRACTICAL APPROACH

When homeopathy works it is amazingly effective. Imagine that your mate or your child wakes up in the middle of the night, doubled over in pain. The choice of the right remedy can transform this situation, and in a few minutes they're out of pain, relaxed, and ready to fall into a peaceful sleep. This is a perfect example of the value of the remedies—they can provide an effective short-term solution until you can call your doctor, dentist, or homeopathic physician in the morning.

Homeopathy works by stimulating the immune response. Homeopathy is also considered a form of energy medicine; acupuncture is another type of energy medicine. Yet researchers still have not been able to explain exactly *how* homeopathy works. The traces of active constituents in a remedy are so minute that they cannot be detected by a conventional microscope. In this respect the constitutents can be compared to subatomic particles, which are also undetectable. Yet few of us doubt the power of the atom or the validity of quantum physics.

Homeopathy meets the two primary criteria required of any medication—safety and effectiveness. Remedies and their application are based on two hundred years of clinical experience, including contemporary research. For example, in the British journal *The Lancet,* a review of more than 85 studies found that in most cases homeopathy was equally effective—or more effective—than other types of medical treatments. In some cases patients treated with homeopathy did twice as well as those who received other types of therapy. Another benefit is that there are almost no known side effects associated with the use of the remedies. (C. Linde, et al. *The Lancet*, vol. 350, September 20, 1997.)

Homeopathy Worldwide

According to the World Health Organization homeopathy is one of the most widely used forms of treatment in the world, second only to herbal therapy. In England members of the royal family have been cared for by homeopathic physicians since the reign of Queen Victoria. In London and Glasgow there are major hospitals that offer homeopathic treatment. Homeopathic remedies can be purchased in almost all drugstores throughout the United Kingdom. Homeopathy is also used extensively in France, Germany, Austria, and Switzerland. In India there are more than 100 homeopathic medical schools. There are also homeopathic medical colleges in Mexico and Brazil, and practicing homeopathic physicians in Argentina.

In the United States, before the advent of antibiotics and modern drug therapy, about 10 percent of American physicians used homeopathic remedies in their practices, and there were homeopathic hospitals and medical schools across the country. Homeopathy earned high praise for its effective use in combating cholera, typhus, and scarlet fever during the epidemics of the nineteenth century. Currently interest in homeopathy is increasing in the United States, in part due to its exceptional safety and its focus on the immune response. These are important advantages, given the increased concern regarding medication side effects, drug costs, and antibiotic resistance.

THE DISCOVERY OF HOMEOPATHY

The homeopathic method was developed by Samuel Hahnemann (1755–1843), a German physician, chemist, and the author of a well-known text on the preparation and use of the standard medicines of his time.

Soon after beginning his career as a physician, he became disillusioned with the practice of medicine. Doctors of the eighteenth century were taught that disease was caused by humors or fluids that must be expelled from the body. To achieve this patients were cauterized, blistered, purged, and bled. Hahnemann protested against these methods, and his colleagues quickly denounced him for heresy. His disillusionment grew when he found himself unable to find a rational treatment for his own daughter when she became critically ill. Consequently Hahnemann gave up the practice of medicine and turned to medical translating for a livelihood. His interest in medicine remained and he persisted in his lifelong goal to discover "some law, whereby the diseases of mankind would be cured."

In 1790 while translating a Scottish medical text, he happened upon information that led to his discovery of the homeopathic method. The text proposed that quinine was an effective treatment for malaria because of its astringent and bitter properties. The explanation seemed implausible to Hahnemann, who knew of other equally bitter substances that were ineffective against malaria.

To test his theory Hahnemann consumed a therapeutic dose of quinine and soon developed all the symptoms of malaria—a chill with exhaustion, achiness, palpitations, and increased thirst. His curiosity was aroused by the similarity between his symptoms and those of malaria, so he allowed the dose to wear off and took a second, and later a third dose, with identical results.

The symptoms Hahnemann had developed corresponded exactly to those of malaria. He reasoned that malaria was cured by quinine not because of its bitter properties, but due to the fact that the drug produces the symptoms of malaria (even in a healthy person). Hahnemann devoted the rest of his life to investigating the principles he had discovered.

One explanation of this phenomenon is that by very mildly intensifying the symptoms of an illness, the disorder is brought to the attention of the immune system. By activating and engaging the body's own natural immune response, the healing process can be accelerated. (Note that when this aggravation occurs, it is exceptionally mild, and usually only lasts for about 15 minutes.)

In essence a well-chosen remedy stimulates the body's own healing processes. Some people find, for example, if they have a cold and they take a homeopathic remedy, they have an overwhelming desire to sleep. They sleep off the cold, while the immune system gets rid of the virus. Other people report that the symptoms just fade away. The remedies work by stimulating the body's natural healing abilities.

TREATMENT OPTIONS

There are three basic types of homeopathic treatment:

- *Acute self-care.* Appropriate for immediate minor concerns such as upset stomach.
- *Acute medical care.* When provided by a physician, homeopathy can be used to address more serious yet immediate conditions.

- *Constitutional prescribing.* Treatment provided by a physician, for more serious long-standing or chronic conditions.

Acute Self-Care

Homeopathic remedies are exceptionally safe, so they can be used for self-care of relatively minor concerns such as indigestion, diarrhea, constipation, vomiting, or other types of digestive episodes. The remedies can also be taken for conditions such as flu or food poisoning, bearing in mind that they are never a replacement for necessary medical care.

The challenge of homeopathy is that it is only effective when you choose the *right* remedy. That means that one must develop a basic understanding of how the remedies work and how to use them. One good way to become informed and skillful at homeopathy is to be seen by a homeopathic physician and learn from experience how the remedies work.

Homepathy can also be self-taught. This often involves a great deal of study and practice and conversation with others who are knowledgeable. Since the remedies are quite safe they can be used on a trial-and-error basis without side effects. However, it is important that self-treatment not be used when a serious condition exists—or when a mild condition persists or recurs—since delaying treatment could result in harm.

The right remedy for any particular situation is selected on the basis of symptoms. Therefore it is essential to have a few good reference books that list symptoms and remedies. In addition one needs the remedies themselves. A home kit of low-potency remedies can be purchased fairly inexpensively and will last for several years. Supplemental remedies are available at a low cost from almost all health food stores. When you travel you'll find that in countries such as Britain, they're also available at most drugstores, even in rural areas.

Acute Medical Care

The homeopathic practitioner uses an approach to acute care that is similar to that used for self-care. However, skilled practitioners base their choice of the right remedy on years of training, study, and experience with patients. If you have an ongoing illness or a serious condition it is important to be seen by a practitioner. For example, if you have Crohn's disease and experience a flare-up, you'll want to be seen by a practitioner rather than self-prescribe.

The homeopathic interview is in-depth and explores physical, mental, and emotional symptoms. (You'll find that most homeopathic physicians are excellent listeners.) However, the purpose of this symptom taking differs from other types of medical care. The goal is to select a remedy that matches and amplifies the symptoms of your illness ever so slightly, drawing it to the attention of your immune system, since the ultimate healer is your own vital force.

When working with a practitioner, you gain the advantage of his or her expertise. That said, if you have chronic illness it is important to work with someone who will monitor your overall progress and not simply focus on each immediate crisis or episode of illness. There is also value in seeking a homeopath who is open to an integrative approach, including the use of nutritional therapy in combination with homeopathy.

Constitutional Prescribing

Homeopathic treatment for more serious or long-standing disorders is best addressed by a practitioner. The approach to these types of conditions is described as constitutional prescribing, which involves the use of subtle remedies that are selected on the basis of symptoms, body type, and personality. Constitutional prescribing is without side effects. It does require a deep understanding of homeopathy and an extensive knowledge of the remedies. Consequently the success of this therapy lies in the skill of the practitioner.

As with any form of treatment it is always important to complement the action of the remedies with good general self-care. The body also needs the raw materials for healing—wholesome food, essential nutrients, rest, fluids, fresh air, activity, and a minimum of stress. This support can maximize the benefits of the remedy and the efforts of your immune system.

Nancy Faass, MSW, MPH, is a writer, editor, and book developer in San Francisco who specializes in complementary medicine in print and on the Web. She is coauthor of *The Germ Survival Guide* and *Boosting Immunity* and developer and editor of *Integrating Complementary Medicine into Health Systems,* voted 2001 Medical Book of the Year. She is coeditor of a book on complementary medicine for health care professionals due out in 2005. Ms. Faass can be reached by e-mail at wordworks@sbcglobal.net.

42

Ayurveda: A Brief Introduction and Guide*

VASANT LAD, AYURVEDIC PHYSICIAN

Ayurveda is considered by many scholars to be the oldest healing science. Ayurvedic knowledge originated in India more than 5,000 years ago and in Sanskrit *Ayurveda* means "the science of life." It stems from the ancient Vedic culture and was taught for many thousands of years in an oral tradition from accomplished masters to their disciples. Some of this knowledge was set to print a few thousand years ago, but much of it is inaccessible. The principles of many of the natural healing systems now familiar in the West have their roots in Ayurveda, including homeopathy and polarity therapy.

ACHIEVING INNER BALANCE

Ayurveda places great emphasis on prevention and encourages the maintenance of health through close attention to the balance in one's life, through right thinking, lifestyle, diet, and the use of herbs. Knowledge of Ayurveda enables us to understand how to create this balance of body, mind, and consciousness according to our own individual constitution. Ayurveda also encompasses specific information on how to make lifestyle changes to bring about and maintain this balance.

Just as everyone has a unique fingerprint, each person has a particular pattern of energy—an individual combination of physical, mental, and emotional characteristics—that comprises his or her own constitution. This constitution is determined at conception by a number of factors and remains the same throughout one's life.

Many influences, both internal and external, act upon us to disturb this balance and are reflected as a change in one's constitution from the balanced state. Examples of these psychological and physical stresses include one's emotional state, work, family relationships, diet and food choices, seasons and

---

*This chapter appears with permission of Vasant Lad, Ayurvedic Institute, Albuquerque, NM, www.Ayurveda.com. © 2005.

weather, and physical trauma. Once these factors are understood, one can take appropriate actions to nullify or minimize their effects and modify the causes of imbalance whenever possible, to reestablish the state of balance harmonious with one's nature and original constitution. Balance is the natural order; imbalance is disorder. Health is order; disease is disorder. Within the body there is a constant interaction between order and disorder. When one understands the nature of disorder, one can reestablish order.

BALANCING THE THREE PRINCIPLE ENERGIES OF THE BODY

Ayurveda identifies three basic types of energy or functional principles that are present in everyone and everything. Since there are no single words in English that convey these concepts, we use the original Sanskrit words *vata, pitta,* and *kapha.* These principles can be related to the basic biology of the body.

All people have the qualities of vata, pitta, and kapha, but one is usually primary, one secondary, and the third tends to be less prominent. The cause of disease in Ayurveda is viewed as a lack of proper cellular function due to an excess or deficiency of vata, pitta, or kapha. Disease can also be caused by the presence of toxins.

From the perspective of Ayurveda, body, mind, and consciousness work together to maintain balance. They are simply viewed as different facets of one's being. Finding the diet and lifestyle appropriate to one's individual constitution can strengthen the body, mind, and consciousness. These are important aspects of our lives over which we have influence. Learning how to achieve greater balance requires an understanding of how each of the three energies of vata, pitta, and kapha influence the body. If you find this approach appealing, you can learn to work with your own inner balance by educating yourself about Ayurveda or working with an Ayurvedic practitioner.

The Vata Constitution

This constitutional type reflects the energy associated with movement and air. Alert and highly active, vata people walk, talk, and think fast. They often have a lean or wiry body type, and can be intense, energetic, or restless. People with a vata constitution tend to have quick minds and usually grasp concepts quickly; they are also known for flexibility and creativity.

Lifestyle Considerations

For those with vata constitutions, the focus is on creating a balance to this intense activity. A balanced lifestyle can provide a sense of grounding and conserve energy. Routine can be very useful in assisting the vata individual to moderate restless energy and minimize nervousness or anxiety. These intense personality types tend to be prone to addiction, so they do best when they avoid sugar, caffeine, and tobacco. Since intensity itself can become intoxicating, relaxation and meditation can be useful in providing balance. A daily oil massage before the bath or shower is also beneficial for relaxation. It is also important for highly active individuals to get plenty of rest.

Diet

People with flexible or creative tendencies often have variable appetites and digestion, so having relaxed meals, at regular times, is important. For those of slender build, the most ideal foods nourish and balance the body—especially warm, cooked foods such as rice, oatmeal, soups, stews, and fresh-cooked vegetables seasoned with oils. Dairy products can be beneficial if well tolerated. They can also use eggs, chicken, turkey, fresh fish, and venison if no specific allergies are present. Although people with a vata constitution are attracted to astringent foods such as salad and raw vegetables, the intake of these foods should be moderated and monitored, especially if there is a digestive disorder. Foods that tend to be most agreeable have sweet, sour, and salty flavors. High-energy people tend to benefit from small meals, three or four times a day, and may snack as needed while maintaining a two-hour gap between each meal.

The Pitta Constitution

This constitutional type reflects the energy associated with heat and fire. Those with pitta-dominant constitutions have a strong metabolism, good digestion, and strong appetites. Their metabolism tends to run hot and they like hot spices, cold drinks, and plenty of food and liquids. This body type may be of medium height and build, with ruddy or coppery skin. Pitta people's sleep is sound and of medium duration. Mentally pitta types are alert and intelligent and have good powers of comprehension.

Lifestyle Considerations

Given their hotter metabolism, their hands and feet stay warm and they tend to perspire easily. Thus pitta people have a lower tolerance for sunlight, heat, and overexertion. There is a tendency to inflammatory conditions such as sunburn, poison ivy, and prickly heat. They feel more balanced when they moderate their exposure to the heat during the summer and do best if they exercise in the coolest part of the day. For people with this constitution, both lifestyle and diet emphasize coolness—cool climate, cooling foods, and avoidance of hot spices.

Diet

General food guidelines focus on countering the tendency to become over-heated, to inflammation or to aggression or hot temper. Therefore animal foods should only be taken in moderation by pitta types. Chicken, turkey, and wild game can be substituted. Sweet dairy products are good if well tolerated and include milk, unsalted or clarified butter, and soft, unsalted cheeses. Yogurt can be used if it is blended with spices, a little sweetener, and water. Barley, rice, oats, and wheat are beneficial carbohydrates for pitta-dominant individuals, as well as chickpeas, black lentils, and mung beans. Most nuts and seeds tend to generate too much body heat; however, coconut is cooling and sunflower and pumpkin seeds are agreeable. Ideally vegetables should form a substantial part of the diet. Spicy foods are minimized, as well as sour, salty, or pungent flavors, and are replaced with sweet, bitter, and cooling foods.

The Kapha Constitution

The water element and placidity or stability are reflected in the kapha constitution. They are often blessed with strength, endurance, and stamina. Physically their bodies and muscles are well developed. They typically have a generous body type and a slow metabolism, so they tend to gain weight easily. People of the kapha type can be disinclined to exercise, although they feel more in balance when they do exercise. Their sleep is deep and prolonged.

Lifestyle Considerations

Psychologically kapha people tend to be calm, tolerant, and forgiving. In balance they often have sweet, loving dispositions and are stable and grounded. Their long-term memory is excellent. Those with a kapha constitution can become restless as the moon becomes full because there is a tendency for water retention (edema) at that time. The winter season, with its rain or snow, dampness, and humidity, is the most important time for people with this constitution to follow the diet and lifestyle guidelines and monitor their balance.

Diet

Kapha people require little animal protein, but chicken, eggs, seafood, and game are agreeable. They should avoid dairy products and fats of any kind. Those with kapha-dominant constitutions need less grain than other constitutions. Buckwheat and millet are optimal grains for them, followed by barley and rice. All vegetables are good for kapha, but one should emphasize leafy greens and vegetables rather than highly starchy root vegetables or those that are too sweet. Generally kapha people can eat raw vegetables, although steamed or stir-fried are easier to digest. Since they do best when they avoid sweets, the only sweetener they should use is raw honey. However, they can use all spices, especially ginger and garlic. Salt is best limited, since it encourages water retention. Tobacco and hard liquor are less likely to be harmful to them than to other constitutional types, given their sturdy constitutions. However, they really do not need alcohol at all. If they do elect to use alcohol, wine is their best choice.

A COMPLEMENTARY SYSTEM OF HEALING

An Ayurvedic approach focuses not on disease but on restoring balance in the individual. This is described in Western medicine as homeostasis. When there is minimal stress and the flow of energy within a person is balanced, the body's natural defense systems will be strong and can more easily defend against disease.

It must be emphasized that Ayurveda is not a substitute for Western allopathic medicine. There are many instances in which the disease process and acute conditions are best treated with drugs or surgery. Ayurveda can be used in conjunction with Western medicine to make a person stronger and less likely to be afflicted with disease. Ayurvedic approaches can also be used effectively to rebuild the body after being treated with drugs or surgery, and in chronic conditions.

We all have times when we don't feel well and recognize that we're out of balance. Sometimes we go to the doctor only to be told there is nothing wrong. From the Ayurvedic perspective an imbalance can be present that has not yet developed into disease—or the imbalance may not yet be recognizable as symptoms of a specific disorder. Yet often imbalances are serious enough to make us notice our discomfort. We may even wonder whether it is just our imagination. This is the ideal time to actively seek to re-create balance in the body, mind, and consciousness.

The Evaluation and Treatment of Imbalances

Ayurveda encompasses various techniques for assessing health. Ayurvedic practitioners carefully evaluate key signs and symptoms of illness, especially in relation to the origin and cause of an imbalance. They also consider the patient's suitability for various treatments. A diagnosis is arrived at through direct questioning, observation, and a physical exam, as well as inference. Basic techniques such as taking the pulse; observing the tongue, eyes, and body; and listening to the tone of the voice are employed during an assessment.

Palliative and cleansing measures, when appropriate, can be used to help eliminate an imbalance, along with suggestions for removing or managing the causes of the imbalance. Recommendations may include the implementation of lifestyle changes: meditation to reduce stress and nurture the spirit, yoga and breathing exercises, massage, a recommended diet, and the use of herbs. In some cases participating in a cleansing program, called panchakarma, is suggested to help the body rid itself of accumulated toxins and benefit more from the various suggested measures of treatment.

In summary, Ayurveda addresses all aspects of life—the body, mind, and spirit. It recognizes that each of us is unique, we all respond differently to the many aspects of life, and each possesses different strengths and weaknesses. Through insight, understanding, and experience Ayurveda can provide a vast wealth of knowledge, both immediate and subtle, for every unique individual.

BASIC PRINCIPLES OF AYURVEDA

- *Everything in your life has an impact on your well-being.* From that point of view, problems with digestion are not simply a matter of digestion. Digestion is also influenced by the basic energy that is dominant in your particular personality (the doshas).
- *The choice of foods and food combinations is important.* Diet is a focal area in the Ayurvedic system because it is relatively easy to change. There are simple things that people can do to enhance their digestion, such as changing their diets and practicing proper food combining. These changes alone can make remarkable differences. Most of us never think about food combining, its impact on digestion, or even the impact of indigestion on the whole system. If the food you eat causes more toxins than your body can eliminate, then naturally you'll have problems.

  Proper food combining and the resulting digestion influence the quality of your blood. The quality of the blood can have a major impact on your physical and emotional balance. Eating foods that your body can thoroughly digest and find calming, and that are nourishing to your individual constitution, will help you to be better able to cope in your day-to-day environment. The ultimate goal of improving digestion is to avoid the buildup of toxins in the body.

- *Hatha yoga is viewed as a way to strengthen your body.* This creates greater flexibility and releases tensions so that you can more fully enjoy your life. A great many problems can be related to a lack of flexibility in the body. If we have strength and flexibility, then we can live better. Within hatha yoga, the system of the three energies can also be related to the yoga postures, using the postures to calm or stimulate. In this way the postures become a means of restoring balance to the body.
- *Cleansing the body can release toxins and improve circulation.* One of the goals of the Ayurvedic physician is to determine where you're out of balance. For many a five-day cleansing cycle is quite beneficial, including daily massage to move the energies and toxins out of areas of stagnation in the body, back into the gastrointestinal track, where they can be eliminated. Cleansing the GI tract is encouraged during this process through a number of specific techniques. In Ayurveda cleansing is a discipline unto itself—the classic practice of panchakarma. We have seen that it can produce remarkable results.

   However, there are cases in which a person may not be strong enough for this cleansing or situations in which the detoxification process may actually worsen the condition. These conditions include dehydration, obesity, or any active infectious disease; cancer of the lungs or testicles, lymphosarcoma, and melanoma, angina pectoris, congestive heart failure, and hypertension; menses, pregnancy, and lactation; and HIV or AIDS. Check with your practitioner before embarking on any cleansing program.
- *Cleansing the mind is an essential element in maintaining balance.* Many of the basic tenets of alternative health grow out of Ayurvedic philosophies, including respect for the importance of meditation and contemplation. For example, there is value in the practice of reviewing your day. Mental and emotional digestion is as important as physical digestion.

   All these habits help us mentally and emotionally process the things we haven't digested. This also has an impact on the body because it is possible to accumulate psychological toxins. For example, the remnants of childhood psychological trauma can act as a form of mental toxin. Therefore it is important to have a process built into our life for reflectiveness. It is essential to have a mechanism for processing and clearing stressful or traumatic experiences. This is a coping skill that can be extremely valuable in the midst of our busy lives.
- *Meditation and visualizations also have beneficial effects on the body.* They can be used to help people uncover areas that are unexamined and process them.

By clearing the mind and body with new coping skills and new self-knowledge, you are provided with the tools to digest new experiences as they come along, as they occur, rather than later. Ayurveda provides the foundation for maintaining physical, mental, and spiritual balance.

Vasant Lad, a native of India, has been a practitioner and professor of Ayurvedic medicine for more than 30 years. He attended Tilak Ayurvedic Medical College in Pune, India, where he later taught and was the residential medical officer at the college hospital. For the past 20 years, he has served as director of a full-time program of study at the Ayurvedic Institute in Albuquerque, New Mexico. Dr. Lad has lectured extensive throughout the United States and has written numerous books and articles on Ayurveda. Dr. Lad's classic books are *Ayurveda: The Science of Self-Healing* (1984) and *The Yoga of Herbs* (1986). He is also the author of *Ayurvedic Cooking for Self-Healing* (second edition, 1997), *Secrets of the Pulse* (1997), and *The Complete Book of Ayurvedic Home Remedies* (1998). His most recent book is the *Textbook of Ayurveda*, Volume 1 (2002).

The Ayurvedic Institute in Albuquerque was founded by Dr. Lad in 1984 to promote the traditional knowledge of Ayurveda, and offers an 8-month studies program, additional advanced study, weekend seminars and intensives, yoga courses, a correspondence course, the traditional cleansing program, and sales of Ayurvedic products and herbs. The institute can be reached at P.O. Box 23445, Albuquerque, NM 87192; by phone at (505) 291-9698; and on the Web at www.ayurveda.com.

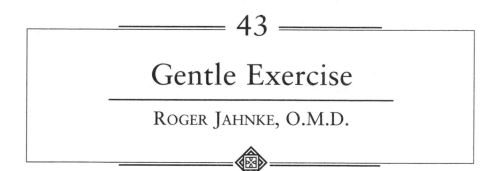

43

Gentle Exercise

Roger Jahnke, O.M.D.

One of the most profound pathways to healing or improved health is appropriate exercise. In the ancient cultures, exercise methods such as yoga, Qigong, and t'ai chi were developed to mobilize healing resources. Qigong from China has long been respected as one of the premier approaches to healing in the world. Yoga from India has also been used as a vehicle for healing for thousands of years. Although we typically think of exercise as vigorous activity for building strength, when the goal is healing, exercise must be modified so that it is less intense. Done correctly, gentle exercise produces and circulates powerful physiological resources for healing.

The lessons that we have learned from ancient Oriental fitness traditions suggest that by slowing and deepening the breath, purposefully and gently moving the body, and focusing the mind, a tremendous health benefit can be gained. Mild fitness practices are at least as valuable as vigorous fitness practices, according to *The Surgeon General's Report on Exercise and Fitness* in 1996. In fact, they may be even better because there's less risk of injury and less need for special equipment. Vigorous exertion spends much of the healing energy that is created by the exercise. Gentle practices such as yoga and Qigong conserve energy. Whenever healing is the goal, energy conservation becomes a major focus.

Research shows that when you're unwell it's important not to exercise vigorously. Free radicals can be produced as a natural by-product of exercise; they're also produced through digestion and many other basic processes. When we're well we have the necessary "cushioning" in the cells to withstand potential damage from free radicals. However, in someone who is less well the body may not be able to clear the free radicals as quickly as necessary, putting them at risk for oxidative stress, which can initiate damage to cells and tissues and even cause disease.

BEGINNING YOUR PROGRAM

Yoga, Qigong, and most of the other exercises discussed in this chapter can be done anytime, anywhere. And each of these practices can be introduced very gradually, paced to your situation. Most of these techniques require no equipment of any kind. Strength training can be done with the use of inexpensive handheld free weights.

We include exercising with weights in this approach because of the spectacular results seen in 80- and 90-year-old people with chronic illness, working with researchers from Tufts University. We felt that if they can do it, you and your doctor might take a serious look at this breakthrough practice.

Check with Your Doctor

If you have chronic illness or if you're over 40, be sure to get a checkup and clearance from a doctor who understands the benefits of exercise before you begin a gentle exercise program. Even then the truth is that nobody is ever going to know as much about your strengths and limitations as you do. So when you exercise be mindful and monitor yourself carefully. Any form of pain is an important message from your body that something may not be right, like the red warning light on your dashboard. With all forms of gentle exercise you must pay attention to the messages from your body and not push yourself. Stay in the zone of comfort. In addition use the messages you get from your body to continually analyze your health and to help you create a personal strategy to solve your health challenges.

The Benefits

When you do a gentle sort of exercise, natural physiological mechanisms are triggered. When people lose their health, some of these mechanisms may become deficient, causing pain and other symptoms. The body's inherent system of self-healing, self-regulation, and self-repair can be stimulated and maximized, using simple and gentle exercise practices.

Oxygen

Perhaps the most important of the body's natural mechanisms of self-repair is the delivery of oxygen. Oxygen is one of the most vital internal healing resources there is. Many people who are suffering from chronic diseases are actually suffering from a kind of oxygen deficiency. There are several reasons why these oxygen deficiencies occur. The lack of activity decreases the circulation of oxygen-bearing blood cells. Or in other cases oxygen deficiency has metabolic causes, due to malfunction of the organs. But when you move gently, deepening the breath and relaxing the mind, oxygen is more effectively delivered to your entire system.

Vigorous and aggressive exercise is typically associated with the delivery of oxygen throughout the body—hence the term *aerobics,* meaning "with oxygen." But it is true that when the person does gentle exercise, it can also be aerobic. We are used to thinking that if we're not vigorously jumping around or using maximal exertion, we're not getting oxygen. That, frankly, is not true. When you go into this deep state of relaxation, along with the movement the body turns on the mechanisms that deliver oxygen into the tissues. Instead of using all the oxygen to operate vigorously active muscles, that oxygen remains within the system to circulate as a healing resource. In addition when you are relaxed the blood vessels expand, carrying more oxygen deeper into the organs and glands.

Cleansing the Cells and Tissues

The second healing benefit of gentle exercise is its positive effect on the lymph system. When you do the deep-breathing practice in combination with gentle motion, it very effectively pumps the lymph. The lymph has two big jobs in the human body. First, it delivers the immune cells to their sites of activity. Second, it eliminates toxins from our system-minimizing pathogens, by-products of metabolism, and any kind of pollution that's gotten into the interior of the system. So when you take that deep breath and when you move the body around gently, you are pumping the lymph, the fluid that eliminates waste products and activates immunity.

Deepening the breath is the key to stimulating the lymph system. The second key activating the lymph is movement—contracting and releasing your muscles. The movement doesn't have to be vigorous. A big part of why gentle exercise is so spectacularly effective is that it effectively turns on the lymph system.

Shifting Out of the Adrenaline Mode

This is important, because the presence of high levels of adrenaline in the human body literally cancels the activity of the immune cells. When you leave the adrenaline bases and migrate to the choline bases, your body has shifted into the relaxation response and the rest-and-repair side of the autonomic function. In this mode your body can produce the neurotransmitters that actually turn on the immune cells. The addition of relaxation to exercise has a positive impact on the effectiveness of the immune cells.

ALMOST ANY EXERCISE CAN BE GENTLE EXERCISE

The whole process that we're describing here typically involves understanding a more gentle approach to exercise. Almost any form of exercise can be modified to become gentle exercise. Vigorous aerobics become mindful low-impact aerobics. Running becomes purposeful walking.

Techniques such as yoga, Qigong, and t'ai chi are very gentle practices, yet highly effective. They typically involve three areas of focus:

- *Moving the body gently,* honoring the limits of a person's vital energy, structure, and physical capacity, and monitoring these limits very carefully.
- *Enhancing the breath* and focusing on it, so that it becomes deep and full, slow and relaxed, compared to the less relaxed, more urgent breathing of more aggressive exercise.
- *Encouraging the mind* and thought patterns toward a state of deep relaxation or meditation as you perform the movements.

With this approach even modified aerobics, swimming, and walking can become a kind of yoga or Qigong. At that point Western exercise and ancient practice merge.

Some people approach exercise as simply a function of the body and don't really factor in the role of the mind. Often we see people exercising on the Stairmaster while reading the paper or riding an Exercycle while watching television. We encourage a different approach. Mindfulness can add a meaningful dimension to exercise. With relaxation and mindfulness, exercise accelerates mind-body interactions. Any increase in your awareness of your body and your health state can be brought to bear on the healing process in different ways—in reporting to your doctor or changing to more healthful behaviors. Mindfulness is an essential component of both yoga and Qigong. The importance of mindfulness is now acknowledged throughout the world of sports, from major-league football and basketball teams who use meditation, to tennis and golf professionals who practice the Zen of the game, and Olympic athletes who use visualization.

It is not unusual for people to believe that more aggressive exercise equals more gain—"no pain, no gain." And yet many are unable to do vigorous exercise due to health limitations. The primary reason for modifying aggressive exercise to gentle exercise is this: When you exercise the body produces a powerful fuel, a healing resource. When you do vigorous exercise you produce that fuel, that vital resource, but because of the vigorous nature of the exercise, most of that fuel is burned and expended by the muscles. When gentle exercise practices are done you still produce that fuel, but instead of spending it on the exertion of exercise itself, your body uses this fuel as a healing resource, literally an inner medicine.

So no matter what kind of exercise you have typically been doing or that you feel you should be doing, consider lightening the exertion a little and slowing the process down. Next engage the breath in a meaningful sort of way, in a kind of rhythmic, deep, slow, relaxed fashion. Finally adjust the mind toward a deep state of relaxation. By clearing the mind and refusing to engage in list making and worry, you curtail the adrenaline-based aspect of your nervous system activity. This activates a whole array of inner healing factors.

WALKING

Walking is one of the most overlooked forms of exercise because people think, "I walk all the time, what's so special about that?" In the 1996 surgeon general's report, walking was considered a preferred form of moderate exercise. Walking is a perfect exercise for those who are not well enough to pursue more vigorous exercise, and perfect for those who have health challenges but are not drawn to more unusual forms of exercise like t'ai chi, Qigong, or yoga.

However, we want to point out that no form of exercise will suit everyone. Even something as universal as walking may not be a match for you in the present. If that's true, it may be a program that you can move into as your health improves. For those readers who can't use walking or who may be using a wheelchair, we would like to direct you to modified Qigong, yoga practices, or other forms of gentle exercise that can be done at home.

Those who can use walking for exercise find that it increases circulation and oxygen levels. If the walker deepens the breath, even while walking slowly, that provides an acceleration of the lymph, which is the detoxification mechanism of the system. It is also possible to modify walking so that it is coupled with deep relaxation or meditation, which activates the healing capacity of the nervous system.

Getting Started

You can walk at a variety of paces. There's slow, purposeful walking, which is a little bit more like Qigong and yoga, and brisk walking that's more like an aerobic activity. There's also race walking, which provides a strong cardiovascular stimulus. For someone who is suffering from a chronic type of disorder, remember that slow, purposeful walking still gives you all the benefits of oxygen, circulation, and stimulation, yet the beneficial by-products of the practice, that fuel or healing resource that we have discussed, are not used up through exertion in the process.

- *Begin slowly and build up. The 90-Day Fitness Program* by Mark Fenton offers an excellent approach to getting started. Walk for five minutes on the first day, and then add just a minute a day. If you do that, in ten days you'll be walking for fifteen minutes, and in a month you'll be walking more than half an hour. By the end of the second month, if you wish, you could be walking an hour a day.

- *Build walking into your life.* Another approach to walking is to build it into your life and your routine, by making it part of the things you must do. To the degree possible group your errands in one location, park your car, and walk. When you're going to an appointment, if you can leave a little early, park a few blocks away (you may have to anyway!) and walk. Take the stairs at work or anywhere you happen to be.
- *Link walking to something you enjoy doing.* If you like a spontaneous approach to life, just remember to include a good walk in your activities each day, or several short walks. If weather inspires you, take joyful walks on sunny days, romantic walks in the rain, or brisk walks in the wind. Bird watchers walk, shoppers walk, lovers walk.
- *Walk with a friend.* This can be one of the best ways to walk and enjoy it. You may have a buddy that you walk with on a regular basis, or friends with whom you go for long walks on the weekends, or whenever you can. Enjoy!
- *Track your progress.* If you value an organized way of doing things, you may want to have a routine that's predictable, and you may find it satisfying to keep a log or a journal. If your doctor says you must walk, get a pedometer so you'll know how far you're actually walking and you can celebrate your goals as you reach them.

Resources

Barough, Nina. *Walking for Fitness: The Low Impact Workout that Tones and Shapes.* DK Publishing Inc., 2003.

Fenton, Mark. *The Complete Guide to Walking: For Health, Fitness, and Weight-Loss.* The Lyons Press, 2001. A comprehensive guide published by *Walking Magazine.*

Fenton, Mark. *The 90 Day Fitness Program.* Perigee, 1995. A great step-by-step method with a journal as well.

Fletcher, Colin, and Chip Rawlins. *The Complete Walker IV.* Alfred A. Knopf, 2003. The definitive hiker's manual.

Kortge, Carolyn Scott. *The Spirited Walker: Fitness Walking for Clarity, Balance, and Spiritual Connection.* HarperSanFrancisco, 1998. Offers inspiration and a clear vision of walking as real exercise.

Malkin, Mort. *Aerobic Walking, the Weight-Loss Exercise.* John Wiley and Sons, 1995. Another perspective on walking as a vigorous approach to exercise.

Just Walking Around

My wife, Rebecca (who also happens to be my best friend), and I have a favorite way of spending free time we call "just walking around." I may ask her on Thursday if she wants to plan something for Saturday, and she may say, "Why don't we just walk around?" That means no plan. It means we'll go for a walk and see where we end up. We could end up window shopping or at the movies, hiking on the beach, or eating at a newfound or old favorite restaurant. So just walking around is a really fantastic combination of getting good (moderate) exercise, the fun of not knowing where you're going but knowing you will be with someone you like, or just being out on your own on a surprise voyage of discovery.

QIGONG

Qigong (pronounced chee-GUNG) is the umbrella of all the traditions of personal improvement and mind-body fitness from the ancient Chinese culture. What we know about these traditions dates back to the beginning of writing in China, around 500 B.C.E. At that time existing documents indicate quite clearly that the Chinese people had already been using these practices for many hundreds of years.

The fact that Qigong and t'ai chi (a form of Qigong) have stood the test of time demonstrates their effectiveness. These gentle fitness practices have been carefully refined over several thousand years. The practice involves the gentle movement of the body with mindful adjustment of the posture. A primary focus is on the breath, usually to deepen and relax the breathing. At the same time, as an essential part of the practice the mind is encouraged to move toward a state of meditation, relaxing and clearing it of details or worries.

The practice can be done literally thousands of ways. By most estimates, there are somewhere between 3,000 and 5,000 variations of Qigong. The various kinds of practice can be categorized by the degree of activity, from the completely quiescent (still practice, standing, sitting or lying down) to vigorously dynamic (slow, full-body movement, or fast as in kung fu). Nonmoving practices are called Qing Gong, and movement practices Dong Gong.

The initial practice, which is done while completely still, can be lying down or sitting. To that practice very gentle and small movements of hands, feet, and shoulders can be added. Next, as vitality improves, the practice can be done while sitting. Later, as strength is building, walking forms of Qigong can be added, logically called Walking Qigong. T'ai chi is, in fact, a beautiful form of Walking Qigong. The most renowned form of Walking Qigong is

What to Do When We Can't Physically Exercise

Lying-down Qigong can be very useful because when we're really unwell, we spend a good deal of time lying down. So we may think, "Well, I can't exercise. I'm in bed lying down." The Chinese would say, "No, not so, you can exercise while you're lying down." "But," you might respond, "I'm not able to move." The Chinese would answer, "External movement is the least important part of the healing exercise. Internal activity is the essence of healing exercise practice."

called Guo Lin, named after a woman in China who had a very serious form of cancer and recovered using Qigong as a complement to her medical treatment. Guo Lin's form is one of the most common Qigong forms that is seen in the parks of China, early in the morning.

Other forms of Walking Qigong include a graceful, philosophical form associated with Taoism called the Wild Goose. Some of the more dynamic forms are called by poetic names: the Crane, Five Elements, Tendon Changing, Vitality, Intelligence. Although some forms of Qigong are highly complex and difficult to learn, others are extremely simple. For example, t'ai chi has 108 movements, which might take anywhere from six months to a year to learn. Whereas there are forms of Qigong that are very beneficial and can be learned in a few minutes. All forms of Qigong, from the simple to the most complex, are improved with regular practice over time.

The body of research from China on Qigong is immense; however, Chinese research techniques have not been as rigorous as those in the United States. The National Institutes of Health (NIH) has funded a number of studies on Qigong and t'ai chi. There have been numerous international scientific congresses on Qigong in China, Japan, Europe, and the United States. The consensus is that Qigong triggers physiological mechanisms with a positive effect on inner healing, including increased oxygen delivery, enhanced immune function and elimination of waste, and improved brain chemistry.

Getting Started

If you find this practice intriguing, you'll want to get a book or a video or both. If the opportunity presents itself, take a class or seek out a private teacher. Simple Qigong practices can be learned and practiced at home. Many hospitals have begun to offer Qigong or modified t'ai chi as a part of their mind-body programming. The YMCA in many communities offers classes. In a growing number of communities it is possible to link up with a practice group either in the park or at the local recreation center. Some of these are offered without charge.

Resources
Books

Cohen, Ken. *The Way of Qigong*. Ballantine Books, 1997.

Crompton, Paul. *T'ai Chi for Beginners*. HarperResource, 2003.

Jahnke, Roger. *The Healer Within*. HarperSan Francisco, 1999.

Jahnke, Roger. *The Healing Promise of Qi*. McGraw-Hill/Contemporary Books, 2002.

MacRitchie, James. *Chi Kung: Cultivating Personal Energy*. Element Books, 1997.

Video

Jahnke, Roger. *Awakening the Medicine Within*. Health Action, 1995; (800) 824-4325.

YOGA

Yoga is a subtle healing practice that originated in India and developed as one of the practices associated with spiritual growth in the philosophy of Vedanta. Hatha yoga is one of the Eight Limbs of Yoga, which also includes breathing practices (pranayama), meditation, and activities of service (karma yoga). Patanjali's *Yoga Sutras*, written around 200 or 300 B.C.E., described yoga, so we know it had been codified by that time. Hatha yoga combines postures, movement, breath regulation, and meditation.

The essence of hatha yoga is the postures, or asanas, that poetically imitate the movements of animals and bear their names (the Cobra, the Lion, the Fish). Each posture is designed to stretch the muscles, flex the joints, and stimulate the internal organs and glands in a different part of the body. When the posture is performed, the body is gradually moved into position through a process of gentle stretching. The position is held without moving, usually for less than a minute, while breathing slowly and deeply, and then the body is returned to a position of rest; lying outstretched or standing quietly.

The postures are designed to strengthen, stretch, and tone muscles and ligaments. In modern exercise terms yoga has come to mean the same thing as stretching; however, because of the links to the breath and mind, yoga is much more than just stretching. The practices also encourage blood circulation while stimulating the secretions of the glands, and encourage the optimal function of the internal organs. For example, the shoulder stand is thought to stimulate the thyroid gland through the gentle pressure of the chin on the throat area. The forward and the backward bend (the Fish) are designed to stretch, align, and strengthen the spinal column and surrounding muscles. A very thorough session of yoga postures can leave one with the sense of relaxation comparable to a good massage.

Getting Started

Yoga can be done with simply the guidance of a well-written book, as long as care is taken not to move too fast, stretch too far, or force the body. There are also good videos and sometimes good TV yoga classes. A live class can also be very encouraging, as long as the teacher doesn't move too fast or too aggressively. Be wary of teachers who say things like "No gain without pain." The idea is to grow into the postures and become more flexible day by day, comparable to adding a minute a day to your walking routine.

Resources

Books

Austin, Miriam. *Cool Yoga Tricks*. Ballantine Books, 2003. Clever ideas on how to modify yoga practice for anyone who finds yoga challenging.

Birch, Beryl Bender. *Power Yoga: The Total Strength and Flexibility Workout*. Fireside, 1995. Astanga yoga, a vigorous form of hatha yoga designed to build strength and stamina, used by the U.S. cycling team.

Iyengar, B. K. S. *Yoga: The Path to Holistic Health*. DK Publishing Inc., 2001. The definitive guide.

Lasater, Judith. *30 Essential Yoga Poses*. Rodmell Press, 2003. Another very aesthetic and accessible guide.

Monro, Robin, and H. R. Nagendra. *Yoga for Common Ailments*. Simon & Schuster, 1990. Pleasing in its simplicity and focus, this book is now out of print, but can be ordered on the Internet or found in libraries.

Payne, Larry. *Yoga Rx: A Step by Step Program to Promote Health, Wellness, and Healing for Common Ailments*. Broadway Books, 2002. Includes a program for digestive disorders.

Sparrowe, Linda. *Yoga*. Hugh Lauter Levin Associates Inc., 2002. A book that conveys the exquisite concentration that can evolve through yoga.

Audiotapes and Videotapes

Audio: *Mindfulness Meditation,* The University of Massachusetts, under the guidance of Jon Kabat-Zinn, offers a set of audio tapes (Series 1 tapes) with hatha yoga exercises. The tapes can be ordered from Stress Reduction Tapes, P.O. Box 547, Lexington, MA, 02420, or by checking their Web site at www.mindfulnesstapes.com

Video: The yoga tapes of Living Arts are available in many health food stores or via their Web site at www.gaiam.com.

Magazines

Shambhala Sun, 1345 Spruce Street, Boulder, CO, 80302-4886, (877) 786-1950, www.shambhalasun.com

Yoga International, 630 Main Street, Suite 300, Honesdale, PA, 18431, (800) 253-6243, ext. 4, subscriptions@yimag.org, www.yimag.org

Yoga Journal, 2054 University Avenue, Suite 600, Berkeley, CA, 94704, (800) 600-YOGA, www.yogajournal.com

Yoga Magazine (from the United Kingdom), c/o Direct Mag, P.O. Box 2165, Williamsville, NY, 14231, (877) 474-3321, www.yogamagazine.co.uk

BREATH PRACTICE

The healing traditions of every ancient culture have included some form of breath practice. This reflects the profound effect of the simple act of breathing. When we consider how the body works, it becomes obvious why these cultures were so interested in breath practice. Every deep breath sets healing in motion.

Boosting immunity. The body and the immune system are maintained in part by the lymph, a marvelous system of clear, colorless fluid that continually bathes the interior of the body in a healing liquid medium.

This system is activated whenever we breathe deeply. As we inhale fully the diaphragm drops, pumping the lymph throughout the body. The lymph is everywhere, delivering immune cells to fight localized infection and washing away the waste products of our cells. These are natural metabolites that would become toxic if they were not removed. With every deep breath the lymph provides internal cleansing and healing. (Since the lymph doesn't circulate when we're inactive, this is a good reason not to become a couch potato!)

Relaxation. When you take a deep breath, you spontaneously relax—twice. This is a kind of built-in miracle. (Note that people who find it difficult to breathe often find it difficult to relax.) In fact, each deep breath provides a number of benefits:

- First, when you take a deep breath you become more conscious. One cannot take a deep breath without becoming more conscious.
- Second, one must relax in order to take a deep breath. This is good.

- Third, you breathe thoroughly and completely.
- Fourth, you exhale, and during the exhalation relaxation spontaneously occurs again. This is exciting. It means that with every deep breath your body actually relaxes twice.

Deep relaxation has an impact on the entire nervous system—especially the automatic (autonomic) mode of the nervous system. When you relax your body shifts into a state of *rest* and *repair,* a chance to recover, rebuild, and restore. It causes a decrease in the adrenaline-driven metabolism that is triggered whenever we're under stress. While the *stress response* is a useful protective mechanism, it's only intended to serve us short term. If we continue to be driven by adrenaline, this can cause undue wear and tear on the body. So breathing and R&R go together.

Getting Started
The Remembering Breath. There are literally hundreds of breath practice methods. One of them we call *the remembering breath.* This practice cultivates a habit that reminds us to periodically take a deep breath. Each breath is triggered by simply remembering to breathe deeply. If you find that you don't remember, build some behavioral cues into your life—hearing the phone ring, walking through a doorway, opening the refrigerator door, or seeing little notes that you place all over the house. You can take a moment to breathe during commercial breaks on television. Any cue can provide a trigger to take a deep breath. Even if you're in a rush to get somewhere, you can take a deep breath without having to stop. On the other hand, taking a deep breath may remind you of the relevance of stopping, even if it's only for a few moments.

Rest and Repair. Another very nourishing breath practice is the long, slow exhalation. Take a deep breath in, hold it for a count of 3, and then exhale slowly through your nose. Let that breath out very, very, very slowly. . . . I mean very slowly. This can take half a minute or more. If you pay careful attention you may sense an internal shift. This is your body moving out of the stress response into rest and repair, shifting into the self-repair mode and setting healing in motion.

The Complete Breath. This means two breaths in, one breath out. Why two breaths in? Because when we normally take one breath in, we tend only to take a partial breath. But if we take two breaths, it becomes a conscious act. You're more likely to become engaged, to really go for it. The next step is to breathe

out slowly through the nose. So breathe in, breathe in, and then breathe out
. . . Slowly . . . Breathe in, breathe in, and breathe out. . . . Slowly . . .

Full-body relaxation. The Jacobsen progressive relaxation method is a variation
of the hatha yoga posture, the Corpse. Take a deep breath and while you exhale,
focus on systematically relaxing a part of your body. You can take your time. For
example, you relax each of your fingers separately, and then relax your arms, and
so forth. This method entails at least thirty-five to forty slow, relaxed breaths.

With any of these breathing practices, you can do some type of movement.
This becomes a form of Qigong, which implies any type of physical movement
performed in a state of deep relaxation, paired with deep breathing. Any form
of meditation or yoga also typically includes *pranayama,* which means
"breath practice." In addition an entire array of new breath practices have
developed tailored to various needs—for chronic obstructive lung disease, for
women in pregnancy, and during childbirth (such as the Lamaze method,
which is timeless because it works!).

Breath practice is the foundation of our capacity to produce the inner
elixir, the healer within. Whether the intent is to heal disease, maximize
health, or engage fully in the moment, the process is always initiated by taking one or several deep, focused breaths. Have you taken a deep breath lately?

Resources

Books

Farhi, Donna. *The Breathing Book*. Henry Holt and Company, 1996.
Jahnke, Roger. *The Healer Within*. HarperSanFrancisco, 1999.
Jahnke, Roger. *The Healing Promise of Qi*. Contemporary/McGraw-Hill, 2003.
Khalsa, Gurucharan Singh, Ph.D., and Yogi Bhajan, Ph.D. *Breathwalk*. Broadway
Books, 2000.
Rosen, Richard. *The Yoga of Breath*. Shambhala, 2002.

Audiotapes

Weil, Andrew, with Jon Kabat-Zinn. *The Andrew Weil Audio Collection:
Breathing and Meditation for Optimum Health*. Sounds True, 2001.

LOW-IMPACT WEIGHT TRAINING

Strength training has been found to produce spectacular benefits and can be
used by people with a wide variety of needs. The practice generally involves
basic exercises with or without small handheld weights, that can involve

either mild or intense exertion. The program was developed by researchers from Tufts University, working with people in their eighties and nineties. The original participants were nursing home residents with severe chronic illness who were able to double their strength in just three months by working with the weights! This approach to weight training has now been in development for more than fifteen years and continues to gain enthusiastic reviews. Strength training has been found to:

- Halt bone loss and even restore bone
- Improve balance
- Help prevent bone fractures from osteoporosis
- Energize
- Trim the body and tighten muscles
- Help control weight
- Improve flexibility
- Revitalize

In our culture it is typical to think of weight training as being something that requires going to the gym and having a lot of special equipment. Clearly this practice is not about buffing up and getting big muscles. In the context of what we're discussing here, it's about using weight training with the goal of mobilizing inner resources. The extent to which you get the increase of muscle mass or muscle strength is really secondary. The most essential improvements result from doing the practices and increasing benefits for the metabolic system. These subtle but important gains include retaining calcium in the bones, stimulating the mobilization of oxygen throughout the blood and the tissues, and building stamina. Weight training also enhances your body's ability to burn fat.

Getting Started

Once you have your doctor's clearance, you may want to gradually work into a weight training program. Really take your time in building up the number of repetitions you do and in building up the amount of weight you're using. The weights used in this program include handheld weights, small free weights, or weights you can strap on your wrists and your ankles to give you a little resistance.

Some people are going to enjoy having an exercise routine or going to the gym. It can also be helpful to keep a log and track your progress. When you're getting started at the gym, you can use their weight training machines without any weight! This still provides the benefits of range of motion, plus the resistance of the weight of the device itself, stimulating your circulation, providing mild stretching, and mildly accelerating your metabolism.

Strengthening the lower back and the abdominals could be one of the most important by-products of gentle exercise, because people with chronic inflammation sometimes have a loss of tone as a result of their illness. Bracing against low-grade pain could alter posture or muscle tone. When tone is lacking it's especially important to begin moderately, to protect muscle and nerve tissue, and avoid new problems. Some gastroenterologists suggest that improving GI tone can make a significant difference in conditions such as motility problems. But it's still best to work all parts of the body, rather than just working the abdominals or the biceps.

If you find yourself craving a less structured approach to life, saying to yourself, "Why should I go to the club? I'm going to rake my backyard," it's helpful to know that both approaches are just fine. What the surgeon general reported in 1996 was that washing your car, weeding your garden, and raking your lawn are all actually mild forms of exercise that generate fitness. Enjoy!

Resources

Nelson, Miriam. *Strong Women Stay Young.* Bantam Books, 2000. This excellent book describes the research by Tufts University, which has revealed that people of any age and fitness level (even those in their 70s and 80s) can use strength training, enjoy it, and gain benefit.

Phillips, Bill. *Body for Life.* HarperCollins, 1999. An excellent guide to weight training.

Phillips, Bill. *Body for Life: Success Journal.* HarperCollins, 2003. A day-by-day journal to inspire and guide your training efforts.

ALEXANDER TECHNIQUE

The Alexander technique is a learning process that teaches individuals to adjust the body position to maximize natural inner resources. The process was discovered when the originator, Mathias Alexander, found that by adjusting the area between the skull and the upper back, he was able to heal a chronic voice condition. Since then millions of people with a wide variety of diagnoses have found that using this method has helped to cure their musculoskeletal problems, as well as more organ-based diseases.

When you sit or stand up straight, arrange your head so that it is atop the spine, relax the shoulders, and then breathe deeply, you have taken one early step in the implementing the Alexander technique. To begin working with this self-care method, look for classes at your community recreation center, local hospital, or through your health plan.

Resources

Brennan, Richard. *The Alexander Technique Manual*. Tuttle Publications, 1996.

Gelb, Michael, and Laura Huxley. *Body Learning: An Introduction to the Alexander Technique*. Henry Holt, 1996.

Robinson, Lynne, and Helge Fisher. *The Mind-Body Workout: With Pilates and the Alexander Technique*. Macmillan UK, 2003.

FELDENKRAIS METHOD

It has been discovered that many of our health challenges are aggravated or even caused by long-term habits of body movement or posture. When these habits and patterns are resolved so that the body functions in the way it was originally designed to function, then aches, pains, and the symptoms of disease can be eased and even healed. The Feldenkrais method is one of the most highly regarded methods for resolving these dysfunctions (usually called neuromuscular patterns).

This health improvement process can involve individual lessons (which looks a little like a bodywork session) or a group instruction (which looks a little like a very gentle yoga class). The goal in both cases is to help the individual to heal old patterns of movement and posture and learn to use the body in ways that resolve pain and heal organ dysfunction.

Resources

Feldenkrais, Moshe. *Awareness through Movement: Easy-to-Do Health Exercises to Improve Your Posture, Vision, Imagination, and Personal Awareness*. HarperSanFrancisco, 1991.

Hanna, Thomas. *Somatics: Reawakening the Mind's Control of Movement, Flexibility, and Health*. Perseus Press, 1998.

Shafarman, Steven. *Awareness Heals: The Feldenkrais Method*. Perseus Press, 1997.

ISOMETRICS

Isometrics involves exercising muscles by pushing against resistance. The advantage to isometrics is that they can be done anytime, anywhere, without special equipment, by most anyone. You'll notice that if you press your left hand down with your right hand, pretty much the same kind of effort is made as if you were lifting a weight with your left hand. So one way to exercise is to use pressure from the hand on different body parts to create the weight and resistance.

Working Your Abs

To strengthen your abdominal muscles through isometrics, lie on your back and assume a position in which you are comfortable, breathing normally. Then act as if you are blowing out a candle. As you do that contract your stomach muscles, so your belly button is moved toward your backbone. Be careful not to contract the muscles you would normally use in doing a sit-up. Simply lie still, contracting the inner abdominal muscles. Hold them contracted and breathe. The action of the breath stretching against the muscles is what creates the exercise. Breathe in that way, pulling your navel toward your backbone, and breathing against that tension of the muscle. This exercise tends to strengthen the inner two layers of muscles in the abdomen. It's also very relaxing!

—Jerry Stine

You can do isometrics lying in bed. For example, to do bicep curls, just press your left hand against your right hand and lift the right hand toward your chin. Then if you want to work the triceps, take the right hand and then press it into the left hand, and resist with the left hand so that way you're working the right tricep. Lift your knee toward your head while pushing downward with your hands to strengthen the thigh.

This form of exercise can be applied to any part of the body. It is a very simple way to mobilize and circulate inner healing resources.

PILATES

Body Control, developed by Joseph Pilates, is the fastest-growing exercise in the world. Pilates was a frail, sickly child who became obsessed with physical fitness and in the process of healing himself, created an eight-point exercise program. The basic Body Control program can be done at home without special equipment. Stretching exercises, however, involve the use of specialized equipment that can be purchased or is available through classes and trainers. This technique is used by the New York City Ballet and the Cincinnati Bengals.

Resources
Books

Crowther, Ann. *Total Pilates: The Unique Step-by-Step Guide to Pilates at Home for Everybody.* Thorsons/HarperCollins, 2003. A pleasing and practical guide to Pilates.

Craig, Colleen. *Pilates on the Ball.* Healing Arts Press, 2001. A unique approach to Pilates using the Swiss exercise ball.

Muirhead, Malcolm. *Total Pilates.* Thunder Bay Press, 2003. A very aesthetic presentation.

Pohlman, Jennifer. *Simply Pilates.* Hinkler Books, 2004. This very affordable package includes a book and a DVD.

Robinson, Lynn, Joseph Pilates, and Gordon Thomson. *Body Control: Using Techniques Developed by Joseph H. Pilates.* Trans-Atlantic Publishing, Inc. 1988. Readers indicate this book is most ideal for people new to Pilates.

Equipment

Pilates equipment for use in your home can be ordered through QVC Home Shopping Channel, (800) 345-1515.

Roger Jahnke, O.M.D., is the author of *The Healer Within* and *The Healing Promise of Qi,* practical guides to the Chinese self-healing arts known as Qigong, which include gentle exercise, breath practice, massage, and meditation. He is an internationally respected teacher and lecturer on Chinese medicine, Qigong, and t'ai chi; senior faculty member at the College of Traditional Chinese Medicine in Santa Barbara; and a founding board member of the National Qigong Association. He has been in the clinical practice of traditional Chinese medicine for more than twenty years. He is a consultant and lecturer on health enhancement and the integration of complementary and alternative medicine. Roger Jahnke provides workshops in t'ai chi, Qigong, and Chinese Medicine. He can be reached through Health Action at (805) 685-4670.

The Health Action Group in Santa Barbara provides training to hospitals, clinics, and corporations nationwide on a wide range of health improvement topics. Health Action can be reached at 243 Pebble Beach, Santa Barbara, CA, 93117, and by phone at (805) 685-4670.

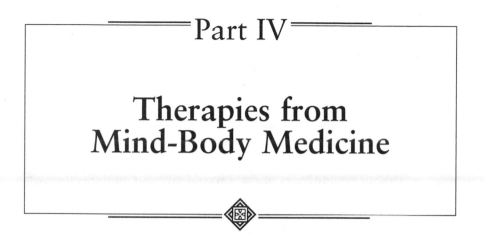

Part IV

Therapies from
Mind-Body Medicine

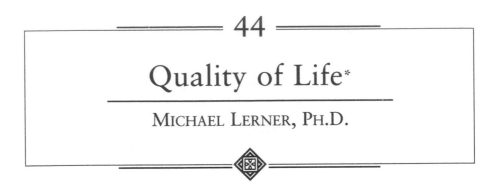

44

Quality of Life*

MICHAEL LERNER, PH.D.

I am often asked, what would I do if I became seriously ill?

I don't know the answer to that question. I do not think anyone can know that unless they actually face the experience. But here are my thoughts.

I would pay a great deal of attention to the inner healing process that I hope a diagnosis would trigger in me. I would give careful thought to what had meaning for me now—what in my life I wanted to let go of and what I wanted to keep.

I would give careful thought to choosing a mainstream physician. I would be looking less for someone with wonderful empathetic skills than for someone who had a reputation for basic kindness who would also be willing to take the time I needed to answer my questions. Above all I would be looking for someone who really stayed on top of the technical aspects of my treatment and who recognized that I was the kind of patient who wanted to share in making the decisions. I would also look for someone who was willing to stick with me if I embarked on alternative therapies.

I would use mainstream therapies that offer what seemed to me a real and meaningful chance for recovery, and I would use them with gratitude and work to augment their effectiveness. But I suspect that I would be somewhat unlikely to undertake experimental therapies or therapies with a low probability of success that were very toxic and would compromise my capacity to live as I chose.

I would use complementary therapies. My first choices would include psychotherapy with a therapist experienced in work with people with chronic illness, a first-rate support group, and a healer with a good reputation. I would deepen and augment my regular nutritional program, and I would strengthen my meditation and yoga practices. I would spend a lot of time in nature, walking in the woods, along the ocean, and in the mountains.

I would unquestionably use traditional Chinese medicine.

---

*This chapter was adapted from the outstanding book *Choices in Healing* by Michael Lerner, Ph.D. (Cambridge, MA: MIT Press, 1997, 4th printing) and is reprinted by permission of MIT Press.

I would explore whether any of the high-tech alternative therapies appeared to have anything to offer me.

I would recognize the months or years of active effort for recovery that lay ahead. I would strive for life, for recovery, with every possible tool and resource I could find. But I would also acknowledge that there may be realistic limits to what can be accomplished.

I would spend time with people I care a lot about, and with books, with writing, with music, with nature, and with God. I would do everything I could do that I had not yet done and did not want to leave undone. I would not waste time with old obligations or conventions, although I would seek to extricate myself from them decently. I would be off into pure life, following its lead.

I can say none of these things with certainty. How can any of us know what they would actually do?

In chronic illness there is no single right choice for all of us, but there are surely right choices for each of us. There are no certain courses of action, but there are certainly educated and wiser choices, as opposed to uneducated ones. The skill is in the movement from ignorance toward knowledge and from knowledge toward wisdom. In wisdom we choose what we are least likely to regret. Accepting the pain and sorrow inherent in the fate we have been given, we can seek also the beauty and the joy.

Michael Lerner, Ph.D., is president and founder of Commonweal (begun in 1976) and the Commonweal Cancer Help Program in Bolinas, California. He received his B.A. from Harvard and his Ph.D. in political science from Yale. After serving as an assistant professor at Yale, Lerner was named a founding associate of the Carnegie Council on Children. He came to California in 1972 and founded Full Circle, a residential treatment center for children with learning and behavioral disorders in Mann County. He has been named a United States–Japan leadership fellow and received a MacArthur Prize Fellowship for his contributions to public health. Michael Lerner is author of *Choices in Healing* (MIT Press, 1997).

45

Meditation in Healing

Madeline Ko-i Bastis, Jon Kabat-Zinn, Ph.D., Nancy Faass, MSW, MPH, Jim Castelli, and H. H. the Dalai Lama

INTRODUCTION

This chapter is offered to readers with gratitude to the authors and publishers included here (see page 421 for complete source information).

When there is chronic illness, it isn't always easy to find something that makes a difference, whether it involves self-care or some type of treatment. For many people with persistent illness, meditation is one of the most important things that can be done to heal the mind and spirit. It is also one of the self-care practices most frequently used by Americans.

In essence meditation involves quieting the mind. This can create a mental space that has been described as "absence of a problem." This can become an important refuge when one is experiencing illness, pain, or other challenges. The ability to shift into a state of pure consciousness can provide a personal retreat, a place of peace.

HEALING MEDITATION

Madeline Ko-i Bastis

When we meditate, each of us enters the same path that the Buddha walked twenty-five hundred years ago. When he was confronted with sickness, old age, and death, he determined to find the way to end suffering. He practiced and found the answer, and so can we. . . .

Regular practice has a calming effect on our lives—we are less likely to react to outer disturbances in ways that are harmful to ourselves and others. Meditation quiets the mind and brings us to a clear space where we feel connected to everyone and everything. We understand, through our own experience, that we *are* everyone and everything. . . .

Meditation practice teaches us to live our lives in the present moment and to know that it is perfect and complete exactly as it is. All we have to do is pay attention. All we have to do is awaken to the present moment. All we have to do is realize that we are perfect and complete exactly as we are. What a relief!

While my own practice is and has for many years been Zen Buddhism, as a counselor I often visited patients who were suffering spiritually, emotionally, and physically. I began to develop a palette of practices to suit their unique experiences and situations. . . . Over the years I have incorporated the following types of [healing] meditation into my work:

- *Mindfulness of breathing,* which focuses on the breath to teach us that everything changes. It can also reduce stress, alleviate physical pain, and help us develop serenity.
- *Walking meditation,* to extend mindfulness to include body awareness. Walking meditation helps us bring attention to our daily activities, whether they are pleasant, unpleasant, or neutral, thereby enriching our lives. Being mindful to the process of our daily lives moment after moment awakes joy. Monitoring an addiction, undergoing chemotherapy, or performing menial chores become an adventure.
- *Metta (loving-kindness),* opening the heart to love and acceptance of oneself and others. Metta speaks to those with low self-esteem, those who cannot forgive, and caregivers who traditionally put their own needs last and burn out.
- *Tonglen (taking and sending),* which teaches us to work with physical and emotional pain and suffering and lessens feelings of isolation.
- *Co-meditation,* originally used to ease a person's death. Co-meditation also releases difficult emotions, relieves stress, and forges a connection between the guide and the recipient.
- *Phowa,* traditionally a meditation for the dying or dead. It can assuage feelings of loss for the bereaved and can easily be adapted as a healing meditation for those who are ill.

THE BASICS OF MEDITATION

To meditate, ideally you want a few basics—quiet and a place to sit. That said, you can meditate anywhere, as the inclination or need arises—on a subway, in an airport, in an emergency room. Meditation in the classic Eastern traditions involves sitting in the half-lotus or the lotus, legs crossed. As long as your back is erect, you can also meditate in a chair or in a kneeling posture (sitting on your feet). One can also meditate lying in bed.

In terms of surroundings, a harmonious space is conducive. Meditating in a natural setting (by a creek or by the ocean) can affirm your link with the Cosmos. Yet no matter where you are, it always simply comes back to the value of this practice.

MEDITATION PRACTICES
JON KABAT-ZINN, PH.D.

The most basic form of meditation involves simply sitting. Just sit. Don't hold on to anything, don't look for anything. Practice being completely open and receptive to whatever comes into your field of awareness, letting it all come and go, watching, witnessing in stillness.

Sitting with the Breath
1. Practice awareness of your breathing in a comfortable but erect sitting posture for at least ten minutes at least once a day.
2. Each time you notice that your mind is no longer on your breath, just see where it is. Then let go and come back to your belly and to your breathing.
3. Over time try extending the time you sit until you can do it for thirty minutes or more. But remember, when you are really in the present, there is no time, so clock time is not as important as your willingness to pay attention and let go from moment to moment.

Sitting with Sound
1. If you feel like it, try just listening to sound when you meditate. This does not mean listening *for* sounds, rather just hearing what is here to be heard, moment by moment, without judging or thinking about them. Just hearing them as pure sound. And hearing the silences within and between sounds as well.
2. You can practice this with music, too, hearing each note as it comes and the spaces between notes. Try breathing the sounds into your body and letting them flow out again on the out-breath. Imagine that your body is transparent to sounds; that they can move in and out of your body through the pores of your skin.

Sitting with Thoughts and Feelings

1. When your attention is relatively stable on the breath, try shifting your awareness to the process of thinking itself. Let go of the breath and just watch thoughts come into and leave the field of your attention.
2. Try to perceive them as "events" in your mind.
3. Note their content and their charge while, if possible, not being drawn into thinking about them, or thinking the next thought, but just maintaining the "frame" through which you are observing the process of thought.

Sitting with Choiceless Awareness

1. Just sit. Don't hold on to anything, don't look for anything. Practice being completely open and receptive to whatever comes into the field of awareness, letting it all come and go, watching, witnessing in stillness.

CREATING YOUR PRACTICE

NANCY FAASS, MSW, MPH

It's important to find a practice that suits your personality and style. One can focus on the breath, on sound, visual symbols, devotional phrases, or on the experience of pure consciousness, merging with the Cosmos. As the sage says, there are many roads. . . . It does not matter how we make the journey. Here are some thoughts to keep in mind as you design your practice.

Is your mind highly restless? Zen meditation can be useful. This involves counting from one to ten—over the course of ten breaths—and then beginning again. Say each number softly in your mind with your inhaled breath. This practice makes it quite obvious when one loses track. The primary focus is on the silence between the numbers.

Are you visual? You may want to arrange and decorate your meditation area. Your practice could involve concentration on a visual symbol, a sacred image, or a candle flame.

Do you learn by listening? You may wish to simply sit and listen to the sounds around you without judgment or attachment, just listening moment to moment, experiencing what you hear as pure sound. Or you may find that you are attracted to the sound of Tibetan bells or to certain forms of chanting or mantra (sacred phrases repeated in rhythm with your breathing).

Are you full of heart? Your practice may be more devotional and could involve prayer or mantra—and a path of service.

Are you highly active? You may find you are most comfortable using a form of moving meditation such as the labyrinth walk. T'ai chi, Qigong, and yoga are considered mind-body activities and at their best always involve a meditative mind-set. Better to do moving meditation than no practice at all.

PRAYING AND PRAYER
JIM CASTELLI

Everyone prays. . . . Whatever the length, language, complexity, or faith of our prayers, they all ultimately have the same purpose: to reach outside of ourselves and touch, perhaps to move, a power greater than ourselves. We pray for mercy, for guidance, for forgiveness, for peace—both global and internal. Every time we pray, we acknowledge that there are things in this life that are outside of our control. Often we pray to bring about change in ourselves as well. Every time we pray, we try to become something more than we are. Just as we strive for "excellence" in our professional lives, we strive for excellence, for improvement, for a way to come closer to that power or spirit in our lives.

Just as we work with our minds in practice, there is also value in working with our perspective on life. Illness has the potential to open our eyes and to provide new insight into joy and suffering, and to increase our empathy with others.

HEALING THROUGH COMPASSION
H. H. THE DALAI LAMA

Compassion doesn't have only mental benefits, but it contributes to good physical health as well. According to contemporary medicine, as well as to my personal experience, mental stability and physical well-being are directly related. Without question, anger and agitation make us more susceptible to illness. On the other hand, if the mind is tranquil and occupied with positive thoughts, the body will not easily fall prey to disease. This shows that the physical body itself appreciates and responds to human affection, human peace of mind.

Another thing that is quite clear to me is that the moment you think only of yourself, the focus of your whole reality narrows, and because of this narrow focus, uncomfortable things can appear huge and bring you fear and discomfort and a sense of feeling overwhelmed by misery. The moment you think of others with a sense of caring, however, your view widens. Within that wider perspective, your own problems appear to be of little significance, and this makes a big difference.

If you have a sense of caring for others, you will manifest a kind of inner strength in spite of your own difficulties and problems. With this strength, your own problems will seem less significant and bothersome to you. By going beyond your own problems and taking care of others, you gain inner strength, self-confidence, courage, and a greater sense of calm. This is a clear example of how one's way of thinking can really make a difference.

One's own self-interest and wishes are fulfilled as a byproduct of actually working for other sentient beings. As the well-known fifteenth-century master Tsongkhapa points out in his *Great Exposition of the Path to Enlightenment*, "The more the practitioner engages in activities and thoughts that are focused and directed toward the fulfillment of others' well-being, the fulfillment or realization of his or her own aspiration will come as a byproduct without having to make a separate effort."

Thus we find that kindness and a good heart form the underlying foundation for our success in this life, our progress on the spiritual path, and our fulfillment of our ultimate aspiration, the attainment of full enlightenment. Hence compassion and a good heart are not only important at the beginning but also in the middle and at the end. Their necessity and value are not limited to any specific time, place, society, or culture. Thus we not only need compassion and human affection to survive, they are also the ultimate sources of success in life.

The material in this chapter was drawn from the following sources:

Madeline Ko-i Bastis, *Peaceful Dwelling: Meditations for Healing and Living* (Boston: Tuttle Publishing, 2000), with permission.
Jon Kabat-Zinn, Ph.D., *Full Catastrophe Living: Using the Wisdom of Your Body and Mind to Face Stress, Pain, and Illness* (Delta/Dell, 1994).
Jim Castelli, *How I Pray* (New York: Ballantine Books, 1994).
Tenzin Gyatso, H. H. the Fourteenth Dalai Lama, *The Compassionate Life* (Boston: Wisdom Publications, 2001), with permission from the publisher.

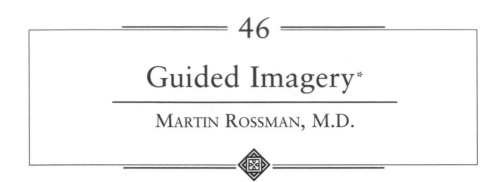

46

Guided Imagery*

MARTIN ROSSMAN, M.D.

Imagery is a way of thinking that involves the senses. The human nervous system codes information in images—and then stores, accesses, and processes the information through those images.

Because of the sensory qualities of imagery, when we imagine an event, the body tends to respond to the images as if they were actually occurring. Examples of this include worry, sexual fantasy, or our reactions while watching a suspenseful movie. Most people are familiar with these experiences and the powerful emotional and physical effects that images can elicit. The mind-body effects of imagery can also be applied beneficially in medicine. For example, imagery can promote relaxation before surgery, reduce post-surgical complications, and speed healing following surgery. It can also induce sleep, relieve pain and nausea, and stimulate immunity.

Imagery is a natural language of the unconscious mind and can provide rapid access to emotional information that may manifest as physical symptoms or behavior. A brief case history follows to illustrate how useful imagery can be as a tool for healing.

A CASE STUDY

When he first came to see me for treatment, 24-year-old Jason wanted to manage his asthma better and perhaps reduce his need for medication. With that goal in mind, I taught him a simple relaxation technique. First, he relaxed the muscles in his body one at a time and imagined himself in one of his favorite places. Next, he used a more specific kind of mental imagery: envisioning his lung passages opening wide and air moving through them freely. By practicing this imagery exercise for about twenty minutes twice a day, he was able to lower his drug dosage and even went for long periods without an asthma attack.

---

*This chapter by Dr. Rossman on imagery originally appeared in *Mind-Body Medicine* (Yonkers, NY: Consumers' Union, 1993). It is reprinted here with the permission of the author.

Then, suddenly, the method stopped working. In fact, sometimes imagery made it harder for him to breathe. Because imagery had once helped him control his asthma so successfully, I suggested that we try a different type of imagery exercise to help him understand what had gone wrong.

After Jason lulled himself into a relaxed state, I advised him to allow an image to enter his mind that would offer a clue to the mystery. He began to see an agitated dwarf dressed like a Roman soldier patrolling the entrance to a tunnel. The dwarf, who called himself Romeo, said he was guarding the roads to Jason's heart. If anyone started to get too close he would close off the tunnel entrance. Jason thought the tunnel reminded him of a bronchial tube. He also pictured many such guards at the "outposts" of his bronchial tubes and saw the tubes all contract and close down in response to a threatened "invasion."

After this exercise, Jason realized that the resurgence of his asthma coincided with the onset of a new romance. His intense feelings for his girlfriend so frightened him that he had been unknowingly using the asthma to keep her away. Because of his illness, he often canceled their dates. And when they were together, she spent much of the time taking care of him, though he really wanted a relationship based on mutual caring. With frustration and embarrassment, he recalled previous budding romances that had been sabotaged by flare-ups of his asthma.

Similarly, he now saw that he had unconsciously used his condition for emotional purposes during childhood. Back then, having an attack meant getting extra care from his mother and the chance to skip activities he disliked, such as gym class and trips to visit relatives.

Breaking the Cycle

To break the cycle, I encouraged Jason to tell Romeo that he appreciated being protected from emotional pain, but that this vigilance was in itself causing pain and physical illness. In his mind, he told the dwarf that he felt ready to risk more intimate relationships, though he still wanted some protection. He began to imagine a series of checkpoints at different distances along the "roads" to his heart and how it felt to allow various people closer. He even envisioned issuing "security clearances" to certain individuals, including his girlfriend. This helped him experience how it felt to allow different levels of intimacy.

After that session, Jason was better able to relax and regulate his breathing. Over the next several months, his asthma did occasionally worsen, but he took those episodes as a sign to pay closer attention to his feelings, especially about his deepening romantic relationship. Within a year, his flare-ups again became rare occurrences.

GUIDED IMAGERY IN HEALING

Jason's case demonstrates two major ways in which guided imagery, as this approach is called, is now used in health care. It can be used actively to help alleviate symptoms, as Jason did by envisioning his bronchial tubes widening. And it can be used receptively, "allowing" images to come to mind to help us understand the emotional meaning our symptoms may have.

The use of inner visions to help the healing process is hardly a new concept. Tibetan Buddhists have been using images in this way since the thirteenth century, if not earlier. The Buddhist approach typically involves meditating on the image of a deity in the act of healing a symptom. Shamanistic practices in cultures throughout the world have employed a similar approach. Only recently, however, has imagery been used by Western physicians and health care providers.

As a primary-care physician treating mostly patients with chronic conditions, I became interested in imagery first as a way to help alleviate my patients' suffering. Since 1972, I have taught imagery techniques to thousands of people. I have seen many people recover from their illnesses after using imagery, and others who have been helped by imagery to lead rewarding lives in spite of their condition.

There are still only a few carefully controlled scientific studies to show precisely how great an impact imagery by itself can have on the body. Such studies are difficult to design and carry out, for several reasons. For one thing, imagery is often used in conjunction with other mind/body techniques such as hypnosis and simple relaxation, making it difficult to separate out the effects of the imagery alone. In addition, the "receptive" imagery techniques are so extremely individualized that it is hard to quantify their effects.

Nevertheless, a small but growing body of clinical evidence strongly suggests that imagery can help people with a wide range of physical illnesses. And some sophisticated physiological studies are pointing the way to understanding just how imagery exerts its effects.

HOW IMAGERY WORKS

The modern use of therapeutic imagery usually entails a 20- to 25-minute session that begins with a relaxation exercise to help focus attention and "center" your mind. If this doesn't adequately ward off distractions, you can also start by inducing a hypnotic state.

Although imagery is often used together with hypnosis, the two techniques are independent and complementary. Put simply, hypnosis is the induction of a particular state of mind, while imagery is an activity. It's perfectly possible to have one without the other, though the combination may be most effective.

In hypnotherapy, specific suggestions are used to relieve physical symptoms, and imagery is generally the most powerful and effective way to provide such suggestions. Rather than simply saying "Your pain is diminishing," for example, a hypnotist may ask you to imagine a painful part of your body feeling warm or going numb. (Imagery itself can also be used to induce a hypnotic state in the first place.)

During a typical session of imagery, you focus on a predetermined image designed to help you control a particular symptom (active imagery) or you allow your mind to conjure up images that give you insight into a particular problem (receptive imagery). Depending on your needs, imagery can be explored on your own, with the help of a book or audiotape, or with a therapist's guidance (see Resources).

Although science has not found the precise basis for imagery's healing abilities, we know enough to make some reasonable speculations about how it works. Visual, auditory, and tactile imagery seem to arise from the brain's cerebral cortex, the seat of higher mental functions, such as language, thinking, and problem solving. (Imagery having to do with smell or emotional experiences may arise from more primitive brain centers.)

When researchers have used a sophisticated technique called positron-emission tomography (PET) to monitor the brain during imagery exercises, they have found that the same parts of the cerebral cortex are activated whether people imagine something or actually experience it. This suggests that picturing visual images activates the optic cortex, imagining that you are listening to music arouses the auditory cortex, and conjuring up tactile sensations stimulates the sensory cortex. Thus, vivid imagery can send a message from the cerebral cortex to the lower brain centers, including the limbic system, the emotional center of the brain. From there, the message is relayed to the endocrine system and the autonomic nervous system, which can affect a range of bodily functions, including heart rate, perspiration, and blood pressure.

Many clinicians believe that the more fully you imagine something, the more "real" it seems to the brain and the greater the amount of information sent to the nervous system. This is one reason it's helpful to use as many senses as possible during guided imagery sessions. (For example, you might imagine lying on the beach, feeling the warm sand, listening to the ocean, and smelling the sea air.) While visualization is certainly the most common form of imagery, and for most people, the easiest, it's not the only one. People who have trouble visualizing may be able to relax by imagining the warmth of the sun, recalling a favorite tune, or conjuring up the aroma of brewing coffee or the taste of freshly baked bread.

THE VALUE OF IMAGERY

Three major qualities of imagery make it particularly valuable in mind/body medicine and healing: It can bring about physiological changes, provide psychological insight, and enhance emotional awareness.

Physiological Changes

Imagery has great potential to affect physiology directly. If you were consciously to try to salivate right now, you probably wouldn't be able to. But notice what happens if you imagine the scene in the exercise below. (This exercise is particularly effective if you close your eyes and have a friend read you the description aloud.)

At the end of this exercise, most people will salivate, especially from the back of the jaws—a simple illustration of imagery's ability to trigger a physiological response. But imagery can also trigger physical reactions that are more subtle than salivation and more important for health. There is preliminary evidence that imagery can have specific effects on the immune system, although the explanation for these findings remains unclear. In several experiments, researchers have looked at the physical effects of imagery combined with other relaxation and stress management techniques, such as the relaxation response, biofeedback, and progressive muscle relaxation. Although these studies did not focus narrowly on imagery, they do suggest it can contribute to a wide range of change in such physiological functions as heart rate, blood pressure, breathing patterns, brain wave rhythms, blood flow, gastrointestinal activity, sexual arousal, and the release of various hormones and neurotransmitters.

An Exercise: Imagine . . .

You are standing in front of a cutting board. Next to it is a good, sharp knife. Take a few moments to imagine the kitchen, the color of the countertops, the appliances, the cupboards, windows, and so on. Also notice any kitchen smells or sounds—the running of a dishwasher or the hum of a refrigerator.

Now imagine that on the board sits a plump, fresh, juicy lemon. In your mind, hold the lemon in one hand, feeling its weight and texture. Then place it back on the board and carefully cut it in half with the knife. Feel the resistance to the knife and how it gives way as the lemon splits. Notice the pale yellow of the pulp and the whiteness of the inner peel, and see whether you have cut through a seed or two. Carefully cut one of the halves in two. See where a drop or two of juice has pearled on the surface of one of the quarters. Imagine lifting this lemon wedge to your mouth, smelling the sharp fresh scent. Now bite into the sour, juicy pulp.

Psychological Insight

Imagery can also help illuminate the connections between stressful circumstances and physical symptoms, where such connections exist. It does this by helping you see the big picture.

When you perceive the world as most people usually do, through logical, linear thinking, you attempt to break it down into small pieces and find the sequences that lead from one piece to the other. Logical thinking is similar to watching a train round the bend: You see one car at a time, with maybe just a little bit of the car that went before it. But imagery puts you in a balloon hundreds of feet above the track, high enough to see the entire train and several miles of track, as well as the town it came from and the city it's going to, the fields through which the train runs, and the mountain range in the distance. You grasp the whole picture and see how each of its parts is related to the rest. In much the same way, imagery can help you perceive connections between physical symptoms and emotional or stressful situations you would otherwise realize.

Here's an example. Two years ago I treated a woman who suffered from chronic arm pain that defied medical diagnosis. During an imagery exercise, she saw the pain as angle irons in her shoulders and metal bars in her arms. She said the images were hard, rigid, cold, and unyielding. When asked for other associations, she immediately thought of her grandfather, whom she had nursed for two years until he died some months before. She wept as she told me she had loved him a great deal, but hadn't been able to have the relationship she wanted with him because he was emotionally hard, cold, and rigid—the very qualities represented in the image of her pain.

I had her use imagery to create a dialogue with her grandfather. In her mind, she expressed all of her feelings to him, and he seemed to soften and thanked her for the loving care. He told her he loved her but wasn't able to express it. They embraced, and a warm feeling began to run through her arms. She had a few follow-up sessions and has been pain-free ever since. The imagery exercises helped her make the connection between her physical pain and its psychological cause, and she was finally able to heal.

Emotional Awareness

The third significant attribute of imagery is its close relationship to the emotions. You can think of the emotions as the means by which thoughts create changes in the body. Fear makes our hearts pound, grief makes us shed tears, and joy leads to laughter. But the natural ways of demonstrating emotions, especially negative ones such as anger and sadness, are often socially unacceptable and are suppressed. People may then find unhealthful outlets for such

An Exercise: Remember . . .

Close your eyes. Take a couple of deep, slow breaths, letting yourself relax as you exhale. Begin to focus inside and recall a room from your childhood. Notice what you see there and any sounds you might hear in the room. Is there an aroma? What else do you notice? Do any feelings come up as you imagine this? Just notice them and let them be there. Then let that image fade, and imagine that you are looking at a very close friend, smiling at you. Notice your friend's smile and his or her eyes. What does this person seem to be communicating?

emotions, such as physical symptoms or behaviors (smoking, drinking, workaholism, and so on) that lead to health problems. Imagery is one of the quickest and most direct ways to become aware of one's emotional state and its potential effect on health. With this in mind, try the exercise above.

Take a few minutes to think about this experience, perhaps writing down some notes about it. How did you feel as you contemplated these two simple images? How much did you write? Notice that it was communicated to you in a second or two through each image. These mental pictures (in whatever sensory mode they appear) are very often worth thousands of words and are a very efficient form of information storage and recall.

APPLYING IMAGERY IN HEALING

Although there is little careful, well-controlled research on the medical benefits of imagery, clinical reports suggest that the technique may help treat a wide range of conditions, including chronic pain, allergies, high blood pressure, irregular heartbeats, autoimmune diseases, cold and flu symptoms, and stress-related gastrointestinal, reproductive, and urinary complaints. Imagery may also help speed healing after an injury, such as a sprain, strain, or broken bone.

Many of these benefits stem directly from the relaxing effects of imagery. In fact, the most common, most useful, and easiest application of imagery in health care is its use in relaxation and stress reduction. Many people find guided imagery the simplest, most natural way to relax. To get a taste of how relaxing imagery can be, try the simple, quick exercise on the next page.

When you return to everyday reality, you're likely to feel calmer, more alert, and refreshed—as if you'd had a much longer rest. This sort of imagery is common to most relaxation techniques, from progressive muscle relaxation to various forms of meditation (see chapter 45).

An Exercise: Transport Yourself . . .

Keep your eyes closed while you take a few deep, easy breaths, and imagine yourself in the most peaceful, beautiful, serene place you can conjure up. Think of a time when you felt relaxed and peaceful—perhaps a walk in the park, a day on a sunny beach, or an evening at a concert—and focus intently on the sights, smells, and physical sensations associated with that event. Focus on this image for about five minutes.

Beyond relaxation, however, active imagery is used—often together with hypnosis—to conjure up positive images designed to alleviate physical symptoms directly. In some cases, these images may have a direct physiological effect. When Jason, the man with asthma, visualized his bronchial tubes opening, he probably began breathing more slowly and deeply without quite being aware of it—changes that would be particularly beneficial for his asthma.

In other cases, imagery may have a beneficial effect on patients even though its effect on their disease can't be determined. The use of imagery in cancer therapy is a good example. In the early 1970s, radiation oncologist O. Carl Simonton and psychologist Stephanie Simonton taught active imagery to cancer patients in the hope that it would help them fight off the disease. (A typical exercise was to imagine the immune system's cells devouring the cancer cells.) Their work received a great deal of publicity and sparked a lot of interest in imagery in general.

In the two decades since the Simontons developed their approach, no definitive, well-controlled study has been done to show whether this kind of imagery improves the overall prognosis for people with cancer. But many people find this kind of imagery helpful, even if it doesn't cure their disease. They report such benefits as relief from anxiety and pain, greater tolerance of chemotherapy or radiation therapy, and a heightened ability to cope with the illness. Imagery helps them to relax and to feel less helpless.

People with cancer or any other illness should not rely on imagery as their sole means of treatment when other, proven methods are available. Still, imagery can be a powerful aid in increasing the effectiveness of medical treatments or in helping people to endure them. Combined with relaxation techniques, imagery has helped people to tolerate such diagnostic and therapeutic procedures as magnetic resonance imaging examinations, bone marrow biopsies, and cancer chemotherapy and radiation. It can also help people prepare for surgery and recover from it.

Inner Harmony through Imagery

At 52, Robert suffered from chronic abdominal pain and indigestion that had been diagnosed as pancreatitis. His doctors had little to offer him but had urged him to follow a low-fat diet, which he had trouble doing. In our imagery sessions, he found an inner adviser who called himself "Moishe." Robert said he looked like a cross between his brother, Morris, and the biblical figure Moses. Moishe, like the doctors, told Robert that he would feel better and give his pancreas a chance to recover if he followed a strict low-fat diet. Robert followed Moishe's advice for several weeks and felt better than he had in years. But when he went on a trip to visit his family, he forgot about his diet. Soon after a meal at a Chinese restaurant, he had a severe episode of abdominal pain and vomiting. He tried to get back in touch with his adviser but had no success.

The next time Robert came to visit me, I guided him through a relaxation process and politely asked Moishe to come and talk with Robert again. Moishe appeared in his imagery, but stood with his head turned away and wouldn't speak. Robert asked him why he was silent, and he replied, "I don't have time to waste. If you're not going to be sincere about this, I'm not going to talk to you." Robert apologized and committed himself again to working toward better health more conscientiously.

Today, two years later, Robert feels working with his inner adviser has been one of the most helpful things he's ever learned. Not only has Moishe helped Robert with his digestive problems, but he was also of great comfort during a very difficult six-month period in which Robert lost the two people closest to him. During that time, Moishe told Robert that he was only an intermediary figure who represented his connection with God. Robert said to me, "Why deal with a middleman?" and now, in his meditations, he feels a sense of inner connection to God. Sometimes he asks questions and receives answers; other times he is satisfied just to enjoy a deep sense of peacefulness.

Another role imagery plays in medical care is to put you in touch with your feelings about your illness. Imagery can be helpful in almost any medical situation that requires problem solving or decision making. By using receptive imagery to explore your emotional reactions to your medical circumstances, you may emerge with a clearer sense of how best to treat an illness or live well in spite of it. You may also better understand how your lifestyle choices may be affecting your health. If your illness is fulfilling some emotional need, coming to terms with that need may ease your physical symptoms.

Receptive imagery treatment may involve a dialogue with images representing symptoms or the illness. During receptive imagery sessions you may also wish to develop an image of your "inner adviser"—an embodiment of your inner wisdom—who can help you understand the emotional meaning of body sensations and symptoms. In my experience, this two-way use of imagery to spur communication between mind and body yields the most profound healing responses.

GETTING STARTED

Depending on the severity of your problem, you may want to try using imagery on your own or with professional help. (For advice on finding help see Resources.) Since imagery may change the body's requirements for medication, it may be best for you to use it under the guidance of your physician, depending on your medical condition. In any case, if you plan to begin an imagery program, it's best to set relatively small goals at first, perhaps aiming simply to learn to relax. Most people can experience relaxation with imagery in a very short time, even during the first session. Once you've mastered that, you can go on to try more complex forms of imagery.

For chronic symptoms, such as pain, you may want to begin by practicing 15 to 20 minutes twice a day for three weeks. This is usually enough to see if the imagery is helpful. For receptive imagery, it often takes two or three sessions with an experienced therapist or instructor to get initial results. It may take longer if you are working on your own or with self-help tapes.

If you use active imagery, keep a daily journal in which you estimate your symptoms' severity day to day. Over several weeks, this will help you determine whether the imagery is having an effect. Similarly, if you are using receptive imagery, it can be helpful to keep a journal of your experiences with imagery, as well as your dreams and emotional reactions.

Until more careful research is done, we don't really know imagery's potential or limitations as a healing tool. Some people seem to respond to it remarkably well, while others don't. Many factors, from your physical condition to your inner resolve, may affect the treatment's success. Experimenting with imagery, however, is easy, safe, and inexpensive. All it takes is the time and willingness to unlock the power of your imagination.

Biographical information for **Martin Rossman, M.D.,** appears on page 94.

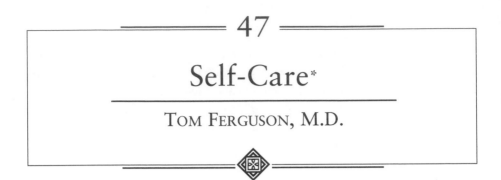

47

Self-Care*

Tom Ferguson, M.D.

We don't mean to imply that everybody should have a self-care plan. If things are going well for you, if you are satisfied with the present pattern of your life and not particularly interested in making changes at the moment, good for you. Keep it up. These guidelines are for those who are interested in making some gentle changes. Remember that the advice that follows has proven useful for some people. But they are ideas to try, not commandments.

The goal-setting exercise that accompanies this article is just that—an exercise. It gives you an opportunity to define a commitment you would like to make to yourself. This is a commitment to yourself, not an irrevocable promise sealed in blood. Think of it as an opportunity to "try on" some new behavior patterns. You are free to go back and revise your goals at any time.

DEVELOPING A PERSONAL SELF-CARE PLAN

1. *Choose a goal that turns you on.* Build on strengths. Cultivate excitement. Starve problems and feed solutions. If you are a smoker and the idea of a regular running program appeals to you, you might find yourself quitting cigarettes about the time your program really steps up. If you have a problem with weight control and you've always been intrigued by meditation, a daily meditation session might be more useful than a whole stack of diet books. Goals that enrich your life are usually more successful—and are certainly a lot more fun—than goals that deprive you of something.

2. *Start by just paying attention.* An excellent way to start an exercise program is to buy a pedometer—a small, watch-sized instrument that records the number of steps you take (available from running, sporting goods, and backpacking stores)—and chart the total miles you walk each

---

*An earlier version of this chapter by Dr. Ferguson appeared online at www.healthonline.com and is included courtesy of the author.

day. A good way to start an eating program is to write down everything you eat for a period of time. To start a smoking program, write down where and when and why you smoke each cigarette. Pay close attention to the ways that other people support desired or undesired behavior in the area you have chosen. Do family members insist on offering you high-calorie goodies? Does everyone else at work light up right after lunch? Don't try to change anything yet, just pay close attention.

3. *Check out your available resources.* Start with your own personal resources. Were you an athlete in high school? If so maybe you can reconnect with some of the habits and practices that kept you in shape back then. Do you love to cook? Maybe you would enjoy developing some nutritious natural-food recipes. Is there a musical instrument or an art or craft that once meant a lot to you? Reconnecting with these areas of interest might be a way to further your own process of self-integration. Have you always had a dream of being a dancer? A painter? A writer? This may be an opportunity to develop these interests.

   What individuals and groups in your community would be the best resources in your chosen area? Who already knows about what you want to know? Are there support groups in your chosen area (Weight Watchers, Alcoholics Anonymous, women's consciousness-raising groups)? Do you have friends who have lost weight, who are runners or meditators? What are the best publications in the area you have chosen?

4. *Brainstorm many possible goals before narrowing them down to one.* If you want to start an exercise program, you might start by brainstorming such goals as swimming the English Channel, walking cross-country across America, running a marathon, running five miles a day, joining (or organizing) a weekly fun run or running support group, running in place for five minutes before your shower each morning, riding your bike to work, taking the stairs instead of the elevator, or taking a fifteen-minute walk after lunch three times a week. Be creative. Feel free to be completely unrealistic. Think of goals that would be fun. Remember, you are just brainstorming. Find your own way to do it. Maybe the best way for you to start an exercise program would be to get a dog and take it for a walk once or twice a day.

5. *Design freedom into your goals.* "I will allow myself to take work breaks to do yoga whenever I feel like it." "I will go to bed early in order

to give myself some quiet time in the morning before breakfast." "I will leave one Sunday a month free to be alone in the woods." "When I go running, I will let myself dance, skip, stop to look at a bird or a flower, or do anything I feel like." These are some goals with built-in freedom.

6. *Reward yourself.* Pay close attention to your successes and the benefits deriving from your new practices. Celebrate your victories. "I ran a whole half-mile today without stopping!" "Doing yoga sure makes my back and shoulders feel good." Think of rewards you might give yourself for reaching short-term and long-term goals. (A hot bath after an evening run, a massage after logging your first hundred miles, dinner and a movie after completing a creative project.)

7. *Ask the support of others, and support them for supporting you.* Pick your support person (or people) carefully. Pick people who accept you as you are, who make you feel good about yourself when you are with them. Tell them that you're working on developing your own self-care plan—you might even show them this article—and ask if they'd be willing to be your support person for the goal you've chosen. Tell them the kinds of things they could do to help support you. Be as specific as you can. Here are some examples: "Serve me smaller portions." "Bicycle along with me sometimes when I go running." "Come with me to the first meeting of a self-help group [or self-care class or workshop]."

   The way to get the best support from a friend is to support her or him for supporting you. "I really appreciated it that you took care of the kids so that I could play my flute." "It was really a help for you to take me into the medical library and show me how to look things up for myself." "It was wonderful when you said every time I wanted a cigarette you'd give me a kiss instead." "I really love it when you compliment me for the weight I'm losing."

   You might also want to consider creating your own imaginary support person. A good description of one way to go about doing this can be found in the book *At a Journal Workshop* by Ira Progoff.

8. *Create a supportive environment.* It may be easier to change your environment than to change your behavior. The easiest way to control your eating is at the place you buy your food. If you have high-calorie, low-nutrition foods around, they'll probably end up being eaten. What goes into your shopping cart goes into your family's bodies. If you're trying to cut down on caffeine, try mixing your present brand of coffee

half-and-half with decaffeinated coffee. Trouble overeating? Put your scale next to your refrigerator. And if your new, smaller portions look too tiny, buy smaller plates. If you're exploring yoga, massage, or meditation, try putting aside a special part of the house—or a special room—for these practices. Does soaking in hot water help you relax? Consider putting in a bigger bathtub. Having trouble finding a good place to run? Join other runners in a campaign for a community running path.

9. *Be aware of feedback and be open to modifying your goal.* How does your new practice make your body feel? How does your awareness change? How does making certain changes in your diet affect the way you feel about mealtime? At what times of day do you find yourself using your new relaxation skills?

   Be aware of negative feedback too. If you've given a chosen practice a good try and it's just not working, give yourself a vacation and reevaluate. Are you trying for too much too fast? Go back to the paying attention and brainstorming stage. You haven't failed; you've gained some useful information. Go back through the goal-setting exercise. Or if it seems right, give yourself a vacation from goal setting for a while.

10. *Remember that your ultimate goal is to discover practices that allow you to experience and develop your own uniqueness.* There are two approaches to developing a self-care plan. One is to imagine the ideal way you think you should be or would like to be. You then focus your attention on all the ways you fail to live up to that ideal. This method is a very effective way of making yourself miserable.

    Method number two is to begin by just tasting your own being, becoming aware of your own body without comparing it to anything or anyone. When you taste a good wine, if you are comparing it to another wine or to how an ideal wine would taste, you will not be able to fully taste the wine you are drinking. If you are reading a book or watching a movie and are too involved in criticizing the plot or analyzing the style, chances are you won't be able to enjoy the story.

    It may be that the most important part of developing a self-care plan is not the things you start doing, but the things you stop doing, a sort of psychological housecleaning, getting rid of some things you don't need anymore. So the best of luck in working toward your own tailor-made self-care plan. And remember that it is you who must be the tailor.

Worksheet for Developing a Personal Self-Care Plan

My main area of interest (such as exercise, weight loss, or coping with an illness):

_____

_____

My main personal strengths and resources in this area:

_____

_____

The best resources for me in this area (people, groups, classes, books, etc.):

_____

_____

Some activities and goals I might choose to help me explore this area (brainstorm!):

_____

_____

I would like to choose an initial activity that I could complete in about ___days/
___weeks/___months:

_____

_____

Within this time limit, the goal I'd most like to set for myself is:

_____

_____

Some small rewards I will give myself for making progress toward this goal:

_____

_____

A big reward I will give myself for reaching my goal:

_____

_____

The people I will ask for support in working toward this goal:

_____

_____

I will contact my support person on_____ (date) to bring them up to date on my explorations in this area:

_____

_____

My commitment again is to accomplish the following activities between now and the following date:

_____

_____

On that date I will give my support person a report on my explorations in this area.

SIGNATURE: _____TODAY'S DATE_____

Tom Ferguson, M.D., is editor and publisher of the industry newsletter *The Ferguson Report: The Newsletter of Consumer Health Informatics and Online Health.* With a medical degree from Yale University School of Medicine, he is a senior associate of the Center for Clinical Computing at Harvard Medical School and an adjunct associate professor of health informatics at the University of Texas Medical Sciences Center, Houston. He founded the journal *Medical Self-Care* and the *Self-Care Catalog,* and has been medical editor for *The Whole Earth Catalog* and a contributor to Bill Moyers's series on mind-body medicine. He is the author of a dozen books on consumer health, and his latest, *Health Online: How to Find Health Information, Support Groups and Self-Help Communities in Cyberspace,* was recently published by Addison-Wesley. Dr. Ferguson is also a consultant to many of the leading companies in the emerging online health industry.

Dr. Ferguson can be reached at doctom@doctom.com. For more information, see his Web site at www.fergusonreport.com.

48

Getting the Support You Need

LEN SAPUTO, M.D., AND NANCY FAASS, MSW, MPH

"No one lives by bread, work, or medication alone. . . . To flourish as an individual, it is necessary to have certain goods in our lives. Just as we need [good nutrition] to be physically healthy, there are values we must have to live well. Experiences of truth, beauty, justice, order, richness, playfulness, and meaningfulness are all food for the soul."

—JOHN SHUMAN, 1998

Many chronic digestive disorders carry with them profound life challenges, as well as obvious physical constraints. Their treatment can make us dependent on the support of health care professionals, as well as on our families and friends. Our lifestyle may become radically altered. The cost of therapy can be devastating. And our relationships may be severely tested.

Ultimately we're all looking for the same thing—all asking the same question—how can we be loved for who we are? When we develop chronic illness, that question may become more difficult to answer. How can we get the support we need if we have lost our health? This is one of the toughest issues in this society—or any other.

Your strategy depends on the needs of your situation. You want to develop an effective suport system, without over-reliance on anyone else. If you feel challenged, then you're being a realist.

WHAT THE RESEARCH SUGGESTS

- *Support matters.* A major study in New York confirmed what we all have suspected—people do better with support. Researchers tracked the progress of more than 700 people with serious illness and found that coping and improvement paralleled the adequacy of social support from family, friends, and others in their lives, even after all the variables were taken into account.

Getting Support

Flo spent all her time in a wheelchair, but she managed to put together a decent support system, since she couldn't leave her apartment. Each day, the meals-on-wheels person brought her lunch, someone else went to the library and got her books, another friend picked up the mail. She had a phone buddy she checked on and friends she talked on the phone with each day, and she visited with her daughter each week.

Marguerite's situation was equally challenging. At 90 she was totally housebound in her cottage. She was able to remain at home through the support of her bridge group. She had a daily visitor, and then once a week the whole group came for a pleasant afternoon of bridge and brought her groceries for the week.

- *The sicker you are, the harder it may be to get support.* If you're really sick and you've been having trouble getting the kind of support you'd like to have, don't blame yourself, because that seems to be the way it is. (This is what researchers have confirmed. Even children get less support if their illness is involved or lengthy. If this is a problem for kids, clearly it's difficult for adults too.)
- *It doesn't matter how many friends a person has, it's the quality of support you get that is important.* Rejoice in the support you *do* have.
- *It's not easy to get support.* One of the reasons support groups have evolved is because people aren't always there for each other. There are many illnesses that tend to dim our charisma, when we need help the most. The programs of Dean Ornish have demonstrated that having support and a sense of community is an important part of healing.

DEVELOP A DIVERSE SUPPORT SYSTEM

If our needs are intense it is important to have a support system that includes a number of people in a variety of roles: family and friends, perhaps volunteers, or people whom we hire for assistance. Religious groups are frequently a good source of assistance. Nurses, physicians, and many other health care professionals are all potential resources to provide support that can help us to heal. If we need help on a daily basis it may require setting up a network that we design to fit our own unique situation.

USING ILLNESS TO HEAL YOUR LIFE

If one has to go through all the trauma of chronic illness, it might as well become an opportunity for growth and change.

The Meaning of Disease: Personal Transformation

When we are ill we want to get well. We don't enjoy being sick. Our most immediate concern is to secure relief from our symptoms and to be "cured" of our illness. We want to operate with a perfect body and to feel good. We seek out health care practitioners who promise to deliver these services and highly value their work. There is nothing wrong with this approach, and it has obvious potential value.

It is also possible to look at the meaning of illness in the context of who we are as unique individuals, determine what the illness represents in our whole life story, and prosper from the journey through it.

Like Pain, Illness Can Be a Signal

Like pain, illness may be a sign that something is deeply wrong in our lives. Just as we usually take pain seriously (and are often sorry if we happen to ignore it), so we may regard illness as a sign that change is needed. Indigenous healers traditionally viewed illness as the reflection of psychological or social dysfunction that has resulted in physical and mental problems.

NOURISHING HEALING PRACTICES

In the tradition of the shaman, the purpose of treatment is to restore the intactness or wholeness of the individual within the context of all aspects of one's entire life. Healing is revered as a sacred journey within.

Changing Our Values

Illness may bring us back to the fundamental values of life, the importance of the people in our lives, and the spiritual aspects of life. When we're sick we tend to become more oriented toward fundamental things. We realize the temporary nature of the material side. Illness can play an important role by awakening us to our spiritual purpose. We are reminded of the significance of our relationships.

Transforming Our External Environment

At times the demands of illness also provide the impetus to make external changes, to find new and practical solutions to basic issues in our life. This may mean changing our environment. It may be necessary to get rid of a toxic

The Joy of Giving

Lenore had a problem, but it didn't slow her down for a minute. She was afflicted with spinal scoliosis to such a degree that it made her frame bent and twisted. Lenore was so gracious, so attractive, bubbly, and positive, that in her presence you immediately forgot about her disability and became swept into her interesting and engaging world. Lenore was a giver. Although she was well past 70, she spent her days shepherding women older and frailer than she to pleasant events—bridge, the theater, choral music, and volunteer work.

Twice Lenore had cared for much older friends with extended convalescences, in each case for more than two years. She shared her spacious apartment with them, putting them up in the study, cooking and caring for them. This capacity to give may have been the source of her boundless energy and the meaningful purpose in her life.

relationship, make a career change, or move to another area. It may mean working as a freelancer or consultant, starting up an at-home business, or involving yourself in meaningful volunteer work with an organization you feel is making a worthwhile difference. It could involve refining a skill you've always wanted to use (fine woodworking, making clothes for homeless children, or taking up calligraphy). It may mean taking the vacation you've always dreamed of, just to get away for a while to catch your breath. Or it could mean developing almost any aspect of your life in a genuinely meaningful way.

Giving Is Easier Than You May Think

No matter what your situation, there's always a little something you can do to help others. If you're housebound, perhaps it's phone work—calling latchkey kids to make sure they're all right, visiting with a housebound senior on the phone each day, or getting out the vote. You may have a skill you can donate—editing the newsletter of an organization you believe in, organizing a neglected project for them, or doing some Internet research. That glow that comes when you've done something worth doing can actually boost your immune response.

Healing through Laughter

Being ill can be depressing. Being depressed can aggravate our illness by suppressing the immune system. And this is compounded further by the fact that it is often difficult to sleep. In addition we may not be able to exercise, which can lead to deepening depression. Anything that can help us lift our spirits is healing.

The healing effect of laughter and positive emotional states has been found to enhance the immune system. Norman Cousins, in his book *Anatomy of an Illness*, described how he used laughter and nutritional therapy to heal from a totally debilitating condition. You may find his experience inspiring and decide to build into your life people and activities that delight you; for example, reading something humorous each day and spending time with friends who are upbeat. Since Dr. Cousins' initial work, the use of guided imagery, hypnotherapy, and a variety of meditative states has also been shown to have a powerful beneficial effect. Our state of mind has a strong influence on the body and its ability to heal.

The Healing Power of Touch

Touch is a basic human need. Infants who don't receive touch may not survive or do not develop normally. We need human contact even more when we are ill. In addition to the soothing aspect of touch, it can unlock painful memories stored in the muscles and tissues of our body, through treatment called somatic therapy. We've all heard of how the mind affects the body through psychosomatic illness. This can work in reverse as well: Treating the body can heal the mind. There are a variety of bodywork techniques that can not only make us feel physically and mentally nourished, but can also do a lot to help our "mind-body" to heal. Mind-body medicine has become a popular approach over the past decade, and therapies like Alexander, Feldenkrais, craniosacral therapy, and many others have been documented to heal the mind-body through manipulation of the body.

The Healing Side of Nature

We have a sacred relationship with nature. In our own individual way we are an integral part of its collective wholeness. Nature too offers a sacred

The Healing Power of Laughter and Touch

Edmund was in the hospital for 99 days (longer than Noah's flood!). For ninety days he was in traction—requiring the patience of both Noah and Job. Inspired by Norman Cousins, he developed a routine that helped him keep his sanity. Every day he rented a humorous movie and spent time reading comedies and uplifting books. He had a massage every evening and also had his barber stop by once a week to keep him trimmed and groomed.

relationship with us. When we accept this invitation, our relationship deepens. Connecting with nature can be very healing—it can be as simple as a walk by a river or smelling the fresh forest rain. These experiences bring us more in tune with our consciousness and spirit. They help us to remember that we are part of all that is, and that it is very nourishing.

Gardening

Activities such as gardening may have profound and lasting effects on body, mind, and soul. In many great religious traditions, gardening is considered a healing and spiritual practice—think of the herb gardens of the European monasteries and the rock gardens of the Asian monasteries. Very simple, very beautiful, yet not elaborate. This is something that can be created without great expense. There are many easy, pleasing ways to garden—for example, organic vegetable gardening using the French intensive method is done in containers, ideal for patios or balconies. Something as basic as pots of herbs lining the windowsill can bring pleasure and provide healing herbs.

Nourish Yourself with Music

Great music, poetry, and art also have the ability to bring us into harmony with nature. The language of tones rhythm, and form allow us to deeply and simultaneously communicate within ourselves and with each other. This resonance creates a sense of unity that can be not only awesome but truly healing. The messages of great composers and artists can transcend the conscious mind, reach us at a soul level, bringing us into more perfect balance. We have all experienced this remarkable phenomenon. The music that nourishes our souls may vary from Bach to African drumming, from choral music to world music.

Creating a Healing Space through Art

The other side of creativity is the opportunity to use our own creative expression. This can put us in touch with intense psychological and creative energy, and enable us to tap a deep vein of power that is difficult to describe. The medium could be anything that is meaningful, anything we enjoy and do well at. The possibilities are endless. If we are ingenious in choosing our medium, money need not be an issue.

In *The Psychology of Chronic Illness,* Robert Shuman, an insightful psychologist who battles multiple sclerosis, suggests that "art can bring the possibility of healing to those living with illness. One purpose of art is to give form to that which is unspeakable, to render coherent the shattered and broken. Just as illness can [negate] experience, art can give it both spirit and flesh. Art is a medicine for the suffering we call illness."

The Power of Music

Jamie had AIDS. As a doctor she was one of the early victims of medicine's "War on AIDS," before they knew how devastating a needle stick could be. At the time there was little to be done about it. The drugs helped, but not that much. But music! She got a Walkman, put together a first-rate collection of tapes, and began immersing herself in a world of music. It didn't heal her, but it transformed the quality of her life.

Support Groups

Getting support has also been a problem for people with conditions such as cancer and AIDS. Over the past twenty years resources for support within these communities have become quite well developed, perhaps because of the life-threatening nature of the illnesses. This has given birth to the highly successful medical support group movement that exists in this country. These groups are often highly valued by patients and praised by researchers for their life-enhancing benefits. The groups seek to provide the emotional and spiritual support that is so important in battling chronic illness, to retain what is most meaningful in life. Some of the support groups are offered to participants with a range of physical conditions, intended for anyone with serious illness, rather than just one diagnosis.

Support is valuable, but be sure that the information you receive is current and correct. Beware that some groups unknowingly perpetuate misinformation about the nature of GI illness and the treatments available. For example, for decades stomach ulcers were thought to be caused by stress. We now know that in many cases they are due to a bacteria, *H. pylori*. It wasn't until an Australian researcher proved the link with the bacteria that medical opinion began to change. There are still many other GI conditions that are consistently misdiagnosed. This is a rapidly changing field with new research that has led to new understandings of the nature of GI conditions. Generally the role of microbial infection continues to be underestimated by the medical community as a frequent cause of GI illness.

Help Online

A recent questionnaire asked 1,000 online patients with serious chronic illnesses about where their most useful information came from: their online support groups, their specialist physicians, or their primary-care doctors. Patients reported that they found online support groups most useful in ten of the twelve dimensions studied. The most impressive take-home lesson was that these online self helpers who often felt overwhelmed, isolated, and discouraged found that Internet resources provided a place where they felt welcomed, valued, and understood.

PRACTICAL MATTERS

- *If your needs are intense consider seeking the help of a volunteer.* Don't overlook or turn down access to volunteer help, because many of the people who are drawn to volunteering are really beautiful people, and it may be that you can get a very special and precious kind of support in that way. Not every volunteer is ideal, however. Others may want to help but may be unable to provide what you really need. Usually you will intuitively know the ones who can be helpful from those who cannot. Follow your inner guidance.
- *Take offers of help seriously.* At least consider them.
- *Consider the value of a good case manager.* If you have access to social services and can find a case manager, it could help you assemble a support system or team. You have to either have money to hire a good case manager (they really do exist) or find a social worker within the system who can help you get linked up. Luck is also a factor in all this.

  If you happen to have chronic illness, do consider getting support from the system. The social work literature says that the role of a good case manager is "the reconstruction and management of social support networks that have been altered or damaged due to illness or inability to cope with chronic illness. Concerns about the efficacy of specific models [and approaches] are not as important as the internal linkages built within each model and the external ties to other institutions and social service organizations forged as a way of synthetically rebuilding a client's social network" (Pescosolido et al., 1995).
- *Don't be shy to seek assistance.* A Swedish study found that people with chronic illness could typically manage at home as long as they had the periodic assistance of a home aide to help with basic chores and errands.
- *Be mindful of where and how you seek support.* Don't join the wrong group or stay in a bad relationship, thinking that it's necessary for your survival. The stress could further weaken your immune defenses.

The Needs of Children

Clearly children need support just as adults do. The research found that teenagers with chronic illness tend to get less support than small children, and that teenagers do better if they have support from peers as well as parents.

Girls tend to have more positive relations than boys. This was the conclusion of a series of seventy interviews with adolescents. Although boys (and men) benefit from support just as much as girls (and women), boys may be less likely to have supports in place or to ask for the assistance they need.

Obviously grandparents can play an important role in providing support to children with special needs. Grandparents have been found in many studies to provide support that complemented that of the immediate family and continued to provide help longer than any other relative. When there are grandparents in the picture who can be helpful, be sure to include them in the planning process to the degree they desire.

ILLNESS OR OPPORTUNITY?

Illness can be looked at as more than physical disability and psychological challenge. It can be seen as an opportunity for spiritual transformation. This is not always easy. Many of us may not feel inclined to engage in this side of our life. In fact, we may even be angered by the suggestion. We may become totally consumed with "putting out the fire" created by the illness, with little energy to search out spiritual transformation! And we may be kept busy just holding on to the shreds of our former life. Most of us consider it asking a lot to make spiritual transformations when we are well!

If there is meaningful interconnectedness of everything in the Cosmos, then there is meaning for illness too. Illness can be viewed from a deeper perspective that considers more than physical misfortune and psychological challenge. It relates to who we are, and is considered in the context of our entire life story and how our life interrelates with the Cosmos. It can be valued as a transformative opportunity that presents the possibility of evolving further on our spiritual path. This is what healing is about. Even though curing the body and healing the soul are not the same, they can occur simultaneously, and are not mutually exclusive.

RELATIONSHIPS

When we are ill restoring our lost dignity and self-respect as human beings is of the utmost importance. Our relationship with ourselves, with those we love, and with God can be mercilessly challenged. We may have difficulty maintaining these vital nourishing relationships at the very time when we need them most.

Here's what the research has to say about chronic illness, support, and relationships:

- *When you have chronic illness and you're in a close relationship, you probably notice (again) that there are advantages and limits to partner relationships.* If the relationship has a strong foundation, you may do better than those without a support system. If there have been problems with communication, illness may amplify them.
- *The quality of the relationship in general probably has an impact on the illness.* If it's a strong relationship with good communication, a person has a better shot at dealing with chronic illness more effectively.
- *On the other hand, toxic relationships can make healing more difficult.* Stress can play a major role in suppressing immune function, so these issues are relevant to the healing process.
- *Chronic illness can place tremendous stress on a marriage.* In general the divorce rate averages about 50 percent. In families where there is a child with chronic illness or a disability, the divorce rate runs about 70 percent. If you find yourself on the losing side of this equation, step back and then move on. Sometimes these apparent losses are a turning point toward a better life.
- *Looking for support? Take a second look.* If you are not getting the support you need from your family and friends, take one more look and see if there is anyone you may have overlooked who could be helpful. You may find that there is a relationship that would work if you adjusted it a little.

  On the other hand, sometimes a relationship is simply unworkable. It's like beating your head against a wall. But sometimes you can shift an aspect of the situation and restore the relationship. It's important to know when to make the effort and when to conserve your energy.
- *Love can only be found if it is looked for.* Look for practical places to invest your energy. Look for people who could be available to you and be supportive. They may not be the people in your life with whom you are closest. But notice where the investment of your energy pays off.
- *Diversify.* We rarely get all our needs met by one person. Sometimes putting together a support system is most successful if we rely on different people to meet different essential needs. This may avoid burning out any one person in his or her attempts to be helpful.
- *When our physical capacity is compromised by chronic illness, our need for nourishing human relationships becomes especially apparent.* At these times we may be less able to care for our own needs and may also be less able to satisfy the needs of our friends and family. Unfortunately fulfilling these needs may be a critically important aspect of maintaining some of these nurturing relationships, and as a consequence, they may disintegrate at the very time that we need them the most.

- *Illness can be viewed as a functional stress test that measures the strength of our relationships.* No one can predict how a relationship will weather the challenges imposed by chronic disease. We do the best we can, and should not be judged by our choices. It is possible for us to continue to learn about improving our relationships. This is our responsibility as human beings.

Doctors report that sometimes a health crisis is the very time when a relationship disintegrates. In some cases, the physically "healthier" partner leaves the relationship. But the one who is ill still has to get on with his or her life and overcome any guilt about what has been left behind. At that point there is often an opportunity for spiritual and personal growth without the limitations of the prior relationship. This may be the point at which true healing can begin. In addition it may provide an opportunity to clear old psychological baggage and emotional habits that may have kept us from relying on our own inner strength. Sometimes the life that follows has higher quality than the earlier existence.

Accessing Healing Relationships

When we are chronically ill our personal challenge is to make changes within ourselves that can empower us to continue to obtain what we need from our relationships. It is risky, and may be wishful thinking, to assume that those around us will change. Ideally, in our deepest and most meaningful relationships, we are loved for who we are, unconditionally, and not just for what we can do or give. For many people there are a few relationships that survive the test of illness. These become exceptionally precious.

Jean Shinoda Bolen, M.D., describes the transformation in our value system that frequently develops from the impact of serious illness in our lives. In this context we transcend a self-centered and materialistic orientation to one oriented to bringing love into our relationships.

The Relationship between Patient and Healer

While the practices of indigenous healers have not been very sophisticated, their strategies leave both the patient and practitioner with a sense of satisfaction and connection. In these systems patients are not looked upon just as a set of symptoms to be treated with a bag of tools. "Being with" a patient supersedes "doing to" them.

Part of the change in your own life may involve finding a health care practitioner who you feel can be more understanding of your situation, or seeking out alternatives that are more congruent with who you are and more compatible with your unique needs. Many people have more than one health care practitioner, supplementing their care with a second therapy such as acupuncture.

Throughout history our ancestors have viewed healing as the return to wholeness. The abstract nature of wholeness makes it a concept that can be difficult to fully appreciate. From a personal perspective wholeness focuses on our human experience, independent from nature. There is obviously great value in the fulfillment of our individual destiny. However, from a broader point of view wholeness is all-inclusive and relates to our interconnectedness with the entire Cosmos. Achieving wholeness from this greater perspective is part of the conscious awakening that our culture is now beginning to experience. In the final analysis healing is about wholeness, and wholeness is about remembering to live centered in love.

For biographical information for **Len Saputo, M.D.,** see page 56 and for **Nancy Faass, MSW, MPH,** see page 386.

49

Support Groups*

REBECCA McLEAN

Humans are social creatures. It's our nature to want to interact and support one another. Groups that form around a common goal or challenge can bring us together for strength and unity. Group members can draw on each other's strengths and celebrate our growth and victories. And the group can help us to hold a positive vision in times of challenge.

A review of the research on social support in the journal *Science* cited sixty-two studies showing that supportive relationships had a positive effect on recovery from chronic illness, infectious diseases, and surgery. Social connection was also shown to improve immune response and heart function. These studies indicate that we tend to function more optimistically when we're supported in a positive environment, connecting in a meaningful way with others.

If you have chronic illness, particularly if it's severe, you may find that you're having difficulty getting the long-term support you need from family and friends. In that case a support group could be helpful. If you find a group where you feel respected and heard, group support can be deeply meaningful.

THE POWER OF GROUP PROCESS

Many of the participants of groups I've facilitated in the Circle of Life program say they found the support group process was life changing for them, and that by meeting weekly with the group they felt their lives changed at an accelerated rate. In addition group participants say they discovered that their primary source of healing lies within themselves. Many of these groups have continued for years after people were in remission, changing the group's identity to "life support" groups!

---

*This chapter is adapted from *The Circle of Life Workbook,* by Rebecca McLean. Reprinted courtesy of the author, Circle of Life (www.circleoflife.net), and Health Action, Santa Barbara, CA.

The Healing Power of Support

Brent joined one of our support groups because he had ulcers and he was finding that his medications were no longer working for him. Brent tended to become highly stressed at work, which was making his ulcers even worse. In the group we went through an assessment process and looked at everyone's strengths and needs. He discovered his strengths were in exercise and relationships. When we explored the places where people wanted to make changes, he felt he was in a rut in his job and needed help with his ulcer diet. First we evaluated his diet, which revealed that he drank a lot of coffee and ate junk food. He was pouring coffee acids into his very sensitive stomach!

His initial action step was to gradually remove coffee from his diet and replace refined foods with more whole grains, like oats and brown rice, and also steamed vegetables. He also realized he was bored with his job and that he drank coffee to feel stimulated. He wanted a better position that would use more of his talents and hold his interest.

His action steps involved going back to college three nights a week to meet the education requirements he needed to get a better job. Once he reduced the stress his ulcer symptoms began to diminish almost immediately, as he decreased the physical stressor (coffee) and the mental stressor (feeling stuck in an unsatisfying job).

Gradually the ulcers began resolving and Brent got a new job. He no longer needs sick days, doctor's visits, or medication. Through the self-inquiry process Brent found his medical problem was being made worse by diet and work stress. Clarifying the problem and taking personal action not only helped to heal his ulcer, it changed his whole life.

A nine-year study published in *The American Journal of Epidemiology* on social networks reported that people with the lowest number of social ties were two to three times as likely to get sick as those with more social connectedness. A series of studies of weekly support groups by psychiatrist David Spiegel, M.D., at Stanford University demonstrated that women with breast cancer who participated in these groups lived twice as long as those who did not. His extensively documented research shows that health support groups create effective, measurable positive health outcomes.

Working within a group can support the process of improvement. A group can provide expanded resources for information, feedback, coping skills, experiences, testimonials, accountability, and support. It can help us grow and improve both by encouraging us and challenging us to stretch.

The Power of Self-Inquiry

Self-inquiry is a master key that opens the door to the discovery of the inner self. Self-inquiry initiates a profound process of awareness. There is a saying: "If you are aware, you are halfway there!"

In the support group work we have found that people often experience great relief simply by identifying their challenges. Without clarity a person can feel powerless and directionless. Self-inquiry consists of posing questions for ourselves and carrying on an inner dialogue. This creates an opportunity to review all that we have learned, read, experienced, or intuited regarding the issue. By consciously inquiring within we often find we have more information than we have realized. Asking questions of ourselves enhances insight, consciousness, and clarity.

This process can create a kind of self-awareness and is also useful in assessing medical issues. We can use self-inquiry to evaluate what we're doing that improves our health, and identify those things that may be moving us in the wrong direction, whether they involve food choices, stress, or whatever. It can help us sort out our level of improvement and whether we need to seek additional medical resources, collect more health information, seek alternative approaches, or implement new heath strategies. It's also important to identify periods when no progress is being made and new solutions are needed.

The Power of Testimonial: Telling and Hearing Stories

We're so incredibly influenced by each other and our stories that the power of testimony is big medicine. When people share how they've implemented self-care practices in their lives or were able to discontinue a damaging behavior, it proves that it can be done. It proves that someone who is no greater than ourselves has been able to achieve a breakthrough.

When someone expresses real insight on how they're getting their life to work, our ears get bigger and our listening deepens! When we see someone with challenges similar to our own making good lifestyle choices and feeling better, there's an automatic sense of inspiration. It gives us the courage and permission to take action ourselves. When we see someone having a breakthrough with their health, their relationships, or in some other area, it reminds us that this possibility is available to us as well. We are each other's mirrors.

We see evidence of the effectiveness of shared experience in the many thousands of success stories from Alcoholics Anonymous. The strength of this movement is built on the power of sharing. Another example of highly effective informal support is the Chinese Cancer Recovery Society, which has millions of members who meet in small groups in parks throughout China. The format of their gatherings includes self-healing practices such as Qigong, having tea together, sharing stories of recovery, and laughter! The impact of the gatherings on members is remarkable.

The Power of Intention: Goals and Readiness for Change

Intention is defined as "having the mind focused on a specific purpose; the course of action one intends to follow; anything intended—an ultimate end." Clarifying one's intention can provide the energy, insight, and information to design a map to one's desired destination.

The Chinese character for intention means "voice of the heart mind," implying both feeling and thought. In China the heart and mind are not viewed as separate, but considered together as one thing. Developing intentions with both heart and mind energy can create goals that reflect our deeper core values.

The terms *intention* and *goal* have similar meanings with subtle differences. Some people associate goals with stress and great effort—something difficult to attain. Focusing on intention can free up the negative connotations often associated with goal setting, yet have the same powerful impact on your process.

Intention and goal setting involve skills worthy of constant refinement. Most people are adrift in an ocean of details. Targeting areas of improvement and purposefully setting goals toward their fulfillment can bring a greater sense of order to the chaos of life. The Circle of Life (see page 457) can be used to enrich the process of goal setting.

An important step in this process involves preparing for change. The Circle of Life includes a useful tool, the Readiness for Change assessment. This tool helps prepare people for change and helps them focus their actions in order to reduce the chances of failure, disappointment, and low self-esteem. The major disappointments in life are often tied to overly ambitious goals that are set in stone or too unrealistic to attain. The weight of such goals can be exhausting. Choosing the most appropriate goals prepares participants for greater success and builds their confidence for taking future action steps as each success reinforces the sense of their own abilities. Over time this useful approach can become internalized, occurring without conscious effort.

Careful assessment and planning is the best way to clarify your intentions and set goals that you can achieve. But even to meet the goal is an effective way to refine or clarify your action steps. When one sets a goal too high, it does not imply failure. It only shows that the particular goal needs to be broken down into smaller, more achievable steps. In some cases old goals must be released and new ones created. Each time we address the process of setting, clarifying, and refining goals, we have an opportunity to hone our skills in a process of continuous improvement.

The Power of Focused Action

An action taken at the right time can mean the difference between easy and impossible. Deciding to quit smoking on the day before your income tax audit may be bad timing. But quitting smoking might be better when the audit is over and you can go cycling to occupy your hands and exercise your lungs. Deciding to start walking every day may be bad timing if it's January in Chicago. But walking outside every day in late April in Chicago is perfect.

It's also helpful for most people to remember that an action step can be broken into smaller, more attainable steps. Taking one small step in the direction of achieving a goal is a setup for success! While we realize this most of the time, when we are mired in chronic illness the burdens can be overwhelming—physical, medical, financial, social, family, relationships, logistics, and quality of life. This may be the time to use this stepwise action approach.

Weight loss is a good example. The goal of losing 25 pounds can be daunting, but if it's broken down into 52 weekly steps, it's much easier to approach. That's less than half a pound a week. Then rather than trying to do it all by dieting, divide up the process. Part of the half pound can come off from eating the right foods, part from exercise, and part by using positive affirmations. Some can be taken off through breathing exercises that accelerate your metabolism, and some from drinking herb teas that improve digestion. That's five different strategies to address the half a pound a week. Stepwise goals reduce problems down to human scale.

The Power Of Affirmation

When we acknowledge the barriers we face, it may become easier to create strategies for overcoming them. We may find our own attitudes, behaviors, and negative internal dialogue are slowing our progress. It's important to be sure we're not self-saboteurs or that someone else in our life isn't unconsciously sabotaging us. One of the most powerful tools for eliminating this internal negativity is the use of positive self-messages, also known as affirmations. Replacing negative self-talk with positive affirmations creates new possibilities and breakthroughs.

Research has demonstrated that carefully constructed affirmations cause shifts in the internal chemistry of the body, particularly brain chemistry and immune function. Dr. Candace Pert, a respected research scientist at the National Institutes of Health, has said, "The body is the outward manifestation of the mind." Simply stated, an affirmative thought or attitude neutralizes a negative thought. Acknowledging the barriers to the fulfillment of your goal can help you to create the affirmations and actions that may ultimately clear the negative energy.

The Power of Accountability

Accountability helps to sharpen the awareness of how we live our lives and how to better manage our time. Accountability, in a safe environment, can have a profound effect on our ability to set more realistic goals and action steps. Accountability gives us support and motivation to keep our commitments to our goals, priorities, and purpose. The objective is to practice external accountability in order to develop a more internalized accountability to oneself.

HOW SUPPORT GROUPS WORK

The goal of the group process is to provide support for participants and give them the opportunity to realize what they need to heal faster. So when we first meet we talk about what it is that everyone wants from the group and what it is that they need in their lives in terms of support. The groups start with a self-inquiry process. I use a diagram I call the Circle of Life, which has twelve major components of life, including self-care, stress mastery, relationship, finances, spirituality, work, and life purpose. First we just look at our lives and evaluate the areas that are strong and those that need support. What do you need? Do you need tools or skills or information or emotional support?

When we don't feel well, it's as if there's a drain on our life energy. It's like being in a boat with holes in it. You know that your goal is to get well so you have a clear destination, but you sense that there's a leak. Sometimes it's a slow leak, but when it becomes a big hole you feel yourself sinking. So you want to find out what is leaking your energy. And sometimes just having an illness itself is a big energy drain, because it takes tremendous energy for the body to heal itself and to cope. Stress may even be one of the causes of the illness. Being closely involved with someone who is extremely negative tends to deepen an illness. So we look at relationships and also identify sources of support.

This assessment process is important. A lot of times when we're not well we tend to feel overwhelmed by everything. So we ask, Where is the drain? What's draining your life force, your energy, your power, your motivation? And what will shift the balance? What strengthens your joy, your health, your peace of mind, your self-acceptance? What supports you? We look at all the different aspects of one's life to see where we need to put the energy.

A Safe Place

It can be nurturing to take part in a support group, where you know other people are having some very similar experiences and where there's no judgment. That's one of the most essential requirements—that you feel you're in a safe environment. The group must be a place where people understand because they're going through a similar experience. When you have safety there's the potential for healing. There's always healing where we feel comfortable, because then we're not using energy to override our emotions, we're not overextending ourselves, and we're not trying to prove anything. We can just be really real.

Steps Toward Healing

The main focus of the group is to acknowledge what's happening in each person's life and where she needs support.

1. First, there's a time of self-inquiry and self-evaluation, looking at your whole life, to ask what gives you energy, what drains your energy. We want to start sealing up the leaks in the boat.
2. After the inquiry process we move forward by focusing on our strengths. When you're sick sometimes that becomes your identity, who you feel you are as a person. And of course that's not the essential you. Even if people are experiencing a major health challenge, they still have their gifts and their strengths. So everyone begins their involvement in the group by sharing their greatest strengths; they may have a spiritual focus or know a lot about nutrition, or have a strong sense of life purpose. By connecting with each other's strengths, we also realize the resources that each member brings to the group, which we can learn and grow from.
3. At that point each person decides where he or she needs support.
4. Then we will draw on the strengths we've seen in each of us to provide support in areas where people need it.

THE CIRCLE OF LIFE

The Circle of Life is the name we have chosen for our approach to the support group process. We use a diagram of a circle that reflects all of the basic aspects of life as a tool for the self-assessment of strengths and needs. The circle serves as a kind of reminder we can come back to, that shows us where we're making progress and where we still need more resources and support. The Circle of Life can be used in a number of ways:

- In a group setting the circle is the gathering of participants, the group or team, that cooperates to improve and support each other. In this context the circle is the contemporary offspring of the ancient council circle or the meeting of the clan. It is also an expression of the breakthrough models for collaboration, such as quality circles, that are being implemented in corporate settings.
- As a self-improvement coaching method, the circle is a method of coaching or mentorship that can be used by individuals, partners, or teams to encourage continuous personal improvement, cycle after cycle.
- As a visual image, which can be used in a process of self-inquiry to assess where we are in each of the major aspects of our lives.

The Circle of Life represents twelve of the primary areas of our existence, focusing on:

Nutrition	Financial health
Exercise and fitness	Play and creativity
Stress mastery	Environment and nature
Self-care	Emotional life
Relationships	Life purpose and service
Work and career	Spirituality and intuition

At the end of the chapter is a copy of the Circle of Life Assessment. We encourage you to explore the value of the circle as a self-assessment tool. You may also want to seek out a certified Circle of Life facilitator in your area.

How to Use this Tool

The Circle of Life can be used in a stepwise journey by assessing where we are, setting goals, and taking action. When we revisit the circle, we have a chance to celebrate successes and set new goals. One of the most powerful concepts in the Circle of Life process is the idea of flexible goal setting, involving a range of goals—working goals, temporary goals, trial goals, and goals that

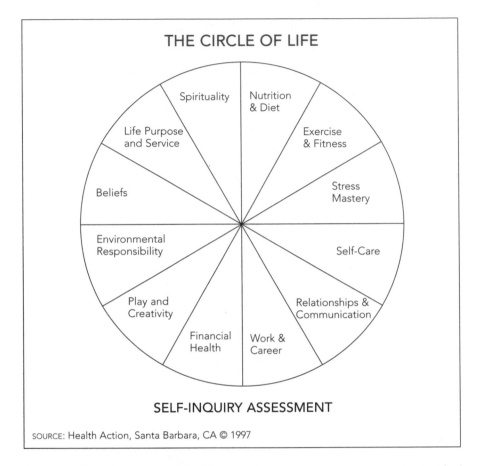

THE CIRCLE OF LIFE

Spirituality

Nutrition & Diet

Life Purpose and Service

Exercise & Fitness

Beliefs

Stress Mastery

Environmental Responsibility

Self-Care

Play and Creativity

Relationships & Communication

Financial Health

Work & Career

SELF-INQUIRY ASSESSMENT

SOURCE: Health Action, Santa Barbara, CA © 1997

give new directions a try. Working goals are constantly changed, clarified, refined, and even retired. These working goals are part of what makes the circle a fail-safe system. When people are encouraged and supported in a continual process of modifying their goals, this provides alternatives to goals that don't seem to be working. The process offers an opportunity to:

- Decide on your intentions and goals.
- Clarify and refine the goals.
- Acknowledge the physical, mental, emotional, situational, and relationship challenges that could keep you from attaining your goals.
- Design powerful positive affirmations (self-messages) that support your intentions.
- Select measurable, attainable action steps.
- Design your action steps, breaking them down to the right size and pace, to guarantee successful outcomes and gradual but assured improvement.

- Set up accountability by stating your action step to the group or to another person.

Setting a goal effectively requires careful and insightful assessment of the situation. Goals that are not carefully set may be too big or even inappropriate—and harder to fulfill. On the other hand, clarifying and refining goals increases the chances for success by providing essential information: obstacles that need to be cleared, possible alternative options, and a realistic expectation of the time it will take to implement improvements and action steps.

The breakthrough secret of the Circle of Life process is remembering that when a goal is broken down into small, realistic action steps and time frames, it may be transformed from a challenging possibility to a manageable probability. And the strength gained from the group, from the circle of support, is literally a joining of energy—an opportunity to share group energy.

Rebecca McLean is the National Director of the Circle of Life Facilitator Certification training. She trains individuals to be facilitators and coaches for support groups in hospitals, clinics, senior programs, schools, parishes, government agencies, and businesses. She also leads weekend group programs at retreat centers and spas.

Ms. McLean has worked in health care for more than 25 years. She has facilitated thousands of group sessions for people with chronic illness, including cancer, HIV, chronic fatigue, MS, and diabetes. Life coaching is another focus of her work, and she has facilitated both group and individuals seeking health, healing, transformation, and joy. Contact her at www.circleoflife.net, rmclean@west.net, (805) 685-4670, or Rebecca McLean, 243 Pebble Beach Drive, Santa Barbara, CA, 93117.

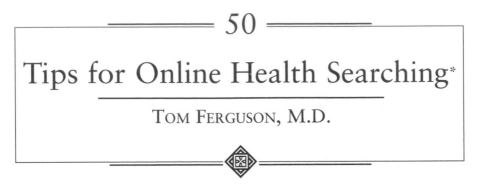

50

Tips for Online Health Searching*

TOM FERGUSON, M.D.

On a typical day more than five million Americans go online looking for health information and advice. Our surveys at the Pew Internet & American Life Project show that more Internet users have sought medical information on the Web than have used it for shopping, stock quotes, or sports scores. Here are a few pieces of advice I often share with lay audiences in my lectures and workshops on online health:

- *Don't search alone.* If the world of online health is new to you or you are dealing with a frightening or poorly understood new diagnosis, ask a Web-savvy friend or family member to sit by your side and show you the ropes the first few times you go online. And even if you are an experienced Web user, you may be able to benefit from the help and support of friends or family members who can help you extend your own search efforts and interpret the things you find.

- *Double-check the information you find online.* Check several sites to make sure they all give the same or similar information. If you still have doubts, post a question at an online discussion group. Or e-mail a question to an online health professional or to the Webmaster of a site devoted to your condition.

- *Be on the lookout for other online patients who share your concerns.* The Web is a wonderful place to look things up—and unlike print sources, it often makes it easy to connect with online authors. If you find a useful Web site, consider sending an e-mail to the Webmaster. And be sure to keep an eye out for online patient-helpers who specialize in your concerns. Patients with the same disease may be able to offer a kind of comfort and commonsense perspective that even your closest friends and family members cannot.

- *If you are dealing with a serious illness, consider joining an online support group.* Knowing that your online friends are walking the same path

*An earlier version of this chapter by Dr. Ferguson appeared in *The Millennium Whole Earth Catalog* and online at www.healthonline.com and is included courtesty of the author.

and are seeking both to give and to receive support helps most online self-helpers feel comfortable in establishing meaningful online relationships based on trust and mutual concern.

- *Use the Net to stay connected with your own intimate network of family members and friends.* The Net can be a powerful tool for staying in touch with those who mean the most to you. Family members, friends, and friends of friends may be able to help in unexpected ways. When you're going through an illness, keeping up with calls from well-wishers can sometimes become a burden. Consider sending out periodic e-mail bulletins to keep loved ones up to date on how you're doing.

- *Use the Internet to get referrals to the doctors and treatment centers you need.* You can frequently use sites devoted to specific diseases to find the top specialists and treatment centers for your condition. You may even be able to correspond directly with leading specialists and researchers by e-mail.

- *Use the Internet to supplement your face-to-face doctor visits, not to replace them.* It isn't always easy to interpret what you find. A frank and open discussion with your physician may help to clear up some of your uncertainties. The best-case scenario is for doctors and patients to work together, as a coordinated team.

- *Tell your doctor what you've found online.* The better you communicate your questions and needs, the better your doctor will be able to respond to them. Be assertive rather than aggressive; express your feelings and your views honestly and openly while showing respect for your health care provider.

- *If some doctors aren't quite ready to become Net-friendly physicians, try to understand.* Many doctors feel so swamped by clinical responsibilities, paperwork demands, and their own pressing financial concerns that it can be difficult for them to see the benefit of spending additional time exchanging e-mails with patients or discussing information you've found online.

- *Apply what you've learned.* The Internet is a two-way street. You can—and I hope you will use the Net to find valuable information and advice for your own health concerns. But once you have your own situation under control, you may well discover that the things you've learned now make it possible for you to provide important help to fellow patients. I would hope that if and when the time is right, you will remember how you were helped and will reach out a helping hand to others.

Biographical information for **Tom Ferguson, M.D.,** appears on page 437.

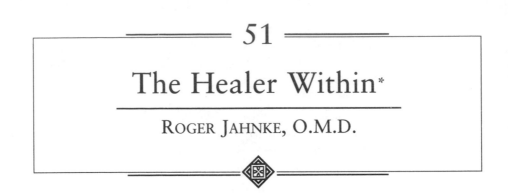

51

The Healer Within*

ROGER JAHNKE, O.M.D.

The marvelous pharmacy that was designed by nature and placed into our being by the universal architect produces most of the medicines that we need.

—NORMAN COUSINS, AUTHOR OF
ANATOMY OF AN ILLNESS AS PERCEIVED BY THE PATIENT

Your body, in cooperation with your mind and spirit, is marvelously blessed with miraculous self-healing abilities. The body is the temple of your life. Mind and spirit are the dwellers within the temple. Mind and spirit maintain the temple. Mind's intelligence and spirit's inspiration vitalize and quicken the body. The three together—body, mind, and spirit—cooperate to produce the most profound medicine ever known in the history of the human race, right within you.

THE BODY'S NATURAL ABILITY TO HEAL

Injuries or illnesses heal naturally when self-healing resources are operating optimally. When you cut yourself the wound heals automatically. When you have a sprain or bruise it heals automatically. When you have a broken bone the physician must set the bone correctly, but then nature heals it spontaneously. The famous sixteenth-century physician Ambroise Pare said, "I administered the treatment, but nature provided the cure."

I had a personal experience of this as a child. Through a series of sports accidents, one of my front teeth was broken off to half its length. While the planning for a cap for the tooth was in process, the tooth actually began to grow. Over six months this tooth grew until it was as long as the other, unbroken front tooth. Some unexplained interaction of forces and elements caused this healing event to occur.

This remarkable gift belongs to every person from birth. It is a wondrous self healing mechanism that has been built into us by the architect of the universe from the beginning of all life. Unfortunately most people have not known about this gift; it has been a secret. Freeing the potential of self-healing in your own life can have marvelous effects. The essential resources for healing, which are naturally occurring within each individual, can be activated purposefully through your own efforts.

When our natural healing ability does not function automatically, it means that something is wrong. Our spontaneous self-healing resources have become damaged or disordered. (So one important aspect of healing is removing any blockages to the functioning of the immune system and restoring it to maximum capacity, while providing the nutritional raw materials the body needs to heal.)

In mild cases these self-healing methods may replace the need for medication—for example, when there is a stress headache, occasional constipation, a cold, aches and pains, insomnia, or anxiety. Even when medicine becomes necessary, self-healing methods complement and support the treatment.

Many techniques and methods for self-healing are quite ancient. Spontaneous self-healing ability is not a dramatic new scientific discovery. Nor is it a New Age phenomenon. There are stories of deep conviction in the Judeo-Christian traditions regarding the healing resources that we have within ourselves. In China and India—and in the ancient Americas, Australia, Africa, and Europe, rich traditions of self-care and self-healing have existed since long before written history. One of the first things I learned about in the study of traditional Chinese medicine was Qi (Chi), which is the name for the medicine within. One of the processes of cultivating the medicine within is called Qigong (Chi Kung).

The naturally occurring self-healing ability of your own body, mind, and spirit is your greatest healing resource. This means that you can reduce your own risk of disease. If you have lost your health and are challenged by illness, you can contribute to your own healing. You can use this healing power as part of any healing process, including the efforts you make in cooperation with your physician to speed your recovery.

THE ESSENCE OF SELF-HEALING

The physician who teaches people to sustain their health is the superior physician. The physician who waits to treat people until after their health is lost is considered to be inferior. This is like waiting until one's family is starving to begin to plant seeds in the garden.

—Yellow Emperor's Classic on Internal Medicine, 500 b.c.e.

Three areas, all based on personal choice and personal action, maximize the activity of our naturally occurring self-healing capability.

- *The first is our choice of attitudes and mental influences.* When we choose to think, believe, and act from a position of power, refusing to be a victim of circumstances, the healer within is automatically strengthened. When we refuse to live under the influence of worry and doubt, the internal medicine is enriched.
- *The second area of choice is lifestyle.* This encompasses nutrition, exercise, rest, relationships, finances, work, spiritual practice, play, water intake, avoidance of alcohol and cigarettes, and so on. From moment to moment each of us personally elects whether to enhance or sabotage the healer within, through our own behaviors and personal choices. In my practice of acupuncture and Chinese medicine I have found that the people who don't take care of themselves are typically the most difficult patients to treat successfully. These are the people who dislike their work, don't take time to play, or have poor self-esteem and communication skills. In such cases, although the acupuncture usually activates the healer within, the person's life situation tends to neutralize their self-healing capacity.
- *The third area of choice is personal self-care.* This involves practices of self-healing and health enhancement methods. Self-care involves gentle movement (such as Qigong or yoga), essential breathing practices, hand and foot massage (as in reflexology), and deep relaxation and meditation practices. These are tools for improving and sustaining the immune system and supporting the function of the healer within. Self-care practices, positive attitudes, and proactive lifestyle complement and enhance each other. I predict that these three areas—attitude, lifestyle, and self-care—will be the foundation on which health care and healing are built in the twenty-first century.

When these aspects of personal choice keep health and healing active in a person's life, they have less need to go to a clinic or hospital. When the healer within is strong and efficient self-healing can progress. Empowered by knowledge and inspiration to take action, each individual becomes the principal source of health, healing, and stress mastery.

The status of attitude, lifestyle, and self-care is noticeable in people's lives. It is fairly obvious when an individual is under the influence of self-doubt, poor nutrition, and a lack of exercise. It is equally obvious when an individual is influenced by enthusiasm, purposeful work, and the regular practice of health enhancement methods. The first person is typically exhausted and frustrated, the other radiant and energetic. One is a victim, the other a leader and a role model. One is part of the problem, the other part of the solution.

ENGAGING THE HEALER WITHIN

Spontaneous remission is the phrase often used in the medical literature to describe cases in which a disease is cured or resolved but no one understands how. In the decades to come the mechanism for spontaneous remission will be vigorously explored and will probably be better understood. For now it is not so important how it happens; it is just enlightening that it does happen.

In situations in which complete healing has occurred, although no one knows exactly how it occurred, it is possible that internal healing resources have been spontaneously activated. In the 1980s the Institute of Noetic Sciences decided to explore the remission concept as a possible strategy to confirm the human capacity for self-healing. Brendan O'Regan, then the vice president of research, began a systematic exploration of the medical literature for references to remission. To everyone's amazement he found an immense number of references: three thousand articles from more than 860 medical journals, in twenty languages. Some of the articles discussed hundreds of cases, so the overall number of cases actually reported in the literature turned out to be in the many thousands.

"We have many cases of remission (one-fifth of all cases) with no medical intervention at all. These are the purest ones, the ones that give us the strongest evidence that there is an extraordinary self-repair system lying dormant within us" (O'Regan, 1995). This historic analysis of the literature on remission from the Institute of Noetic Sciences is a powerful confirmation of the healer within.

To accelerate our naturally occurring healing capability is actually quite easy. Once we replace the idea that health improvement comes only from external sources with the knowledge that healing can come from the healer within, the practice of self-healing methods is simply logical.

> *There must be some primal force,*
> *but it is impossible to find.*
> *I believe it exists, but cannot see it.*
> *I see its results, I can even feel it,*
> *But it has no form.*

—CHANG T'SU, PHILOSOPHER, POET, FOURTH CENTURY B.C.E.

Biographical information for **Roger Jahnke, O.M.D.,** appears on page 412.

52

The Proactive Patient

Nancy Faass, MSW, MPH

DECIDING ON YOUR NEXT STEP

In order to get well, it's important to identify the resources you need.

- A diagnosis or more information?
- A second opinion on your treatment or pending surgery?
- A plan for self-monitoring to find out what's working and what isn't?
- Support to carry out a complicated regimen?

WORKING WITH A GOOD PROFESSIONAL

Even doctors don't treat themselves. Seek out a health care professional who is knowledgeable and highly informed. You want someone who understands your condition through experience and training—and also intuitively.

It's important that you work with a practitioner with whom you have a meaningful dialogue—who listens to you, answers questions, offers advice, and discusses options. It is essential to work cooperatively with him or her in sorting out your problem. It is the interplay, the feedback between the practitioner's insight and yours, that may uncover the solution to your illness.

You may also find it important to work with more than one practitioner. They must know the generalities of your condition—the therapies used to treat it and the typical response. But it's utterly impossible for them to predict how your particular body will respond. Since they cannot be with you every hour of every day, and you probably couldn't afford it if they could, you become their eyes. It will be up to you to observe your responses, to see when the shifts toward healing occur. Find ways to record what is needed to measure change in your condition—keep a log, a food diary, or a journal. You must be the one to watch for downturns and report on how you turned them around, or how aspects of your illness refused to be remedied. It's important to catch each problem soon after you begin to slide away from health, to keep you on a healing path.

The Challenges of Chronic Illness

Once there was a great man who was loved by millions for the beautiful music he created. He had friends all over the world and an adoring wife with whom he was very close. One day he came home, walked up the stairs to his room, closed the door, and did not come down for a year. His wife pleaded with him (through the door) to return to his work, to join her for dinner. She reminded him that his audiences missed him. But the man could not be dissuaded. A year later he resumed his work and his family life, and pronounced himself cured of the illness so frustrating, so humiliating, he would not even discuss it—digestive disease.

Does this story have a familiar ring? Have you ever wished you had the resources to simply close the door on life because you too have digestive illness? If so you are not alone. Ninety million Americans suffer with digestive disease, according to the National Institutes of Health. Worldwide, about three million people die each year from GI infection and diarrhea-related conditions. A large percentage of them are children.

For many, digestive illness can be so limiting that they become unable to work, to socialize, or to carry on the simplest activities of the day, to do things most of us have so taken for granted. Even in their mildest form, digestive disorders are confining. Imagine something important that you want to accomplish and then imagine trying to do it well while suffering from diarrhea or constipation. Could you deliver a speech effectively? Negotiate a contract powerfully? Get your work done rapidly? Could you flirt? Have fun at the beach . . . or anywhere?

Yet digestive illness is beyond the range of polite social discourse—and therefore an illness for which it can be difficult to rally support. If you broke your arm you could get tremendous sympathy and encouragement. Everyone would ask what happened, sign your cast, offer you advice, and wish you well. And next week they would want to know how you were doing. In contrast, it's difficult to imagine, for example, discussing a colonoscopy, even with family members. And research shows that for some people these issues are so taboo, they would literally rather die than discuss them with their doctor.

If you have chronic digestive illness this book was written for you. Our goal is to provide you with all the important, safe, and effective new resources that are now available in integrative medicine and coming into the fore. Soon, we expect that nutritional medicine (healing through nutrition) will be broadly available, and your own family doctor or internist will be using the new lab testing and nutrients for your healing.

But your illness is now, limiting each day as the clock ticks away. So we want to place these resources at your disposal, for your consideration. We wish you well.

STATING YOUR OWN TRUTH

Create an alliance with your doctor and become a powerful team—go for a balance between respecting your doctor's advice and not abandoning what you believe to be true from your own experience. Tactfully, politely, state your own truth, your perceptions, your experience.

If you have approached your relationship with your doctor or practitioner in this spirit and it isn't working, you may want to bring along a patient advocate on your next office visit or bring your mate or your best friend. If that doesn't change the dynamic, it's time to seek a second opinion.

WHAT YOU CAN DO FOR YOURSELF

You have to want to get well—no one else can make that commitment for you. Be as realistic as you can, because denial will cheat you of the information you need to heal. Never give up hope. Positive thoughts can be healing, and despair may aggravate your condition.

- *Educate yourself.* Make use of books, the Internet, Medline, your public library, and the medical library, as well as the media.
- *Get copies of your own records.* Legally you have a right to them. Remember that ultimately you will experience the impact of all medical decisions about your care far more than anyone else involved.
- *Become highly self-observant.* To the degree that you can, come out of denial so you can accurately discern what's going on with your body and your situation. This can be harder than it sounds. As much as you can, reconnect with your body so that you can feel where there's pain and when things aren't working. This information is vital to the healing process.
- *Consider making just one change at a time—one change a week.* This will help you determine what is most effective for your unique body, chemistry, and genetics. For example, of the thousands of nutrients and herbs on the market, what helps you thrive? Which cause reactions? What can you afford? Which work only short-term and which can be taken long-term?
- *If you want to take an herb, begin slowly and check with your practitioner.* Are you taking a drug? Again be mindful. Check with your pharmacist to avoid multidrug interactions. Use informed judgment, common sense, an open mind, and healthy skepticism in all you do.
- *Ask for what you need.* Advocate for yourself impartially, as objectively as possible. Be assertive but not aggressive. Take good care of yourself.

GETTING A SECOND OPINION

Integrative medicine is based on the same scientific information used in mainstream medicine. The same science forms the basis for understanding and diagnosing illness but the therapies are frequently different. They are milder and more natural, and therefore slower acting, involving healing through nutrition, herbs, or even lifestyle.

The emphasis is also different; it involves another way of looking at the same information. One example is that in treating GI illness, practitioners of complementary medicine place more emphasis on treating GI disorders due to bacteria, yeast, parasites, and viruses. It continues to surprise us that this emphasis should come from the alternative side, since Western medicine is based on an understanding of pathogenic microbes and the use of antibiotic (antibacterial) medications. Yet mainstream labs and doctors continue to overlook the issue of infection and consider it simply a problem of underdeveloped countries, rather than a frequent aspect of digestive illness in our overcrowded big cities.

Integrative medicine offers a range of strategies that can be helpful in treating digestive disorders, including:

- *Immune support.* Complementary practitioners focus on supporting the immune system. This means providing the raw materials the body needs to heal—good nutrition and nutritional supplements, clean air, water, and food, rest and relaxation, and gentle exercise.
- *Functional medicine.* This approach focuses on restoring proper function to organs and cells. It can also involve minimizing toxins, eliminating allergenic foods, and restoring GI processes using nutritional supplements.
- *Complementary therapies.* Acupuncture unblocks the energy and circulation in the body and stimulates the vital force. Homeopathy also focuses on stimulating the vital force, using minute doses of nontoxic remedies.

When to get a second opinion? If you find that you're not getting well or if your doctor is scheduling you for major surgery and you're not sure that's what you want, get a second opinion from a doctor who practices integrative medicine—nutritional, functional, orthomolecular, or naturopathic medicine. To find an integrative physician check the Resources for organizations that provide practitioner referrals. Here are a few places to start:

- The American College for the Advancement of Medicine (nutritional medicine)
- The American Academy of Environmental Medicine
- Bastyr University (for trained naturopaths)

- The Institute for Functional Medicine
- The Society for Orthomolecular Health-Medicine (nutritional medicine)

BEGIN WHERE YOU ARE

When we get sick, we want to know what is wrong and what we can do about it. This is the basis of rational treatment. However, in some cases this is not possible.

In functional medicine, for example, you do not need a firm diagnosis to take the first steps toward healing. This is the value of functional testing, which evaluates impaired function rather than tissue damage and pathology. This emphasis makes it possible to focus on restoring function. Nutrition, acupuncture, and homeopathy can also promote healing in situations in which the diagnosis is unclear. As you know from this book, there are many other effective strategies for healing and many excellent resources.

MAKE PEACE WITH YOUR ILLNESS

Love your body; respect all the parts and functions of you, even when they don't seem glamorous. If you can, take high pleasure in the food you eat, and respect the importance of keeping your body clean and clear. Appreciate the intricacies of your body, value the importance of your stomach acid and mucus, and treasure all the other seemingly mundane miracles that make your life possible each day. These are the mechanisms through which your body works. Respect and honor them. Remember that you are your own best advocate.

If I am not for myself then who will be for me?
If I am for myself alone, then what am I?
If not now, when?

—HILLEL

Biographical information for **Nancy Faass, MSW, MPH,** appears on page 386.

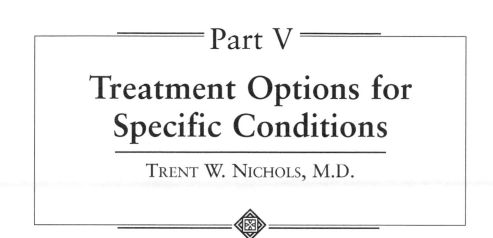

Part V

Treatment Options for Specific Conditions

Trent W. Nichols, M.D.

TREATMENT OPTIONS DIRECTORY

Bacterial Overgrowth / *See* chapter 21

Cancer of the Colon / 473

Cancer of the Pancreas / *See* Pancreatic Cancer

Candida (Yeast Overgrowth) / 477

Celiac Disease (Sprue) / 481

Cirrhosis / 485

Constipation (Chronic) / 488

Crohn's Disease / *See* Inflammatory Bowel Diseases (IBD)

Diarrhea (Chronic) / 494

Diverticulosis and Diverticulitis / 499

Dyspepsia—Without Ulcers / 502

Disorders of the Esophagus / *See* Reflux and Heartburn—GERD

Fibromyalgia / 504

Fissures / 510

Fistulas / 511

Food Allergies / 512

Gallstones / 512

Gastritis / 517

Heartburn / *See* Reflux and Heartburn—GERD

Hemorrhoids / 520

Hepatitis (Chronic) / 523

Indigestion (Chronic) / *See* Dyspepsia—Without Ulcers

Inflammatory Bowel Diseases (IBD): Ulcerative Colitis and Crohn's Disease / 526

Irritable Bowel Syndrome (IBS) / 532

Lactose Intolerance / 537

Liver Disease / 538

Malabsorption / 544

Pancreatic Cancer / 546

Pancreatitis / 548

Parasites/Parasitic Infection / *See* chapter 21

Pruritus Ani / 551

Reflux and Heartburn—GERD (Gastroesophageal Reflux Disease) / 551

Strictures and Structural Conditions / 557

Ulcers/Ulcer Disease / 560

Ulcerative Colitis / *See* Inflammatory Bowel Diseases (IBD)

Viral Bowel Disease / *See* chapter 22

BACTERIAL OVERGROWTH

See chapter 21

CANCER OF THE COLON

Malignant tumor of the large intestine: A malignant growth that invades surrounding tissue may spread throughout the body, and can potentially reoccur. Cancer of the colon can be fatal.

Causes

The incidence of gastrointestinal cancer has been associated with diets high in fat and sugar and low in fiber. In societies that traditionally have a low incidence of colon cancer, such as the Japanese, it has been found that when people begin to eat a Westernized diet of refined foods and high fat, the prevalence of colon cancer increases and becomes comparable to that of industrial nations with diets of refined foods.

Increased fat intake has been found to be a factor because fats are subject to free radical damage. Saturated fats stimulate at least one gene that promotes inflammatory messengers (prostaglandins) shown to initiate the cancer process.

Certain illnesses tend to be associated with increased risk for colon cancer:

- IBD (inflammatory bowel disease).
- Ulcerative colitis of more than ten years' duration.
- Crohn's disease.
- Inflammation that lasts for an extended period of time.
- Genetic factors.
- Breast cancer.
- Obesity, inactivity, and constipation.
- The presence of polyps: Patients with numerous polyps have such a high rate of colon cancer that by age 30, almost all have diagnosed colon cancer. The two primary medical interventions for this condition have been colon removal at a young age or the use of a drug (sulindac, Clinoril) that inhibits the production of an overly reactive immune response by the prostaglandins. Aspirin also decreases the risk of colon cancer. Cigarette smoking can be a factor in both polyp development and the incidence of colon cancer, so it is important to stop smoking.

People with constipation and slower colonic transit time are more prone to colon cancer. Therefore take constipation seriously and seek professional help if you find this condition has lasted for more than one month.

Early Detection

Routine screening for polyps is an excellent preventive measure and should include direct examination of the colon via colonoscopy. Polyps are benign nubbins that grow in the colon. The development of cancer is believed to occur about ten years after polyps begin developing. If the polyps are removed the potential for cancer is decreased. Therefore routine screening and periodic polyp removal are important. This early intervention, which should begin at age 50, has the support of about half the medical insurance companies in covering the expense of the examination.

Hemoccult blood testing of the stool looks for hidden blood in the stool. Given the increased risk of colon cancer this should be done yearly after age 20. However, this test is not always totally accurate. If there is a family history of colon or breast cancer or if there is a positive result on the test for blood in the stool, colonoscopy should be performed, and then periodic screenings should be begun.

Flexible sigmoidoscopy is another useful form of monitoring, done every three years from age 40 on. This provides direct examination of the lower two feet of the colon and should be done for both men and women. This can be performed by your primary-care physician. However, reliance on this examination alone is unwise, since it misses two-thirds of the colon. An air-contrast barium enema may be added, but this combination is not as accurate as colonoscopy.

Early Intervention—Signs and Symptoms

- Rectal bleeding or blood in stool
- Abdominal pain
- Weight loss
- Iron deficiency anemia

Testing

- Stool test for undetected blood (fecal occult blood test—hemoccult).
- Sigmoidoscopy.
- Barium double-contrast enema (X-ray).
- Colonoscopy.
- Virtual colonoscopy (a new CT scan X-ray of the colon, enhanced by computer analysis).
- Blood tests for those who have a history of colon cancer. Testing for carcinoma embryonic antigen (CEA) can reveal an antigen that is a by-product of active cancer. A fecal test for markers of colon cancer is now available, but testing is more than $1,000 and is not usually reimbursed by insurance carriers.

Mainstream Treatment

Prevention and early intervention are still the most important aspects of treatment. The removal of polyps usually interrupts the cancer sequence. Most polyps are initially benign. If polyps are detected early enough, abdominal surgery can be prevented. Polyps are usually removed with a wire snare and cautery during colonoscopy, so this type of surgery usually doesn't require an incision. In cases in which the polyp is too large or the malignancy is too advanced to be removed by snare, surgery through an incision in the abdominal wall is necessary and removal of a section of the bowel is indicated. This procedure, called resection, is used to treat 50 percent of colon cancer; the other 50 percent require adjunct chemotherapy, or in the future will be treated with immunological therapy. Radiation is not generally helpful except in cases of anal-rectal (anorectal) carcinoma. One of the more promising forms of chemotherapy appears to be the drug Campostar. Two new drugs have been approved for advanced colorectal cancer—the monoclonal antibody cetuximab (Erbitux) and the angiogenesis (blood vessel)-inhibiting monoclonal antibody bevacizumab (Avastin).

Surveillance with yearly colonoscopies is essential for those in remission. This is vitally important to detect reoccurrences or new cancers at the earliest stage possible.

Complementary Treatment

In individual cases nutritional therapy has been found useful. Even for people undergoing conventional treatment, excellent nutrition can offer a significant benefit by supporting the body and immune function.

Resources for integrative treatment include the Cancer Treatment Centers of America in Zion, Illinois; Tulsa, Oklahoma; and other cities. These centers have perhaps the broadest experience in this area. They use mainstream approaches such as surgery, radiation, and chemotherapy. They complement these therapies with the use of nutrition, guided imagery, massage, and behavioral therapy.

Other respected centers that use nutrition and alternative therapies include the Block Center in Evanston, Illinois, and the Geffen Cancer Center in Vero Beach, Florida. Some patients have excellent experience with this approach, and in other cases the cancer can not be halted, but for some of these quality of life is improved. Clearly no therapy works for everyone.

Some of the specific alternative-therapy programs that have also been used include the Gerson diet, the Kelly method used by Dr. Nicholas Gonzales in New York City, and the macrobiotic diet as described by Michio Kushi.

Vitamin therapy has been a promising component of nutritional treatment. Specific nutrients found to be important in prevention include vitamins C, D, and E, and the minerals calcium, selenium, and other trace minerals. Research has found that cancer prevention (for example lung cancer in smokers) has not been effective when a single nutrient alone was used in supplement form. Therefore we highly recommend the full complement of vitamins and minerals from natural sources. Since we are all affected by stress and pollution, most people benefit from supplemental nutrients.

Two useful books on this topic are *The Definitive Guide to Cancer* by the Burton Goldberg Group (Future Medicine Press, 1997) and *Choices in Healing* by Michael Lerner (MIT Press, 1997).

Treatment in Development

- Experimental treatment using toxins from the bacteria pseudomonas has been utilized in combination with antibodies in tumor therapy in some cases; this treatment has been evaluated by the National Cancer Institute (NCI). You can call the NCI and get information on new research and new clinical trials. This information is also available on the World Wide Web at www.nih.gov on the page for NCI.
- Urso, used in the treatment of gallstones, has been found to prevent colon cancer; this substance, used in Chinese medicine, is derived from bear bile. It is now available in prescription form under the names Urso or Actigall. Urso tends to decrease secondary bile salts, which are potentially carcinogenic to the body.
- Anti-angiogenesis is a mechanism that contains the spread of cancer, decreasing the metastases of tumors by cutting down on the blood supply to the tumor.

Prevention

- Exercise
- Not smoking
- Avoid sugar and fat, and eat fewer calories and refined carbohydrates
- Increase intestinal motility with fiber, fruits, and vegetables or motility enhancers such as cellulose (FiberCon), bentonite, or aloe vera in capsule form
- The use of probiotics to promote motility and decrease inflammation
- Caltrate, a calcium supplement, has been shown in one study to reduce the incidence of colonic polyps if taken daily

Take any inflammatory condition seriously.

Preventive Diet

For general prevention, good nutrition has been proven to be essential. A preventive diet should include fiber and antioxidants from both fresh foods and a good-quality supplement. Alkalinizing your diet through salads and low-starch vegetables, alkaline water, and liquid chlorophyll (DeSoussa's) is generally health promoting, although not specifically cancer preventive. (See chapter 32—First Aid for Inflammation.) What the research does show is that people who eat fresh fruits and vegetables have about 50 percent the risk of cancer of those who do not.

Flaxseed oil (an omega-3 oil, used as a supplement and for salads) and olive oil (a monounsaturate) can be helpful in preventing the stimulation of the body chemicals that cause inflammation (prostaglandins). Calcium supplements also appear to be preventive, by apparently toning down the genetic mutation that can play a role in cancer (K-*ras*). With this in mind, it is also important to maintain a balanced intake of calcium and magnesium. Antioxidants in general have an important preventive effect that has been proven. Be sure to take antioxidants and trace minerals either individually or in a formula that includes copper, zinc, manganese, and selenium.

Avoid diets that are low in calcium and vitamin D, high in phosphates (such as sodas), and high in fat. Regular aspirin use can help prevent polyps, but is known to cause leaky gut and GI bleeding. Ask your integrative practitioner for Kaprex from Metagenics as an alternative. B complex vitamins are extremely important in minimizing the production of the metabolite homocysteine, which is also carcinogenic.

CANCER OF THE PANCREAS

See Pancreatic Cancer.

CANDIDA (YEAST OVERGROWTH)

Candida is a form of yeastlike fungi normally found in the digestive tract that can overgrow and become too numerous in the intestines; the most frequently occurring species is *Candida albicans*. It can be pathogenic when it becomes too populous, crowding out the beneficial bacteria. This overgrowth can be caused by prolonged use of antibiotics, the use of steroids (prednisone), taking birth control pills, severe infection, or major immunosuppression (such as in AIDS). (A checklist of additional candida causes and symptoms appears in chapter 2.)

The most frequent symptoms of candida include fatigue, irritability when hungry, headache, depression, brain fog, bloating and gas, diarrhea, constipation, itchy bottom or vagina, urinary frequency, sore throat and mouth, severe athlete's foot or fungal toenails, chemical sensitivity, cravings for sugar or alcohol, and food sensitivity.

Causes

- Antibiotic therapy—one of the most frequent causes
- In women elevated hormones due to pregnancy, hormone supplementation, or birth control pills
- Use of prednisone or other immunosuppressant medication
- Mercury from amalgam fillings is a suspected factor
- Depressed immune function in combination with a highly sweet and starchy diet
- Frequent exposure to a high-mold environment
- Parasitic infection
- Candida is particularly prevalent in conjunction with AIDS

There is now medical coding for candidiasis of the colon, which indicates that candida is now recognized as a cause of illness throughout the body. Until recently it was viewed as a disorder primarily of the esophagus and the vagina. Doctors are now beginning to view it as a legitimate health condition throughout the rest of the body.

Yeast in the digestive tract can produce toxins that can promote a variety of symptoms. They also produce alcohol as a by-product in the process of breaking down starches (which can cause brain fog and autointoxication). They can promote an increase in pathogenic enzymes (called proteolytic or protein-digesting enzymes) that allows the candida to invade the tissue elsewhere in the body, as is often seen in cases of AIDS and other conditions of immunosuppression. The journal *Medical Hypothesis* has reported on research suggesting that chronic candidiasis can be associated with some cases of chronic fatigue syndrome.

Diagnosis and Testing

Stool testing typically involves evaluation by microscope or culturing and growing the yeast (for example, a 24-day culture). Species include *Candida albicans* and *Candida glabrata*. Microscopic exam of stool produces information on the type of candida (whether the infection is due to dividing forms, which are considered more disease producing and pathogenic than nondividing forms). Evaluation for candida overgrowth can also be performed through a blood test, which measures antibodies produced by the immune system in its efforts to control the candida.

Some labs also test the yeast to see which antifungals and herbs destroy it (sensitivity testing). (See the resource section for information on medical laboratories.)

Many commercial and hospital labs do not consider yeast to be a problem and do not report it on stool exams.

Mainstream Treatment

- Nystatin, a prescription antifungal medication, is available in capsules, liquid, powder, gels, and a troche (a lozenge). However, when tested for susceptibility, most strains have been resistant to this antifungal and we have not prescribed it in the last five years.
- Diflucan (fluconazole) is another class of medication; it can be very useful but expensive.
- Nizoral (ketoconazole) can be useful but may have accompanying liver toxicity. However, in situations in which a yeast condition is resistant to all the previously mentioned drugs, the risks of ketoconazole may be worth it. Before beginning this medication consider getting the functional-medicine liver detox test. (See testing—chapter 17.) It is also recommended that you get a liver enzyme profile periodically during the therapy to be sure the drug is not causing damage. An additional treatment option for those with resistant yeast is miconazole, available only from compounding pharmacies. (See Resources for information on compounding pharmacies.) Major systemic treatment that supports immune function could be helpful; ask a physician practicing functional/nutritional medicine about such treatment.

Complementary Treatments

Herbs can be alternated with drug therapy or used individually:

- Available from the health food store—garlic oil in capsule form or fresh; oil of oregano; *Pseudo winteracolorata;* grapefruit seed extract (Nutritibiotic); berberine (barberry extract); pau d'arco; tea tree oil. General immune stimulants include echinacea and goldenseal.
- From physicians' offices and compounding pharmacies—Tanalbit; SF-722 (undecylenic acid) by Thorne, in capsules and topical form; combination formulas such as AC Formula by Pure Encapsulations; Candacin by Metagenics; Kolorex by Forest Herbs (available from Lifespan Institute); and gentran violet used as a topical.
- From Chinese medicine—Ganoderma, also called Ling-Zhi (lingshi), is a mushroom imported from China, which tends to removes toxins, may stimulate immunity, and seems to have antibacterial and antifungal properties.

Diet

A diet very low in refined carbohydrates with no sugar is key in gaining control of this condition. Moderate complex carbs and fruit. Avoid foods with fermented content, such as vinegar or pickles. Refer to *The Yeast Connection* by William Crook, *The Body Ecology Diet* by Donna Gates (B.E.D. Publications, 1996), and *Depression: Cured at Last* by Sherry Rogers.

All these authors recommend minimizing the use of antibiotics and prednisone to the degree possible, staying off sweets and starches (simple carbohydrates such as sugar, pastas, and breads), and eating complex carbohydrates in moderation. Avoid any product that contains brewer's yeast or baker's yeast, and minimize other fermented products. Avoid sodas and fruit juice; instead, develop the taste for spring or mineral water, lemon water (hot or cool), and herb tea (hot, iced, or even room temperature).

Nutrients

Take probiotic supplements to restore the friendly flora. This is key. Treatment is not meant to totally rid the body of candida—this is impossible. Rather the goal is to keep the flora in balance and avoid overgrowth. Probiotics, periodically taken, can help maintain this balance. This is important, because yeast can become pathogenic when they overgrow.

Blood sugar and insulin swings tend to be associated with yeast conditions, in part because of deficiencies in the trace minerals chromium and vanadium. These two minerals can be supplemented in capsule form as chromium and vanadyl sulfate and can help with insulin sensitivity and insulin resistance. If there is a significant overgrowth, also supplement trace minerals and/or ask your doctor to measure trace mineral levels, prescribe supplements, and monitor them. Mineral testing is available from commercial reference laboratories or Doctor's Data through a prescription from your doctor. Antioxidant vitamins A, C, and E are important, as well as alpha-lipoic acid (which is a metabolic antioxidant).

Risk factors: Diabetics tend to be more prone to yeast overgrowth because of the tendency for high blood sugar. Some people who consume too much alcohol may actually have alcohol cravings driven by the yeast. People who eat a highly sweet or starchy diet with lots of yeast products may have a greater tendency to yeast overgrowth. Soft drinks and commercial fruit juice are also high in sugar and can promote these imbalances.

Complementary Therapies

- Acupuncture can enhance immune function and assist the body in combating the overgrowth of yeast and then keep the yeast population in balance. NAET therapy also appears to be useful against yeast and fungal sensitivities.

- Mind-body therapies can help with stress management, which allows the immune system to recoup and cope with the overgrowth.
- Allergy testing: Allergic responses to candida can be detected through antibody testing, available from Immunosciences. (See chapter 21 for additional information on candida and chapter 24 on restoring and rebalancing flora.)

CELIAC DISEASE (SPRUE)

Celiac disease, also known as celiac sprue, is a chronic problem of malabsorption that results from an allergic response to gluten, which is a protein found in wheat. Sprue leads to malabsorption and a deficiency of nutrients. This is due to the shrinkage and destruction of the microstructures in the GI lining that absorb nutrients from our food—the microvilli and the villi on the lining of the small intestine. This condition also often causes diarrhea; however iron deficiency, osteoporosis, weight loss, irritable bowel syndrome, and even constipation may be the only apparent symptoms. Celiac sprue is now considered the most prevalent genetic disease in the United States, affecting about one of every 160, according to a nationwide study conducted by Dr. Fasano and associates.

Celiac disease or sprue is a condition that is frequently overlooked or misdiagnosed. Sprue often occurs as a latent condition and is found in about 25 percent of diabetics. This is a genetic disorder that is inherited, and is common in Ireland and northwestern Europe. It is rare among Asians, people of Jewish heritage, and African Americans. Latent sprue (hidden gluten allergy) may occur in as much as 10 percent of the population. It is frequently associated with blood group O and occasionally in type A blood.

Problems due to sprue actually occur at the level of the cell. Research has found that sugar residues (lectins) on the cell surface selectively bind the microscopic particles of wheat that are toxic (gliadin fractions). This explains why extremely tiny amounts of wheat or gluten can set off this condition. Avoiding sprue symptoms means far more than just avoiding bread or even wheat. It means not eating any prepared or processed food to which wheat or gluten have been added. It is important to maintain a strict diet because a number of more serious illnesses can occur as the result of an untreated sprue condition.

Associated Diseases

There are a large number of associated conditions. Of these the most common is type I diabetes. Neurological disorders that can also result from the malnutrition of sprue include peripheral neuropathy, abnormal myelinization of the spinal cord, and night blindness. In rare cases encephalopathy can occur—a toxic brain syndrome due to sprue and B vitamin deficiency that can lead to coma, because insufficient nutrient absorption is taking place. One of Dr. Fasano's studies suggests that gliadin may actually act on the brain by interfering with the binding sites (opiate receptors) for B-casomorphine (endorphins). Other serious complications that can occur in rare cases include increased incidence of lymphocytic cancer. Incidents of hypocalcemia have also been reported (tetany), as well as increased incidence of fractures and collapsed vertebrae.

Symptoms

Typical symptoms include chronic diarrhea, abdominal pain, gas, bloating, and other signs of malabsorption; weakness; weight loss; failure to thrive; and chronic sensitivity to starches and foods that contain grains. In 10 percent of people with sprue, a bumpy itchy rash (dermatitis herpetiformis) occurs. Sprue can also cause infertility or delayed menarche, chronic fatigue, anorexia, frequent bruising due to vitamin K deficiency, and many conditions related to malabsorption, such as anemia. Seizures, depression, and schizoaffective disorder are also possible.

Children with sprue develop a characteristic appearance with thin, wasted extremities, a bloated abdominal area, and loose stools. Low levels of vitamins D and K can lead to softening of the bones (osteomalacia). Protein malabsorption can lead to loss of muscle mass, weakness, and generally impaired development. Deficiency of lactase (the enzyme for milk digestion) can be associated. Sprue also causes the most extreme form of leaky gut. Testing shows that when particles are released in a sprue condition, the lining of the GI tract is so damaged that extremely large molecules leak through. This can cause all the symptoms associated with leaky gut syndrome, including allergies, increased burden on the liver, and a range of health conditions (see chapter 7).

Causes

Celiac disease is caused by specific antibodies (antigliadin and antiendomysium antibodies). It is often linked to other autoimmune disorders and may be a factor in the overstimulation of the T cells and the immune system in general. The offending substance is wheat protein, which contains gluten components (glutamine and gliadin). Other grains besides wheat that contain gluten include barley, rye, and oats. For some, rice and corn are tolerated staples.

This is typically an inherited autoimmune disorder. Sprue is associated with specific genetic patterns and tissue types. If the gene for sprue is present and the T cells are overstimulated by gluten in the diet, a clone of T cells is produced. This can bring on sprue symptoms, and a destructive immune response can occur. For those with the gene this may occur after exposure to a virus, following surgery, or with some other type of stressor.

Testing

Testing for the gliadin antibody used to be considered a general screen. Since this test is also positive in some other diseases, it has been mostly replaced by the following evaluations:

- The most highly sensitive blood test for this condition is the antiendomyseal antibody. Another test is the tissue transglutamase antibody, which is more specific.
- HLA typing is available, and the two genes necessary for the disease are DQ2 and DQ8.
- Tests for 24- or 72-hour fecal fat, which measure all the fat in the stool over a one-hour period to determine the level of fat absorption, are of historical benefit only.
- Small-bowel biopsy is the gold standard in order to observe the lack of villi under the microscope. This exam is performed at the three-month follow-up to check on the progress of healing. However, variability in pathologist interpretation of the biopsy is a problem. A training program has been developed at the University of Maryland Center for Celiac Research to address this concern.

Mainstream and Complementary Treatment
Diet Therapy

Working carefully with a dietitian, using diet diaries and other approaches to help track food intake and symptoms, can be exceptionally helpful. Nutritional counseling is vital, because overcoming this condition requires reading every label, even on apparently innocent products such as chewing gum, medications, and vitamins. The diet for sprue requires careful monitoring for life. The good news is that when patients stick to the diet, no other therapy is usually needed, and they typically do very well. However, patients who cheat on their diet continue to suffer and need the assistance of a dietitian. National support groups such as the Celiac Sprue Association, Celiac

Disease Foundation, and American Celiac Society are very helpful in meal planning and providing information on sources of nongluten flour and foods. Many health food stores now carry a range of gluten-free products and grain substitutes. *Living Without* magazine is a great resource as well.

Some patients may also need steroids (prednisone). Nutritional supplements can be beneficial in many cases, such as the peptide preparation Seacure and the amino acid L-glutamine, as well as vitamins, enzymes, and other nutrients.

The Gluten-Free Diet

A whole-food gluten-free diet is the most important single factor in treating this condition. A gluten-free diet eliminates all wheat, oats, barley, and related grains. Patients are later biopsied again to determine if the villi are growing back. Once off the offending foods, the villi should return, along with the restoration of many functions.

Patients who don't respond to these therapies may require the elimination of all food containing amylopectin (all carbohydrates containing disaccharides, eliminating sugar, starch, lactose, and all the grains). Foods not permitted include most grains: wheat, barley, corn, rye, oats, rice, buckwheat, millet, triticales, bulgur wheat and wheat germ, spelt, and quinoa. Various root vegetables, legumes, and other carbohydrates may also be restricted, such as potatoes, yams, parsnips, chickpeas, bean sprouts, soybeans, mung beans, fava beans, garbanzo beans, amaranth flour, and even cottonseed grain substitutes, and seaweed. See *Breaking the Vicious Cycle* by Elaine Gottschall (Kirkton Press, 1994), which also contains delicious recipes.

Supplements

- Nutritional therapy also involves probiotics, L-glutamine, and bromelain.
- An enzyme supplement (either a plant-based enzyme formula that includes protease and amylase or enteric-coated pancreatin) can be used to support digestion until healing is well progressed.
- Permavite powder from Allergy Research Group (see Resources); also trace minerals; folic acid; vitamins A, B complex, B_6; gamma-orazinol; Robert's Formula; and Seacure.
- Herbs include DGL, nettles, and aloe vera (liquid or gel).

Complementary Therapies

Complementary therapies include acupuncture to allow the body to heal fully. Also consider the usefulness of stress management and gentle exercise, as well as Reiki or massage therapy.

On a gluten-free diet symptoms typically abate in six months, and some people see major improvement in three to four months. The most important factors are getting an accurate diagnosis and then avoiding all food containing gluten.

CIRRHOSIS

Also see Liver Disease.

Cirrhosis is a chronic liver disorder involving damage to liver cells and scarring of liver tissue (fibrotic tissue), decreased blood flow, and the development of abnormal nodules that interfere with liver function. Symptoms include jaundice, ascites (the accumulation of fluid in the body cavity), and eventually liver failure.

Classification is based on evidence from microscopic evaluation of biopsied tissue. In micronodular cirrhosis, the tissue is found to have small nodules under the microscope. As the liver regenerates, recovering from the damage of oxidative stress and chronic inflammation, a harmful band of scar tissue can develop around the regenerating nodule.

Major Causes

- Alcoholism. Among people with alcohol addiction, almost half eventually develop cirrhosis. Both genetics and lifestyle appear to be factors in the development of this condition. This condition constitutes about 50 percent of cirrhosis cases. Women have a greater susceptibility to this condition because their livers are smaller.
- Chemical and drug overload can overwork the liver's capacity, causing scarring.
- Viral hepatitis B and C, chronic active hepatitis, and autoimmune hepatitis.
- Autoimmune conditions include biliary cirrhosis, which can result from bile duct obstruction, and sarcoidosis, a condition that resembles tuberculosis that can cause cirrhosis.
- Genetic factors also play a role in cirrhosis, and include:
  - Excess deposits of the mineral copper in the liver (Wilson's disease)
  - Excess iron deposits in the liver
  - An enzyme that inhibits the enzyme trypsin, sometimes causing cirrhosis and respiratory disease (alpha-antitrypsin deficiency)
  - Cystic fibrosis, which can cause enzyme deficiencies leading to cirrhosis
  - Glycogen storage disease, a rare inherited condition

- Obesity or elevated blood lipids are often associated with NASH (non-alcoholic fatty liver disease).
- Heart failure can cause blood to pool in the liver; this congestion can cause cirrhosis.
- Idiopathic—cause unknown, now thought to be caused largely by NASH (fatty liver).

Symptoms
- Enlargement of the parotid gland in the cheek
- Weight loss and muscle atrophy
- Weakness, fatigue, nausea, vomiting
- DuPuytren—contractures of the palm or reddening of the palm
- Fluid in the belly that causes swelling of the abdomen (ascites)
- Swelling of the legs (edema), pain over the liver
- GI bleeding from varices (abnormal enlarged veins, due to impeded circulation), which develop in the area of the esophagus, around the navel (umbilicus), or in the area of the anus (hemorrhoids)
- Jaundice
- Arterial spiders—red marks on face or chest and neck
- Enlarged breasts in males (gynecomastia), because cirrhosis changes the metabolism and affects hormone levels, increasing estrogen and decreasing testosterone
- Diminutia—chest and pubic hair are decreased in males, again due to the hormonal imbalance

Testing
- Physical exam to detect an enlarged or tender liver
- Early intervention is possible through alternative functional testing—the liver detox profile (see chapter 17)
- Conventional liver test (which assesses enzyme levels) and looks for elevated transaminase and bilirubin, and a decrease of albumin in the blood
- Antibody tests for hepatitis B and C
- ANA Test (antinuclear antibody) for autoimmune hepatitis, which untreated can cause cirrhosis
- AMA Test (antimitochondrial antibodies) for antibodies associated with biliary cirrhosis (in about 90 percent of cases)
- Serum iron levels—test for elevated levels of iron in the liver (hemochromatosis)
- Ultrasound can demonstrate nodules in the liver
- CT scan can confirm diagnosis by recording density of the scar tissue

- Liver biopsies tend to be accurate in 98 percent of cases when done by laparoscopy, but tend to be too expensive and invasive
- Needle biopsy (without laparoscopy) is about 75 percent accurate

Mainstream Treatment

- Rest and repair—minimize exposure to chemicals and other toxins (see chapter 23).
- Drug and alcohol abstinence.
- Viral hepatitis B and C are treated with interferon, an antibody that increases the immune response to fight the infection, and ribravirin, an antiviral. See Hepatitis for more details.
- Hemochromatosis can be treated by extensive blood draws to decrease the iron load.
- Wilson's disease—penicillamine, zinc acetate (Galzin), and Tetra-thiomolybdate remove copper by chelating it, drawing it out of the liver.
- Autoimmune conditions are treated with corticosteroids or nutritional medicine.
- Biliary cirrhosis is treated with bile salts such as Urso and Actigall, with or without the addition of the drug methotrexate to calm the immune system.
- Colchicine, used for gout, has been found helpful in alcoholic cirrhosis because it helps reduce scar tissue.
- Liver transplantation is effective in 70 percent to 80 percent of cases. Unfortunately there are often not enough livers to go around.

Complementary Treatments
Nutrition and Vitamins

- Good nutrition is essential—a diet lower in fat, high in protein (70 to 90 grams protein daily) and complex carbohydrates
- Antioxidants
- SAM—S-adenosyl-methionine, a specific biochemical that acts as a powerful free radical squelcher, is particularly useful for liver disease and related conditions
- The amino acid family of nutrients
- Decrease copper in copper-excess forms of cirrhosis
- Be sure to avoid supplements that contain iron in iron-excess forms of cirrhosis

Herbs

- Silymarin (milk thistle) is known as a potent liver healer
- Dandelion

- Chinese herbs such as schizandra, especially for hepatitis B and C
- Systemic Formulas—L-Liver and also Systemic Formula #5, which acts as a stabilizer
- Turmeric is a secondary herb (less potent but helpful)

(See also chapter 37 on herbs. Check the section on liver-support herbs.)

Complementary Therapies

- Acupuncture
- For detailed treatment information, see Liver Disease, with additional information on supplements, acupuncture, detoxification, chelation therapy, and new treatments

Resources

Jeffrey Bland, Ph.D., *The 20-Day Rejuvenation Diet Program* (McGraw-Hill, 2000). This book provides insight into liver function and its role as one of the most important organs of the body, including recent research and information on how to optimize liver function.

CONSTIPATION (CHRONIC)

Constipation is defined as a decrease in the frequency of bowel movements accompanied by prolonged or difficult passage of stool. It is a symptom complex, not a disease. In other words it is a dysfunction of the body and can be caused by a number of diseases or imbalances.

There is no rule for the optimal number of daily or weekly bowel movements. However, for research criteria, two or fewer bowel movements a week is considered constipation.

Mainstream Diagnosis and Testing

- Obstructions from colon cancer or stricture must be ruled out through examination by colonoscopy or barium enema. The minimal direct exam should include the lower sigmoid colon by sigmoidoscopy.
- Colonic transit time is a useful supplementary test. Transit time is the length of time from when food is taken in until a bowel movement occurs—this can range from 4 hours to 72 hours or longer. In this test the patient ingests a number of radiopaque pellets, which are visible on an X-ray; the tiny pellets are taken in a capsule. During the duration of the test, X-rays of the abdomen are taken periodically until all the pellets have passed or until about a week has elapsed, whichever comes first.

- Since low thyroid production can be a cause of chronic constipation, lab testing of blood for thyroid status is a useful initial screening.
- Stool analysis. Sometimes stool volume and frequency can be measured, especially in hospitals. The stool can be weighed and the moisture calculated.
- The pelvic floor EMG, which is considered anal-rectal manometry. EMG (electromyogram) uses a sensor to provide information on the dynamics of the colon as well as the sphincter relaxation and pelvic floor function.
- A defogram is a special type of X-ray that records a bowel movement, also called a defecatory exam. The video-proctogram is an X-ray video that provides information on the workings of the lower colon. It can measure the anal-rectal angle, sphincter contraction, and the activity of the muscles used in evacuation.
- Physicians who suspect laxative overuse sometimes order a stool exam to detect the presence of laxative preparations. A stool evaluation with phenolphthalein is a dye test that can detect the presence of Ex-Lax. Magnesium from milk of magnesia is measured in a blood sample. To save time and money, be honest with your doctor about your habits so you can work together to solve your problem.
- Slowed transit time (colonic inertia). This condition, which is surprisingly common, has a genetic basis and is often passed from mother to daughter. These patients, when examined by colonoscopy, typically have long, redundant (looping) colons. This condition is also associated with mitral valve prolapse, a type of heart murmur. They may also have fingerprints that show arched patterns on the fingertips.

  Often women who are postmenopausal and thin tend to have this condition. Since many women gain weight after menopause, doctors conjecture that those who are thin and have constipation may have this constellation of symptoms (constipation due to slowed motility, and lack of appetite because the stomach does not empty completely).

Complementary Testing

- The Comprehensive Digestive Stool Analysis (CDSA) from Great Smokies Diagnostic Laboratory, based on stool samples, provides a profile of fat absorption and bacterial flora. It also rules out parasites and includes information to some extent on how well food is and is not digested.
- Stool testing for parasites, bacteria (both aerobic and anaerobic), or yeast overgrowth by a lab that specializes in this type of testing.

  Constipation often accompanies infection by parasites. For example, in a survey of 670 patients in 1996, the Parasitology Center found that patients reported constipation as a symptom associated with *E. histolytica* in 26 percent of cases, with *E. coli* in 13 percent, and with *Blastocystis hominis* in 16 percent. Another survey, performed by Leo Galland, M.D., in his New York City practice, reported that of 100 patients with giardia, 40 percent indicated constipation with no diarrhea as a symptom.

- Stool testing should be performed by a lab that has the special expertise necessary for good detection, such as a university lab or a private lab such as IPD (the Institute of Parasitic Diseases).
- Testing for bacterial overgrowth by checking antibodies (our immune defenses) in a bowel flora antibody test (Immunosciences Lab, Inc.).
- Testing for the overgrowth of bacteria through chemical markers called organic acids (Great Plains Lab and Metametrix). (See also chapter 21 on microbes and bad bugs.)
- Magnesium-calcium levels. Inadequate levels of magnesium in the body can also cause constipation. Therefore testing for magnesium levels is also an important initial evaluation. Elevated calcium levels can also be a cause of constipation. These tests are usually performed on blood.
- Profile of nutrient status to detect any major deficiencies that might be causing constipation. Vitamins Diagnostics and Spectra-Cell in Texas provide general screening tests for a range of nutrients. (See Resources.)

Mainstream and Complementary Treatments

Treatment primarily consists of increasing liquids and fiber. Both mainstream and complementary practitioners favor these solutions. Note that both medical traditions also identify laxative overuse as a problem (over-the-counter products *and* herbs).

Minimize the intake of sweets; fruit juices should be kept to a minimum and diluted half with clear water. The best choices include spring or mineral water, lemon water (hot or cold), and herbal tea (hot or iced).

Fibers include soluble fibers, such as:

- Psyllium seed (available in health food stores under a variety of brand names and in drug stores as Metamucil, which typically contains added sweetener). Psyllium is helpful to some, but even as a fine powder can cause problems if there are allergies or major inflammation.
- Wheat bran is helpful to some because of its iron content, but too rough for those with inflammation, and potentially harmful to those with celiac sprue, an allergy to wheat protein.
- Oat bran and baby oat bran are favored by some, and are known as a reducer of cholesterol, but will cause reactions in those with overgrowth of bacteria, yeast, or parasites, which thrive on starches and sugars (carbohydrates).

- Flaxseeds can provide a good source of fiber. They can be used in several ways:
  - Sprinkled on food, they have a nutty flavor (try about two tablespoons)
  - They can be eaten in the morning as a kind of aromatic cereal—pour boiling water over 2 to 4 tablespoons of the seeds, then cover and let steep for about five minutes
  - If whole flax are too irritating the seeds can be ground into a powder that can be added to juice, milk, or food—whatever is tolerated
  - If inflammation is extreme try a more mucilaginous substance such as slippery elm or aloe vera
- Cellulose is a nonsoluble fiber helpful in some cases. In pharmacies it is available as Fiber Con, and from nutrient companies is found in Permavite, which contains cellulose and glutamine in a formula of supportive nutrients available from Allergy Research Group.

Mainstream Treatments

Medications and therapeutics include:

- Betalactulose (Chronulac), an absorbable sugar that promotes bowel movements. Available by prescription only.
- Calcium polycarbophil (Equalactin) holds liquid in a spongelike action that encourages motility; it also increases hydration of the stool.
- Magnesium can be useful, including milk of magnesia. Magnesium chloride is also available in an enteric-coated tablet as Slow Mag. Magnesium stimulates muscle contraction and peristalsis throughout the intestines and hydrates the stool.
- There is prokinetic medication that stimulates the smooth muscles of the colon by stimulating the serotonin receptors in the GI tract (tegaserod, Zelnorm).
- Miralax is a PEG (polyethylene glycol) osmotic agent that pulls water into the colon.

Surgery

- Sometimes surgery is performed in cases of severe constipation, which we call colonic inertia, when there is no motility of colon. Some patients have had subtotal or total colectomy. We are hoping that in the future this type of treatment can be avoided through magnetic therapy (Magnetic Molecular Energizer), which may regenerate the enteric nervous system that supplies the colon.

- Sphincterotomy involves the removal of a strip of the muscle from the lower sphincter when there is an outlet-obstruction problem, which can be diagnosed with the radiopaque markers and EMG tests. This surgery removes a centimeter-wide bit of muscle from the upper sphincter and 8 centimeters from the distal rectum.
- Impaction can require a nonsurgical medical procedure in the emergency room. Be sure to monitor a tendency toward constipation and see the doctor before the situation becomes serious.

Complementary Treatments
Diet
- Fiber is essential. Include fresh fruits and vegetables, but monitor for carbohydrate intolerance.
- Alkalinize the body. A salad a day can provide additional wholesome fiber. If inflammation is a problem, try butter lettuce or juice your vegetables). (See chapter 30 for more on alkaline diets.)
- Increase omega-3 fatty acids (flaxseeds, flax meal, or 1 tablespoon flax oil per day), make the effort to get off laxatives, and retrain the bowel. Flaxseeds can be ground in a coffee grinder to create a powdered meal or prepared by steeping, covered, in boiling water for five minutes.

Nutritional and Herbal Supplements
- Avoid frequent use of senna or cascara sagrada because they tend to lead to laxative abuse.
- Aloe vera, as a laxative can be quite helpful in the short term. Try two capsules at bedtime. Some people also respond to the juice or gel.
- Yellow dock is a mild herbal laxative that can also be used in combination with aloe vera. Again, consider all laxatives temporary measures.
- Magnesium is useful, but in high doses is known to cause "a precipitous cleanse"—the very rapid propulsion of the stool when it finally works, which can be unpredictable and as much as six hours later—so use it at a time when you don't need to leave home. This can also be true of cascara sagrada, aloe, or any nutrient or herb with a laxative effect.
- Sometimes a lot of vitamin C can be useful. Vitamin C can be taken in high doses of up to 10 grams a day. Taking vitamin C "to bowel tolerance" means taking 1,000 or 2,000 mg every two hours until diarrhea occurs. That indicates the maximum dose. At that point scale back from that dose and try it at the more moderate level for several days to determine if symptoms improve. Do not remain on these high doses indefinitely, due to the occasional potential for kidney stones.

- MSM (methyl-sulfonyl-methane) works well for constipation in some cases; this is a mild mineral supplement of a sulfur derivative in capsule form.
- Slippery elm is a soothing natural fiber somewhat like flaxseed that creates a gelatinlike substance and encourages motility; available in capsules or bulk.
- Bentonite clay can be helpful for periodic cleanses. As it moves through the body it mechanically absorbs material from the lining of the GI tract, so it is believed to draw and remove some of the bacteria or parasites adhering to the GI lining. However, it also absorbs minerals, so monitor your weight to be sure you are getting enough nutrients. Sonne #7, also sold as Arise and Shine, is a highly respected brand of bentonite. Important: Be sure to take enough liquid with it or constipation could become worsened, and it could even cause impaction.
- Take probiotics. Better bowel flora increases motility. Types of flora that seem to provide a good response include: *Lactobacillus acidophilus* (DDS strain by Natren); bifidobacteria (Custom Probiotics), and soil-based protolytic bacteria (Primal Defense). After antibiotics consider taking the beneficial yeast *Saccharomyces boulardii* or other probiotics.

Colonics and Enemas

Some people will need periodic enema therapy, but we do not recommend it indefinitely. Enemas mean that natural function has not resumed. If there is infection present, reinfection can occur and can also be spread to other members of the household when they come in contact with microscopic remnants of fecal matter.

Sometimes people really do feel benefit from a colonic session. However, periodically people are infected through colonic therapy. Since the procedure is quite invasive for a nonsurgical treatment, it is important that cleanliness be paramount and that disposable speculums and tubing be used.

Conventional medicine uses a liquid preparation to clear the colon in preparation for GI examinations. These liquids can be taken as an emergency measure. They are called CoLyte, Nulytely and GoLytely and are available from pharmacies with a prescription from your doctor. They can be used with the monitoring of your physician until normal function returns. They can also be taken during a detoxification regimen.

Complementary Therapies

- EMG biofeedback and pelvic flow retraining.
- Gentle exercise such as Qigong, t'ai chi, and yoga. Exercise with machines that work the abdominal muscles (the abs) or do gentle crunches with

knees bent to protect the back and sciatic nerves. Walking is useful, although surprisingly, it does not help everyone.

- Acupuncture
- Energy work on the abdomen for irritable bowel. Abdominal massage can be used in some cases if it helps. If not explore other therapies.
- Magnetic therapy can be used, in which one wears a large magnet (the back flex) on the abdomen or sleeps on a magnetic sleep pad.

CROHN'S DISEASE

See Inflammatory Bowel Diseases (IBD).

DIARRHEA (CHRONIC)

An abnormally frequent discharge of semisolid or fluid fecal matter from the bowel. Diarrhea is a symptom rather than a specific disease. It can result from deranged motility, or from infection by bacteria or parasites, or from chronic inflammation. Diarrhea can cause additional problems, such as the malabsorption of nutrients and the inability to absorb water from the colon.

Causes
- Bacteria can trigger diarrhea; offenders include bacteria that cause food poisoning, such as toxigenic *E. coli,* salmonella, shigella, and campylobacter, as well as staphylococcus and *Clostridium difficile.* These bacterial infections are often described as food poisoning.
- Following antibiotics, an overgrowth of yeast or toxic bacteria can cause diarrhea.
- Viruses include rotavirus, Norwalk agent, and enteric adenovirus, which often accompanies colds, with symptoms that resemble flu.
- Parasitic infections—microscopic parasites that can cause infection include giardia, and amoebas such as *E. histolytica* and *D. fragilis,* cryptosporidium, cyclospora, microspora, and *Blastocystis hominis.* Larger parasites such as *Taenia solium,* a pork tapeworm, can also be a cause of diarrhea.
- Travelers diarrhea—parasitic infections and bacteria such as toxigenic *E. coli* and cholera can cause diarrhea in travelers to foreign countries where sanitation and food preparation may expose travelers to pathogens, particularly those for which no immunity has been developed. Tropical pathogens tend to be more virulent and harmful than those of temperate climates. Exposure to many of these microbes occurs here in the United States as well—and probably more frequently than we suspect.

- Marine toxins—ciguatera toxins in fish poisoning from jack fish, mackerel, and other sources.
- Tuberculosis can affect the GI tract through raw, unpasteurized milk.
- Changes in the intestinal tract due to surgery—removal of a portion of the small or large bowel or intestinal bypass.

Diarrheal infections are typically contracted through food, water, or fecal/oral transmission from food handlers (for example, in restaurant food); from people in contact with stool, such as day care workers; transmission in school or institutional settings; from eating spoiled food (don't keep any food longer than two to three days); and from intimate contact with someone who already has an infection.

Symptoms

- Watery diarrhea, abdominal cramping, heavy fatigue/malaise, fever.
- Bloody diarrhea can be caused by amoebas, campylobacter, salmonella, shigella, and toxigenic *E. coli*. If you have bloody diarrhea, see a doctor as soon as possible.

In general, diarrhea tends to be self-limiting. Self-medicate if diarrhea is not bloody, your temperature is below 102°F, and your immunity is strong. Keep fluids up and replace electrolytes; Pedialyte, available in most drugstores, is a good source. If diarrhea persists beyond seven days, be sure to see a doctor.

Diagnosis

- Antibody testing can be exceptionally helpful (see Immunosciences Lab on page 570 under Resources).
- Stool cultures. Three samples are best, each taken 48 hours apart. Many labs are not trained in the detection of these microbes. Send to a university lab or a lab with specialized expertise, such as the Parasitology Center (see page 569 under Resources).

  Stool cultures should include testing for yeast, which can play a role in diarrhea. Patients with heavy overgrowth of yeast can develop toxigenic diarrhea and may have ongoing inflammation. In severe chronic cases colonoscopic or sigmoidoscopic exam with biopsy is necessary to identify the inflammation.

Mainstream Treatments

- Rest. In severe cases of diarrhea it may become essential to rest the gut with parenteral intravenous nutrition.

- Medications. Antibiotics can be given for persistent diarrhea to eradicate pathogens: ciprofloxin (Cipro), ampicillin (Amoxicillin), or other broad-spectrum antibiotics, as well as metronidazole (Flagyl). Calcium polycarbophil (Equalactin) is used for loose but not watery diarrhea. The choice of medication is based on either:
  - Sensitivity testing in the lab (which identifies the drugs that will destroy the pathogen)
  - A review of the current medical literature on Medline to identify the medications currently successful against a particular microbe, compared with your history of response to drugs
- Drugs to slow motility. Imodium or Lomotil are sometimes used to slow motility and decrease water secretion, but they should not be used until *after* you have had a stool culture. The diarrhea is the body's way of washing pathogens out of the GI tract. Slowing motility when there is a pathogenic infection blocks the body's way to remove the pathogen. Slowing motility can prolong the infection.
- Antitoxin drugs. The medications Questran or cholestyramine are drugs that bind the toxins produced by pathogens such as *C. difficile*. Drugs are currently in development for the toxins produced by cholera bacteria and toxigenic *E. coli*.
- Oral gamma globulin. Immune antibodies are found in preparations from the health food store, such as colostrum, and in UltraFlora Plus, available from Metagenics (a concentrate of immune globulin protein available through physicians). These preparations may be used in cases of diarrhea from infectious agents, because they interfere with adherence of the microbe to the GI wall.
- Probiotics, beneficial bacteria, are now more widely accepted as a resource to reduce the occurrence of diarrhea from foreign travel or from antibiotic therapy. New types of probiotics are coming on the market that seem to be heat stable. If these products prove to be as good as their promise, they could be used when traveling as a preventive measure.

Complementary Treatment
Remove the Cause

- Remove any pathogenic microbes (bacteria, yeast, parasites).
- Remove any foods from the diet that may be causing an allergy, sensitivity, or intolerance, or that are difficult to digest or absorb. (See chapters 8 and 20 on allergies.)
- As a rule, stop dairy products and wheat. If diarrhea or sensitivities continue, seek comprehensive allergy testing. With a dairy allergy diarrhea

can sometimes wash away the source of lactase, the enzyme that digests milk. In some cases the body's ability to produce the enzymes to digest milk does not return, or at least not immediately. With a wheat allergy or celiac disease, diarrhea can be a primary symptom.

Replace Digestants

- The secretion of digestive enzymes can be compromised by microbial infection. Missing enzymes can be supplemented through a multiple enzyme formula. It may also be necessary to supplement hydrochloric acid production with betaine hydrochloride. If impairment is significant, a useful strategy is to support pancreatic function with pancreas glandulars. Another secretion that can become depleted over time includes intrinsic factor (a protein essential for the absorption of vitamin B_{12}). (For more about the importance of B_{12} deficiences, see chapter 33.)

Restore Flora

- Restore beneficial flora (particularly acidophilus). Good bacteria include acidophilus, bifidobacteria, *Saccharomyces boulardii* (a beneficial yeast available from Pure Encapsulation and Thorne). Real cultured yogurt tends to be good for those who are dairy tolerant (for example, the brand Brown Cow, which includes bifidus cultures).

Repair

Repair refers to nutritional support for healing and regenerating the GI mucosa. A list of beneficial nutrients follows; select those most relevant to your needs or work with your physician in designing an individualized program in response to testing for deficiencies.

- Vitamin A or beta-carotene for the differentiation, growth, and function of the GI lining.
- A good multivitamin.
- Vitamin B5 (pantothenic acid), which stimulates protein synthesis.
- Vitamin C, which helps in collagen formation.
- Vitamin E (alpha-tocopherol), an important antioxidant essential to the integrity of GI mucosal cell membranes.
- Zinc plays a vital role in immne support and is involved in enzyme function, in the structure of cell membranes, and in replication of cells, so it's important in the repair of the GI lining and works with vitamin A.
- Trace minerals to minimize inflammation.

- Pepto-Bismol—the mineral bismuth—or the generic version helps prevent bacteria from adhering to the wall of the gut. Take 20 minutes before meals.
- L-glutamine, an amino acid, is the preferred fuel for the small intestinal lining cells (enterocytes); take it with trace minerals as cofactors to optimize the L-glutamine.
- Inulin in capsule form stimulates the production of butyrate by the friendly flora. Inulin has an insulin-like activity that helps the transfer of glucose across the cell membrane.
- Butyrate nourishes the lining cells of the large intestine (colonocytes).
- Short-chain fatty acids (omega-3s), flaxseed, and cod-liver oil act as anti-inflammatories.
- Omega-6s—black currant seed oil, borage oil, and primrose oil cut down on inflammation. (See information on fatty acids, chapter 25.)
- Glutathione, taken with the precursors N-acetyl cysteine and cysteine, which all provide molecular fuel for detoxification pathways.
- Bioactive peptides like Seacure help with the rebuilding process.
- UltraClear Sustain, which is rice based, or other rice-based protein powders to provide additional nourishment while minimizing allergic responses.
- Colostrum supplement. If you are milk tolerant, colostrum is a supplement that contains antitoxigenic antibodies (IgG) extracted from cow's milk. If well tolerated this product tends to speed healing.

Herbs

Anti-inflammatory herbs that are mild and mucilaginous include aloe vera, slippery elm, and flaxseeds (ground). They may supplement the mucous action of the gut. Products that contain pectin also promote mucous action, firm the stool, and provide soluble fiber. Primary herbs helpful with diarrhea include ginger (in capsules, liquid tincture, or tea), garlic, oil of oregano (in capsules), black tea (for its astringent properties), dried oak bark (use in powdered form, as a tea), tea tree, fenugreek, and psyllium. Secondary herbs include red raspberry leaf, bayberry root bark, goldenseal and cinnamon in small doses, geranium root, carob, chamomile, and marshmallow root.

Complementary Therapies

- Homeopathic treatment is well documented to be a significant strategy against diarrhea, and has been successful even against cholera. If you are extremely or chronically ill and want to use homeopathy, have the remedy prescribed for you by a well-trained homeopathic physician. This is especially important if your fever is greater than 102°F, if you have bloody diarrhea, or if your condition has persisted for more than seven days. If the episode seems mild give your vital force a boost with one of these noninvasive remedies. However, should your symptoms grow worse or persist, be sure to call your doctor immediately.

- Acupuncture, if you can leave home.

DIVERTICULOSIS AND DIVERTICULITIS

Diverticulosis consists of pockets that occur in the wall of the colon, in which the wall is stretched and bubbled due to a rupture (herniated tissue). It occurs primarily in the descending colon (the sigmoid), which is on the left side of the body.

When the muscle of the colon wall is weakened, the pressure can produce a hernia in the wall of the gut, particularly in places where the blood vessels penetrate through the muscular wall. This has been found to be due to imbalanced pressure in the colon, which can result from a diet low in fiber.

Diverticulitis occurs when there is infection and inflammation in the pockets or herniated sacs.

Half the U.S. population over 40 have one of these conditions. They are diseases of Western civilization, believed to be due to the refined diet of industrial nations, low in fiber and high in sugars. It has been observed that people in non-Western cultures eating a high-fiber diet have no incidence of this disease.

Causes

This condition can result not only from poor diet, but also is associated with processes that occur in the body due to aging. As we age there is a change in the ecology of the gut bacteria, with a loss of the beneficial bacteria (lactobacillus and bifidobacteria). As a result, when refined sugar and starches are eaten an overgrowth of harmful bacteria can occur. This can cause an increase in bloating and gas, which raises the pressure in the colon.

Pancreatic enzymes also decrease as we age, so starches and sugars are digested less efficiently, another contributor to bloating, gas, and increased pressure. Decline in good quality collagen can occur with aging or poor nutrition. Note that many people have both irritable bowel and low-grade diverticulitis—bacterial overgrowth can be a common feature of both conditions. Delayed food allergies may be another element in triggering diverticular spasm. Not drinking enough fluid is another factor.

Symptoms

Diverticulosis often causes no symptoms whatsoever. Nonspecific complaints can be associated with it, such as constipation or diarrhea, abdominal pain, or gas and bloating.

Diverticulitis occurs when there is a high degree of inflammation. Features of this inflammation may include detectable pain, occasionally a fever or bleeding, and a change in bowel habits. Testing will show a high sedimentation rate, a reflection of the level of active antibodies in the bloodstream and therefore the degree of inflammation. Sometimes this can produce the symptoms of appendicitis, called left-sided appendicitis.

Diverticulitis with bleeding should be considered a medical emergency.

Testing
- Testing for sedimentation rate.
- CBC—a white blood cell count to check for the presence of infection and other markers of illness.
- A physical exam to check for tenderness in the abdomen.
- Other testing may include the barium enema, a CT scan, or a colonoscopy. Note to doctors: In the barium enema process, Swedish research has found that methyl-cellulose enemas are more useful in the diagnosis of diverticulosis.
- Helical CT scans offer increased sensitivity in the detection of inflammation.

Mainstream Treatments
Antibiotics such as Cipro and Flagyl are given orally if the condition is mild, or intravenously if it is severe. There may be a need to be treated with nystatin afterward. It is essential that all antibiotic therapies are followed with probiotics, taken for several weeks.

When there is recurrent or frequent diverticulosis, a partial colectomy may be indicated, especially in cases where there is continual bleeding or when the condition is severe and the patient is not responding to treatment. Provide support to the immune system before considering surgery.

For mild conditions, antispasmodic drugs such as hycosamine sulfate (Levsin-SL) or dicyclomine (Bentyl) have been found helpful. Robinul Forte can be used every 8 to 12 hours.

Diet
Eliminate sugar and other refined sweeteners and starches that might feed bacteria (such as pastas, bread, potatoes, and corn [see chapter 31]). The earlier approach to this condition was to eliminate high-fiber foods that might get caught in the diverticular pockets, such as seeds, corn, and nuts. However, we now recommend a high-fiber diet, which does not appear to trigger the inflammation because it does not feed the harmful bacteria. In addition be sure to drink enough water (at least 6 to 8 glasses a day) so that stool does not become too dry, which could then become caught in the diverticular pockets.

Nutrients

For inflammation consider the use of:

- Trace minerals (zinc, copper, manganese, and magnesium can become significantly depleted)
- Vitamin C and the other antioxidants
- A multiple-enzyme product, plus additional bromelain
- Cod-liver oil or fish oil (in lemon flavor liquid or in capsules), which contains vitamin A (also DHA and EPA)
- UltraClear Sustain, a powdered low-allergenic dietary supplement from Metagenics
- Butyrate, an essential fatty acid and an effective colon fuel
- Inulin, which helps the body produce butyrate (found in Jerusalem artichokes)
- Butyrate enemas, which have been effective and can be obtained from a compounding pharmacy (see Resources)

Herbal Remedies

- Complementary therapies to control the inflammation include herbal combinations that decrease the harmful gut bacteria, such as Tanalbit
- Aloe vera (juice, capsules, or gel intended for internal use only) as an anti-inflammatory; slippery elm; psyllium; powdered flax meal (but not the whole seed); Seacure; or garlic oil in capsules
- In mild to moderate cases, antispasmodic herbs such as peppermint, spearmint, deglycrrhizinated licorice (DGL), and hawthorn may also be helpful
- In some cases, curcumin

Complementary Therapies

- Massage. Visceral manipulation seems helpful in painful types of diverticulosis; this can be done by a physical therapist. Shirley Trickett recommends solar plexus massage in her book *The Irritable Bowel Syndrome and Diverticulosis: A Self-Help Plan* (Thorsons, 1990, pp. 106–107). Chi ne sang is a helpful form of visceral massage. Both approaches should be focused on maintaining peristalsis.
- Exercise. Use yoga, gentle exercise, or walking to promote good muscle tone and peristalsis.
- Stress reduction. Hypnosis, self-hypnosis, and other stress-reduction techniques are helpful, because of the inflammatory nature of this condition.
- Acupuncture has been specifically used for both diverticulosis and diverticulitis. Specific acupoints for diverticulosis and diverticulitis, especially

in the mild form, are included in textbooks on acupressure and acupuncture. In mild cases self-applied acupressure can be used, or Acu-Stim can be performed with a small electromagnetic unit. The Solitens is a medical device that could be ordered with a prescription from a physician, from Nikken—(888) 264-5536 (order number 1322). A good guiding text is K. Serizawa, *Tsubo*, 2nd ed. (Japan Publications, 1995).

DYSPEPSIA—WITHOUT ULCERS

This diagnosis describes any upper GI conditions that typically include indigestion or heartburn and ulcerlike symptoms without evidence of an ulcer. In nonulcerative dyspepsia, there is no localized inflammation or ulcerated crater visible in an endoscopic exam. There is no clear cause, but there is evidence of dysfunction. Nonulcerative dyspepsia is also called NUD. Symptoms include belching, bloating, pain, or discomfort after eating. Dyspepsia may be a catch-all category for a number of frequently occurring subtle conditions.

Diagnosis

This disease is defined by ruling out organic disease. Likewise this diagnosis is applied if no reflux of the esophagus and no *H. pylori* infection are detected. Previously, *H. pylori* infection was suspected to be the cause, but recent studies have shown that treating this form of dyspepsia as if it were an *H. pylori* infection produced no improvement.

Conventional Testing

- A viral infection of the intestinal tract can cause a motility disorder. Symptoms of diarrhea, flatulence, bloating, or other GI symptoms may follow the infection. Titers for antibody response to the virus can confirm this (Immunosciences Lab).
- Acid levels are tested to rule out hyperacidity and peptic ulcer disease. A gastric capsule or nasogastric tube can measure the acidity (pH) with a pH meter.
- Abnormal gastric pacemaker evaluated by EGG. Nonulcer dyspepsia may be a motility disorder of the stomach in some cases. A study of nonulcerative dyspepsia by Ken Koch, M.D., at Penn State Medical Center, in which this author participated, involved the following: An electrogastrogram (an EGG, the equivalent of an EKG of the stomach) was used to evaluate patients with symptoms of nausea or bloating. It was found that these patients often had an abnormal gastric cycle. There is normally a "housekeeping" rhythm of the stomach of 3 cycles per minute. These are electrical and muscular waves that help the digestion and churning of

food into smaller particles. In these patients there were often cycles that were too slow (1 to 2 cycles per minute) or too rapid (6 to 10 per minute). Therapy for this consisted of low-dose cisapride (Propulsid), or metoclopramide (Reglan) a prokinetic medication of 5 mg to stimulate stomach motility. Diabetic patients with delayed emptying were given doses of 10 to 20 mg.

- Small bowel motility evaluation at a tertiary-care or major medical center may be required in some patients.

Functional Testing

- Flora balance. Any motility disorder changes the flora balance, which can also affect the intestinal transit. Check through a Comprehensive Digestive Stool Analysis (see chapter 17).
- Bacterial overgrowth of pathogenic organisms can also occur following antibiotic therapy or steroid therapy. This can be confirmed by testing for organic acids, which evaluates the by-products of the bacteria. Available from Metametrix Laboratories and Great Plains Lab.

Mainstream Treatment

- Low-dose Reglan or cisapride, prokinetic agents that promote motility
- Multiple small meals
- Stress reduction
- Antinausea medications

Nutritional Therapy

- Remove infection by microbes (typically with prescription medication in combination with or alternating with herbal remedies).
- Detect and remove any offending allergic foods through careful self-monitoring for reactivity or blood testing for allergies (see chapter 20).
- Replace digestants (see chapter 24).
- Restore flora (see chapter 24).
- Repair GI lining with nutrients and anti-inflammatories (see chapter 32).
- Nutrients include pyridoxal phosphate, a form of vitamin B_6, found to help with nausea, available from Lifespan Institute (LifespanProducts.com). Be sure to take a vitamin B complex supplement as well.
- Include a balance of vitamins, minerals, and magnesium.
- Pepto-Bismol—the mineral bismuth may be helpful in cases where there is an undetected *H. pylori* infection.
- Herbs that might help include: peppermint, licorice and DGL, aloe for inflammation, ginger for nausea, slippery elm.

Complementary Therapies

- Acupuncture can be used to treat nausea and possibly normalize the gastric pacemaker rate.
- Magnet therapy uses a strip over the pacemaker area of the stomach that entrains the rate and normalizes pacemaker function.
- Stress reduction to allow the immune system to participate in healing, including yoga, hypnotherapy, biofeedback, exercise, and music therapy. These can be helpful as stress reducers, which can bring about indirect improvement, since stress makes everything worse.

DISORDERS OF THE ESOPHAGUS

See Reflux and Heartburn—GERD.

FIBROMYALGIA

Fibromyalgia Syndrome (FMS) is commonly associated with the presence of widespread pain and tenderness. It is often accompanied with fatigue, stiffness, and decreased muscle endurance. This pain is accentuated when pressure is applied to specific tender points. Fibromyalgia syndrome is the formal diagnosis when 11 out of 18 of these specific tender points are found.

Diagnosis
Essential Characteristics

- Chronic, generalized aches, pains, or stiffness
- Absence of other systemic conditions to account for these symptoms
- Multiple tender points at specific locations

Additional Criteria

- Disturbed sleep
- Generalized fatigue or tiredness
- Swelling, numbness
- Pain in the neck and shoulder area
- Chronic headaches
- Irritable bowel symptoms

Conventional medical therapy consists of antidepressants, reassurance, and in some cases physical therapy with trigger point injections or spray and stretch treatments.

Causal Factors

Conventional medicine has clearly linked disturbed sleep and depression to fibromyalgia. However, since fatigue and muscle pain are symptoms found in so many conditions, it appears that there are multiple causes of fibromyalgia. In each case the approach must be tailored to the symptoms, history, and test results of the individual patient. Causal factors that have been explored in the medical literature, in order of the amount of research, include:

- Neck injury or physical trauma
- Infection due to mycoplasma bacteria
- Hormone deficiencies: growth hormone, cortisol, and DHEA
- Yeast infection—*Candida albicans*
- Excessive levels of nitric oxide
- Phosphate buildup in the muscles
- Genetic tendency to poor vitamin B_6 metabolism, resulting in lower levels of B_6
- Heavy metal toxicity
- Additional factors identified in research on fibromyalgia: low thyroid, underactive adrenal, low vitamin B_{12}, GI parasites, and depression

Neck Injury or Physical Trauma

Investigators note that many fibromyalgia patients have a history of neck trauma or an auto accident associated with the onset of their symptoms. Research recently presented at a Physical Medicine Conference at the NIH reported the following: A pain clinic neuroradiologist, evaluating the MRIs of fibryomyalgia patients, noticed that many had an undetected break in the discs, primarily in the neck (Carolyn McMakin, M.S., D.C., Portland, Oregon). Dr. McMakin has successfully treated many of these patients with micro-current at specific biological frequency.

A recent study of fibromyalgia confirmed the presence of biochemical markers for pain and inflammation in these patients. Findings included higher levels of a neurotransmitter (Substance P) in pain pathways and circulating inflammatory chemicals (cytokines) in their cerebrospinal fluid.

Infection

Several types of infections have been associated with fibromyalgia:

- Mycoplasma. This species of bacteria, which is much smaller than typical bacteria, lives inside the body's cells as a virus would. Mycoplasma has been implicated in chronic fatigue syndrome experienced by some Gulf

War veterans. These infections also appear to be associated with fibromyalgia (Garth Nicholson, Ph.D., San Diego). Through lab work his research has identified mycoplasma infections in approximately one-half of the fibromyalgia patients tested, and in arthritis patients as well.

- Lyme disease. It is also believed that as many as 25 to 40 percent of long-term Lyme patients develop fibromylagia-like symptoms. Both Lyme *(Borrelia burgdorferi)* and mycoplasma are difficult to diagnose and are therefore often missed.
- Other infectious agents associated with fibromyalgia include human herpes virus 6 (HHV6), chlamydia bacteria *(Chlamydia pneumoniae),* the mononuleosis virus (Epstein-Barr), fifth disease (parvovirus B19), and hepatitis C.

Hormone Deficiencies

Some fibromyalgia patients show test results that indicate significant hormone deficiencies.

- Human growth hormone. Severe deficiencies of this hormone, necessary for healing and tissue regeneration, were found in one subset of patients.
- DHEA. Investigators have also found that DHEA (dihydroepiandrosterone, a precursor of the hormones estrogen and testosterone) and cortisol were significantly lower in fibromyalgia patients when compared to patients without illness. DHEA is an adrenal, steroid-type hormone that is secreted in response to chemical stimulus from the pituitary gland.
- Cortisol. The levels of this adrenal hormone were also significantly lower, suggesting the value of adrenal support and possibly thyroid supplementation as well.
- Thyroid. Functional hypothyroidism, a relative inability to convert T4 (the precursor thyroid hormone), to T3 (the active thyroid hormone), is often present and may be associated with cold hands and feet, and low body temperatures of 97.4 or below (taken in the underarm before getting out of bed).
- Hormonal replacement therapy. This approach is often needed in premenopausal and menopausal fibromyalgia patients. Hormone replacement is now possible with natural, plant-based supplements (sterols) available by prescription from special compounding pharmacies. These phytonutrients have advantages over earlier forms of herbal therapy, because they can be custom-formulated for each patient. This is a viable alternative to animal-derived hormone medications.

Yeast Infection—Candida albicans

Candida albicans and other yeast have also been implicated in fibromyalgia. Testing using the CDSA (Comprehensive Digestive Stool Analysis from Great Smokies Diagnostic Laboratory) often reveals overgrowths of fungi in these patients. In addition higher levels of tartaric acid are sometimes found in the urine of fibromyalgia patients. Tartaric acid (associated with *Candida* infections) is an inhibitor of the Krebs cycle. This is the process of energy production within every cell in the body—so compromises in these processes could be a factor in fatigue symptoms.

Antifungal medications used to address the candida overgrowth of fibromyalgia patients were also found to significantly reduce the tartaric acid in these patients' urine. Other nutrients found to reduce tartaric acid include malic acid and magnesium. The virulence of *C. albicans* may be related to its ability to induce inflammation through immune messenger chemicals, such as cytokines.

Excess Nitric Oxide

An overexpression of nitric oxide is another of the current causal theories concerning fibromyalgia. These elevated levels of nitric oxide appear to be caused by an error in the signaling of immune messenger chemicals. When too much nitric oxide is expressed, then the inflammatory process (cytokines) is initiated. This can result in muscle pain that resembles the kind of aches associated with a cold or the flu. Excessive nitric oxide could either be caused by an overly active immune system or by the presence of undetected, smoldering infection.

Excessive nitric oxide can cause oxidative stress. The part of the cell most sensitive to this stress is the mitochondria, the source of energy within the cell. When the mitochondria become impaired symptoms of muscle stiffness and fatigue can result.

Phosphate Buildup in Muscle Tissue

Another possible causal factor in some patients is excessive phosphate accumulation, which presents as hard and swollen muscles. An endocrinologist, (Paul St. Armand, M.D. Marina del Rey, CA; www.guaidoc.com) first discovered this link after observing that some fibromyalgia patients have a high amount of dental tartar on their teeth. Since dental tartar contains accumulate phosphate, the doctor reasoned that there might be phosphate buildup in the bodies of these patients. Dr. St. Armand found that guaifenesin helps dissolve excessive phosphate that accumulates in the hard and swollen muscles of fibromyalgia patients.

- Guaifenesin is now available as an over-the-counter medication.
- This therapy is only successful if the patient also follows a diet free of sal-icylates (a substance found in aspirin and certain foods).
- It is also important that a diet low or moderate in carbohydrates be fol-lowed (low on the Glycemic Index). For more resources on this diet, see *The Formula, Atkins for Life,* or *The South Beach Diet.*

Genetics and B₆

Some patients with fibromyalgia have vitamin B_6 deficiencies. One of the genetic characteristics sometimes seen with B_6 deficiency is "Morton's foot" (in which the second toe is longer than the big toe—or is at least the same length). (Devin Starlanyl, M.D., *Fibromyalgia and Chronic Myofascial Pain Syndrome: A Survival Manuel,* chapter 7.) We have measured vitamin B_6 stores in patients with Morton's foot, and our lab work had a similar finding.

Another hypothesis is that patients with Morton's foot have an inability to metabolize vitamin B_6 (pyridoxine hydrochloride) into its active form as pyri-doxine 5 phosphate (Carl Pfeiffer, M.D., Ph.D., the Princeton Brain Bio Institute). Supplementation with vitamin B_6 (in the form of P5P) is essential for the metabolism and synthesis of serotonin and collagen. P5P is vitamin B_6 in a more bioavailable and highly metabolized form, and is available as a supple-ment from health food stores, from Pure Encapsulations, and from Lifespan Institute. Patients with a B_6 deficiency also appear to have hypermobility of joints, and this has also been noticed in some fibromyalgia patients.

Heavy Metal Toxicity

Toxicity due to mercury or tin (in dental fillings), antimony, nickel, and other metals can poison the cells and tissues. Testing for these exposures requires special expertise, most often provided by doctors or clinics of environmental medicine and by environmental dentists. Toxic exposures should be evaluated through a physical examination, 24-hour urine collection, and in some cases hair analysis or provocative testing after chelation. When having mercury fill-ings removed, be sure you are working with a dentist who has specialized training. If the mercury is accidentally reintroduced to the body, this can cause damage to the brain and the liver.

Additional Factors

Causal factors that have been linked to fibromyalgia, identified in the research of Dr. Jacob Teitelbaum, include low thryoid, underactive adrenal, fungal overgrowth, low vitamin B_{12}, bowel parasites, and depression. (For more information, see the work of Dr. Teitelbaum, M.D., in his exceptional resource, *From Fatigued to Fantastic* [Avery/Penguin Putnam, Inc., 2001].)

Additional Therapies

- Ultrasound and other physical therapies have been found to be helpful.
- Acupuncture has proven to be an excellent therapy for some patients, to relieve pain and stiffness and increase stamina.
- Improving liver detoxification with Medi Clear, Ultra Clear, Adva Clear, or Ultra Clear Plus has been successfully employed in many of these patients. Several nutritional therapies using CoQ_{10}, alpha lipoic acid, and milk thistle have also been successful. These nutrients support the liver and the body's mitochondria.
- Testing for intestinal permeability (leaky gut syndrome), because intestinal hyperpermeability results in increased absorption of food antigens, foreign compounds, and even bacteria that have to be detoxified.
- Improving digestive health is a sound general approach, developing an individualized program using the "4 Rs":
    - Remove bad bugs, allergens, and toxins
    - Replace enzymes, bicarbonate, and betaine hydrochloric acid (HCl)
    - Restore digestive flora and increase fiber
    - Repair with vitamins A and the mineral zinc, pathothenic acid (B_5), B_6, and L-glutamine.

    This approach will support proper GI friendly flora and restore the integrity of the gut lining and normalized bowel movements, thus breaking the cycle of increased oxidative stress and liver detoxification abnormalities.
- Identify food allergies through an elimination diet or diagnosis through a blood test; this may also be needed by some patients with fibromyalgia.
- Glutamine, an amino acid that is the preferred fuel of the small intestinal cells, is helpful.
- Seacure, extracted from fish protein, provides growth factors for intestinal cell repair. These nutrients can be used effectively in combination, which has been evaluated by the author in a controlled clinical trial.
- Electromagnetic therapy has, in our experience with the Magnetic Molecular Energizer (MME), been likewise encouraging. Twenty-four out of twenty-six patients with fibromyalgia improved with MME treatment. See www.amripa.com for more information and case histories.

Lifestyle Approaches

- Minimizing use of NSAIDS (nonsteroidal anti-inflammatories). These over-the-counter medications tend to relieve pain in the short term, but long-term usage has been found to cause leaky gut, increased oxidative stress, and liver detoxification problems.
- Magnetic mattress pad. A double-blind placebo-controlled randomized study in patients with fibromyalgia using a magnetic mattress pad especially

of the type manufactured by Magnetico has found that patients experience an approximately 25 percent decrease in pain (total tender-point pain intensity) over a six-month period. This study was performed at the University of Virginia and published in the *Journal of Alternative and Complementary Medicine* in 2001.

- Avoidance of excessive A/C electromagnetic radiation from household appliances. Many patients with fibromyalgia, when scanned with a gauss meter, have an unusual distribution of normal electromagnetic current within the body, suggesting a blockage of D/C current (personal observation by the author). This suggests benefit in limiting exposure to electrical currents, for example, working at a flat panel display computer monitor (LCD), rather than a conventional monitor. Avoid heating pads and electric blankets. Fibromyalgia patients seem to be more sensitive to the electromagnetic field from appliances, television sets, and computers. Acupuncture, which is intended to balance the electromagnetic meridians of the body, can also be effective. (For more information see the books of Devin Starlanyl.)
- Support groups. Dr. Devin Starlanyl's Web page, which connects to a number of support groups, is also very good. See www.sover.net/~devstar/.
- Exercise. We recommend stretching and flexibility exercises and/or aerobic conditioning when possible. For patients whose fatigue is too severe to exercise, massage is an option worth considering to promote circulation in the muscles. In cases of extreme fatigue, consider breathing exercises (see chapter 43 for information and resources).

As you can see, there is no magic bullet for this disorder, but these therapeutic approaches have been successful in patients with fibromyalgia, particularly when the underlying causal factor(s) can be identified and the most effective forms of treatment can be matched to the cause and the needs of the individual patient.

FISSURES

A fissure is a cut in the skin lining the anal canal, usually in the internal portion of the canal, but occasionally in the anal opening. Its symptoms are pain and bleeding, in some cases following constipation.

Possible causes for fissures include anal trauma or extreme constipation with large stools that tear the skin. Chronic anal fissures are another class; when they persist for more than a month, this indicates a problem of increased sphincter pressure, which implies the need for surgical treatment.

Diagnosis

Anoscopy can find the tear in the bottom of the anal area. However, examination under anesthesia is often necessary. Anal-rectal manometry (EMG) can be used to measure pressure in the case of sphincter problems.

Medical Treatment

- Warm sitz baths
- Astringents
- Ointments
- Topical low-dose nitroglycerin to relieve spasm of muscle
- Stool softeners
- Injection therapy
- Cauterizing the area with silver nitrate stick (performed by a physician as an office procedure)
- Chronic fissures may require a surgical excision to remove a portion of the sphincter muscle (sphincterotomy)

Herbal Therapy

For mild cases take gotu kola or aloe vera, in conjunction with medical treatment.

FISTULAS

Fistulas are defined as one or more tracts that drain from the anal canal, which most often occur in Crohn's disease, but can also be due to trauma, syphilis, TB, radiation therapy, anal cancer, chlamydial infection, or anaerobic bacterial infection. Symptoms include drainage of pus from the area.

Medical Treatment

- Surgical incision and drainage
- For Crohn's disease, treatment with metronidazole or infliximab (Remicade) (which contains tumor necrosis antibodies, in a therapy targeted at the immune system, and requires an intravenous infusion), which is costly
- Cases of chlamydia are treated with Bactrim

Herbal Therapy

Treatment is with cleansing herbs, such as gotu kola, aloe vera, chaparral (now off the restricted list), red clover, or goldenseal (not to be taken for more than three weeks at a time).

FOOD ALLERGIES

See also chapters 8 and 20 on allergies.

Allergy symptoms occur in many forms and may include headaches, irritability, inappropriate weight gain, skin problems, aching joints, diarrhea, or abdominal complaints.

Diagnosis

- Elimination diet
- IgG food allergy testing for delayed symptoms
- IgE testing for immediate food allergy

Treatment

- Identify and remove the allergen from the diet, replace digestants, restore flora, repair the GI tract.
- Medication: Cromolyn sodium (Gastrochrom) can be taken before meals to block the release of histamine (from the mast cells, which are immune-reactive cells).
- Supplements: Bioflavonoids such as quercetin, vitamin C, and proanthanols such as grape seed tend to reduce allergic reactivity. MSM tends to decrease histamine release, the cause of many allergic symptoms.

Complementary Therapies

- Allergy therapy (see chapter 20).
- NAET therapy. In *The NAET Guidebook*, Debi Nambudripad, Ph.D., discusses applied kinesiology for use in allergy elimination. This is a specialized approach that involves using acupuncture and acupressure and is most often used by acupuncturists.
- Hyposensitization, also known as provocative neutralization, or immunotherapy with diluted concentrations of the allergic substance.
- Homeopathy, if it is provided by a knowledgeable practitioner, can be helpful in treating allergies.

GALLSTONES

The gallbladder is the reservoir for bile, which is a natural solvent within the body that helps to emulsify fats and digest them. Bile is a body chemical made from cholesterol that links with fat to assist in its transport from the digestive tract through the bloodstream and into the cells for absorption.

The bile can clump into solid, stonelike formations that may lodge within the bile ducts, either as gallstones or as a sludgelike material that can interfere with the functioning of the gallbladder. An acute inflammation of the gallbladder (cholecystitis) can result due to the blockage, and sometimes requires immediate surgery. In addition when there is defective functioning, the gallbladder doesn't empty as well. This means there is poorer digestion of fats because of insufficient bile secretion.

Incidence and Risk Factors

- Rarely occurs before age 20.
- A gene has been identified that makes people more susceptible to gallbladder disease.
- Northern Europeans may have a higher incidence.
- Gallstones occur primarily in females, especially those who have been pregnant.
- Gallstones seem to accompany obesity.
- Rapid weight loss, particularly in previously obese women, puts them at higher risk.
- Those who consume a high-fat diet have the highest incidence. This is because consuming a great deal of fat saturates the bile, making it more likely to form stones. For example, in the Pima Indians of California, 70 percent have gallstones because of heredity and a diet high in saturated fats and starches. However, Pima Indians in Mexico, who are similar genetically, have a low incidence due to the difference in diet. Heredity is not destiny.
- Bacteria are implicated in the development of gallstones. They apparently can initiate the core formation of the stone, called the nidus.
- A gallstone with a different chemical makeup than that typically found in gallbladder conditions is associated with sickle-cell anemia and hemolytic anemia. This form is not cholesterol based.

Signs and Symptoms

- Abdominal pain in the upper right area of the abdomen under the liver. The pain can radiate around to the back, especially the right shoulder blade. The pain is associated with eating fatty foods. Sometimes it may be just a dull ache or a sensation of bloating after meals.
- Attacks of severe pain, with blockage, fever, and jaundice, can occur from the blocking of the bile ducts into the gut.
- Problems with motility of the bile duct and the gallbladder may be the issue, a condition that may be improved by taking drugs or nutrients that promote motility, such as magnesium or olive oil taken in small amounts to avoid a rapid gallbladder flush and a lodged stone.
- Gallstones with no symptoms—about half of the patients with gallstones

will have no symptoms (asymptomatic) and are typically diagnosed through a routine screening.

- When there is long-standing untreated gallbladder inflammation, gall-bladder cancer can occur.

Diagnosis

- Ultrasound of the gallbladder has been the standard for several decades.
- The biliary scan utilizes a radioactive material that is then excreted from the liver into the gallbladder. This test can be helpful in diagnosis when the ultrasound does not show a gallstone but the symptoms are present. The scan measures emptying time using a hormone called CCK, which stimulates emptying of the gallbladder. Doctors also monitor for pain during the test as a symptom. This delay in emptying is often misinterpreted as a symptom of gallbladder disease, especially in cases of irritable bowel syndrome. The customary solution is the removal of the gallbladder, only to have the symptoms return in a month or two. If gallbladder removal is recommended based on delayed emptying, we encourage you to seek a second opinion from a gastrointestinal motility expert.
- ERCP is a multifaceted procedure involving the endoscope and an injection of dye into the gallbladder, which makes it possible to detect gallstones in the ducts. If stones are detected it is possible to open the ducts surgically to remove the stones.

Surgery

- Surgery is now frequently used to remove the gallbladder (cholecystectomy). Laparoscopic removal of the gallbladder is the most frequently performed procedure. This surgery is delicate and complicated and should be performed by a surgeon highly familiar with this specific operation. After laparoscopy stones may recur in the remaining ducts. At that point the ERCP procedure can later be used to remove stones, using endoscopy for stone extraction.
- The disadvantages to removing the gallbladder are that bile salts are no longer concentrated in the gallbladder, which can result in a form of diarrhea referred to as bile diarrhea. When bile comes directly out of the liver the small intestine must adapt, which it eventually does. However, post-cholecystectomy syndrome diarrhea can last for six to twelve months after surgery. Of those who have their gallbladder removed, 25 percent will have some symptoms following surgery. Questran is a bile resin that may help with this type of diarrhea.
- Post-cholecystectomy syndrome can often trigger or worsen irritable bowel syndrome.

- Alternative surgical treatment—lithotripsy—is infrequently done. In this treatment sound waves are used to smash the gallstone, while the patient is under anesthesia, similar to the procedure for kidney stones.

Nonsurgical Therapy

- Shock wave therapy. This form of treatment uses high-frequency sound waves to fragment the stones. Bile salt is administered afterward to dissolve the small pieces.
- Contact dissolution. Another method called contact dissolution can also be used to dissolve gallstones. The doctor inserts a catheter through the abdomen under CT scan guidance and then injects a special drug directly into the gallbladder. In many cases the stone disappears within a few hours. Contact dissolution and shock wave therapy are still considered experimental, but are options for a patient who is not a surgical candidate.

Medication

- Urso and Actigall are the two primary drugs used in gallbladder therapy. Surgery is a more frequently used option because drug therapy can take up to two years and not fully dissolve all the stones. Small amounts of Urso (originally bear bile from Chinese medicine) or aspirin have been found to protect against the development of gallstones, by reducing the saturation of the bile.
- If you are being treated for Lyme disease with IV Rocephin, take Urso to prevent gallbladder sludge.

Complementary Treatments

Naturopaths do a gallbladder flush, typically using olive oil. This approach appears to work better for sludge or in very moderate cases. If you have not had a scan and do not know the size of the stone, do not do an olive oil gallbladder flush, because the stone could be released and then lodged in one of the ducts of the system, requiring emergency surgery.

Prevention

Diet

- Low-fat, high-fiber diet
- Vegetarians have a much lower rate of gallstones than nonvegetarians
- Coffee drinking in moderation has been shown to decrease the incidence of gallstones
- Avoid rapid weight loss

Nutrients

- Vitamin C and other major antioxidants
- As a preventive, low-dose aspirin has been found to reduce the incidence of stones
- Phosphatidyl-choline; choline and inositol
- Magnesium sulfate; trace minerals, but if there is jaundice, avoid supplements with copper
- Pancreatic enzymes, particularly lipase, which digests fats
- Gallbladder flush using olive oil—have a scan first and have the flush performed under a doctor's supervision
- Psyllium
- Taurine may prevent cholesterol stones

Herbs

- Silymarin is highly recommended
- Red beet (fresh or powdered in capsules)
- Pancreatin (pancreatic enzymes to promote digestion)
- Peppermint, alfalfa, ginger, fennel
- L.V.R. Formula is also a very helpful herbal combination from Pure Encapsulations
- Dandelion root leaf can be used as a mild diuretic
- Bladderwrack is moderately helpful with weight loss
- Compounded fennel and wild yam can be very useful in combating flatulence
- Turmeric, oregon grape, bupleurum, and coin grass may reduce gallbladder inflammation and relieve liver congestion

Hormones

In women this condition is often associated with hormone changes in midlife or pregnancy. If this is a major problem, get your hormone levels checked, particularly by a physician who practices nutritional medicine or is knowledgeable about herbs and nutrition, to address both issues at once.

Complementary Therapies

- Acupuncture therapy involves a specific gallbladder meridian that can be stimulated for treatment
- Homeopathic treatment does not dissolve stones, but can help with the symptoms

GASTRITIS

Gastritis is defined as an inflammation of the stomach lining, and it can either be acute or occur as a long-term chronic condition.

Causes

- *Helicobacter pylori* bacteria
- A decrease in the number of cells that produce essential digestive acids (associated with autoimmune conditions and the presence of overly reactive T cells)
- Drug-associated sensitivity to nonsteroidal anti-inflammatory drugs (NSAIDs) or arthritis drugs
- Cause unknown (idiopathic)

This condition is fairly common, seems to accompany aging, and occurs in almost 4 percent of those age 21 to 30 and in more than 16 percent of those over 70. Some facts to consider:

- Autoimmune gastritis, *H. pylori* infection, and sensitivity to NSAIDs are strongly associated with genetic predisposition.
- Gastritis is more common in patients of Scandinavian origin.
- *H. pylori* infection can cause thinning of the stomach lining (atrophy) and the loss of acid-producing cells. This predisposes people to gastric cancer later in life.

Symptoms

- Bloating, bad taste in the mouth, poor digestion, diarrhea; in some cases, no symptoms.
- Pernicious anemia (vitamin B_{12} deficiency) or megaloblastic anemia (a type of anemia in which the red cells become enlarged and are more fragile).
- Vitiligo (skin discoloration) is sometimes associated with autoimmune gastritis.
- Flatulence.
- Chronic fatigue.
- Stroke (in the central nervous system). Malabsorption is associated with gastritis and low acid production. The nutrient deficiencies (such as vitamin B_{12}) that result from malabsorption can ultimately lead to stroke. This is especially true if elevated homocysteine levels also occur (due to inadequate vitamin B_6 and folic acid, malabsorption, or genetic abnormalities). Vitamin B_{12} levels may also decrease when there is bacterial overgrowth. The use of antibiotics can be helpful in correcting these overgrowths, but it is also important to restore flora and moderate carbohydrates.

- Untreated chronic vitamin B_{12} deficiency from pernicious anemia can cause major cognitive problems, mental confusion, and disorientation. If this goes untreated, it can lead to demyelinization of the spinal cord, which causes significant sensory, motor, and neurological problems.

Diagnosis and Treatment

- Endoscopy of the stomach reveals the appearance of the stomach wall; in gastritis, it may appear thin or inflamed.
- Multiple biopsies can also demonstrate the presence of inflammation when gastritis is present. In the early stages of gastritis, metaplasia occurs, involving the transformation of the stomach lining cells into another, less functional type of cell. When this occurs gastric glands lose their function and are no longer able to produce hydrochloric acid, which is essential for digestion. In addition intestinal lining cells invade the stomach region. This can be a precancerous condition.
- Measurement of acidity. A nasogastric tube is swallowed and a hormone (pentagastrin) is injected to stimulate acid, and the pH is measured.
- In most cases of autoimmune-related gastritis, the body develops an antibody targeted against the acid-producing cells of the stomach (parietal cells). Tests are available that can detect this antibody.
- Another test is available that identifies the antibody erroneously targeted against intrinsic factor (the essential body chemical needed for the absorption of vitamin B_{12}). The antibody that attacks intrinsic factor is usually present in autoimmune gastritis.
- Testing for vitamin B_{12} levels in serum, as well as folic acid (see chapter 33 for more information).
- Testing for pepsinogen 1, a peptide that rises in patients lacking the hormone that stimulates essential acid secretion (gastrin).

Treatment of Gastritis Caused by H. pylori or Autoimmune Conditions

- Replace acid with a betaine hydrochloride supplement
- *H. pylori* is treated with antibiotics and proton pump inhibitors to eradicate the infection
- Vitamin B_{12} can be supplemented by injection or sublingual tablets or drops

Treatment of Gastritis Resulting from NSAIDS or Arthritis Medication

Superficial erosions occur in the stomach lining. This condition is treated by:

- Reducing acid with H2 blockers or proton pump inhibitors. Prevacid has been approved for this indication.

- Avoiding NSAIDs or arthritis medication.
- Taking Cytotec, a medication that acts as a protection against the erosion of the gastric lining, and can be taken in combination with the NSAIDs or arthritis medication.

Nutritional Therapies
- Juice therapy (especially cabbage juice)
- Aloe vera
- DGL (deglycyrrhizinated licorice)
- Bitters or gentian to stimulate acid production
- Betaine HCl

Diet
- Individualize diet
- Consult *Eat Right 4 Your Type* (Peter D'Adamo, Putnam, 1996)
- Try monomeals (eating a single food at a sitting, which tends to be more digestible) taken over the course of the day; become informed about food combining, which means eating protein or starch with vegetables, but avoiding a meal that includes large amounts of protein *and* starch eaten together
- Testing for food allergy or the elimination diet (see chapter 20)
- Vitamins—low hydrochloric acid means poor absorption; therefore all vitamins and minerals need to be supplemented

Herbs
- Peppermint oil, turkey rhubarb root, fresh goldenseal (not to be taken for more than three weeks at a time), vegetable glycerin, fennel seed
- Rice bran oil may normalize production of gastric acid; slippery elm eases inflammation; marshmallow root is soothing; butter burdock root is an antispasmodic

Complementary Therapies
- Acupuncture.
- Homeopathy.
- Massage and energy work: solar plexus massage, Reiki, Qigong.
- Soothing therapies to supplement other treatment: aromatherapy, music therapy (the Mozart effect—relaxation promotes digestive secretions).
- Moderate exercise; active exercise cuts back on acid secretions. (See chapter 43 for information on breathing exercises, walking programs, and therapeutic approaches to exercise.)

HEARTBURN

See Reflux and Heartburn—GERD.

HEMORRHOIDS

Hemorrhoids are enlarged and protruding blood vessels in the anal area, with weakened prolapsed walls, either inside the anal canal or outside in the tissue surrounding the anus.

Typical symptoms include bleeding or blood in the stool. Swelling or protrusion of the hemorrhoids can occur. Clotted external hemorrhoids are very painful and can cause swelling and discomfort when sitting.

Possible causes include overactivity or a motility disorder such as diarrhea or constipation. The internal sphincter muscle can spasm in abnormal muscle contractions and aggravate a potential condition. Persistence of congenital hemorrhoidal bands can also be a factor.

Collagen problems can also play a role, and may occur during pregnancy, from heavy lifting, from sitting a lot, due to a vitamin deficiency (possibly B complex vitamins), or as a result of aging. The condition may also involve a lack of tone in the blood vessel, surrounding muscle, and connective tissue.

Diagnosis

Examination is performed with a slotted anoscope (which is a short tube inserted into the anal canal), with or without a fiber-optic light, which can show the hemorrhoids or anal lesions more clearly. Sigmoidoscopy or colonoscopy should be performed to rule out other causes of rectal bleeding.

Mainstream Medical Treatment

Therapies such as warm sitz baths, anal/rectal cleaning, and hydrocortisone suppositories are often helpful. A high-fiber diet and supplementary fiber such as Konsyl or Metamucil are frequently prescribed. (See Constipation for other suggestions on fiber.) Caution: The over-the-counter drug Preparation H contains mercury and can be dangerous if used on a prolonged basis, because of the tremendous potential for the absorption of mercury from the anal canal.

Outpatient Surgical Treatment

- Internal rubber band ligation, utilizes a rubber ring stretched over a cone and fitted on a firing apparatus. When placed over the hemorrhoid and released, it encircles the tissue and stabilizes it.
- Infrared photo coagulation involves placing a light wand over the base of the hemorrhoid. The instrument superficially cauterizes and seals the

blood vessel. This method has a high success rate and is generally the best technique for internal hemorrhoids.

- Electrocoagulation is a similar technique that uses electrocautery to cauterize the tissue, but it takes considerably more time and in the author's opinion does not work as well as rubber band ligation or photo coagulation.
- CO_2 lasers are used in outpatient treatment, for both internal and external hemorrhoid excision and removal. Local anesthesia and occasionally stitches are required. This is typically the most successful technique for external hemorrhoids.
- Cryosurgery is not used as frequently now because it has a long recovery period.
- Injection sclerosing therapy is also used less often because it involves an injection of chemicals that can leave ulcers or hard fibrotic scar tissue.

Surgical Treatment

- Blood clots (thrombosis) of external hemorrhoids are treated by surgical removal (excision) and can be performed through laser surgery in the doctor's office or manually with a scalpel. Local anesthesia is required.
- Total surgical removal (hemorrhoidectomy) is reserved for prolapsed hemorrhoids that cannot be reduced by internal repositioning or other techniques (fourth-degree hemorrhoids). Very swollen, clotted external hemorrhoids may also require complete surgical removal. This is performed under local or general anesthesia in the hospital. However, scarring or stricture of the anal canal can occur and interfere with bowel movements, which may require periodic anal dilation to stretch the strictured area. Postoperative pain may be severe in some patients.

Topical Preparations

- Anurex is a suppository chilled in the refrigerator and placed in the anal canal, which reduces inflammation.
- Anusol hydrocortisone suppositories are used to reduce inflammation.
- Rowasa suppositories contain mesalamine, which is often helpful in the treatment of inflammatory bowel disease and is also helpful in treating hemorrhoids.

Diet

- People with low-fiber diets have more hemorrhoids, so a high-fiber diet is recommended. Psyllium or cellulose, if tolerated, or other fiber supplements are often beneficial.

- Avoid constipation; keep up with liquid intake. Perhaps keep a chart to be sure you're consuming enough.

Nutrients
- Vitamins C, A, and E
- Bioflavonoids such as Pycnogenol may strengthen the vessel wall
- CoQ_{10} is a protectant of the engine of our cells (the mitochondria)
- Trace minerals for chronic inflammation—copper, zinc, and manganese

Herbs
- Anti-inflammatories such as aloe (which can be taken internally and also applied externally) and slippery elm
- Ginger, gotu kola, red beet, bilberry, collinsonia, taken orally
- Witch hazel pads (Tucks) are available as astringent wipes and are reported to decrease inflammation
- Geranium root and plantain as a topical astringent

Homeopathics
- If your hemorrhoids are serious, see a well-trained homeopathic physician for either an immediate or long-term remedy. Homeopathic remedies, well chosen, can be a potent cure for hemorrhoids.
- Use *Aesculus* for burning hemorrhoids with a sensation of a lump in the anus that feels worse when walking and *Hamamelis* for large bleeding hemorrhoids with a raw feeling.
- For more information on homeopathic first aid, see the section on hemorrhoids in chapter 41.

Acupuncture
This can often numb the area and decrease pain by unblocking the meridians. Some people with hemorrhoids or other rectal conditions get excellent results with acupressure. A wonderful book that guides the reader through the process with easy-to-find landmarks is K. Serizawa's *Tsubo* (2nd ed., Japan Publications, 1995). These same points also work well with electroacustim.

Exercise
- Refrain from heavy lifting and super-vigorous exercise.
- Moderate exercise is okay, but check with your doctor and let the level of discomfort guide you.
- If you are able to exercise moderately, this will help to increase tone and improve bowel movements.

- Kegel exercises can be helpful. If your condition is severe, ask your doctor to arrange biofeedback (pelvic floor EMG), which can be exceptionally helpful when retraining muscles.

HEPATITIS (CHRONIC)

For detailed treatment information please see Liver Disease.

Hepatitis is inflammation of the liver from a variety of infectious agents and other causes. Here we will focus primarily on hepatitis caused by infection.

Causes

- Viruses identified as hepatitis A, B, C, D, and E; new strains continue to be identified.
- Epstein-Barr virus, which causes hepatitis, also causes infectious mononucleosis.
- Cytomegalo virus can infect the liver.
- Bacterial infections such as tuberculosis and typhoid (caused by salmonella).

Symptoms

Symptoms are similar in all forms, but the potential for liver failure is greater in some forms. Typically flulike symptoms are accompanied by fever, chills, nausea, vomiting, aching in joints and over the liver, and occasionally jaundice. Some people may experience intense symptoms.

Viral Hepatitis A

- Transmission: through food handling, exposure to stool, or contaminated food or water.
- Severity: acute and usually mild, rather than chronic; one form can be fatal if not treated.
- Incubation period is 2 weeks to 48 days, with acute inflammation that eventually goes away and does not become chronic. A fulminant form is occasionally seen, requiring treatment comparable to dialysis or transplantation, and if not so treated can be fatal.
- Prevalence: The potential for epidemics of viral hepatitis A is found most often in the third world or in environments where there are crowded conditions or poor sanitation. In these areas 50 percent or more of the population test positive for hepatitis antibodies, but often the majority have no symptoms. In Taiwan and the region that was formerly Yugoslavia, which have the highest degree of exposure, 90 percent of adults tested have hepatitis antibodies. Among those who have

been exposed and therefore test positive, the majority of people have no symptoms. Switzerland has the lowest percent of antibody-positive adults.

- Nursing homes and day care facilities are high-risk environments. Fecal/oral exposure also occurs in residents of long-term care institutions, such as those in mental institutions and prisons.

Hepatitis B

- Transmission: most often occurs through needle sharing and intimate sexual contact.
- Severity: most often acute; 25 percent of cases become chronic and are at risk for liver failure. In such chronic cases people may experience fatigue, but more commonly have no symptoms and are only diagnosed when they are having their blood tested or are donating blood and are rejected.
- Incubation period: 28 to 160 days.
- Prevalence: worldwide. More carriers have been exposed to viral hepatitis B than any other type of hepatitis, and 5 percent of the world's population are carriers.
- More male than female, more tropical, more urban.
- In Southeast and Central Asia, exposure is as high as 80 percent, almost half acquired in the perinatal period around birth.
- Specifics on transmission: In the United States, the prevalence is 12 percent. Hepatitis B can be contracted from blood transfusions, contaminated needles, needle sticks, and sexual contact. Even tattoo wells have been implicated, and manicure instruments can transmit the virus. The bodily fluids in which hepatitis B is transmitted are saliva, blood, tears, and semen. During the mid-1980s, blood transmission accounted for the majority of infections of hepatitis B. Now that blood is screened for both HIV and hepatitis B, blood transmission is rare.
- Prevention: The same type of precautions against HIV are also appropriate for hepatitis B.

Hepatitis C

- Transmission: primarily thought to be through blood transmission, such as transfusions.
- Severity: 50 percent of the cases are acute; 50 percent become chronic with the potential for liver failure.
- Incubation period: from blood can be 5 to 26 days; the intermediate form has a 6- to 12-week incubation period.
- Prevalence: found worldwide.

- Specifics on transmission: primarily through blood products, especially through multiple transfusions or banking blood/platelet factor transfusions. When blood banks pool or concentrate blood the risk increases. Periodically hepatitis C is transmitted in waterborne epidemics in India and other tropical areas. Sexual transmission and infection from contaminated tattoo instruments are less likely, but still possible.
- Symptoms: same as hepatitis B. Chronic hepatitis can cause an enlarged liver, which can lead to chronic fatigue syndrome, cirrhosis, and liver failure, diagnosed by elevated enzymes in the blood picked up by traditional liver testing (GGT [Gamma-glutamyl transpeptidase] or ALT, AST).

Hepatitis D

- Severity: The D virus can cause deterioration of the liver.
- Prevalence: Hepatitis D, or Delta Agent hepatitis, is only associated with hepatitis B infections. This condition is often found in the Mediterranean region or the Middle East, where as many as 40 percent of hepatitis B virus carriers have been exposed to hepatitis D. It is sometimes epidemic in isolated communities in South America.
- Incubation period: 20 to 50 days.
- Transmission: It can occur from needles, sexual contact, or transfusions. A person can acquire hepatitis D infection at the same time he or she is infected with the hepatitis B virus (this is called co-infection). A person with hepatitis B can be infected with hepatitis D virus at any time after acute hepatitis B virus infection (this is called super-infection). The combination of hepatitis B and D can be more serious than hepatitis B alone and is more likely to cause serious chronic hepatitis and cirrhosis.

Hepatitis E

- Prevalence: Hepatitis E is similar to hepatitis A and is acute rather than chronic. Although hepatitis E is unusual in the United States, the virus has produced large outbreaks in India and Pakistan and South and Central America. It occurs primarily in middle-aged or pregnant women.
- Incubation period: 40 days.
- Transmission: It is acquired by direct contact with an infected person's feces or indirect fecal contamination of food, water supply, raw shellfish, hands, or utensils when sufficient amounts of the virus enters the mouth.

Mainstream and Alternative Treatment

See Liver Disease for specific information.

Herbs

- For healing and strengthening: silymarin (milk thistle), St. John's wort, leptotaenia (lomatium), schizandra
- Systemic Formulas L-Liver, Systemic Formula No. 5, Systemic VIVI Lomatium Formula
- See the section on liver support in chapter 37, on herbal remedies

INDIGESTION (CHRONIC)

See Dyspepsia—Without Ulcers.

INFLAMMATORY BOWEL DISEASES (IBD): ULCERATIVE COLITIS AND CROHN'S DISEASE

IBD is a chronic inflammatory condition of the large or small intestines that occurs in two forms:

- Ulcerative colitis, which affects the colon, but just the lining
- Crohn's disease, an inflammatory condition that can affect all layers of the intestine or even the entire length of the digestive tract from the mouth to the anus

The causes of IBD are still generally unknown. In fact there may be a number of different causes for these conditions. Consequently treatment that works for one person may not work for the next. These are extremely complex, challenging illnesses. Causal factors suggested by researchers include:

- Possible abnormal overgrowth of bacteria in the GI tract or reaction to viral infections such as measles virus in the wall of the GI tract (in the lining cells).
- Possible contributing disorders such as tuberculosis, or pleomorphic bacteria that have no cell walls and therefore are extremely difficult to detect.
- Disordered immune processes (or autoimmune condition). Both ulcerative colitis and Crohn's are considered immune disorders.
- Genetics appears to be a major factor, as these illnesses tend to run in families. This is especially true of Crohn's disease. For example, it occurs frequently among the Ashkenazi Jewish people and also people from the British Isles, particularly Ireland.
- Stress and inflammation play a role in this disorder.
- Other factors include altered GI flora, delayed food allergy (such as IgG-related sensitivities [see chapter 20]), and diminished blood flow to colon.

- Decreased blood supply (ischemia), such as seen in the elderly. Those on medications that inhibit circulation are more likely to contract this condition.
- Anti-inflammatory drugs, particularly NSAIDs, are implicated in these two disorders because these medications can increase gut permeability.
- Increased oxidative stress and decreased antioxidants may be factors, since this implies lowered cellular defenses.

There are links between immune disorders, IBD, and conditions such as rheumatoid arthritis. This means that when the immune system becomes overly active in our defense, our immune response can actually be toxic to us and cause leaky gut syndrome and overstimulation of the immune system with illnesses such as arthritis, dermatitis, inflammation of the colon (colitis) or lower portion of the small intestine (ileitis), and eye inflammations of the iris (iritis). Inflammatory processes and damage due to immune overresponse is similar in these GI conditions and in rheumatoid arthritis.

Causes of Crohn's Disease

- Heredity is clearly associated with Crohn's disease, and it is observed to run in families. Relatives with no symptoms may still have small patches of inflammation seen in a colonoscopic examination and increased gut permeability. However, within a family, some members will develop inflammation and symptoms and others will not.
- Bacterial overgrowth after antibiotic therapy can promote symptoms of inflammation and bring on attacks of Crohn's disease.
- A change in intestinal permeability can also trigger symptoms.
- Food allergies have been directly implicated. Elemental diets (synthetic liquid diets) consisting entirely of powdered soy or rice-based drinks with added nutrients are designed to minimize allergies. This diet tends to be as effective in Crohn's as steroids and can put the patient in remission.
- Autoimmune disorders that have been associated with Crohn's disease include: food allergies, rheumatoid arthritis, eczema, asthma, and hives.
- Viruses, bacteria such as yersinia, and other forms of bacterial overgrowth can break down bile acids and produce secondary bile salts, which can trigger inflammation.

Symptoms of Crohn's Disease

- Intestinal scarring from chronic inflammation can cause stricturing and narrowing of the gut, resulting in obstruction and requiring surgery.
- Diarrhea, abdominal pain, weight loss, rectal bleeding, and/or bloody stools.

- Limited growth, excessive weight loss, or in rare cases even weight gain. An overgrowth of bacteria or candida can drive an appetite for sweets and starches, causing excessive weight gain and triggering symptoms.
- Fever of unknown origin.
- Crohn's typically manifests in young people in their preteens or teens. The other age group most likely to develop Crohn's is people in their seventies.
- In the intestinal tract active Crohn's is seen as patchy intestinal inflammation.
- Symptoms can occur throughout the entire GI system, such as fistulas (draining sores in the rectum, bladder, and vaginal tract, or on the skin).

Symptoms in other parts of the body, seen in Crohn's but also in ulcerative colitis, include:

- Skin ulcerations and/or swollen, sore red nodules under the skin (erythema nodosum).
- Iritis (inflammation of the iris).
- Mouth ulcers: superficial ulcers in the interior of the mouth, on the gums, and on the tongue.
- Polyarthritis (aching and swelling of small joints throughout the body)— for example, in the hands or feet, in the elbows or the collarbone, and in the knees.

Ulcerative Colitis

Inheritance is not as clear as in Crohn's, although some genetic factors have been discovered. Genetic models of the inheritance patterns suggest that ulcerative colitis is probably caused by one major gene that has yet to be identified. Symptoms are usually limited to the colon: primarily diarrhea, abdominal pain, discomfort, and bleeding. Weight loss and obstructive symptoms are rare.

Seasonal flare-ups of both Crohn's and ulcerative colitis often occur in the spring and fall. One explanation favored by the author is that the balance between repair factors and inflammation is tipped because intestinal DNA replication is diminished in those seasons.

Lab Tests for Crohn's and IBD

Although these are two distinct conditions, both conventional and functional lab testing is the same for colitis and Crohn's.

Conventional Lab Testing

- Stool testing for white cells as an indication of infection
- Elevated sedimentation rate (reflects the level of antibodies and indirectly the level of inflammation)
- Colonoscopy of the entire colon or enteroscopy of the small intestine
- Specialized X-ray of the small intestine, called enterocylsis
- Video capsule (M2A)
- Contrast barium enemas of the colon and the ileum (lower small intestine)

Functional Lab Testing

- Antibody testing for bacteria, viruses, or other pathogens.
- Comprehensive digestive stool analysis—Great Smokies Diagnostic Lab.
- Lactulose-mannitol urine test for intestinal permeability. This test is very important in Crohn's and is also relevant in ulcerative colitis. (See chapter 7 on permeability.)
- IgG blood tests for delayed food allergy (see chapters 8 and 20).
- Organic acids test to check for markers of elusive bacteria.
- Testing for vitamin profiles or antioxidant status to indicate any significant nutrient deficiencies that might be affecting general immunity.
- Blood testing for trace minerals: low copper, zinc, manganese.

Mainstream Treatment for Crohn's Disease and Ulcerative Colitis

- Steroids (prednisone or budesonide [Entocort EC]) are prescribed or used in combination with 5-ASA medications—in the class of mesalamine, drugs such as Pentasa or Asacol or sulfasalazine (Azulfidine). Colazol (balsalazide) appears to be more potent in some patients with ulcerative colitis. Mesalamine is a derivative of salicylic acid and is thought to be the active component of sulfasalazine (Azulfidine), a combination of a sulfa drug and salicylic acid. Mesalamine works as an anti-inflammatory agent and is used in treating ulcerative colitis and Crohn's disease.
- More recent drugs include chloroquine (Plaquenil), an antimalarial drug that calms the immune system.
- Major immunosuppressants—azathioprine (Imuran) or the parent drug 6-MP.
- Ciprofloxin (Cipro) is an antibacterial that tones down the immune system.

Surgical Treatment

- Resection (removal) of the entire colon in ulcerative colitis is considered to be a cure for life. This conventional wisdom isn't always true for all people, as the author has seen a number of patients who continued to have lesions elsewhere in the body.

- Resection may be necessary for the scarred section of the bowel in Crohn's that hasn't responded to medical therapy and has either led to obstruction or to recurrent bleeding.

Ulcerative colitis may become so severe that a removal of the entire colon may be necessary, or in the case of Crohn's, removal of a section of the small intestine (referred to as surgical resection). However, we try to minimize this removal, particularly since in the case of Crohn's, removal often doesn't cure the disease. In most cases the disease process is driven by an overreactive autoimmune response, and when the intestinal tissue is removed, the process simply occurs in other tissue.

Recent Controversial Treatment

- Crohn's: Some people respond to anti-TB therapy (atypical tuberculosis in some patients is suspected as a cause).
- T-cell apheresis reduces the load of T cells through a process like dialysis, which can help in severe conditions, and has been performed at Baptist Memorial Hospital in Memphis, Tennessee. Adacolumn Apheresis System is also currently undergoing clinical trials in the U.S.
- Patients with Crohn's who also had bone marrow transplants or AIDS (situations that reduce T cells) have had a remission of Crohn's because of the decreased number of T cells in the body. This tragic correlation points to the relationship between immune system activity and these severe intestinal inflammations.
- Leukine, a macrophage colony stimulator, is currently undergoing clinical trials at the time of this book's publication. It appears very promising for Crohn's patients.
- Interleukin and antisense therapy, which turn off the body's signals that promote inflammation. Antisense therapy appears to be quite effective by enema in cases of ulcerative colitis, and as intravenous treatment for Crohn's disease.
- Remicade and TNF-alpha antibodies (infliximab)—turns off tumor-necrosis for Crohn's fistulas in about 70 percent of patients. Intravenous maintenance therapy is usually needed in moderate to severe cases of Crohn's disease. Some patients with ulcerative colitis also respond, but insurance usually does not pay for this therapy as a treatment for colitis. Complications include drug reactions, TB, and progression to non-Hodgkin's lymphoma and Hodgkin's disease in patients with more severe disease activity in a few cases, because the immune system's ability to fight cancer is suppressed.

- Newer 5-ASA medications such as balsalazide (Entocort EC), which is probably better absorbed in the colon, squelches free radicals and turns on manganese superoxide dismutase, a protective enzyme in the mitochondria (the energy center of the cell).
- In Europe copper superoxide dismutase made from recombinant DNA has been experimentally used with success in treating Crohn's and rheumatoid arthritis.

Dietary Therapy

- Enteral and parenteral nutrition are used in treating Crohn's in cases of severe weight loss, chronic diarrhea, or intestinal obstruction. Providing supplemental nutrients can be helpful in many conditions, ranging from mild to severe, and as an adjunct to drug therapy.
- Disaccharide elimination diets. See Elaine Gottschall's *Breaking the Vicious Cycle* (Kirkton Press, 1994).
- Food elimination diets. Research has found that many people with inflammatory bowel disease have major food allergies, including problems with wheat, milk, or citrus. If the allergy is a causal factor, removing the trigger food can make a significant difference.
- Major nutrients—the amino acid L-glutamine to decrease gut permeability, omega-3 fish oils to restore vitamin A levels for antibody production, and Seacure peptides for repair factors.
- Friendly flora are underappreciated in GI function. Support flora with FOS (fructo-oligosaccharide) in those who can tolerate carbohydrates. The major strains are lactobacillus and bifidobacteria. Also consider mutaflora, a form of beneficial *E. coli* from Germany.
- *Saccharomyces boulardii* is a beneficial yeast that is especially useful during and after antibiotic therapy.
- Many of these nutrients are found in UltraClear Sustain, a powdered nutritional supplement from Metagenics, available by prescription.
- Inulin, an active constituent of the Jerusalem artichoke, increases short-chain fatty acids (butyrates) and is useful for those who cannot tolerate fiber.
- Glycoamines found in Mannitec, a glucose and amino acid combination.

Herbs

- According to many naturopaths, a useful herbal formula for mild to moderate conditions is Robert's Formula. Bastyr University also has its own herbal formula.
- Aloe vera (liquid); capsules are also helpful but have a laxative effect, so do not take if diarrhea is present. This herb is typically taken at bedtime.

- Slippery elm or ground flaxseed.
- Cat's claw as a natural infection fighter. Garlic capsules can be helpful, but beware of irritation.
- Alfalfa, peppermint, hawthorn, or valerian may relieve spasms.

Complementary Therapies

- Acupuncture.
- Sublingual oral allergy therapy most often provided by physicians in environmental medicine.
- NAET therapy. This is a specialized approach to allergy elimination most often used by acupuncturists, and involves acupuncture and acupressure.
- Gentle exercise. Increase blood flow to the digestive tract through walking, low-impact aerobics, t'ai chi, Qigong, or yoga. Be careful not to overdo it—aggressive exercise could stimulate bloody diarrhea.
- Mind-body therapies. Stress reduction, relaxation, self-hypnosis to modify the immune process, support host defenses, and provide adrenal relief.
- Biomagnetic therapy is a noninvasive treatment just coming into the fore that may be used for treating IBD in the future.

IRRITABLE BOWEL SYNDROME (IBS)

In this condition intestinal function is compromised and the dysfunction can occur in the small intestine or the colon, or both. It can be characterized by abdominal discomfort or pain, bloating, mucus in the stools, and irregular bowel habits. IBS is typically a gut motility problem involving either constipation or diarrhea, or an alternation between these two extremes. It may also involve low-grade inflammation that is not detected in evaluations but plagues the patient (termed subclinical inflammation). Pain is sometimes associated with this condition, but is less frequently seen.

Causes

At present the cause is not well understood. *IBS* may actually describe a number of different conditions or diseases and is something of a catch-all term. Studies have been unable to demonstrate any single physical abnormality that reliably identifies IBS. Current thinking suggests that extended antibiotic use or infection by parasites, bacteria, or viruses may be major factors. It may involve:

- Immediate allergies (IgE), delayed food allergies (IgG), or food sensitivities. Research has detected increased numbers of mast cells, associated with allergic responses (see chapter 8).

- Overgrowth of bacteria in the small intestine (see chapters 6 and 21).
- Infection, including undetected parasites or viruses (see chapters 15, 21, and 22).
- Increase in immune activity, evidenced by an increase in white blood cells (lymphocytes), which would imply the presence of low-grade inflammation (found in research studies).
- Hormonal imbalance.
- Genetic factors.
- Psychological trauma or depression.
- Imbalance of the autonomic nervous system, which controls many aspects of gut function, including motility, so it can cause both diarrhea and constipation.

IBS is a chronic disorder that occurs in at least 15 percent of the general population—and twice as many females are affected as males. Among people with digestive problems who are seen by a gastroenterologist, typically 40 percent have IBS. It tends to be a chronic problem, with symptoms that come and go over a period of months, years, or even over a lifetime. The symptoms of IBS often present for the first time early in life; for half of those affected, problems begin before the age of 30.

Diagnosis

Since so many different kinds of conditions are grouped under IBS, a thorough history and chronology of the condition can be quite important. With so many possible causes and diagnoses, it is essential to identify the history of trigger events, such as prior antibiotic therapy, traveler's diarrhea, or food intolerance.

A recent article in *The Journal of the American Medical Association* implicated bacterial overgrowth in these conditions. Currently, IBS is considered a stress disease. It is noteworthy that stomach ulcers were once viewed as a stress-related condition, until the Australian researcher, Barry Marshall, identified *H.pylori* bacteria as a major causal factor.

Testing

Traditional lab testing is generally not helpful in the diagnosis of IBS except to exclude diseases such as cancer of the colon or small intestine, ulcerative colitis, or Crohn's disease. Testing for blood in the stool (Hemoccult testing) should be done, as well as a sigmoidoscopy (with biopsy) to exclude conditions such as inflammatory bowel disease or amoebic colitis.

Here are some functional lab tests that may be helpful:

- Antibody testing to detect parasites, harmful bacteria, viruses, or yeast
- Stool testing for parasites
- Food allergy testing in the blood for IgE and IgG allergies
- Intestinal permeability testing (lactulose/mannitol test)
- Comprehensive Digestive Stool Analysis to assess digestion and identify yeast or bacterial imbalance
- Liver detoxification challenge
- Oxidative stress evaluation to determine levels of toxic free radicals in the body
- Breath testing to identify bacterial overgrowth; this test can also be used to determine lactose intolerance
- Testing for the ionized calcium/magnesium ratio to find mineral imbalance (useful in cases of constipation-predominant IBS) can be obtained through tertiary hospital labs
- EXA testing to measure minerals within the cell (intracellular electrolytes), available through IntraCellular Diagnostics, Inc.

Treatment

The overall strategy is the "4 Rs" program. (See chapter 19.)

- Remove infective microbes—bacteria, parasites, yeast, or viruses—as well as foods in the diet that may trigger inflammation
- Replace digestants (behaine hydrochloride, digestive enzymes, and bicarbonate, as needed)
- Restore beneficial bacteria in the digestive system
- Repair GI damage with vital nutrients

Diarrhea-Predominant IBS

Two patterns are evident in this condition:

- Lactose intolerance, which requires the avoidance of lactose-containing foods, or in some cases, supplementing with lactase.
- Food hypersensitivity or delayed food allergy, which requires the discovery and removal of the offending allergenic foods, and nutritional support for healing the mucosa. Elimination diets or rotation diets can be helpful once the food allergies have been discovered.

Provocative neutralization allergy therapy shows promise in desensitizing patients with food or other allergies. Digestible powdered-food supplements of rice protein concentrate have proven to be an excellent element in the hypoallergenic diet for many patients (except those who are unable to tolerate carbohydrates). Other nutrients important in healing the GI mucosa include vitamins A, B$_5$ (pantothenic acid), B$_6$ (which should be taken with the entire B complex), and C; the mineral zinc; and the amino acid L-glutamine. Choice of dietary fiber may require assessment or trial and error, particularly if inflammation appears to be present. Other considerations are the elimination of dietary irritants and stimulants, possibly including some spices, alcohol, and tobacco. It is also important to consider the connection between stress and increased tone of the sympathetic nervous system (the *stress response*), which can speed up motility, causing diarrhea, cramping, or spasms. If inflammation is present a blended food diet can be useful, using the blender or a mini–food processor.

Constipation-Predominant IBS

This type of IBS may be due to the inadequacy of fiber or fluids, as well as regular exercise. Dysbiosis due to parasites or bacteria accompanied by constipation may also be a factor.

- Fiber may be added to the diet in small amounts (5 grams per week) and gradually increased to 25 to 30 grams per day. Insoluble and nonallergenic fiber can enhance the growth of friendly flora. Do not include psyllium or wheat fibers, but consider the use of cellulose fiber or ground flaxseeds, or aloe vera in capsules.
- High-quality bentonite clay may be used as long as it is not continued for extended periods of time. Be sure to drink lots of fluid with bentonite or it can cause impaction. Sonne No. 7 (also marketed as Arise and Shine) is a quality product.
- Chronic lack of magnesium in the diet may also be a factor. Supplement the diet with foods high in magnesium when possible, as well as magnesium supplement (citrate, chloride, maleate, or glycinate). If there is alternating diarrhea with constipation, magnesium glycinate is preferable.
- Monomeals (the use of a single food at a meal) may also be helpful.

IBS with Pain or Gas and Bloating

Gas and bloating can result whenever there is incomplete digestion.

- There may not be sufficient hydrochloric acid or digestive enzymes; supplement with betaine hydrochloride and quality enzymes (either vegetarian or animal-based enzymes) such as the Wobenzyme or Zywobin Forte by Ecological Formulas (see Resources).

- Gas and bloating can also result from the overgrowth of opportunistic flora (dysbiosis) and fermentation of starches.
- Lactose intolerance or food allergies may be a cause.
- Supplement with acidophilus and bifidus if dysbiosis is a factor. FOS products may also be taken to support the friendly bacteria. However, since FOS is a natural sweetener, it may cause increased gas, so start with small doses.
- Provide sufficient short-chain fatty acids, found in flaxseed oil and in whole and ground flaxseeds, foods, and supplements with inulin such as UltraClear Sustain, and foods such as Jerusalem artichoke and dandelion greens. Research has found that olive oil appears to be the most stable of the cooking oils; whenever possible, purchase organic oils stored in dark glass bottles.
- Abdominal pain may be caused by excessive gas production, impacted stool, or muscle spasms. Antispasmodic medications or calmatives such as peppermint, spearmint, and hawthorn berry may be helpful, and potentially the use of 5HT3 medications. Zelnorm is now available for constipation-predominant IBS in women. Magnesium supplements can also be quite helpful for this type of constipation, taken at an individualized dose. (Begin with one and gradually increase the dose on days when you will be at home most of the day, as too much magnesium can cause a sudden bowel movement.)

Complementary Therapies

- Diet. In some forms of IBS, allergies, sensitivities, or food intolerance may be issues. Consider an elimination diet to identify trigger foods or general conditions such as carbohydrate intolerance. (See chapters 8 and 20 on allergies, and chapter 31 on managing carbs and blood sugar.)
- Nutrients. Anti-inflammatory nutrients can be beneficial, such as vitamin A, L-glutamine, and Seacure. If a viral condition underlies the problem, consider Monolaurin capsules from Ecological Formulas.
- Herbs. Soothing herbs such as aloe vera (liquid, gel, or caps), flaxseed meal, slippery elm, or marshmallow; if infection is present, a wide range of anti-infectives can be beneficial. (See the chart on herbs at the end of chapter 21 on clearing bad bugs.) Herbs that address spasm (antispasmodics) include alfalfa, peppermint, valerian, and hawthorn. (Also see chapter 37 for information on antibacterial and antimicrobial herbs.)
- Acupuncture. This can strengthen immune response and support the body in fighting infection; if there is undetected inflammation present (subclinical inflammation), acupuncture can be helpful in calming it.

- Homeopathy. This can be useful in situations with complex, difficult-to-diagnose symptoms and has an excellent historical track record with GI conditions. See a highly skilled practitioner.
- Mind-body therapies. If there is a history of sexual or physical abuse, psychotherapy and support groups can be extremely helpful. Relaxation techniques, stress management, hypnotherapy, and biofeedback have also been found beneficial.

LACTOSE INTOLERANCE

Inability to digest milk is often due to a missing enzyme—lactase—needed to break down the natural sugar in milk, called lactose. This condition is different from a food allergy. When there is an allergy to dairy products the body produces antibodies against milk protein, which triggers the activity of the immune system with reactive body chemicals such as histamines. Symptoms of lactose intolerance include gas and bloating and/or diarrhea.

Note that some people are also unable to digest casein, the protein in milk and dairy products. Casein is also found in many nondairy foods. Supplementing with lactase does not support the digestion of casein.

Incidence

- Lactose intolerance is the most common disorder of carbohydrate digestion in humans in the world. Most adults worldwide are unable to digest milk, with the exception of some peoples from Northern Europe.
- Age is an important determinant. Children with a genetic predisposition to lactose intolerance show symptoms around the age of five to seven.
- Inherited lactase deficiency that manifests at birth is a rare occurrence.
- After diarrhea or GI viral infection (enteritis), lactase is often lacking in the regenerated microvilli and appears to be depressed for a longer period than any other metabolic process. In some cases the body's ability to produce lactase is permanently impaired and it must be supplemented on a permanent basis.

Diagnosis

- Home testing for lactose intolerance. In the morning on an empty stomach, drink one or two glasses of milk. If there is an intolerance, diarrhea or gas will be evident.
- Breath test. This consists of measuring hydrogen excretion after drinking milk. The test is available in most hospital labs and in some gastroenterologist's offices. It reflects fermentation by colonic bacteria from

nonabsorbed lactose. Since milk is normally broken down and absorbed in the small intestine, if undigested milk reaches the colon and is fermented, it implies malabsorption of lactose (milk sugar). The fermentation releases hydrogen gas, which explains how lactose intolerance can cause gas and bloating.

- Lactose tolerance test. This consists of drinking 15 grams of milk and then measuring blood lactose, which shows how much has been absorbed into the system. In someone who is lactose intolerant, there is very little absorption of this milk sugar, and this will be reflected in the testing levels.
- If a small bowel biopsy is already being performed a sample can be taken to check for lactose intolerance done in conjunction with other diagnostic testing. It checks for the presence of the enzyme that digests milk—lactase (found in the brush border of the microvilli).
- Blood tests for IgG or IgE antibodies can be ordered from labs that do anitbody allergy testing (ELISA). (See Resources.)

Treatment

- Lactose-free diet.
- Lactase enzyme replacement—taking a supplement containing lactase, such as a lactase enzyme supplement from the health food store or Lactaid from the drugstore, before milk or dairy-containing foods are ingested.
- Cheeses that are almost completely lactose free include Swiss, sharp cheddar, Edam, and Jarlsberg.
- Note that if you are allergic to milk protein, you will still have some reactivity to milk or dairy products, even when lactase is supplemented. Symptoms of an allergy to milk protein are highly individual and can range from GI symptoms to respiratory problems (frequent colds), achy muscles, fatigue, or any of a number of other problems. This allergy can be checked in blood or saliva.
- Herbs: For symptomatic relief, ginger, peppermint, gentian, and possibly aloe vera gel.

LIVER DISEASE

Liver disease can range from mild inflammation, jaundice, or minimal scar tissue to conditions as serious as scarring or nodules that can lead to cirrhosis and liver failure. When the flow of blood through the liver is impeded by scarring, portal hypertension occurs. As a result collateral blood vessels may develop; these are enlarged veins at the lower end of the esophagus (called varices), around the navel, or around the rectum (as hemorrhoids). Hemorrhaging can develop due to high blood pressure within the liver (portal hypertension). As the liver becomes less functional, its ability to perform routine duties is impaired:

- Protein synthesis cannot be maintained.
- Toxins are passed on to the rest of the body and the brain, causing brain fog and confusion.
- Fluid can seep out of the arteries and veins into the body cavity, causing generalized edema. When serum albumin declines, this edema (ascites) occurs.
- Decreased circulation can cause a buildup of bile, bilirubin (a breakdown product of red blood cells), and other biochemicals in the liver.

Common Liver Conditions

- *Hepatitis and Fatty Liver (NASH, or Nonalcoholic Steato-Hepatitis):* Some people who are overweight and have a metabolic syndrome also have some degree of liver inflammation—hepatitis. There can be other causes of fatty liver and hepatitis as well. (For more specific information see Hepatitis [Chronic].)These conditions are diagnosed through testing that checks for higher levels of an enzymes called transaminase. The testing also measures markers for fibrinogen, a sign of scarring in the liver. The degree of scarring tends to parallel the severity of liver disease. This condition has now become the fifth leading cause for liver transplants in the United States.
- *Nonalcoholic Fatty Liver (NAFL):* Some people with these disorders may not have discernable symptoms. Their lab tests come out normal, despite weight gain, metabolic syndrome, and impaired liver function. In these cases elevated enzymes and possible scarring are not detected in routine blood tests, despite the presence of hepatitis.

  NAFL is of real concern. Often these conditions are not detected until they become so serious that more extensive testing is required—an ultrasound, a CT scan, an MRI, or a liver biopsy. Since this type of testing is seldom performed in a yearly checkup or a screening, these liver conditions may go undetected until the patient is quite ill with established cirrhosis.
- *Cirrhosis due to hemochromatosis:* This genetic condition causes the body to store too much iron, which can overload the liver, eventually causing scarring (also referred to as fibrosis). This scarring inhibits the liver's ability to synthesize protein (which is essential to build or repair tissue). It also interferes with disposal of red blood cells. Old red cells are replaced frequently because they are constantly knocking into things and

getting beaten up and damaged. One of the liver's many important jobs is to replace old red blood cells, dispose of the discarded ones, and excrete the waste (bilirubin) into the bile.

Patients with liver disease should be seen by a gastroenterologist or hepatologist. Severe liver disease can result in confusion, extreme jaundice, and eventually liver failure. In severe cases hepatic coma or encephalopathy can occur.

Primary Causes of Liver Disease

- Viral hepatitis—currently five viruses have been identified, and there may be additional strains
- Chronic alcohol overconsumption
- Obesity with fatty liver
- Pregnancy can sometimes cause fatty liver
- Medication toxicity—the most frequently occurring is unintentional overdosing with acetaminophen (Tylenol)
- Industrial or environmental toxins—causing damage through acute or chronic exposure
- Accidental poisoning from substances such as mushroom ingestion
- Hemochromatosis—excess iron concentrated in the liver
- Wilson's disease—excess copper concentrated in the liver
- Crigler-Najjar syndrome and Gilbert's disease—hereditary conditions that cause jaundice
- Blood clot (thrombosis) in either of the main veins going into the liver—veno-occlusive disease, clotting in the splenic vein, or Budd-Chiari syndrome, clotting in the hepatic vein

Mainstream Testing

- AST-ALT—measures liver enzymes that indicate liver inflammation (transaminases). These tests are relatively sensitive. The GGT is even more sensitive for early stage conditions, but not every liver profile includes this test.
- Bilirubin—a breakdown product of red blood cells that can cause jaundice if not cleared.
- Total protein albumin—a decrease in albumin shows protein synthesis is diminished.
- Immune testing for antibodies as follows:
    - Hepatitis A, C, D, and E testing for an antibody and antigen
    - Hepatitis B testing for the B core antibody and antigen and B surface antigen

- DNA polymerase (a marker for active hepatitis B)
- Antibodies for IgG (reflects chronic conditions, past exposure) and IgM (reflects acute current conditions)

- Blood tests to measure for iron overload (serum iron) and copper overload (ceruloplasmin).
- Alpha-antitrypsin—identifies deficiencies associated with early emphysema, which also result in liver disease.
- Liver biopsy is the best way to tell if chronic liver disease is present. This is done as an outpatient with a very fine needle under ultrasound guidance. When the biopsy is examined under the microscope, scar tissue (cirrhosis) and evidence of viral infection can be seen if inflammation is present.
- Imaging using the MRI or CT scan can show the presence of scar tissue, an enlarged liver, or one that is shrunken and atrophied. Patients with liver disease this serious should be managed by a hepatologist or a gastroenterologist rather than a general practitioner.

Functional Testing

- Comprehensive Digestive Stool Analysis (CDSA) to check for dysbiosis and bacterial translocation (labs that provide this testing include Great Smokies Diagnostic Laboratory, Doctor's Data, and Meridian Valley Laboratory)
- Liver detoxification profile from Great Smokies Diagnostic Laboratory
- Intestinal permeability evaluation, because increased permeability places an exceptional load on the liver and also reflects elevated cytokines, a marker for inflammation
- Evaluating the acupoints on the ear (auricular acupuncture) can provide useful diagnostic feedback

Environment

- Minimize all over-the-counter drugs, especially Tylenol.
- Minimize exposure to gasoline, fumes, solvents or other chemicals that might burden the liver. Avoid alcohol in any form.

See chapter 23 for in-depth information on minimizing toxins.

Treatment

- Hospitalization and liver washout are required when there is overwhelming hepatitis (fulminant form). The liver may need artificial cultured liver cells, in a procedure comparable to dialysis.

- Specialized diet.
- Actigall or Urso is derived from bear bile, learned from Chinese medicine to be beneficial. Used as an immunomodulator, this substance rids the liver of secondary bile salts, which tend to be toxic.
- Prednisone may prep the patient for treatment with alpha-interferon therapy (antiviral medication).
- Alpha-2b interferon, by injection, is used to stimulate the immune system in cases of hepatitis B and C. Used as aggressive therapy in chronic condition to prevent cirrhosis. Retreatment may be required.
- Alpha-2b interferon (Pegasys, PegIntron) plus ribavirin (Copegus, Rebetol) is used as combination therapy for initial treatment or retreatment. Ribavirin inhibits the virus from replicating and improves response rate in more than half of patients.
- Amantadine, an anti-influenza drug, may be useful in treatment of viral hepatitis.
- As many as 25 experimental compounds are undergoing clinical trials for use in the treatment of hepatitis C as this book goes to press, including mistletoe extract.
- At the time of this writing, little is known about therapy for hepatitis D and E.

Nutrition

- Monitor fat-soluble vitamins in chronic liver disease and use water-soluble vitamin E. Vitamins A, E, and any other fat-soluble vitamins can be toxic to the liver in high amounts.
- All antioxidants and trace minerals tend to be depleted because of inflammation. Do not supplement copper or iron, since poor circulation can elevate these minerals. Alpha Lipoic Acid is favored by many nutritionists.

Herbs

- Silymarin (milk thistle), according to Italian and Chinese data, is effective for most forms of hepatitis. However, introduce silymarin gradually. With one form of liver disease, there is reactivity even to silymarin.
- Other herbs for healing and strengthening: schizandra, an herb from Chinese medicine that has antiviral and immune-stimulating effects; St. John's wort; leptotaenia (lomatium).
- Systemic Formula L-Liver; Systemic Formula No. 5; Systemic VIVI—Lomatium Formula.

See chapter 37 on herbs, the section on liver support.

Complementary Therapies

- Minimize the load on the liver.
  - Medications. Under the supervision of an integrative physician, simplify your regimen of medications. The goal is to minimize the amount of drugs and chemicals your liver is required to break down.
  - Toxins. Also minimize the amount of chemicals you are exposed to at work and at home that may be overworking the liver. (See chapter 9 on sources of toxins, and chapter 23 on avoiding toxins.)
- Detoxify the liver. See chapter 26 on detoxifying and repairing the liver. If you have cirrhosis or liver disease this process must be done under the supervision of a doctor. Integrative physicians tend to have the dual training relevant to a nutritional approach to liver treatment, performed in a medical context.
- Chelation therapy. For copper overload, penicillamine, zinc acetate, or tetrathiomolybdate is given as an oral supplement to remove some of the metal from the body. For those with iron overload, a form of chelation therapy is used when patients can't have blood drawn to reduce iron levels.
- Treatment for alcoholism. There are two programs that have a history of high success rates in treating alcoholism:
  - The multivitamin approach developed by Joan Mathews Larson in Minneapolis, described in her book *Seven Weeks to Sobriety* (Fawcett Columbine, 1997).
  - Acupuncture detoxification has been pioneered by Dr. Michael Smith in New York. Practitioners across the country are trained in this method. Ask acupuncturists in your area about the availability of this technique. The clearinghouse for this type of information is NADA, the National Acupuncture Detox Association at (888) 765-NADA.
- New treatments. MME treatment (based on technology comparable to the MRI) is currently available at six centers. The device is under research protocol seeking FDA approval; it has a history of being used in mainstream environments, with applications in tissue regeneration. (See chapter 39.)
- Homeopathy. Useful in mild, persistent hepatitis. Work with an experienced practitioner.
- Energetic therapies. Qigong or t'ai chi, and yoga. Use gentle massage or Reiki, but not vigorous massage. If the spleen is enlarged be sure to check with your doctor before beginning exercise or even vigorous massage, because rupture is possible.
- Mind-body therapies. Because hepatitis is immune modulated, imagery and stress reduction are useful.

MALABSORPTION

Causes of poor or altered absorption of nutrients include:

- Intestinal viral or bacterial infection or overgrowth of bacteria
- Celiac disease—genetic intolerance of the gluten (protein) in wheat
- Severe allergies
- Insufficiency of pancreatic enzymes due to conditions such as infection, cystic fibrosis, alcoholism, or pancreatic cancer
- The strength of our immunity and our body's ability to repair gut-lining tissue
- B_{12} or folic acid deficiencies (it is important that adequate levels of both be maintained)

Patients may have one or more of the following symptoms: weight loss, loose stools, diarrhea, flatulence, stools that float (possible from poor digestion of fats and starches), or cramping.

Mainstream Testing

- The hydrogen breath test is one of the best tests for evaluating bacterial overgrowth.
- Testing for lactose intolerance and celiac disease is important.
- Pancreatic tests—pancreatic stimulation to measure the amount of bicarbonate secreted after stimulating the pancreas with the hormone secretin.
- The d-xylose test measures malabsorption by indicating whether simple sugar molecules are completely absorbed in the small intestine. This is also a good test for bacteria overgrowth.
- The lactulose-mannitol test can be used to detect situations in which absorption is poor, in addition to measuring leaky gut (the passage of large molecules through the gut wall).
- Testing for the level of bacteria through urine, serum, and breath testing.
- If endoscopy is being performed a sample of bacteria can be taken at the same time by enteroscope (small bowel endoscope) to measure the level of bacterial overgrowth.
- Biopsy of the small bowel through upper endoscopy or by a tethered capsule. This is one of the best ways to determine the cause of malabsorption.
- X-rays of the small bowel, to indicate the pattern of the mucosa, which reflects whether there is damage to the lining and the villi.
- NG enteroclysis—a nasogastric tube is used to X-ray the duodenum and jejunum, and diluted barium is utilized to provide detailed images of the small intestine.

- Video capsule (M2A) is being used to visualize the lining of the small intestine.
- A CT scan can pick up a diverticulum, an abscess, or even a fistulous tract as is sometimes seen in Crohn's disease, causing bacterial increase (dysbiosis) and therefore malabsorption.

Stool Samples

- Quantitative, 72-hour fecal fat (three-day) collection in which a standardized amount of fat is included in the diet and then measured in the stool to show whether the fat is being absorbed.
- CDSA (Comprehensive Digestive Stool Analysis) provides multiple information including: profile of absorption of various types of fats, fiber, acidity, friendly flora and pathogenic bacteria, parasites, and yeast. (See chapter 17 on testing, and chapter 21 on clearing bad bugs. Labs that offer this test include Doctor's Data, Great Smokies Diagnostic Laboratory, and Meridian Valley Laboratory. See Resources for contact information.)
- Biological terrain assessment (BTA) involves the analysis of acidity (pH) in blood, urine, and saliva. This test also measures electrical resistance in body fluids, which reflects oxidative stress and malabsorption of minerals. Accuracy of this testing remains anecdotal.

Diet

In this area of treatment mainstream and complementary therapies are in agreement. Diet is determined by the cause of the disorder, and the diet must be individualized in each case. For example, with celiac disease the primary approach is to avoid gluten. In specific food allergies it is essential to avoid the offending food and usually also do an elimination or rotation diet. (See chapters 8 and 20 on allergies.) Raw foods and/or juices can be helpful if tolerated because they contain their own enzymes. The Vita-Mix is useful for food processing because it retains some of the fiber and pulp in the juice. Sampson and Champion juicers have also received good reports from doctors and patients.

Nutritional Therapy

- Remove the cause of the malabsorption, such as gluten intolerance or food sensitivities.
- Replace the missing factors, such as enzymes, hydrochloric acid, or bicarbonate.
- Restore probiotics with lactobacillus and/or bifidobacteria, and support with inulin and FOS (fructooligosaccharides) if tolerated.

- Repair by providing L-glutamine, glycine, and other essential nutrients to rebuild the GI lining; Seacure to provide healing peptides; trace minerals such as zinc, copper, and manganese; anti-inflammatories such as flaxseed oil (omega-3 acids); antioxidants to repair tissue and protect against oxidative stress.

Complementary Therapies

- Herbs. Include dandelion, aloe, ginger, gentian.
- Acupuncture. To balance the meridians and improve tone in the GI tract.
- Gentle exercise. Any movement that simulates peristalsis, such as Qigong, yoga, Pilates, walking, or other therapeutic movements.
- Massage therapy. To enhance energy from the fatigue of malabsorption.
- Magnetic therapy. Magnetic sleep systems are believed to improve enzymatic action in the body. The back flex can be worn in the day, over the abdomen, to enhance circulation.

Short-Bowel Syndrome

A complex condition typically caused by malabsorption that usually accompanies removal of a significant amount of small intestine. Short-bowel syndrome can result from surgery due to Crohn's, cancer, or the clotting of an artery in the digestive tract. This condition often requires intravenous nutrition (hyperalimentation). In some centers, small bowel transplantation is used to address these chronic conditions.

A new resource for patients is a center near Boston that uses nutrition to improve regrowth of gut tissue. By supplementing glutamine and growth hormone, they are able to improve patterns of absorption and regrow some tissue while improving absorption in existing tissue. They can be reached at the Nutrition Restart Center, Hopkinton, MA, 01748; (800) 867-6761.

PANCREATIC CANCER

Pancreatic cancer is now the fifth leading cancer in the United States for both men and women, and appears to be increasing in number as the population grows older. People who have had pancreatitis are more prone to pancreatic cancer. Risk factors include cigarette smoking, alcohol consumption (particularly beer), gallstones, a diet high in animal fats, and diabetes.

Symptoms

Abdominal pain that is vague and dull in the middle of the abdomen, occasionally going through to the back. Weight loss with poor appetite, occasionally with an aversion to meats and a metallic taste in the mouth. Other major symptoms include diarrhea, weakness, vomiting, jaundice, abdominal mass, migratory thrombophlebitis (recurring blood clots in the leg and pelvic veins), and GI bleeding.

Diagnosis

- Lab testing. Ca 19-9 is the name of a cancer antigen that can be detected through a test based on blood type. Approximately 85 percent of all pancreatic cancers will have this marker, which is a carbohydrate produced by the cancer cell.
- A CAT and MRI scanning. For the CAT scan the tumor must be at least 2 cm to be visualized.
- Ultrasound is not as accurate as the scans.
- ERCP may be performed and samples taken of pancreatic fluid for the examination of cancer cells or markers that may indicate obstruction of the pancreatic duct.
- MRCP is an MRI that uses contrast to image the ducts in the pancreas and may be helpful in some cases.
- Biopsy under imaging. Needle biopsy under CAT or MRI guidance is often needed to provide diagnosis.

Treatment

- Surgical removal of the pancreas (resection) is possible only in about 50 percent of cases, those that present with jaundice. Surgical removal is often not possible because detection occurs too late and the pancreas is located so close to other vital organs. Prognosis is usually very poor in those patients with pancreatic cancer that cannot be resected, with a life span of 6 to 12 months at best.
- Chemotherapy, especially with gemcitabine.

Complementary Treatment

- Nutritional adjunctive therapy is receiving good reports; this approach uses antioxidants and organic fruits and vegetables, and appears to prolong life and increase quality of life when combined with chemotherapy (NOAT—Nutritional Oncology Adjunctive Treatment, Philadelphia, Pennsylvania). There are various other alternative treatments that include diet therapy, such as the Gerson diet and the work of Dr. Nicholas Gonzales in New York (see Cancer of the Colon for additional information).

- Essiac tea contains five herbs, including burdock root, which has been shown to have anticancer properties. To be used only in combination with adjunctive chemotherapy and nutritional therapy, because it doesn't work as a stand-alone cancer therapy.
- Detoxification.
- Acupuncture for pain control and nausea.
- Subtle energy therapy, such as Reiki.
- Massage therapy, which improves lymphatic drainage and detoxification.
- Qigong, gentle exercise known for its beneficial effects on lymphatic drainage.
- Guided imagery.

PANCREATITIS

Inflammation of the pancreas usually results from the blockage of the ducts of the pancreas, causing the enzyme-rich juices of the pancreas to build up inside this organ, breaking down its own tissue, self-digesting (auto-digesting) because the function of the enzymes includes the digestion of protein.

Incidence and Causes

- Gallstones are the cause of pancreatitis in about 50 percent of patients in industrial nations.
- Alcoholism is also associated as a causal factor of pancreatitis in men. If gallstones aren't detected by an ultrasound, they are still suspected if there is pain and no evidence of alcoholism. In that case biliary drainage to clear minute gallstones and biliary sludge can be helpful and is performed through upper endoscopy.
- Malnutrition due to protein deprivation is a primary cause in underdeveloped countries.
- Familial pancreatitis occurs as an inherited condition.
- Abnormal structure of the ducts. The pancreatic duct may not be fully developed, or there may be an accessory duct that takes over for the missing duct. When the structure of the duct is malformed, it is called pancreas divisum, and frequent pancreatitis can be associated.
- Scarring of the pancreatic outlet can occur, called stenosis. Obstruction can result from the scarring due to chronic inflammation. It can be treated by opening the sphincter of the duct, using a specially developed endoscope in a procedure called ERCP (endoscopic retrograde cholangiopancreatography). Pressure measurements can also be taken. MRCP may also be helpful.

Additional factors in pancreatitis include:

- Diabetes, which makes people more prone to gallstones, due to chronic inflammation and the presence of proteins within the body that have aged too rapidly from high blood sugar.
- A number of medications have been associated as causal factors in pancreatitis, such as 5-ASAs, tetracyclines, sulfa drugs, Imuran, valproic acid (for seizures), and diuretics (such as thiazides).
- Estrogens. The body's own natural estrogens are known to cause this condition in rare cases.
- Bacterial infections and viruses, such as Reye's syndrome and mumps, can cause pancreatitis. Other microbial triggers include AIDS, cytomegalovirus, Coxsackie B, campylobacter, and mycoplasma.
- Elevated calcium levels in conditions such as hyperparathyroidism.
- Extremely high triglycerides (blood lipids/fats).
- Trauma, such as an accident that damages the pancreas.

Signs and Symptoms
- Abdominal pain that is severe, steady, dull, or boring, generally in the middle of the abdomen and under the ribs
- Abdominal distention
- Fever or vomiting
- Mild jaundice due to biliary obstruction
- Fluid in the lining covering the lungs
- Shock, or in severe cases coma

Diagnosis
- Blood tests for the presence of enzymes leaking from the pancreas into the bloodstream—particularly amylases (which digest starches) or lipases (which digest fats).
- Ultrasound of the pancreas, which will show swelling.
- Abdominal CT scan will show dilation of the duct, hemorrhage, or necrotic areas where cysts and abscesses are occurring.
- Chest X-ray may show fluid in the lining of the lungs (pleural effusion), which indicates the spread of the inflammation from the abdomen into the lung space.
- ERCP. This is an endoscopic dye test used in conjunction with an X-ray. This procedure could cause mild inflammation, but it can also be therapeutic because it can be used to remove gallstones if they are found to be present.

Treatment

- There is no known drug treatment for this condition, although in Europe it is treated, with marked reduction of mortality, using intravenous selenium.
- Hydration using NG tube feeding or intravenous rehydration to replace fluids and rest the gut.
- Pain control, such as with Demerol.
- Terbutaline, used in asthma treatment and given by injection early on in pancreatitis, has been successful in unpublished research by a Penn State surgical team.
- Surgery may be necessary to remove the abscess or improve drainage.

Prevention

- Abstinence from alcohol. Since alcoholism is linked with gallstone formation and pancreatitis, people who overconsume alcohol will want to seek treatment. Alternative therapies with an excellent success rate include acupuncture detoxification and nutritional therapy. See Joan Mathews Larson's program in *Seven Weeks to Sobriety* (Fawcett Columbine, 1997). Both approaches have success rates ranging from 50 percent to 90 percent, even in long-term conditions.
- Avoidance of fatty foods.
- Supplementation with pancreatic enzymes to rest the pancreas.
- Use of Urso or Actigall (ursodeoxycholic acid) to prevent gallstones.
- Use of statin drugs to treat elevated triglycerides.

Complementary Treatment

- Prevention of gallbladder disease by preventing gallstones. Use silymarin and Urso and observe a low-fat diet.
- Herbs like grape seed extract, bromelain, aloe vera in liquid or capsules, dandelion, licorice (in capsules, extract, or tea).
- Turmeric root is an anti-inflammatory; silymarin can be used to heal the liver and minimize sludge in the system.
- Chinese herbal medicine has been found to reduce mortality from 9 percent to 3 percent in severe pancreatitis. See a knowledgeable doctor of Oriental medicine.
- Acupuncture for pain relief and prevention of gallbladder disease.
- Homeopathy may be helpful for chronic, recurrent gallbladder disease.
- Mind-body therapies for pain control; see *Full Catastrophe Living* by Jon Kabat-Zinn (Delta-Dell Books, 1990) and *Turning Suffering Inside Out* by Darlene Cohen (Shambhala, 2001).

PARASITES/PARASITIC INFECTION

See chapter 21.

PRURITUS ANI

Pruritus ani is defined as an itchy anus. Some of the potential causes are:

- Food allergies
- Poor hygiene
- Pinworms, candida, parasites, and possibly other GI infections (for example, with cyclospora parasitic infections, in one study 20 percent of patients reported pruritus ani)

Diagnosis

- Diagnosis depends on direct inspection with an anoscope
- Inflammation and redness are visible around the anus
- Antibody panel for parasites (Immunosciences Lab)
- Stool sample for yeast, pinworms, and parasites (O&P—ova and parasites)
- Allergy testing for IgE- and IgG-related allergies—ImmunoLabs in Fort Lauderdale and Great Smokies Diagnostic Lab

Diet

Do a first-stage elimination diet, avoiding coffee, citrus, spicy foods, and wheat. If there is no improvement within a month, you can put these foods back in your diet one by one and carefully observe your initial response. Use this opportunity to monitor for other allergy symptoms as well (see chapter 20). Use the same herbs as those for hemorrhoids.

Topical Treatment

- Sitz baths or showering
- Maintain hygiene through the use of witch hazel pads (Tucks)
- Suppositories by prescription (Rowasa), hydrocortisone (Anusol-HC)

REFLUX AND HEARTBURN—GERD (GASTROESOPHAGEAL REFLUX DISEASE)

Acid reflux is a condition in which stomach acid is regurgitated up into the esophagus, causing damage to the lining of the esophagus. This condition is also known as gastroesophageal reflux disease (GERD). A survey of normal hospital employees found that 7 percent experience heartburn daily and 15 percent experience it monthly. A European study found that pregnant women are the most likely to have daily heartburn—48 percent to 78 percent of those surveyed.

Symptoms

Although reflux causes heartburn, by definition it also involves damage to the esophageal lining. Heartburn can be so intense it can cause anginalike chest pain. A wide range of symptoms are seen in patients with reflux. Common concerns include:

- Chest discomfort or pain over the breastbone
- Wheezing
- Asthma at night (nocturnal)
- Hiccups
- Stricture or bleeding ulcers in the esophagus
- Hoarse voice
- Damage to vocal cords
- Chronic cough

Take heartburn and reflux seriously. Reflux is important, because it can evolve into esophageal cancer. All people will have occasional symptoms of heartburn over the course of their lives. Heartburn and reflux are two of the most common GI ailments seen in a general medical practice. In fact about half the people with chest pain who see a doctor are found to have heartburn and reflux. However, since it's better to be safe than sorry, whenever there is a question, definitely get your heart checked as soon as possible.

Causes

1. Incomplete closing at the junction between the esophagus and stomach of the lower esophageal sphincter (LES), which may be weakened due to a number of causes: age, pregnancy, or hormones. A drop in pressure can be caused by certain foods, including peppermint, alcohol, and fatty foods, affecting the function of the sphincter.
2. Hiatal hernia. About half the people with heartburn and reflux have a hiatal hernia, a defect in the diaphragm muscle that allows part of the stomach to rise into the chest cavity. This makes it more difficult for the sphincter between the esophagus and the stomach to close properly. The incomplete closing of the sphincter can be due to the loss of muscle tone in the lower sphincter or to changes in pressure. Those with larger hiatal hernias are more likely to have significant reflux.

3. Incomplete esophageal clearing. We all regurgitate a little, but in people with serious reflux, the esophagus does not fully clear the regurgitated stomach acid. Anything that affects saliva secretion can make reflux worse. Insufficient saliva can be an important factor, since saliva helps clear acid from the esophagus. Low saliva levels may be due to:
   - Dehydration from a low intake of fluids
   - Drying medications, including antihistamines and tricyclic antidepressants
   - Diseases such as Sjögrens syndrome, where there is a defect of saliva production
4. Slowed movement of food in the esophagus (insufficient esophageal motility) due to aging, medications, or diseases that affect the muscles and interfere with muscle contractions (such as multiple sclerosis, scleroderma, and Parkinson's).
5. Delayed or slowed emptying of the stomach. If your stomach is full all the time or if there is delay in emptying, there can be more reflux. Reflux can be aggravated by conditions such as diabetes or medications that delay gastric emptying (these medications include calcium channel blockers and anticholinergics). One-fourth of patients with reflux have delayed gastric emptying. Dysbiosis is another suspect and is gaining recognition because of the brain-gut axis connection. Due to the abnormal gut ecology, the small intestine pacemaker is affected, which then slows stomach emptying, and so on. Food allergies are also suspect.

Preventive Factors

- Improve the quantity of mucus production. Use interventions that increase the flow of saliva, such as chewing gum, deglycyrrhizinated licorice (DGL), or aloe vera juice or gel.
- Sufficient blood supply to the esophagus. Try ginkgo biloba or niacin (which both mildly dilate blood vessels). Also try yoga, which can moderately stimulate blood flow.
- Get assistance to quit smoking, because it decreases the mucous barrier, reducing the protection to the lining of the esophagus. Smoking also decreases muscle tone of the junction and decreases the secretion of bicarbonate from the duodenum, which neutralizes stomach acid.
- Cut the intake of foods that decrease sphincter pressure or irritate the esophagus: mint (which is a smooth-muscle relaxant) and irritants such as spicy foods, alcohol, coffee, and some oils.
- Improve dysbiosis with probiotic supplements. If yeast is present, use antifungals. An elimination diet to detect allergies may also be beneficial. (See chapter 20.)

Diseases Associated with Reflux

- Diabetes can affect motility.
- Obesity places pressure on the abdomen and creates the potential for hiatal hernia, and changes emptying time.
- Pregnancy—the pressure of the fetus at the base of the esophagus and the increased production of hormones that cause muscle relaxation.
- Neuromuscular disorders that affect coordination throughout the body, including the esophagus, and interfere with swallowing and sphincter pressure, such as Parkinson's, multiple sclerosis, muscular dystrophy, and Alzheimer's.

Diagnosis

- Physical exam is often not helpful, although occasionally the doctor can hear gurgling of the stomach in the chest, which is the symptom of a large hiatal hernia.
- An upper barium X-ray is often too sensitive, and may pick up variations that do not cause problems.
- A double-contrast X-ray is more helpful because it is able to define the esophageal mucosa and lining better than single-contrast X-rays.
- Upper endoscopy is performed to look for damage from reflux, to define hiatal hernias, and to biopsy lesions.
- Measuring esophageal pressure is done by evaluating esophageal motility. This technique uses pressure sensors contained in a small tube that is swallowed and then pulled up and down through the various sphincters. Esophageal pressure determinations are not commonly done, but can be very helpful in difficult cases.
- Ambulatory pH testing consists of swallowing a small tube with a probe to measure acidity. The patient walks around with a small data recorder that measures acidity (pH), and when it drops below a certain level, acid is suspected of regurgitating up into the esophagus. The recorder can also mark symptoms periodically at the patient's request, which can be evaluated with the pH record at a later time.
- A nuclear-medicine scan uses radioactively labeled material or food. When reflux occurs the material regurgitated from the stomach into the esophagus can be scanned with a nuclear-medicine device to measure the amount of reflux.
- Severe complications can be handled through outpatient endoscopy, which can treat the strictures with dilation or a balloonlike mechanism to stretch them.
- Fundoplication is a technique that is performed with the laparoscope. The lower esophageal sphincter can be tightened by laparoscopic fundoplication.

- Several new endoscopic therapies are now FDA approved. These include the Stretta, which uses radio frequency via a balloon placed into the esophagus to thicken the lower esophageal sphincter and the Endocinch, which uses a sewing procedure to again tighten the lower esophageal sphincter. The Enteryx uses injection of a biopolymer into the wall of the esophagus at the sphincter to tighten the junction. None of these procedures have been proven to be effetive past one year of therapy.

Medications

- A therapeutic trial of antacids for two weeks is often prescribed by primary-care physicians. If this brings about an improvement the condition may be reflux. The risk is that more serious conditions may be overlooked, such as an erosive condition or Barrett's esophagitis, which is precancerous.
- Proton pump inhibitors have generally replaced the histamine blockers for serious reflux conditions. These are medications that block the production of acid by inhibiting the proton pumps of the stomach, specialized cells (chief cells) that produce stomach acid through a molecular pumping action. Medications most frequently used include lansoprazole (Prevacid) esomeprazole magnesium (Nexium), rabeprazole (Aciphex), pantoprazole (Protonix), and omeprazole (Prilosec), which was the first.
- Cisapride (Propulsid) helps empty the stomach and tighten the lower esophageal sphincter (LES). Cisapride was withdrawn from the market because it caused cardiac irregularities but is now available under a limited access protocol.
- Histamine blockers are now used less, they are primarily used for short-term therapy—typically two weeks or four treatments. They include cimetidine (Tagamet), ranitidine (Zantac), nizatidine (Axid), or famotidine (Pepcid).
- H2 blockers are available as over-the-counter medications at half the prescription dosage—Pepcid AC, Tagamet HG, Zantac 75, or Axid AR. Doctors are now seeing patients who have been self-medicating with these over-the-counter meds, but who actually have more serious conditions such as strictures, erosive or Barrett's esophagitis, episodes with asthma, or false-alarm cardiac conditions. The use of these widely available medications may delay more appropriate diagnosis and treatment.

Over-the-Counter Medications

- Minimize antacids, which may cause aluminum toxicity.
- Minimize bicarbonate, which can change acid balance problems or cause too much alkalinity.

- Alginic acid (Gaviscon) can be beneficial because it creates a barrier that floats on the stomach acid, so that acid doesn't enter the esophagus. However, it is high in sodium, so minimize sodium in your diet (for delicious salt substitutes, see chapter 30).

Lifestyle Changes
- Quit smoking. We all now recognize what a battle this addiction can be. Seek medical support, knowing that if you quit, your health risks will drop over time to almost normal.
- Consider a weight-loss diet. Some good, tasty, easy-to-follow diets can be found in *The formula, Atkins for Life,* and *The South Beach Diet.*
- Avoid tight clothing across the abdomen (such as tight belts, girdles).
- Eat smaller meals more frequently.
- Don't eat close to bedtime.
- Eat slowly, and relax after a meal.

Diet Changes
- Avoid fatty foods.
- Cut down on fats and simple sugars.
- Drink fluids with meals, because they help gastric emptying.
- Avoid spicy foods and highly acidic foods.
- Use an elimination diet for delayed food allergies (see chapter 20). Take probiotics and/or antifungals for yeast overgrowth or dysbiosis (see chapter 6).

Nutrients
- Magnesium is important for muscle contractions and relaxation. Review your intake and ask your doctor about your optimum level. Generally there is too much calcium in our diet, which causes magnesium depletion. Phase in magnesium gradually since it can cause a sudden bowel movement.
- Trace minerals. Low levels of copper, zinc, manganese, and selenium correlate with inflammation.
- Bioactive peptides with anti-inflammatory action, such as Seacure, have received positive reports.

Herbs
- Avoid mint in candy, herb teas, or any other form.
- Aloe vera liquid and gel have anti-inflammatory action; try them whenever you have heartburn. Slippery elm is another soothing herb.
- MSM (methyl sulfonyl methane) is a therapeutic mineral supplement that is getting good reports.

- Noni juice—the juice from a tropical tree with herbal properties.
- Licorice DGL seems to help mucus, and has been found effective in numerous studies.

Complementary Therapies

- Acupuncture. This seems to be more effective for this condition than acupressure. There are specific points that help gastric emptying that can be treated using a small portable electromagnetic acupuncture device, such as the Acu-Stim. These devices are available from Nikken with a prescription from your doctor. (*See* Resources.)
- Homeopathy can be useful. See a well-trained homeopathic physician.
- Magnetic sleep systems. The use of a magnetic mattress or large magnet over the offending area may improve the tone of the sphincter muscle or help the stomach's emptying by retraining of the gastric pacemaker. At present these reports are anecdotal, from physicians and patients.
- Exercise. It is good for heartburn to exercise: walking, running, yoga.
- Stress reduction.

Complications

- Barrett's esophagitis can be a precancerous condition. Treatment is proton pump inhibitor and periodic surveillance via upper endoscopy with multiple biopsies.
- Dysphagia (difficult or painful swallowing) is an alarm that most often suggests the presence of cancer. It is important to evaluate the condition through an endoscopic examination and a biopsy.
- Alcohol overconsumption is associated with reflux because it lowers the pressure in the esophagus and sphincters. It also creates the risk of esophageal varices, varicose veins in the area of the esophagus that can cause symptoms of dysphagia.

STRICTURES AND STRUCTURAL CONDITIONS

Esophageal Stricture

This disorder involves a narrowing of the esophagus, a condition that may be present from birth, in tissue structures described as webs or rings within the esophagus. It may be caused by inflammation due to reflux, which can scar the tissue or be caused by tumors.

In general symptoms include difficulty swallowing or getting food stuck after eating, especially dense or dry foods such as beef or chicken; in some cases pain may be prominent or there may be heartburn. In other cases the condition may be painless.

Diagnosis and Treatment

- The upper GI barium swallow can be quite useful in diagnosing these conditions. The test can be done in real time, so that the technician can observe the esophagus during the test to evaluate the transit time of food or whether contractions are occurring. The contractions are found in conditions described as corkscrew esophagus, rosary bead esophagus (with spasms caused by acid reflux), stricture (a narrowed area), or when a tumor is present.

- Endoscopy allows the physician to view the tissue directly with a scope. This procedure can also be therapeutic, because the tissue can be dilated with a balloonlike attachment or other scoping techniques. When the passageway is expanded, the scar tissue is stretched and the correction may need only periodic attention, or may even be permanent. Biopsies can also be performed to assess tumors or inflamed tissue.

- Manometry involves the measure of pressure in the esophagus to detect excessive increases or decreases. This information can be used, for example, to diagnose low pressure of the esophageal sphincter, a form of stricture that can result when the acid or bile from reflux actually scars the esophagus. A high-pressure condition, called achalasia, is also possible, in which the muscles are too tight due to increased muscular tension. Esophagomyotomy may be performed in cases that do not respond to other forms of therapy. In this surgery a strip of muscle is removed from the lower sphincter to prevent the muscle from tightening excessively. Cancerous tumors of the esophagus often have to be removed by surgery, or in some cases can be removed by laser through the endoscope.

Other Treatment

Medication can be used to relax spastic disorders of the smooth muscles of the esophagus, including sublingual long-acting nitrates (amyl nitrate or nitroglycerin) or calcium channel blockers such as nifedipine (Procardia) or diltiazem (Cardizem) that affect smooth muscles. Medication is useful in cases that are not true strictures but rather narrowing due to spasm. Antidepressants such as trazodone (Desyrel) may be helpful, because they improve communication between the brain and the autonomic/cholinergic nervous system. These conditions are comparable in some ways to an irritable bowel syndrome of the upper esophagus.

Other Structural Problems of the GI Tract

Gastric volvulus occurs when the stomach twists upon itself. This condition is due to a hernia of the diaphragm, causing the stomach to ride up through the diaphragm area and get caught. Sudden severe pain with vomiting can accompany this condition. This is to be considered a medical emergency. It is diagnosed through a barium swallow and typically corrected through surgery. However, in some cases it is self-correcting when a nasogastric tube is inserted and changes the gastric pressure. At that point the stomach may naturally return to the proper position.

Chronic Ulcer Disease with Stricture

Chronic duodenal ulcers can cause the narrowing of the outlet of the stomach, termed duodenal stenosis. The symptoms include nausea, vomiting, inability to eat a full meal, and history of chronic ulcer disease. Often dilation of the pylorus with the scope may correct this condition. Diagnosis is made by both upper GI X-ray series and endoscopy to rule out the presence of cancer in any form.

If the ulcer is active it is important to address it, using proton pump inhibitors, H2 blockers given intravenously, and a nasogastric tube to remove the fluid in the stomach. In some cases the narrowed area of the pylorus can be dilated using an endoscope with a balloon inserted through the scope, which often corrects this condition. In rare cases surgery is necessary. Again it is important to rule out gastric cancer.

Intestinal Obstruction

Obstruction typically occurs in the small intestine following surgery, due to scar tissue from prior operations. It can also be caused by Crohn's disease. Diagnosis is made by X-ray, CT scan, or endoscopy.

Symptoms can include intermittent or acute abdominal pain or distention. In some cases just resting the bowel takes care of the problem. In other cases surgery, nasogastric tubes, and IVs are helpful. The long tube or the nasogastric tube may be used to remove fluid from the small intestine or the stomach. Again it is important to rule out tumors. It is necessary to correct electrolyte imbalance and replace fluids as needed.

Complementary Therapies

Because these conditions are mechanical, they typically require surgical or mechanical intervention rather than alternative therapies. Acupuncture is probably the only alternative to be explored. For example, in the case of achalasia, using an electromagnetic TENS unit on relevant acupuncture points can lower the pressure, and in some cases that is sufficient to restore functioning.

Stricture of the Colon

Strictures of the colon are typically caused by ulcerative colitis or Crohn's disease and are evidenced by the inability to have normal bowel movement or having very small bowel movements. Diagnosis is by barium enema or colonoscopy. Therapies include balloon dilatation and biopsy to rule out cancer, or surgery.

Chronic Intestinal Pseudo-Obstruction

This condition occurs when there is ineffective intestinal motility, characterized by symptoms of chronic intestinal obstruction. The colon is dilated and there is no motility. This condition is accompanied by chronic constipation, distention and bloating, slow transit, and an absence of bowel sounds.

The acute form can require surgery. The chronic form may be due to muscular dystrophy, nerve degeneration, visceral neuropathy, Schuster's syndrome (a hereditary condition with digital arches and chronic constipation, with or without chronic fatigue syndrome), Parkinson's disease, brain or spinal cord tumor, chronically low parathyroid function (hypoparathyroidism), or dysfunction on a cellular level. Decompressive colonoscopy can be very helpful to remove as much fluid and air as possible from the colon. In some cases this procedure is so successful, surgery is unnecessary.

Poor motility has become quite common in our society, due to the increase in GI surgeries and the use of narcotic painkillers and antipsychotic medications, which can drastically slow motility. Patients using these medications should take a significant amount of fiber and fluids. Many of these conditions are reversible if you catch them early enough. Avoid the long-term use of laxatives, which may work initially but cause poor tone of the colon muscle and in the long term make the problem worse. Cholinergic drugs are now being used to treat this condition.

ULCERS/ULCER DISEASE

An ulcer is a lesion in the lining of the stomach or the first part of the small intestine (duodenum). Researchers have found ulcers to be caused by infection due to the bacteria, *Helicobacter pylori (H. pylori)*. Researchers once believed ulcers resulted from hyperacidity and stress.

In humans *H. pylori* was considered a harmless resident of the stomach and GI tract. Dr. Barry Marshall, an Australian researcher, investigated the bacteria in the early 1980s. When his request for a grant to do further research was rejected, to prove his point he ingested a test tube of *H. pylori* bacteria and days later developed a major case of stomach ulcers. He was evaluated, treated with antibiotics that resolved his symptoms and infection, and the rest is history.

Gastric ulcers in the elderly are worrisome because of their association with cancer and for this reason should be endoscoped and biopsied.

Symptoms

- Chronic abdominal pain in the area of the stomach.
- Pain that occurs after eating (postprandial), when the stomach is empty, at 11 A.M., 4 P.M., 10 P.M., and 1 to 2 A.M. This is most common for duodenal ulcers, which are relieved by antacids or eating.
- Frequent heartburn that may resemble reflux.
- Symptoms that may be intermittent or even be silent and are apparent only after GI bleeding; this is more characteristic of ulcer disease caused by the use of NSAIDs.
- Nausea and vomiting. Prolonged vomiting is rare, unless a stricture or obstruction is present.
- GI bleeding.

Causes

Peptic ulcer disease is like being on a teeter-totter—it is a matter of balance between protective factors and ulcerative factors, as well as exposure to infection.

- Exposure is more frequent in certain environments, such as medical care facilities. Among medical students positive titers for *H. pylori* (reflecting exposure to the infection) increase by 33 percent over the course of their medical education.
- Animals such as cats can be carriers. *H. pylori* bacteria are also associated in the body with gingivitis (gum disease).
- Old water systems and piping have been found to harbor *H. pylori*.
- Factors that compromise the protective mucous barrier: smoking, alcohol, NSAIDs (nonsteroidal anti-inflammatory drugs), stress (including physical stressors such as surgery, burns, or traumatic injury), decreased blood flow.
- Seasonal variations of ulcer disease. Repair is less active in the spring and fall because growth factors, cell turnover, and DNA for intestinal repair are the lowest when we are adapting to the change in season.

Diagnosis

- Upper endoscopy.
- X-ray—upper GI barium series (contrast or double-contrast, which involves air and barium).
- A therapeutic trial is often recommended with H2 blockers for two weeks, but some patients may have acid reflux. If a gastric ulcer is present this treatment will be masking the symptoms and may allow more serious complications to develop. With OTC availability of H2 blockers such as Pepcid AC and Tagamet HB, there will be a greater tendency for this kind of problem.

- Testing for *H. pylori* antibodies in a blood draw, finger stick, saliva test, or breath test. Unless the test is measuring IgM antibodies in response to a current infection, the test may show the presence of *H. pylori* bacteria but still doesn't necessarily indicate the presence of an active ulcer infection.

Mainstream Treatment

For ulcers caused by *H. pylori* infection:

- Triple therapy—two antibiotics such as amoxicillin and clarithromycin, plus a proton pump inhibiting drug such as lansoprazole (Prevacid) Prevpak to lower stomach acid. Aciphex, amoxicillin, and clarithromycin used twice a day for 7 days has been recently approved.
- Another triple therapy combination is bismuth-metronidazole-tetracycline (Helidac).
- Remember to take probiotics with antibiotic therapy, such as acidophilus or live-culture yogurt.

For ulcers not caused by *H. pylori* infection:

- Proton pump inhibitors such as omeprazole (Prilosec), lansoprazole (Prevacid), esomeprazole magnesium (Nexium), rabeprazole (Aciphex), or pantoprazole (Protonix)
- H2 blockers such as cimetidine (Tagamet), nizatidine (Axid), famotidine (Pepcid), or ranitidine (Zantac) in prescription strength

Surgery

In cases of extensive bleeding.

Diet

Diet therapy has fallen out of vogue, but earlier was the only therapy available. This typically consists of all soft food, including milk and cream (not great for daily-intolerant people or those with cholesterol problems). When there is a great deal of inflammation, some relief can be gained by blending foods—the small jar attachment to a blender or a mini–food processor can be invaluable in this regard. Fresh juices can also be helpful if tolerated, but care must be taken not to take in too much carbohydrate (carrot juice, for example, is quite sweet).

Complementary Therapies

- Nutrients. Vitamins A and E to promote mucous membrane healing; copper, zinc, manganese tend to be depleted in chronic inflammation; rice bran extract—gamma-oryzanol.

- Juices. A cabbage juice regimen has anecdotal reports of benefit with ulcer conditions.
- Herbal therapies. Deglycyrrhizinated licorice (DGL), aloe vera, slippery elm, grape seed extract, citrus seed extract, ginger (tea or capsules).
- If *H. pylori* is detected through lab work, consider garlic oil in capsules, grape seed extract, gentian, goldenseal (for no longer than three weeks, to protect the microflora).
- Plautonol is a Japanese nutraceutical found to inhibit growth of *H. pylori.*
- Sublingual SOD is a supplement that works on superoxide dismutase (SOD) and is a free radical squelcher.
- Gum mastic is another inhibitor of *H. pylori,* taken in combination with olive leaf extract and colloidal silver, one dropperful in a cup of water (all of these supplements are available from Allergy Research Group—see Resources).
- Acupuncture. With chronic problems; there are specific points that are useful that can help with pain and nausea and assist gastric emptying.
- Homeopathy.
- Energy exercise. Yoga, t'ai chi, and Qigong.
- Mind-body therapies. Meditation and stress reduction.

ULCERATIVE COLITIS

See Inflammatory Bowel Diseases (IBD).

VIRAL BOWEL DISEASE

See chapter 22.

Resources

DIRECTORY

Resources on Digestive Health / 564
- Books / 564
- Research Services for Patients / 565
- Referrals to Practitioners / 565
- References for Practitioners / 566
- Web Sites / 566
- National Associations / 567
- Compounding Pharmacies / 567
- Sources of Nutrients / 568
- Laboratory Testing / 569

Herbs and Botanical Resources / 570

Environmental Medicine Resources / 572

Resources on Parasitic Infection / 573

Resources on Bioelectromagnetism / 574

Chinese Medicine Resources / 575

Guided Imagery Resources / 576

Healing Mind and Body / 577

RESOURCES ON DIGESTIVE HEALTH

Books

Berkson, D. Lindsey. *Healthy Digestion the Natural Way*. John Wiley & Sons, 2000.

Bland, Jeffrey, Ph.D. *Genetic Nutritioneering*. McGraw-Hill, 1999.

Bland, Jeffrey, Ph.D. *The 20-Day Rejuvenation Diet Program*. McGraw-Hill/Contemporary Books, 1999.

Bock, Kenneth, M.D., Steven Bock, M.D., and Nancy Faass. *The Germ Survival Guide*. McGraw-Hill/Contemporary Books, 2003.

Braly, James, and Jim Thompson. *Food Allergy Relief*. McGraw-Hill/Contemporary Books, 2000.

Crook, William, M.D. *Yeast Connection Handbook*. Professional Books, 1999.

D'Adamo, Peter, and Catherine Whitney. *Eat Right 4 Your Type*. Putnam Publishing Group, 1996.

Gach, Michael. *Acupressure's Potent Points: A Guide to Self-Care for Common Ailments*. Bantam, 1990.

Galland, Leo, M.D. *Power Healing*, 2nd ed. Random House, 1998.

Gates, Donna, and Linda Schatz. *The Body Ecology Diet*. B E D Publications, 2002.

Gershon, Michael, M.D. *The Second Brain*. Perennial, 1999.

Gittleman, Ann Louise. *Guess What Came to Dinner?* 2nd ed. Avery/Penguin Putnam, 2001.

Golan, Ralph, M.D. *Optimal Wellness*. Wellspring/Ballantine, 1995.

Gottschall, Elaine. *Breaking the Vicious Cycle*. Kirkton Press, 1994.

Haas, Elson, M.D. *The New Detox Diet*. Celestial Arts, 2004.

———. *The Staying Healthy Shopper's Guide*. Celestial Arts, 1999.

———. *Staying Healthy with Nutrition*. Celestial Arts, 1992 (new edition, revised and referenced, 2005).

Hammond, Christopher. *The Complete Family Guide to Homeopathy*. Element Books, 1995. (Possibly the best book ever written for consumers on homeopathy. Out of print, but available on the Web.)

Jahnke, Roger. *The Healing Promise of Qi*. McGraw-Hill/Contemporary Books, 2002.

———. *The Healer Within*. HarperSanFrancisco, 1999.

Levin, Buck. *Environmental Nutrition*. Hingepin Pub, 1999.

Lipski, Elizabeth. *Digestive Wellness,* 2nd ed. McGraw-Hill/Contemporary Books, 1999.

Lockie, Andrew, M.D., and Nicola Geddes, M.D. *Complete Guide to Homeopathy,* 2nd ed. DK Publishing, 2000.

Rogers, Sherry, M.D. *Detoxify or Die*. Prestige Publishers, 2002.

Ross, Julia. *The Diet Cure*. Penguin USA, 2000.

Rossman, Martin, M.D. *Fighting Cancer from Within*. Owl Books, 2003.

———. *Guided Imagery for Self-Healing*. H. J. Kramer, 2000.

Saputo, Len, M.D., and Nancy Faass. *Boosting Immunity.* New World Library, 2001.

Teitelbaum, Jacob, M.D. *From Fatigued to Fantastic*. Avery/Penguin Putnam, 2001.

Research Services for Patients

The Heath Resource, Inc., 933 Faulkner Street, Conway, AR 72034, (800) 949-0090, moreinfo@theheathresouce.com, www.thehealthresource.com.

Integrative Medical Solutions, Brian Bouch, M.D., c/o Hill Park Clinic, 245 Kentucky Street Suite A, Petaluma, CA 94952, (707) 773-0333, medsolv@svn.net, personalized medical research and advocacy service.

World Research Foundation, 41 Bell Rock Plaza, Sedona, AZ 86351; (928) 284-3300, www.wrf.org.

Referrals to Practitioners

American Academy of Environmental Medicine, 7701 E. Kellogg, Suite 625, Wichita, KS 67207, (316) 684-5500, www.aaem.com.

The American Association of Naturopathic Physicians, 3201 New Mexico Avenue NW, Suite 350, Washington, DC 20016, (866) 538-2267 or (202) 895-1392. Directory mailed for $5, or by accessing www.naturopathic.org.

American Chiropractic Association, 1701 Clarendon Boulevard, Arlington, VA 22209, (800) 986-4636, www.amerchiro.org.

American College for Advancement in Medicine, 23121 Verdugo Drive, Suite 204, Laguna Hills, CA 92653, (800) 532-3688 or (949) 583-7666, www.acam.org. For practitioner referral, send an envelope with two stamps to the above address.

American Holistic Veterinary Medical Association, 2218 Old Emmorton Road, Bel Air, MD 21015, (410) 569-0795, www.ahvma.org.

Bastyr University Referral Line, 14500 Juanita Drive NE, Kenmore, WA 98028-4966, (425) 823-1300, www.bastyr.edu. Referrals to naturopathic physicians.

Environmental Dental Association, (800) 388-8124. For book orders call EDA at (858) 586-1208. To receive a list of alternative dentists, send a self-addressed stamped envelope with 60¢ postage. Enclose $5 and mail to EDA, P.O. Box 2184, Rancho Santa Fe, CA 92067.

Institute for Functional Medicine, 4411 Pt. Fosdick Drive NW, Suite 305, P.O. Box 1697, Gig Harbor, WA 98335, (800) 228-0622, www.functionalmedicine.org. Referrals to physicians and practitioners who have taken functional medicine training.

National Center for Homeopathy, 801 N. Fairfax Street, Suite 306, Alexandria, VA 22314, (703) 548-7790 or (877) 624-0613, www.homeopathic.org.

Orthomolecular Health-Medicine, 2698 Pacific Avenue, San Francisco, CA 94115, (415) 922-6462.

References for Practitioners

Bland, Jeffery. *Clinical Nutrition.* Institute for Functional Medicine, 2004.

Feldman, Mark, Lawrence Friedman, Bruce Scharschmidt, and Marvin Sleisenger, eds. *Sleisenger and Fordtran's Gastrointestinal and Liver Disease.* 7th ed. W. B. Saunders, 2002.

Functional Medicine Updates, Institute for Functional Medicine, Gig Harbor, WA; (800) 843-9660. Monthly medical updates on audiotape, as well as publications, regional workshops, and yearly conferences.

Murray, Patrick, and others. *Medical Microbiology.* 4th ed. Mosby, 2002.

Tuberose.com. Good reference Web page on liver detoxification processes.

Werbach, Melvyn R., M.D. *Nutritional Influences on Illness.* 2nd ed. Third Line Press, 1996.

Web Sites

About.com, about.com/health/

Dr. Andrew Weil's Web site, www.drweil.com

Great Smokies Diagnostic Laboratory, www.gsdl.com

Health Medicine Forum, www.healthmedicine.org

Health Online, www.healthonline.com

Health World, www.healthy.net

Institute for Functional Medicine, www.functionalmedicine.org

PubMed, www.ncbi.nlm.nih.gov/PubMed/. Enter the key word you wish to search

Medscape, www.medscape.com

WebM.D., www.webMD.com

One of the resources doctors use is Medline, the online database of the National Library of Medicine at the National Institutes of Health. Medline is now accessible to the public as well, at www.nlm.nih.gov. To search millions of medical journals in an instant, go to Medline Plus and follow the instructions. You can make sure you're searching the right key words by checking the library's special MeSH headings.

National Associations

American Liver Foundation, 75 Maiden Lane, New York, NY 10038, (800) 465-4837 or (212) 668-1000, www.liverfoundation.org. Information on liver disease, hepatitis, and gallbladder disease.

Crohn's & Colitis Foundation of America, 3386 Park Avenue South, 17th Floor, New York, NY 10016, (800) 932-2423, www.ccfa.org.

Digestive Disease National Coalition, 507 Capital Court NE, Suite 200, Washington, DC 20002, (202) 544-7497, www.ddnc.org.

Gluten Intolerance Group, 15110 10th Avenue SW, Suite A, Seattle, WA 98116, (206) 246-6652, www.gluten.net.

National Colorectal Cancer Research Alliance (NCCRA), www.eifoundation.org/national/nccra/splash. Free CD for consumers and professionals on Colorectal Cancer Education (for PCs or Macs).

National Digestive Diseases Information Clearinghouse, 2 Information Way, Bethesda, MD 20892, (800) 891-5389 or (310) 654-3810, www.digestive.niddk.nih.gov.

Compounding Pharmacies

Referrals to Compounding Pharmacies

International Academy of Compounding Pharmacists, Sugar Land, TX 77487; (800) 927-4227 or (281) 933-8400, www.iacprx.org.

Professional Compounding Centers of America (PCCA), Houston, TX 77099; (800) 331-2498 or (281) 933-6948, www.pccarx.org. To locate the nearest specialty compounding pharmacy near you, contact the PCCA.

Specific Pharmacies

Abbott's Compounding Pharmacy, Berkeley, CA, (800) 327-6842 or (510) 548-8777, www.abbotscompounding.com.

College Pharmacy, Colorado Springs, CO, (719) 262-0022, www.collegepharmacy.com.

Wellness Pharmacy, Homewood, AL, (800) 227-2627 or (205) 879-6551, www.wellnesshealth.com.

Women's International Pharmacy, Madison, WI, (800) 699-8144 or (608) 221-7800, www.womensinternational.com.

Sources of Nutrients
Companies that Sell to Both the Public and to Health Care Professionals

Allergy Research Group/Nutricology, 30806 Santana Street, Hayward, CA 94544, (800) 545-9960 or (510) 487-8526, www.allergyresearchgroup.com. An outstanding line of nutritional supplements.

Lifespan Institute, San Rafael, CA, (415) 479-3552. Nutritional supplements, testing, and consulting available to the public. A source of pharmaceutical-grade tryptophan: www.GotTryptophan.com, and a Web site with nutritional solutions for fatigue and stress-related problems: www.LifespanProducts.com.

Seacure from Proper Nutrition, Inc., 739 Hoffecker Road, Pottstown, PA 19465, (800) 555-8868, www.seacure.biz. Available to the general public and physicians. Next-day shipping is available if desired.

Tyson Nutraceuticals, 12832 Chadron Avenue, Hawthorne, CA 90250, (800) 799-3233 or (800) 318-9766, www.tysonnutraceuticals.com. A complete line of amino acids, vitamins, minerals.

Vitamin Express, San Francisco, CA, (800) 500-0733, www.vitaminexpress.com. Mail-order service, discounted prices, providing both familiar and specialty brands.

Vitamin Research Products, 3579 Highway 50 East, Carson City, NV 89701, (800) 877-2447, www.vrp.com. Custom line of vitamin products.

The Vitamin Shoppe, 2101 91st Street, North Bergen, NJ 07047, (800) 223-1216, www.vitaminshoppe.com. Discounted mail-order service, providing familiar brands.

Companies that Sell to Physicians and Pharmacies Only

InterPlexus, Inc., 6613 S. 192nd Place, K103, Kent, WA 98032, (800) 875-0511, www.interplexus.com. Specialty products, including those for immune support.

Marco Pharma International, P.O. Box 489, Twin Lakes, WI 53181, (800) 643-4221, www.internatural-alternative-health.com. A variety of German imports, including enzymes.

Metagenics, 100 Avenida La Pata, San Clemente, CA 92673, (800) 692-9400, www.metagenics.com. Products formulated by Jeffrey Bland, Ph.D., including UltraClear and Sustain.

Pure Encapsulations, 490 Boston Post Road, Sudbury, MA 01776, (800) 753-2277, www.purecaps.com.

Thorne Research, P.O. Box 25, Dover, ID 83825, (800) 228-1966 or (208) 263-1337, www.thorne.com. A wide range of products and specialty formulas.

Tyler Encapsulations, Integrative Therapeutics, Inc., 9775 SW Commerce Circle, C5, Wilsonville, OR 97070, (800) 931-1709, www.integrativeinc.com. Specialty products.

Laboratory Testing
Information for the Public and for Doctors

BioHealth Diagnostics, 2929 Canon Street, San Diego, CA 92106, (800) 570-2000, www.biohealthinfo.com and www.biohealthcenters.com. Lab test panels and consultation.

Great Plains Laboratory, 11813 W. 77th, Lenexa, KS 66214, (913) 341-8949, www.greatplainslaboratory.com. Testing for organic acids, implicated in digestive disorders, autism, ADHD, and other conditions.

Great Smokies Diagnostic Laboratory, 63 Zillicoa Street, Asheville, NC 28801, (828) 253-0621, www.gsdl.com. Testing for digestive concerns, intestinal permeability, and markers of infection; genetic testing and evaluations for liver function and oxidative stress.

Immuno Laboratories, 6801 Powerline Road, Fort Lauderdale, FL 33309, (800) 231-9197 or (954) 691-2500, www.immunolabs.com. Food allergy testing for both immediate and delayed allergies and sensitivities (IgE and IgG).

Lifespan Institute, San Rafael, CA, (415) 479-3552, www.LifespanProducts.com. A broad range of functional testing available to the public.

The Parasitology Center, Inc., 903 S. Rural Rd., #101–318, Tempe, AZ 85281, (480) 767-2522, www.parasitetesting.com. Laboratory testing for the detection of human parasitic infections and toxicities from neurocutaneous syndrome (see chapter 15).

SpectraCell Laboratories, 7051 Portwest Drive, Suite 100, Houston, TX 77024-8026, (800) 227-5227 or (713) 621-3101, www.spectracell.com. Testing for vitamins, minerals, fatty acids.

Information for Health Care Professionals Only

BodyBio, 45 Reese Road, P.O. Box 809, Millville, NJ 08332, (888) 320-8338, www.bodybio.com. Analysis and consultation on essential fatty acids and blood chemistry.

Diagnos-Techs, Inc., 6620 S. 192nd Place, Building J, Kent, WA 98032, (800) 878-3787, www.diagnostechs.com. A wide range of testing for digestive disorders, as well as for hormone function.

Doctor's Data, P.O. Box 111, West Chicago, IL 60186, (800) 323-2784, www.doctorsdata.com. Laboratory profiles for gastrointestinal and liver health, amino acid status, and toxic exposures.

Immunosciences Lab, Inc., 8693 Wilshire Boulevard, Suite 200, Beverly Hills, CA 90211, (310) 657-1077, www.immuno-sci-lab.com. Evaluations of gastrointestinal status and immune function, as well as testing for parasite, bacteria, and viral antibodies.

Meridian Valley Laboratory, 801 SW 16th, Suite 126, Renton, WA 98055, (425) 271-8689, www.meridianvalleylab.com. Full-service lab and allergy tests.

Metametrix Clinical Laboratory, 4855 Peachtree Industrial Blvd, Suite 201, Norcross, GA 30092, (800) 221-4640, www.metametrix.com. Lab evaluations, including allergies, detoxification, dysbiosis, hormones, oxidative stress.

National Medical Services, 3701 Welsh Road, Willow Grove, PA 19090, (800) 522-6671 or (215) 657-4900, www.nmslab.com. Reference lab used by hospitals and labs across the country, and which provides specialized testing including heavy metals.

Vitamin Diagnostics, Inc., 2 Industrial Drive, Suite A, Keyport, NJ 07735, (732) 583-7773. Testing to determine the levels of vitamins, minerals, and essential fatty acids in the body.

HERBS AND BOTANICAL RESOURCES
Timothy Kuss, Ph.D.

Herbal Products

Quality herbs that have been gathered fresh can be obtained from Eclectic, Gaia, New Chapter, and other companies and are found in health food stores. Exceptional herbal formulas that are also available from health professionals include PhytoPharmica and Systemic Formulas.

East Earth Trade Winds, P.O. Box 463151, Redding, CA 96049, (800) 258-6878, www.snowcrest.net/eetw/. Chinese herbal formulas.

Eclectic Institute, 36350 SE Industrial Way, Sandy, OR 97055, (800) 332-4372, www.eclecticherb.com. A source of quality wild-crafted, organic freeze-dried fresh herbs and tinctures.

Gaia Herbs, 108 Island Ford Road, Brevard, NC 28712, (800) 831-7780 or (828) 884-4242, www.gaiaherbs.com. A source of quality herbal concentrates and tinctures.

Herbs for Kids, 1441 W. Smith Road, Ferndale, WA 98248, (800) 232-4005, (800) 541-1356, www.herbsforkids.com. Pesticide-free and alcohol-free glycerites for children.

Infinity Health, 1100 West Littleton Blvd., Suite 360, Littleton, CO 80120, (800) 733-9293 or (302) 703-3772, www.infinityhealth.net. A wide range of single herbs and combination remedies, including Nature's Answer and Systemic Formulas.

New Chapter, 22 High Street, Brattleboro, VT 05301, (800) 543-7279, www.newchapter.info. Herbal formulas to address inflammation and provide antioxidants and immune support.

PhytoPharmica, 825 Challenger Drive, Green Bay, WI 54311, (800) 376-7889 (consumers), (800) 553-2370 (retailers), www.phytopharmica.com. Quality standardized herbal extracts.

Finding an Herbalist

Seek the advice of a trained herbalist whenever possible. The small expense can turn into a great savings by using the proper herbs for your own unique situation. Look in the yellow pages of your local phone directory under *Herbalist,* or contact the American Botanical Council.

Herb Associations

American Botanical Council, 6200 Manor Road, Austin, TX 78723, (512) 926-4900, www.herbalgram.org.

American Herbalists Guild, 1931 Gaddis Road, Canton, GA 30115, (770) 751-6021, www.americanherbalistsguild.com.

Herb Research Foundation, 4140 15th Street, Boulder, CO 80302, (303) 449-2265, www.herbs.org.

Books and Publications

Castleman, Michael. *The New Healing Herbs,* 2nd ed. Bantam, 2002.

Duke, James A. *The Green Pharmacy Herbal Handbook.* Rodale Press, 2000.

HerbalGram, American Botanical Council, www.herbalgram.org.

The Herb Quarterly, EGW Publishing Company, (925) 671-9852, www.herbquarterly.com.

Hoffmann, David. *The New Holistic Herbal,* 3rd ed. Element Books, Ltd., 1991.

Landis, Robyn, with K.P. Khalsa. *Herbal Defense.* Warner Books, 1997.

Mowrey, Daniel B., Ph.D. *The Scientific Validation of Herbal Medicine.* McGraw-Hill, 1998.

Murray, Michael T. *The Healing Power of Herbs.* Prima Lifestyles, 1995.

Werbach, Melvyn, M.D., and Michael T. Murrary. *Botanical Influences on Illness,* 2nd ed. Third Line Press, 2000.

Herbal Study Programs

Bastyr University, Distance Learning Program, Seattle, WA, (206) 517-3549, www.bastyr.edu.

East-West School of Herbology (herbalist Michael Tierra), Santa Cruz, CA, (408) 336-5010, www.planetherbs.com.

Sage Mountain Home Study Herbology Course (herbalist Rosemary Gladstar), P.O. Box 420, East Barre, VT 05649, (802) 479-9825, www.sagemountain.com.

The School of Natural Healing (herbalist John Christopher, N.D.), Springville, UT, (800) 372-8255, www.schoolofnaturalhealing.com.

Western States Chiropractic College, Botanical Medicine for Health Professionals, 2900 NE 132nd Avenue, Portland, OR 97230, (800) 641-5641.

ENVIRONMENTAL MEDICINE RESOURCES
Jeffry Anderson, M.D.

Books

Ashford, Nicholas, and Claudia Miller. *Chemical Exposures: Low Levels and High Stakes*. John Wiley & Sons, 1998. The definitive text, meaningful to both general audiences and professionals.

Audesirk, Teresa, Gerald Audersirk, and Bruce Byers. *Biology, Life on Earth*, 6th ed. Prentice Hall, 2001. The biology of life on our planet, including good information on the dynamics of the cell.

Colborn, Theo, Dianne Dumanoski, and John Myers. *Our Stolen Future*. Plume, 1997.

Rogers, Sherry A., M.D. *Tired or Toxic?* Prestige Publishers, 1990. Possible links between disorders such as chronic fatigue and the effects of environmental toxins.

Steingraber, Sandra. *Living Downstream*. Vintage, 1998.

Wallace, Robert. A. *Biology, the World of Life*, 3rd ed. Pearson-Addison Wesley, 1998.

Organizations

American Academy of Environmental and Integrative Medicine, 7701 E. Kellogg, Suite 625, Witchita, KS 67207, (316) 684-5500, www.aaem.com. Resources for professionals and the public: conferences and training, books and audiotapes, and referrals to physicians.

The American Environmental Health Foundation, 8345 Walnut Hill Lane, Suite 225, Dallas, TX 75231, (800) 428-2343, (214) 361-9515, www.aehf.com. Sponsors research and scientific symposiums for professionals. Books, abstracts, and audiotapes on treatment strategies. Environmentally safe products for the home and personal care.

Chemical Injury Information Network, P.O. Box 301, White Sulphur Springs, MT 59645, (406) 547-2255, www.ciin.org. Research services, advocacy, referrals, and educational materials, including a monthly newsletter and more.

Books and Journals for Professionals

Alberts, Bruce, and others. *Molecular Biology of the Cell,* 4th ed. Garland Science, 2002.

The Journal of Nutritional & Environmental Medicine. Official journal of the American, British, and Australian enviornmental organizations. Taylor & Francis Group, Inc.

Klaassen, Curtis D. *Casarett and Doull's Toxicology, the Basic Science of Poisons,* 6th ed. McGraw-Hill Professional, 2001.

Rea, William, M.D. *Chemical Sensitivity. Vols. 1 to 3.* Lewis Publishers, 1998.

Toxicology and Industrial Health. Arnold Journals.

RESOURCES ON PARASITIC INFECTION
Omar Amin, Ph.D.

Books (of interest to professionals and consumers)

Ash, L. R. and T. C. Orihel. *Atlas of Human Parasitology.* American Society for Clinical Pathology Press, 1997.

Bogitsh, B. J., and T. C. Cheng. *Human Parasitology.* Academic Press, 1998.

Garcia, L. S. *Diagnostic Medical Parasitology.* Washington, D.C.: American Society for Microbiology, 2001.

Gillespie, S. H. and P. M. Hawkey. *Medical Parasitology: A Practical Approach.* Oxford University Press, 1995.

Gittleman, A. L. *Guess What Came to Dinner.* Avery/Penguin Putnam, Inc., 2001.

Mahon, C. R. and G. Manuselis, Jr. *Textbook of Diagnostic Microbiology.* W. B. Saunders, 2000.

Weintraub, S. *The Parasite Menace.* Pleasant Grove, UT: Woodland Publishing, 1998.

Journals

American Journal of Public Health, Annals of Tropical Medicine and Parasitology, Comparative Parasitology, Folia Parasitologia, Helminthologia, International Journal for Parasitology, Journal of Parasitology, Parasitology, and *Systemic Parasitology.*

Professional Resources

Dr. Omar Amin, Ph.D., Director, Parasitology Center, Inc., 903 S. Rural Road, #101-318, Tempe AZ 85281, www.parasitetesting.com. The laboratory provides analysis for specimens of parasites and yeast. Educational services and consultations regarding infections and management, including herbal and allopathic protocols. Dr. Amin also provides training in parasitic detection and laboratory protocols.

Amin, O. M. *Parasitic Infections in Humans: Diagnosis and Pathology: A Five-Part Video Set.* The Center for the Improvement of Human Functioning, 1997. To order contact the center in Wichita, KS at (800) 447-7276.

Professional Organizations

American Society for Microbiology, Washington, DC, (202) 737-3600, www.asm.org.

American Society of Parasitologists, Iowa City, IA, (319) 335-1061, http://asp.unl.edu.

American Society of Tropical Medicine and Hygiene, Northbrook, IL, (847) 480-9592, www.astmh.org.

British Society for Parasitology, www.mri.sari.ac.uk/bsp.

CDC (Centers for Disease Control), Division of Parasitic Diseases, www.dpd.cdc.gov/DPDx/.

Helminthological Society of Washington (D.C.), www.gettysburg.edu/~shendrixhelmsoc.html.

Stanford University, BioNet, www.bio.net.

RESOURCES ON BIOELECTROMAGNETISM
Trent W. Nichols, M.D.

Books

Becker, Robert, and Gary Selden. *The Body Electric: Electromagnetism and the Foundation of Life.* William Morrow, 1998.

Blank, Martin, ed. *Electromagnetic Fields: Biological Interactions and Mechanisms.* American Chemical Society, 1995.

Lawrence, Ronald, M.D., and Paul Rosch. *Magnet Therapy: The Pain Cure Alternative.* Prima Lifestyles, 1998.

Null, Gary. *Healing with Magnets.* Carroll and Graf, 1998.

Polk, Charles, and Elliot Postow, eds. *CRC Handbook of Biological Effects of Electromagnetic Fields,* 2nd ed. CRC Press, 1995.

Rosch, Paul J., M.D., and Marko Markov, eds. *Bioelectromagnetic Medicine.* Marcel Dekker, 2004.

Advanced Magnetic Research Institutes

AMRI of California, 27652-B Camino Capistrano, Laguna Niguel, CA 92677, (949) 367-0877, www.amri1.com.

AMRI of Michigan, 43393 Schoenherr Road, Sterling Heights, MI 48313, (586) 254-7711, www.amri-mi.com.

AMRI of Pennsylvania, Center for Nutrition and Digestive Disorders, 195 Stock Street, Suite 211B, Hanover, PA 17331, (717) 632-0300, www.amripa.com.

AMRI of North Carolina, *Dayspring Medical Center,* 217 Dayspring Way, Mocksville, NC 27028, (336) 492-2874, www.amri-nc.com.

AMRI of Washington, *Tahoma Clinic,* 801 SW 16th, Suite 121, Renton, WA 98055, (425) 264-0059 ext. 260, www.tahoma-clinic.com.

CHINESE MEDICINE RESOURCES
Efrem Korngold, O.M.D.

In the United States there are more than ten thousand certified or licensed practitioners of acupuncture and herbal medicine. There are at least two dozen schools of Chinese medicine, offering three- and four-year programs that graduate hundreds of new practitioners annually. There are also numerous state and national organizations of Chinese-medicine professionals, researchers, and educators.

Books

Beinfield, Harriet, and Efrem Korngold. *Between Heaven and Earth: A Guide to Chinese Medicine.* Ballantine Books, 1992. Available in hardcover and paperback.

Pitchford, Paul. *Healing with Whole Foods,* 3rd ed. North Atlantic Books, 2003.

Sources of Referrals and Information

The Association of Acupuncture and Oriental Medicine (AAOM), 909 22nd Street, Sacramento, CA 95816, (916) 451-6950, www.aaom.org.

The Acupuncture and Oriental Medicine Alliance (AOMA), 6450-43rd Ct., N.W., Suite B, Gig Harbor, WA 98335, (253) 851-6896, www.aomalliance.org.

The Council of Colleges of Acupuncture and Oriental Medicine (CCAOM), 7501 Greenway Center Drive, Suite 820, Greenbelt, MD 20770, (301) 313-0868, www.ccaom.org. The Web site includes information on selecting an acupuncturist.

The National Certification Commission for Acupuncture and Oriental Medicine (NCCAOM), 11 Canal Center Plaza, Suite 300, Alexandria, VA 22314, (703) 548-9004, www.nccaom.org.

Sources of Books and Chinese Herbal Products

Blue Poppy, 5441 Western Ave., #2, Boulder, CO 80301, (800) 487-9296, (303) 447-8372, www.bluepoppy.com. Books, audiotapes, and videos, and other resources on acupuncture and Chinese medicine.

K'An Herb Company, 6001 Butler Lane, Scotts Valley, CA 95066, (800) 543-5233. Available to health care professionals.

Redwing Books, 202 Bendix Drive, Taos, NM 87571, (800) 873-3946, www.redwingbooks.com. Books and information on acupuncture and Chinese medicine.

Shen Nong Herbs, 1600 Shattuck Avenue, #125, Berkeley, CA 94709, (510) 849-0290. Available to both the general public and to professionals.

GUIDED IMAGERY RESOURCES
Martin Rossman, M.D.

Books and Audio Tapes

Rossman, Martin, M.D. *Fighting Cancer from Within.* Owl Books, 2003.

———. *Guided Imagery for Self-Healing.* H. J. Kramer, 2000.

———. *Preparing for Surgery* (compact disc). Sounds True, 2004.

Weil, Andrew, M.D., and Martin Rossman, M.D. *Self-Healing with Guided Imagery* (set of 2 compact discs). Sounds True, 2004.

Resources and Training (for the public and professionals)

The Academy for Guided Imagery, 30765 Pacific Coast Highway, Suite 369, Malibu, CA 90265, (800) 726-2070, www.interactiveimagery.com. Imagery-related tapes and videos for the public and professionals. Training for health professionals to use guided imagery, including certificate programs and conferences.

The Institute of Transpersonal Psychology, 1069 E. Meadow Circle, Palo Alto, CA 94303, (650) 493-4430, www.itp.edu. The institute offers training in the many uses of imagery, including its applications in healing.

HEALING MIND AND BODY
Len Saputo, M.D., and Nancy Faass, MSW, MPH

Books

Benson, Herbert, Ph.D. *The Relaxation Response.* HarperTorch, 1976. A classic, still in print and still a best seller, reflecting essential insight.

Bolen, Jean Shinoda. *Close to the Bone.* Scribner, 1998. Using illness as a means of opening the heart and as a door to personal transformation.

Cohen, Darlene. *Turning Suffering Inside Out.* Shambhala, 2002. True wisdom on coping with chronic pain.

Cousins, Norman. *Anatomy of an Illness.* Bantam, 1991. Using laughter and nutrition to heal the body; an account of Cousins' personal experience in self-healing.

The Dalai Lama. *An Open Heart.* Little, Brown and Company, 2001. This is a rich and nurturing book on applying spirituality in everyday life; in healing our relationships, we may heal ourselves.

Kabat-Zinn, Jon, Ph.D. *Full Catastrophe Living: Using the Wisdom of Your Body and Mind to Face Stress, Pain, and Illness.* Delta Books, 1990. A wealth of resources for self-healing, including hatha yoga, mindfulness meditation, pain management, and stress reduction.

———. *Wherever You Go, There You Are.* Hyperion, 1995. The essentials of meditation.

Ko-i Bastis, Madeline. *Peaceful Dwelling: Meditations for Healing and Living.* Tuttle Publishing, 2000. Meditation as a tool for dealing with illness and suffering.

Lerner, Michael, Ph.D. *Choices in Healing.* MIT Press, 1996. A comprehensive, practical (and inspired) resource for coping with cancer or other types of chronic conditions.

Myss, Carolyn. *Why People Don't Heal and How They Can.* Three Rivers Press, 1998. An expanded understanding of the nature of illness and the value and relevance of addressing illness on many levels.

Remen, Rachel Naomi. *Kitchen-Table Wisdom.* Riverhead Books, 1997. Remarkable true stories, shared wisdom that humanizes the face of illness.

Shuman, Robert. *The Psychology of Chronic Illness.* Basic Books/HarperCollins, 1996. Insight into the nature of chronic illness and resources for healing, written by a wise and honest psychologist who has personally experienced illness.

Singh Khasa, Dharma, M.D. *Meditation as Medicine.* Fireside, 2001. The applications of yoga and meditation in healing, including a focus on specific conditions.

Smith, Jean, ed. *Breath Sweeps Mind.* Riverhead Books, 1998. A superb introduction to meditation.

Index

Absorption, 58, 69, 146
  celiac disease, 482
  essential fatty acids, 146, 221
  folic acid, 295, 297
  nutrients, 14–15, 25, 28–29, 351, 370
  paracellular/transcelluar, 60
  toxins, 206, 229
  weight loss, 80
  See also Malabsorption
Acetylcholinesterase (AChE), 206
Achlorhydria, 124
Acid reflux. *See* Reflux
Actigal, 550
Acupuncture, 360–62, 480–81, 484
  electroacupuncture, 359, 361–62
  mind-body therapy, 464, 469, 470
  Qi, for restoring, 380–81
  smoking and alcohol cessation,
    110
  See also individual conditions
Adenovirus, 190
Adrenal function, 12, 155, 157, 245,
    305, 308–9
Adrenaline, 66, 89, 90, 302, 397, 399,
    406
Advanced Magnetic Research
    Institutes (AMRI), 363–65
Aging process, 17, 58, 106, 108, 262,
    295–96, 349
AIDS, 49, 51, 54, 58, 81, 128, 150,
    321, 393, 444, 478, 530, 549
AIDS wasting syndrome, 321
Albumin, 317
Alcohol, 243–44, 265
  drug interactions, 318–19

esophagus, 312
free radical stress, 109–10
gastritis, 239, 243, 313
microcirculation, 351
pancreatitis, 548, 550
ulcers, 242, 314
See also Liver disease
Alexander, Mathias, 409
Allergies, 8–9, 16, 65–72
  blood tests, 142, 170–71, 503, 529,
    538
  diagnostic testing, 141–43, 165,
    170–72, 481
  diet, 166–68
  digestive enzymes, 168–69
  digestive rehabilitation, 224
  food, 512
  homeopathy, 512
  IBS, 534–35
  nervous system, 64, 67
  protein triggers, 69–70
  stress, 72
  therapy, 512
  treatments, 71–72, 166–69, 171–72,
    512
  wheat/gluten intolerance, 29, 38, 64,
    71, 155, 158
Allergy Research Group, 100, 211,
    220, 225, 484, 491
Aloe, 300, 333, 492, 536
Alpha-antichymotrypsin, 156
Alzheimer's disease, 18, 105, 326, 352,
    353, 364, 554
American Academy of Environmental
    Medicine, 99, 204, 469

American Celiac Society, 484
American College for the
  Advancement of Medicine
  (ACAM), 99, 469
American Journal of Epidemiology, 451
American Water Works Association, 193
Amin, Omar, 137
Amino acids, 101, 237–38, 299–300,
  337
Amoebas, 130, 156, 176, 181, 346, 494
Amoebic dysentery, 176
Anal/perineal area viruses, 191–92
Anderson, Jeffry, 86
Anderson, Scott, 31
Antibiotics, 52–53
  bacteria resistant, in dental amalgam,
    82
  candida, 21, 477
  cautions in using, 326–27
  diarrhea, 494, 496
  diverticulitis, 500
  as first treatment, 179
  flora eradication, 14, 33, 47, 51–52,
    218
  in food, 74, 197
  gastritis, 517, 518
  ulcers/ulcer disease, 560, 562
Antibodies, 29–30, 33, 35, 37
  DHEA levels, 307
  diagnostic testing, 126–29, 490,
    500, 529, 540
  H. pylori, 562
  IgA, 38, 39, 40, 71, 127
  IgG, 66, 135, 141–43, 151, 170,
    191, 498, 538, 541
  IgM, 127, 191
  level reductions, 255–56
  list, 39
  microbial, 128
  role, 128
  SIgA, 30, 35–41, 71, 154–55,
    157–58, 224–25

tumor therapy, 476, 511
  See also individual conditions
Antidotes, 171–72
Antigens, 29–30, 33, 35, 304
Antioxidants, 107–10, 151–52, 232,
  235–38, 487
Appendectomy, 35–36
Arthritis, 17, 18, 54, 60, 62, 81, 147,
  361
Aspirin
  cancer, 473, 477
  detoxification, 234, 245
  gallstones, 515, 516
  herbal therapy, 328, 337
  intestinal bleeding, 37
At a Journal Workshop (Progoff), 434
Atkins for Life (Atkins), 354
ATPase, 84
Attention deficit disorders
  (ADD/ADHD), 57, 63, 81, 115,
  135, 179
Autism, 57, 64, 104, 115, 125, 135,
  179
Autoimmune disorders, 17, 81, 115,
  128, 295, 307, 482–83, 485, 517,
  527
Ayurveda, 387–94, 391–92
Ayurvedic Institute in Albuquerque,
  394

Bacteria, 130–37
  anaerobes, 179–80
  antibiotic-resistant, 74, 82
  detecting, 130–37
  HSOs, 216
  IBS, 180
  overgrowth, 297, 473
  treatments, 181–88
Bacteroides, 51
Baker, Sidney MacDonald, 143
Barium enema, 121, 474
Barium swallow, 120

Bassett, Andrew, 363, 364
Bastyr University referral line, 99, 469, 531
Beaumont, William, 87–89
Becker, Robert, 363
Bentonite clay, 234–35, 476, 493, 535
Berberine, 342–43, 479
Beta-glucuronidase, 81, 148
Betaine hydrochloride, 27, 163, 168, 187, 210–11
Betaine (TMG), 301–2
Bevacizumab, 475
Beyond Probiotics (Gittleman), 216
Bicarbonate, 25, 28, 71, 124–25, 163, 165, 169, 209, 544–45, 553, 555
Bifidobacteria, 42, 44, 214, 216
Bile salts, 43, 476, 487, 514, 527, · 542
Biliary cirrhosis, 318, 485, 487
B-interferon, 43
Biochemical individuality, 3–4, 138, 145, 153
Bioelectromagnetic therapy, 359–64
Bioflavonoids, 220
Bland, Jeffrey, 110–11, 163, 321, 488
Blastocystis hominis, 133, 137, 176, 177
Block Center, 475
Blood sugar
  benefits of stable levels, 271
  diabetes, 270–71, 354
  Glycemic Index, 272–79
  hypoglycemia, 85, 240
  insulin, 4, 97, 209, 211, 265–66
  levels, 85, 163, 270, 273, 279, 290, 338
  managing, 269–80
  pancreas, 211
  See also Insulin
Blood tests
  Coxsackie virus, 190
  hemoccult, 474

homocysteine levels, 353
progesterone levels, 310
toxic exposure, 205, 206
See also individual conditions
BodyBio Corporation, 221
Body Ecology Diet (Gates), 480
Body Electric: Electromagnetism and the Foundation of Life (Becker), 363
Bonlie, Dean, 363
Botanicals, 5
Brain function
  ammonia build-up, 85
  bicarbonate secretion, 125
  digestive system overload, 115
  liver connection, 319, 321
  metabolic profile, 159
  peptides, effect on, 84
Breaking the Vicious Cycle (Gottschall), 163, 484
Bromelain, 484
Burton Goldberg Group, 476
Butyrate, 31, 42, 52, 81, 163, 226, 300
  n-butyrate, 148

Cadmium, 74, 80
Caffeine, 239, 244–45, 263, 312, 389, 435
Calprotectin, 147, 210
Cancer
  aspirin, 473, 477
  chemical toxins, 205
  chemotherapy, 475
  flora, 43
  nicotine, 242
  oxidative stress, 105
  radiation, 475
  toxins, effect on, 85
  See also individual conditions
Cancer Treatment Centers of America, 475

Candida albicans (yeast overgrowth)
antibodies, 478
blood tests, 150
causes, 478
diagnostic testing, 135, 149–51, 213, 478–79, 135, 149–51
diet/nutrition, 260, 262, 278, 480
flora balance, 42, 46–47, 178–79, 278
herbal therapies, 262, 338, 340, 344, 345
prevention, 183–84, 186
questionnaire, 19–21
self-testing for, 19–21
symptoms, 477–78
therapies, 223, 480–81
treatments, 479
Carbamates, 206
Carbohydrates, 239–41, 269–80
Carcinoma embryonic antigen (CEA), 474
Carnitine, 299–300
Celiac Disease Foundation, 483–84
Celiac disease (sprue), 29, 76, 481–85
antibodies, 482
blood tests, 483
diabetes, 482
diagnostic testing, 483
diet/nutrition, 483–84
genetics, 481
leaky gut syndrome, 482
supplements, 484
treatments, 483
Celiac Sprue Association, 483
Cellular immunity, 35, 36–37
Cellulose, 163, 219, 220, 476, 491, 521, 535
Center for Nutritional and Digestive Disorders, 104
Centers for Disease Control (CDC), 18, 130, 134, 175, 193
Central Institutional Review Board, 364

Cetuximab, 475
Chelators, 238
Chemicals, 73–79, 202–8, 245–46
Children
ADHD, 63–64, 179
allergies, 38, 71
brain-injury, 319, 321
cancer, 43
celiac disease, 482
digestive illnesses, death and, 467
enteroviruses, 190
flora, 44, 45, 179
herbal supplements, 339, 343, 347
L. plantarum, 217
PCM, 255–56
support for, 439, 445–46
toxic exposure, 201, 204, 207
Chinese Cancer Recovery Society, 453
Chinese medicine, 366–81, 373–77
acupuncture, 368, 369, 380
benefits, 380–81
body constituents and, 366–67
books on, 381
diminishing digestive function, 373–74
disharmony, disease and, 367–68
herbal, 336, 343, 369, 479, 488, 550
Qi, 366–73, 375, 377, 378–81, 463
self-care, 374–77
three pillars of health, 370–71
tongue diagnosis, 371–72
Urso, 476
Chlordane, 202
Chlorophyll, 285
Choices in Healing (Lerner), 476
Cholecystokinin (CKK) 69, 84
Cholesterol, 43, 85
Chronic fatigue syndrome, 18, 82, 190, 482
Chronic illness
challenges, 467
coping with, 10–11

digestive rehabilitation, 218, 223–24
duodenal ulcers, 559
fibromyalgia, 190
intestinal pseudo-obstruction, 560
microcirculation, 349–52
treatments, 146, 282
viral infections, 181
See also Liver disease
Chronic intestinal pseudo-obstruction, 560
Chymex Test, 71
Cimetidine, 325
Circadian Prescription (Baker), 143
Circle of Life, 450, 453, 455, 457–59
Circle of Life Assessment, 457–58
Cirrhosis, 485–88, 539–40
diet/nutrition, 487
genetics, 485
herbal therapy, 487–88
treatments, 487–88
See also Liver disease
Clinical Nutrition (Bland), 111
Clostridium difficile, 53, 216, 326
Cohen, Darlene, 550
Colchicine, 487
Colitis, 65, 74
Colon
bacteria, 33, 35, 146
cancer, 52, 76, 85, 147, 148, 156, 473–77
diagnostic testing, 121–24, 135, 474
diet/nutrition, 477
function, 29
nutrients for repair, 300–301
spastic, 50
stricture, 559–60
therapy, 493
treatments, 475–76
viruses, 191
Colonoscope, 121, 474, 475
Colostrum, 214–15, 224–25

CoLyte, 493
Commensals, 137
Comprehensive digestive stool analysis (CDSA). *See* Diagnostic testing
Constipation, 65, 69, 77, 114, 282–83, 488–94, 560
acupuncture, 493
diagnostic testing, 488–90
diet/nutrition, 492–93
exercise, 493–94
herbal therapy, 492–93
treatments, 490–92
Copper deficiency, 291, 292
Corticosteroids, 326
Cortisol, 157–58
Cortisone, 308–9
Coxsackie virus, 190
Crohn's disease, 494, 526–34
allergies, 65, 224
antibodies, 530
appendix removal, 36
B_{12} deficiency, 296, 297
causes, 527
diagnostic testing, 147, 529, 533–34, 545
fistulas, 511
genetics, 63, 526
herbal therapy, 334, 338
ileum, 35
leaky gut syndrome, 58, 63, 97, 149
obstruction, 559
short-bowel syndrome, 316, 546
stress, 87–88, 380
symptoms, 528
toxins, 74, 76, 81
treatments, 170, 216, 226, 326, 529–31
Cryptosporidium, 46, 77, 127, 131, 133, 156, 175, 177, 494
Crypts, 60, 127
CT scanning, 122–23
Cyclospora, 130–31, 134, 176

Cystic fibrosis, 485
Cytokins, 60
Cytotec, 519

Daoust, Jim, 355
Daoust, Joyce, 211, 224, 355
DDT, 202
Definitive Guide to Cancer (Burton
    Goldberg Group), 476
Deglycyrrhizinated licorice (DGL), 325
Dementia, 296, 298, 352, 353
Dental toxicities, 136
Depression: Cured at Last (Rogers),
    480
Depression, 76, 81, 85, 137, 157–58
*Detox Diet: How-to and When-to
    Guide for Cleansing the Body of
    Toxic Substances, Updated*
    (Haas), 240
Detoxification, 16, 229–38
    chemicals and heavy metals, 233
    defined, 229
    liver-clearing products, 99
    overloading, 231–32
    phases, 102–3, 108
    sauna therapy, 233–34
    self-help, 98–101
    supplements for, 319
    toxins, 85, 95–97, 98, 114–17
    treatments, 233–34, 236
    vitamin A, 294
Detoxification Healing (Baker), 143
DHEA, 55, 155, 157–58, 306–8,
    310–11
Diabetes
    celiac disease, 482
    gallstones, 549
    insulin, 278, 355
    pancreatic cancer, 546
    reflux, 553, 554
    sugar, dietary, 211, 262
    vitamin deficiencies, 292, 293, 319

weight gain, 97
yeast overgrowth, 480
See also Blood sugar
Diagnostic testing, 120–25, 153–60
    AChE levels, 206
    anaerobes, 180
    antibody, 126–29, 170–71, 180, 486
    barium enema, 121, 474
    barium swallow, 120
    CDSA, 50, 55, 125, 146–48, 180,
        182, 188, 210, 489, 545
    CEA, 474
    Chymex Test, 71
    Coca Test, 165
    colonoscope, 121, 474, 475
    cortisol levels, 157–58
    CT and MRI, 122–23, 359, 363,
        486, 500, 539, 541, 545, 547,
        559
    DHEA, 157–58
    digestive health, to determine,
        209–10
    elastase levels, 147
    endoscopic ultrasound, 122
    endoscopy, 121
    esophageal motility test, 124, 554
    fecal fat analysis, 210
    functional, 4–5, 125, 138, 139–40,
        152, 154–55
    gluten, reactions to, 158
    Health Profile, 6–9
    homocysteine levels, 4, 100, 103,
        301–2, 352–53
    hydrochloric acid and bicarbonate
        measurements, 124–25, 210
    intradermal, 171
    iodine deficiencies, 356–57
    laporoscopy, 123–24, 487, 514, 554
    metabolic profile, 159–60
    minerals, 480
    M2A Capsule, 122
    nitric oxide, 156–57

organic acids, 180

oxidative stress, 151–52

Pentagastrin, 124

physical exams, 55, 289, 392, 486, 500, 508, 554

progesterone levels, 310

pruritus ani, 551

red blood cell membrane fatty acid test, 221

sigmoidoscopy, 474

solvents, 207

starch levels, 163

toxicological assays, 205

ultrasound, 122, 486, 509, 514, 539, 547, 549

virtual colonoscopy, 121–22

See also Antibodies; Blood tests; *individual conditions*

Diarrhea, 69, 294, 297, 482, 494–99, 531

  acupuncture, 499

  diagnostic testing, 495

  herbal therapy, 498

  homeopathy, 498

  therapy, 498–99

  traveler's, 46

  treatments, 495–98

Dientamoeba fragilis, 134, 137

Diet

  acid-alkaline balance, 267–68

  Ayurveda, 389–90, 391

  biorhythm, 266–67

  carbohydrates, 234, 269–80, 353–55

  cheating, 277

  dining out, 276–77

  elimination, 141–43, 166–67, 553

  exercise, 249–50

  food combining, 266

  Gerson, 475

  Glycemic Index, 265–66, 274

  healthy basics, 257–68

  hyperalimentation, 546

  immune system, effects on, 255–56

  Kelly method, 475

  liquid, 235

  low-fat, 271, 430, 550

  microbiotic, 475

  ratio of nutrients, 276

  rotation, 72, 167–68

  20-Day Rejuvenation Diet Program (Bland), 111, 488

  vegetarian, 237, 261, 302

  water, 257, 292

  what to avoid, 262–65

  See also individual conditions

Diflucan, 479

Digestion

  allergies, effect on, 68

  balance, 13–14

  communication within, 82–84

  consequences of poor digestion, 16–18

  eating on the go, 377

  enzymes, 33

  essential fatty acids, 221

  food temperature, 375–76

  good, factors in, 376–77

  nutrients for repair, 291–92, 313–14

  overload, 115–16

  process, 26–29

  protective barriers, 24–31

  Qi, 366–73, 375, 377, 378–81, 463

  rehabilitation, 218, 223–24

  related illnesses, 112–17

  stress, 88, 91

Dioxins, 74, 76, 85, 194, 197, 203, 207

Disease, defined, 153

Diverticulosis and diverticulitis, 121, 499–502

  acupuncture, 501–2

  diagnostic testing, 500

  diet/nutrition, 500–501

  herbal therapy, 501

therapy, 501–2
treatments, 500
DNA, 29, 82, 85, 105, 145–46
Doctor's Data, 180
Drugs
  cautions, 323–27
  cost, 321
  damaging effects, 245–46
  5-ASA, 316–17
  functional medicine, 2, 4–5, 99, 104,
    111, 138, 140, 153–54
  H2 blockers, 325
  NSAIDs, 246
  and nutrition combinations, 312–22
  preventive medicine, 138–40
  side effects, 318–19
  See also Aspirin
Dysbiosis, 14, 49–55
  allergies, 71
  fermentation, 52
  IBS, 536
  leaky gut syndrome, 55, 63
  putrefactive, 51–52
  stress, 53
Dysentery, 80, 176, 284, 339
Dyspepsia
  acupuncture, 504
  diagnostic testing, 502–3
  diet/nutrition, 503–4
  indigestion, 27
  therapy, 503–4
  treatments, 503
Dyspepsia (without ulcers), 291, 292,
  332, 502–4

Eat Right 4 Your Type (D'Adamo),
  264
E. coli, 38, 42, 44, 46, 176, 213
Edison, Thomas, 322
Elastase, 147
Electroacupuncture, 359, 361–62
Encephalopathy, 482

Endocrine function, 53, 83, 140
Endorphins, 360, 361, 482
Endoscopic retrograde cholangiopan-
  creatography (ERCP), 547,
  548–49
Endoscopic ultrasound, 122
Endotoxins, 229
Entamoeba hartmanii, 176
Entamoeba histolytica, 131, 133–35,
  176, 489
Enteroviruses, 190
Environment. *See* Toxins
Environmental Working Group
  (EWG), 75, 193, 197
Enzymes, 163
  antioxidant, 152
  beta-glucuronidase, 81, 148
  calprotectin, 147
  digestive, 27–28, 33, 146, 148,
    168–69, 211, 221
  elastase, 147
  EPX, 147
  GI tract repair, 220
  glutathione, 80
  lactase, 264, 482, 534, 537, 538
  liver, 101
  pepsin, 88
  proteases, 52
  supplements, 212
  toxic, 35, 43
  trypsin, 485
  See also Pancreas
Eosinophil Protein X (EPX), 147
Epithelial growth factors, 226
Epithelium, 27, 32, 84
Epstein-Barr virus, 191
Esophagus, 504
  achalasia, 290, 361
  Barrett's esophagitis, 312, 313, 555,
    557
  cancer, 85, 312, 552
  incomplete esophageal clearing, 553

motility, 124, 326, 553, 554
nutrition, 312
peristalsis, 24
sphincter, 242, 312, 552, 554, 555, 557
stricture, 557–58
therapy, 312
treatments, 362
varices, 243, 486, 538–39, 557
See also Reflux
Essence, 366–67, 370, 402, 403, 416
Essential fatty acids, 221–22, 226, 299
Excito-toxins, 70
Exercise, 249–50, 432–33
aerobic, 233–35, 249–50
Alexander technique, 409–10
antioxidants, 109
benefits, 10, 396–97
breath practice, 405–7
Feldenkrais method, 410
free radicals, 151
gentle, 395–412
isometrics, 410–11
leaky gut syndrome, 57, 60
Pilates, 411–12
Qigong, 401–3, 493, 543, 563
stress, 109
t'ai chi, 395, 398, 399, 401, 412, 420, 532, 543
walking, 399–404, 417, 454
Walking Qigong, 401–2
weight training, low-impact, 407–9
yoga, 403–5, 493, 563
"Experiments and Observations on the Gastric Juices and the Biology of Digestion" (Beaumont), 88

Faass, Nancy, 386
Failure to thrive, 29, 482
Famotidine, 325
Fasano, Alessio, 481–82

Fats
intake, 43, 51, 100, 300, 473, 550
monounsaturated, 260, 262
polyunsaturated, 235, 303
saturated, 303, 473, 513
trans, 302–3
See also Oils
Fenton, Mark, 399
Ferguson, Tom, 437
Fermentation, 52, 81, 83, 86
FFP Laboratories, 357
Fiber, 53, 163, 219, 302, 327, 473, 490–91, 492, 535
Fibromyalgia, 504–10
Fighting Cancer From Within (Rossman), 94
Fissures, 510–11
Fistulas, 511, 528, 530
Flatulence, 48, 76, 77, 147, 177, 258, 301, 333, 346, 371, 501, 517, 544
Flaxseed, 222, 283, 303–4, 477, 491
Flora, 14, 31
Candida albicans, 178–79
destruction of, 81
diagnostic testing for, 213
enhancing, 99–100
FOS, 163, 215, 300, 342
friendly, 42–48
harmful, 49–55
healthy diet, 261–62
restoring, 212–15, 219
Fluoride, 73–74
Folic acid, 289–90, 294–298, 300–302
Folic Acid (Baker), 143
Food and Drug Administration (FDA), 75, 197, 346, 363, 364, 543, 555
Food-combining theory, 72
Foods
additives, 70
antioxidants, 107–10, 151–52, 232, 235–38

chelators, 238
fast/junk, 264–65
healing, 235–37
organic, 9, 55, 78, 99, 110, 145, 197–99
raw, benefits, 236
temperature, 375–76
Food sensitivities. *See* Allergies
Formula, The (Daoust), 272, 276, 355
40-30-30 Fat Burning Nutrition (Daoust), 211, 224, 355
Framingham Study, 4
Free radicals, 17–18, 101, 102, 105–10, 114, 151–52, 216
Fructo-oligo-saccharides (FOS), 163, 215, 300, 342
Full Catastrophe Living (Kabat-Zin), 550
Functional medicine practitioner, 153–54
Functional Medicine Updates (audio series), 111
Furlong, John, 152

Galland, Leo, 222
Gallbladder disease, 123–24, 512–16, 550
acupuncture, 550
cancer, 514
herbal therapy, 550
homeopathy, 550
Gallstones, 476, 512–16, 518, 550
acupuncture, 516
diabetes, 549
diagnostic testing, 514
diet/nutrition, 515–16
herbal therapy, 335, 337, 516
homeopathy, 516
therapy, 515, 516
treatments, 514–15
Gamma linolic acid (GLA), 222
Ganoderma, 479

Gas/bloating. *See* Flatulence
Gastric volvulus, 558–59
Gastritis, 239, 243, 244, 313, 517–19, 592
acupuncture, 519
diagnostic testing, 518
diet/nutrition, 519
genetics, 517
herbal therapy, 286, 332, 333, 519
homeopathy, 519
therapy, 519
treatments, 518–19
Gastroesophageal reflux disease (GERD). *See* Reflux
Gastronoma, 124
Gates, Donna, 480
Geffen Cancer Center, 475
Genetic Nutritioneering (Bland), 111
Genetics
coding, 9
diagnostic testing, 9, 97, 99, 144–46
DNA, 29, 82, 85, 105, 145–46
errors, 145–46
free radicals, 105
health factors, 9
highly sensitive individuals, 76
HLA typing, 483
leaky gut syndrome, 63, 67
make-up, 9, 41, 78, 138, 144
mercury exposure, 82
predisposition to disease, 5, 14, 96–98, 145, 148, 152
Type I allergies, 66–67
German Commission E, 337, 344
Giardia, 42, 46, 58, 130, 134–35, 137, 156, 173, 177, 294
Gilbert's syndrome, 97, 318
Gittleman, Ann Louise, 216
Glenn, John, 362
Gliadin, 482
Glutamine, 170, 299–300
Glutathione, 232, 301–2

Gluten intolerance, 29, 64, 155, 158, 286, 481, 482–83
Glycemic Index, 211, 265–66, 272–79, 355
Glycogen storage disease, 485
Goldenseal, 342, 343
GoLytely, 493
Gonzales, Nicholas, 475
Gottschall, Elaine, 163, 484
Great Exposition of the Path to Enlightenment (Tsongkhapa), 421
Great Smokies Diagnostic Laboratory, 152, 178, 180, 182, 204, 489, 507, 529, 541, 545, 551
Guided imagery, 422–31
Guided Imagery for Self-Healing (Rossman), 94
Guo Lin, 402
Gut-associated lymphoid tissue (GALT), 35, 38, 40

Haas, Elson, 246–47
Hahnemann, Samuel, 383–84
Health Action Group, 412
Heartburn. See Reflux
Heart disease, 4, 43, 85, 101, 105, 145
Heart failure, 393, 486
Heidelberg capsule, 124, 210
Helicobacter pylori. See H. Pylori
Hemorrhoids, 192, 298, 301, 520–23
    acupuncture, 522
    diet/nutrition, 521–22
    exercise, 522–23
    herbal therapy, 337, 338, 522, 551
    homeopathy, 522
    treatments, 520–21
Heparin, 352
Hepatitis, 58, 335–36, 343–44, 523–26, 540
    A, 523–24, 540, 542
    acute, 317
    antibodies, 523

autoimmune, 97, 486
B and C, 344, 486–88, 506, 524–25, 542
D and E, 525
diagnostic testing, 540–41
diet/nutrition, 542
environment, 541
Epstein-Barr virus, 191
herbal therapy, 335, 336, 343, 344, 526, 542
homeopathy, 543
leaky gut syndrome, 58
NASH, 539
therapy, 543
toxic, 318
treatments, 541–42
Herbal therapy, 328–47
    antibacterial, 342–43
    antimicrobial, 338–42
    antiparasitic, 346–47
    antiviral, 343–44
    antiyeast, 262, 338, 340, 344–45
    Chinese, 336, 343, 369, 479, 488, 550
    combination remedies, 347
    digestion, promoting, 332–33
    guidelines, 328–32
    intestinal healing, 333–35
    Robert's Formula, 431, 484
    slippery elm, 282, 285–86, 335, 338, 493
    See also individual conditions
Herpangina syndrome, 190
Herpes viruses, 189, 192
Hiatal hernia, 68, 120, 552, 554
HIV, 15, 193, 212, 321, 393, 459, 524
Hodgkin's disease, 36
Homeopathy, 382–86, 522
    See also individual conditions
Homeostatic soil organisms (HSO), 216

Homocysteine levels, 4, 100, 103, 301–2, 352–53
Hormones
  adrenal, 157–58
  cortisone therapy, 308–9
  DHEA, 155, 157–58, 306–8, 310
  gallstones, 516
  genetic errors, 145
  glucagon, 120
  levels, 155, 157, 305–6
  liver disease, 96
  peptide stimulation, 69
  progesterone, 310–11
  role of, in healing, 305–11
  secretin, 125
  thyroid, 103
  toxins, 116, 139
H. pylori, 17, 124, 137, 313–14, 325, 502, 517
H2 blockers, 325
Human Genome Project, 97, 144–45
Hydrochloric acid (HCl), 27, 31, 116, 168, 209
  measurements, 124–25
  poor digestion, 52
  as protective barrier, 25–27, 33
  supplemental, 27, 31, 116, 168, 209
  See also Betaine hydrochloride
Hyperacidity, 124, 291–92
Hyperalimentation, 546
Hyperpermeability. *See* Leaky gut syndrome
Hypersensitization, 16
Hypochlorhydria, 124
Hypochlorite, 106

IBS. *See* Irritable bowel syndrome
Idiopathic, 486
IgG ELISA test, 142
Immune system
  checklist, 255–56
  damage from toxins, 76, 80
  defenses, 32–41
  digestive role in, 29–30
  importance, 378–79
  influences on, 5, 9–10, 40
  malfunctioning, 54
  overstimulation, 81
  parasitic damage to, 133
  protective immunity, 13
  suppression, 18
  toxins, 112
  See also Blood sugar
Immunocytes, 157–59
Immunoglobulin A (IgA), 38, 39, 40, 71, 127
Immunoglobulin G (IgG), 66, 135, 141–43, 151, 170
ImmunoLabs, 551
Immunosciences Laboratory, 180
Indigestion. *See* Dyspepsia
Inflammation, 17, 61, 63
  diagnostic testing, 156–57
  essential fatty acids, 221
  first aid for, 281–87
  progesterone therapy, 310–11
  reducing, 220–21
  treatments, 281–87
Inflammatory bowel diseases (IBD), 44, 49, 57, 156, 190–92, 206, 316–17, 320, 380, 526–33
  acupuncture, 532
  diagnosis, 533
  diagnostic testing, 156, 528–29, 533–34
  diet/nutrition, 316, 320, 531
  genetics, 526
  herbal therapy, 531–32
  stress, 91
  symptoms, 527–28
  therapy, 316–17, 532
  treatments, 529–31, 534
  ulcerative colitis, 58, 74, 76, 81, 97, 104, 131, 216, 315, 563

viral bowel disease, 191
See also Crohn's disease
Institute for Functional Medicine, 99,
    110–11, 140, 470
Institute of Noetic Sciences, 465
Institute of Parasitic Diseases (IPD), 490
Insulin, 4, 97, 209, 211, 265–66
    resistance, 355–56
    See also Diabetes
Intelligence, 24–25
Interactive Guided Imagery, 94
Intestinal permeability, treatments,
    219–20
Intestines
    herbs for healing, 333–35
    nutrients for, 292–93
    permeability, 231
    viruses, 190
Intrinsic factor, 163, 313
Inulin, 163, 316
Iodine deficiencies, 356–57
Iron, 42, 217, 301–2, 320, 485–87,
    539–42
Irritable bowel syndrome (IBS), 18, 65,
    74, 76, 180, 309, 532–37
    acupuncture, 536
    constipation predominant, 535
    diarrhea-predominant, 534–35
    diet/nutrition, 536
    4 Rs treatment program, 534
    herbal therapy, 536
    homeopathy, 537
    lactose intolerance, 534, 536
    with pain or gas and bloating, 535–36
    supplements, 535
    therapy, 536–37

Jahnke, Roger, 412
Jeffries, William McKinley, 309
Jones, David, 321
*Journal of American Medical
    Association*, 180, 323

Kabat-Zin, Jon, 550
Kaminski, Mitchell, 321
Koch, Kenneth, 362
Korngold, Efrem, 381
Kunin, Richard, 192
Kushi, Michio, 475
Kuss, Timothy, 347–48

Lactase, 264, 482, 534, 537, 538
Lactobacilli, 42, 46, 48, 216
Lactobacillus acidophilus, 43, 44, 213,
    214
Lactobacillus bulgaricus, 43, 214
Lactobacillus DDS, 216
Lactobacillus glutamine, 225, 283–84,
    484, 536
Lactobacillus plantarum, 214, 217
Lactoferrin, 214, 215, 216–17, 225
Lactose intolerance, 43, 139, 214,
    215, 264, 287, 300–301, 537–38
    antibodies, 498, 537
    diagnosis, 537–38
    diagnostic testing, 139, 537–38
    IBS, 534, 536
    incidence of, 537
    treatments, 538
Lad, Vasant, 394
Lancet, The (journal), 382
Laporoscopy, 123–24
Larson, Joan Mathews, 550
Lawrence, Ronald, 362
Leaky gut syndrome (hyper-
    permeability), 15, 57–64
    allergies, 16, 66–68, 71, 85, 169–70
    autoimmune complications, 62
    conditions contributing to, 57–58
    describing, 58–60
    diagnostic testing, 99, 149
    essential fatty acids, 221
    genetics, 63, 67
    liver stress, 61–62
    malabsorption/malnutrition, 86

nutrients for, 169–70
supplements, 224–28
toxins, effect on, 85, 97
treatments, 169–70
Lerner, Michael, 415, 476
Levin, Alan, 65
Lifespan Institute, 12, 568
Lifestyle, 5
  attitude, 253–54
  Ayurveda, 389–90
  choices, 464
  diet/nutrition, 248–49
  exercise, 249–50
  free radicals, 105–6, 110, 115
  importance, 10–11
  liver disease and, 95
  rebalancing, 248–54
  reflux and, 556
  sleep, 250, 252
  toxins and, 9, 78, 95–96
  treatment and, 2–3, 5–6, 138, 146,
    155, 159, 188
Ling-Zhi, 479
Linus Pauling Award, 321
Liver disease, 538–39
  alcohol, 58, 96–98, 228, 485, 543
  biochemical production, 108
  blood tests, 486, 539, 541
  brain connection, 319, 321
  causes, 540
  chronic, 317, 320
  detoxification, 16, 95, 97–99,
    101–2, 108, 114, 152
  diagnostic testing, 99, 486–87,
    540–41
  diet/nutrition, 100–101, 301–2,
    317–21
  digestive role, 30–31
  drug interactions, 318–19
  herbal therapy, 335–37
  NAFL, 97–98, 100, 299, 486, 526,
    539, 540

NASH, 486, 539
  as protective barrier, 30–31
  reducing stress on, 231
  support, 231–32
  treatments, 320
  viruses, 191
  See also Cirrhosis; Detoxification;
    Hepatitis; Leaky gut syndrome
Living Without (magazine), 484
Lugol's Solution, 357
Lupus, 17, 54, 76, 81, 128
Lymph tissue, 33
Lynn, Paul, 287
Lysosomes, 39
Lysozyme A, 156

Macrophages, 30, 36, 38, 80
Magnesium, 221, 319, 490, 491, 492,
  535
Magnetic molecular energetics (MME),
  363–64, 491
Magnetic resonance imaging (MRI),
  122–23, 363, 539, 547
Magnetism, 360
*Magnet Therapy, the Pain Cure
  Alternative* (Rosch and Lawrence),
  362
Malabsorption, 65, 84, 158, 544–46
  celiac disease, 481, 482
  deficiencies, 25, 297
  diagnostic testing, 544–45
  diet/nutrition, 100–101, 545–46
  gluten intolerance, 158
  irritation, chronic, 29
  leaky gut syndrome, 63, 67, 246,
    297
  magnesium deficiency, 320
  malnutrition, 63, 80
  parasites, 133, 176
  short-bowel syndrome, 546
  stroke, 517
  supplements, 101

therapy, 546
toxins, 75–76
Malnutrition, 40, 63, 80, 83, 548
Manganese, 316–17
M cells, 36
McLean, Rebecca, 459
Measles, 190–91
Medical Hypothesis (journal), 478
Medicine. *See* Drugs
MegaNutrition for Women (Kunin), 192
MegaNutrition (Kunin), 192
Mental disorders, 63–64
Mercury, 73–75, 98
    amalgams (dental), 54, 74–75, 77, 80, 82, 136, 201–2, 205
Meridian Laboratory, 180
Metabolic profile, 159–60
Metabolic syndrome, 97, 355
Metametrix and Great Plains Lab, 180
Methionine, 302
Methylation, 353
Microbes, 127, 130–37, 173
Microcirculation, blood tests, 352
Microcirculation, 4, 349–52
    diagnostic testing, 351–52
    therapy, 351–52
    treatments, 351–52
Microsporidia, 177
Microwave therapy, 362
Milk/dairy intolerance. *See* Lactose intolerance
Miller, Joseph, 171
Mind-body therapy, 87, 398, 442, 481, 537, 543, 550
    breath practice, 405
    imagery, 92–94, 422–31
    massage, 475, 484, 543, 548
    meditation, 416–21
    proactive patient, 466–70
    self-care, 432–37
    self-care choices, 464

self-healing support, 462–65
    See also Acupuncture; Exercise; Stress
Mitochondria, 84, 98, 112, 115
Monolaurin, 191, 192
Monosodium glutamate (MSG), 70, 95
Montezuma's revenge. *See* Diarrhea
Motility, 46, 69, 82–84, 120, 123–24
Mouth
    anatomy, 24
    Chinese tongue diagnosis, 371–72
    indicators of nutritional health, 289–90
    ulcers, 189, 528
    viruses, 189–90
MSM (therapeutic sulfur), 170, 221, 226, 286
M2A (mouth to anus) capsule, 122
Mucosa, 29, 53, 55, 80, 82–83, 157, 158, 187–88, 225–26
Mucous membranes, 290

N-acetyl cysteine (NAC), 220, 225, 318
N-acetyl-glucosamine (NAG), 226
NAET Guidebook (Nambudripad), 512
Nambudripad Allergy Elimination Technique (NAET), 481, 512
Nambudripad, Debi, 512
Nat Cell Thymus, 225
National Cancer Institute (NCI), 476
National Institutes of Health (NIH), 359, 402
N-butyrate, 148
Nervous system
    allergies, 64, 67
    chemical effects on, 70, 84, 116
    digestive system overload, 115
    mercury effects on, 74
    mucosal cell communication, 83
    stress, 91
    sympathetic, 89–90

Neurocutaneous syndrome (NCS), 136
Neurological problems, 18
New Detox Diet: The Complete Guide to Lifelong Vitality (Haas), 240
Nichols, Trent W., 104
Nickel, 80, 81
Nicotine, 239, 241–43
90-Day Fitness Program (Fenton), 399
Nitric oxide, 156–57
Nitrosamines, 81
Nizoral, 479
Nonalcoholic fatty liver, (NAFL), 97–98, 100, 299, 486, 526, 539, 540
Nonalcoholic steato-hepatitis (NASH), 486, 539
Nonsteroidal anti-inflammatory drugs (NSAIDs), 54, 58, 163, 228, 239, 246, 325, 517, 518, 519, 527
Nulytely, 493
Nutrition
    AIDS patients, 321
    antioxidant rich foods, 235–38
    and drug combinations, 312–22
    mineral deficiencies, 25
    parenteral feeding, 315–16
    for repair, 288–304
    support, 31, 44, 50, 53, 55, 113
    therapy, 2–5, 41, 315–16, 475
    therapy, combined with drugs, 312–22
    treatments, 186–88
    See also Diet
Nutrition Restart Center, 316
Nystatin, 479

Obstruction, 367, 559–60
    biliary cirrhosis, 318, 485, 487
    intestinal, 488, 492, 531, 559–60
    pancreatic duct, 547, 548, 549
Oils
    cod liver, 222, 291, 293, 299

fish, 222, 293, 299
flaxseed, 222, 283, 303–4, 477
herbal, 479
omega, 222, 238, 286, 299, 304
vegetable, 303
Omeprazole, 325
Oral tolerance, 40
O'Regan, Brendan, 465
Organic foods, 9, 55, 78, 99, 110, 145, 197–99
Organochlorines, 206–7
Organophosphates, 206
Oxidative stress. *See* Free radicals

Pancreas, 28
    care, 211
    CDSA, 147
    digestive communication, 82, 84
    enzymes, 27, 71, 106, 147–48, 169, 187, 211, 236, 499, 516, 544, 550
    glandular, 211
    improving function, 210
    nutrients for, 292
    secretions, 25, 28, 124–25, 209
Pancreatic cancer, 85, 477, 544–48
    diabetes, 546
    diagnostic testing, 547
    herbal therapy, 548
    treatments, 547
Pancreatitis, 58, 292, 430, 548–50
    blood tests, 549
    diagnostic testing, 548, 549
    diet/nutrition, 550
    familial, 548
    treatments, 548, 550
Paracellular/transcellular absorption, 60
Parasites, 173–78, 551
    cryptosporidium, 77, 131, 175, 177, 494
    detecting, 130–35, 137, 177–78

diagnostic testing, 50, 55, 135, 177–78, 182, 204, 489
eradication, 218–19, 223
giardia, 42, 46, 58, 130, 134–35, 137, 156, 173, 177, 294
sugar, 224, 239–41, 292
symptoms questionnaire, 21–23
waterbourne, 130–31, 173, 174, 196–97
Parasitic infections, 18, 22, 23, 59, 115, 130–35, 147, 551
characteristics, 132–33
constipation, 489, 493, 535
diarrhea, 494
herbal therapy, 339–40, 347
list of, 132
microscopic, 176–77
prevalence, 175
risk factors, 133
symptoms, 175–76
treatment, 137
Paristology Center, 131–32, 137, 176, 178, 184, 489, 495
Parkinson's Disease, 18
Pentagastrin, 124
Peptic ulcer disease, 76, 120, 295
Peptides, 69–70, 83–85, 96, 220, 225, 226, 284–85, 378
Permavite powder, 220, 484
Pert, Candace, 378, 455
Pew Internet & American Life Project, 460
Peyer's patches, 36
Pharmax Group, 48
Phosphatidal choline, 226
Physicians, integrative, 4, 5, 98, 104
Pilates, Joseph, 411
Pilla, Arthur, 363
Plummer, Nigel, 48
Pneumocystis, 321
Poliomyelitis, 190

Polycyclic aromatic hydrocarbons (PAHs), 85
Polyps, 121, 122, 147, 473, 474, 477
Positronemission tomography (PET), 425
Power Healing (Galland), 222
Prednisone, 317
Primary sclerosing cholangitis (PSC), 97
Probiotics, 14, 44, 48, 100, 116, 148, 163
See also Supplements
Progoff, Ira, 434
Prostaglandins, 221, 291, 299, 337, 473, 477
Protein calorie malnutrition (PCM), 40
Pruritus ani, 551
Pseudomembranous enterocolitis, 326
Psychology of Chronic Illness (Shuman), 443
Pulsed electromagnetic fields (PEMF), 362–63
Putrefaction, 51–52, 81, 83, 86

Qi, 366–73, 375, 377, 378–81, 463
Quercetin, 220, 226

Ranitidine, 325
Readiness for Change assessment, 453
Receptors, 64, 68–69, 79–80, 83
Red blood cell membrane fatty acid test, 221
Reflux, 242, 313, 378, 504
causes, 552–53
diagnostic testing, 554–55
diet/nutrition, 553, 556
heartburn, 520, 551–57
herbal therapy, 556–57
homeopathy, 557
lifestyle, 556
medications, 555–56
prevention, 553

symptoms, 552
therapy, 557
Reiki massage therapy, 484, 543, 548
Relaxation. *See* Mind-body therapy
Resection, 475
Rinkel, Herbert, 171
Rogers, Shirley, 480
Rosch, Paul, 362
Rosenbaum, Michael, 41
Rossman, Martin, 94
Rotavirus, 190

Sacchromyces boulardii, 214, 216
S-adenosyl-methionine (SAM), 487
Safe Uses of Cortisone (Jeffries), 309
Salmonella, 46
Salt, 261
Saputo, Len, 56
Sauna therapy, 233–35
Schizophrenia, 57, 81
Science (journal), 450
Seacure, 69, 170, 220, 225, 281–85,
    484, 498, 509, 531, 536, 546, 556
Sears, Barry, 211, 224, 355
Secretory immunoglobin A (SIgA), 30,
    35–41, 71, 154–55, 157–58,
    224–25
Selye, Hans, 89, 308
Septicemia, 48
Seven Weeks to Sobriety (Larson), 550
Shen, 366–67, 370
Short-bowel syndrome, 316, 546
Shuman, Robert, 443
Sick-building syndrome, 75–76, 202–3
Sigmoidoscopy, 121, 474
Simonton, O. Carl and Stephanie, 429
Single nucleotide polymorphisms
    (SNPs), 145–46
Sleep, 250, 252
Small intestine, 28, 156, 191
SNACCs (sugar, nicotine, alcohol,
    caffeine, or chemicals), 239, 249

Society for Orthomolecular Health-
    Medicine, 192, 470
*Solving the Puzzle of Chronic Fatigue
    Syndrome* (Rosenbaum), 41
Sphincterotomy, 492
Spiegel, David, 451
Spontaneous remission, 465
Sprue. *See* Celiac disease
Standard Process, 211
Stenosis, 548
Stine, Jerry, 12
St. Martin, Alexis, 87–89
Stomach acid. *See* Hydrochloric acid
    (HCl)
Stomach cancer, 17, 242
Stomach viruses, 190–91
Streptococcus thermophilus, 43,
    214
Stress
    allergies, 72
    detoxification, 16
    digestive response to, 87–90
    dysbiosis, 53
    effects, 88, 91
    environmental, 109
    exercise, 109
    fight-or-flight response, 89–90
    flora balance, 46
    hormone therapy, 310–11
    IBD, 91
    managing, 379–80
    modern, 90
    oxidative, 12, 102, 105–10, 114,
        151–52
    reduction therapy, 10, 40, 91–92,
        93, 170, 251–53
    relaxation response, 92–93
    sympathetic system, 158
    See also Mind-body therapy
Stressors, 47
Strictures and structural conditions, 121,
    488, 521, 552, 554, 555, 557–61

diagnostic testing, 558
therapy, 559
treatments, 558
Sucralfate, 325–26
Sugar, 239–41, 269–80
Superoxide dismutase, 216
Super Supplements (Rosenbaum), 41
Supplements
    amino acids, 237–38
    antioxidant, 237
    antioxidant protection, 110, 151, 157
    B₁₂, 298
    bicarbonate, 209, 212
    bitters, 212
    butyrates, 226, 300
    cholesterol, 43
    colostrum, 214–15
    DHEA levels, 157, 311
    enzymes, 212, 484
    essential fatty acids, 222, 238
    flora, 48
    folic acid, 297–98
    GI cleansing, 116
    GI tract repair, 219
    HCl, 27, 31, 116, 168, 209,
        210–11, 535
    homocysteine levels, 100
    hormone, 311
    indigestion, 27
    iodine, 357
    iron, 320, 487
    magnesium, 535, 536
    metabolic function, 160
    pancreatic enzyme levels, 147
    Permavite powder, 220, 484
    probiotics, 213, 215, 216–17, 480,
        484
    selenium, 294–95
    stomach acid, 31
    See also Herbal therapy; Vitamins
Support, 434, 438–49
    groups, 444, 450–59

    online, 444–45, 460–61
    proactive, 466–70
    self-healing, 462–65
*Surgeon General's Report on Exercise
    and Fitness*, 395
Syndrome X, 97, 355

T cells, 17, 35–38, 107, 128, 190,
    197, 482
Testing. *See* Diagnostic testing
Therapy
    behavioral, 475
    bioelectromagnetic, 359–64
    compassion, 420–21
    cortisone, 308–9
    drug and nutrition combinations,
        312–22
    enemas, 493
    guided imagery, 422–31, 475
    microwave, 362
    mind-body, 87, 92, 398, 442, 481,
        537, 543, 550
    NAET, 481, 512
    nutraceuticals, 323–24
    nutritional, 315–16, 475
    prayer, 420
    quality of life, 414–15
    sauna, 233–34
    tissue regeneration, 362–64
    vitamin, 188, 476
    water, 253
    See also Acupuncture; Herbal
        therapy; *individual conditions;*
        Support
THMs, 73–74
Thymus extracts, 225
Tight junctions, 58, 61, 85–86, 226
Timmins, William G., 160
Tin, 74
Toxins, 73–86
    absorption, 114
    cancer, 85

chemicals, 73–79, 202–8, 245–46
cosmetics, 200–201
dental toxicities, 136, 201–2, 204
detoxification, 116–17
diagnostic testing, 203–6
domino effect, averting, 230–31
environmental, 9–10, 53–54, 203–4
in food, 195, 197–98
in home and garden, 198–200
metals, 70, 73, 78–82, 204–5, 206
minimizing exposure, 193–208
neurotoxic pollutants, 81, 84, 207
occupational/industrial, 203
organochlorines, 206–7
organophosphates/carbamates, 206
PCBs, 73–74, 76, 85, 194, 197,
    202–3, 207
pesticides, 70, 73–76, 205, 206
sick-building syndrome, 75–76,
    202 3
solvents, 207–8
sources, 229–30
toxic overload, 95–104, 114–15
vitamin A, 293
in water, 73–74, 193–95, 196
See also Detoxification
Transcutaneous Electrical Nerve
    Stimulation (TENS), 361–62
Traveler's diarrhea, 46
Treatments
    antidotes, 171–72
    Ayurveda, 391–93
    bacterial infections, 181–88
    chronic pain, 360–62
    ERCP, 547, 548, 549
    4R support program, 162–63, 509,
        534
    functional, 139–40, 153–60
    GI tract repair, 218–28
    individualized approach, 3
    integrative, 2, 4–5, 98, 181, 282–83
    MME, 543

referrals, 469–70
resection, 475
second opinions, 469–70
viral illness, 191–92
See also Homeopathy; *individual
    conditions;* Nutrition
Trimethylglycine (TMG), 353
Turning Suffering Inside Out (Cohen),
    550
20-Day Rejuvenation Diet Program
    (Bland), 111, 488
Type 1 and 2 Allergy Relief Program
    (Levin), 65

Ulcerative colitis. *See* Inflammatory
    bowel diseases
Ulcers/ulcer disease, 560–63
    alcohol/nicotine, 242, 314
    caffeine, 244
    cause, 124, 170, 181
    crack cocaine, 246
    diet/nutrition, 224, 286, 291, 303
    herbal therapy, 334, 335, 337–38,
        345
    mouth, 189, 528
    peptic ulcer disease, 76, 120, 295
    stress, 89, 444
    therapy, 362
    treatments, 326, 333
UltraClear Sustain, 315–16, 319, 321
University of Maryland Center for
    Celiac Research, 483
Urso, 476, 550
U.S. Environmental Protection Agency,
    193

Vegetarians, 237, 261, 302
Venereal warts, 191–92
Videoscope, 28
Villi, 28–29, 221–22
VIP, 69–70
Viral activation, 82

Virtual colonoscopy, 121–22
Viruses, 189–92
Vitamin Diagnostics, 180
Vitamins, 238, 261
  A, 38, 41, 71, 169–70, 191, 225, 256, 290, 293–94
  antioxidant supplements, 151
  B₁₂, 81, 295–97, 301, 518, 544
  B complex, 294
  C, 165, 189, 232, 237, 298, 492
  D, 292, 298–99, 482
  deficiencies, 290, 293–96, 482
  E, 107, 108–9, 288–89
  K, 31, 33, 482
  therapy, 188, 476
Vojdani, Aristo, 129

Waldeyer's ring, 190
Walleczek, Jan, 364

Wall Street Journal, 130
Walter Reed Army Research Center, 346
Weight gain, 96, 97, 271
Weight loss, 80, 354, 454, 513, 528, 544
Wheat intolerance, 29, 38, 71, 481, 482
Williams, Roger, 3
Wilson's disease, 485, 487
World Health Organization, 383

X-rays, 50, 120–24, 360, 549

YMCA, 402
Yoga Sutras of Patanjali, 403
Yogurt, 43, 214

Zinc, 169, 226, 292, 300
Zone, The (Sears), 211, 224, 272, 276, 355